VOLUME SIXTY NINE

ADVANCES IN
PHARMACOLOGY

VOLUME SIXTY NINE

Advances in
PHARMACOLOGY

Emerging Targets & Therapeutics in the
Treatment of Psychostimulant Abuse

Edited by

LINDA P. DWOSKIN

Associate Dean for Research
Endowed Professor in Pharmaceutical Education
Department of Pharmaceutical Sciences,
College of Pharmacy
University of Kentucky, Lexington, KY, USA

Serial Editor

S. J. ENNA

Department of Molecular and Integrative Physiology,
Department of Pharmacology, Toxicology and Therapeutics,
University of Kansas Medical Center, Kansas City,
Kansas, USA

Managing Editor

LYNN LECOUNT

University of Kansas Medical Center
School of Medicine, Kansas City, Kansas, USA

AMSTERDAM • BOSTON • HEIDELBERG • LONDON
NEW YORK • OXFORD • PARIS • SAN DIEGO
SAN FRANCISCO • SINGAPORE • SYDNEY • TOKYO
Academic Press is an imprint of Elsevier

ELSEVIER

Academic Press is an imprint of Elsevier
525 B Street, Suite 1800, San Diego, CA 92101-4495, USA
225 Wyman Street, Waltham, MA 02451, USA
32, Jamestown Road, London NW1 7BY, UK
The Boulevard, Langford Lane, Kidlington, Oxford, OX5 1GB, UK
Radarweg 29, PO Box 211, 1000 AE Amsterdam, The Netherlands

First edition 2014

Notice
No responsibility is assumed by the publisher for any injury and/or damage to persons or
property as a matter of products liability, negligence or otherwise, or from any use or
operation of any methods, products, instructions or ideas contained in the material herein.
Because of rapid advances in the medical sciences, in particular, independent verification of
diagnoses and drug dosages should be made

British Library Cataloguing-in-Publication Data
A catalogue record for this book is available from the British Library

Library of Congress Cataloging-in-Publication Data
A catalog record for this book is available from the Library of Congress

ISBN: 978-0-12-420118-7
ISSN: 1054-3589

For information on all Academic Press publications
visit our website at store.elsevier.com

Printed and bound in United States in America
14   15   16   10 9 8 7 6 5 4 3 2 1

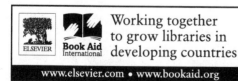

Working together
to grow libraries in
developing countries

www.elsevier.com • www.bookaid.org

CONTENTS

PREFACE

Despite the considerable progress in understanding the biological basis of drug abuse, no pharmacotherapeutics have been approved by the FDA for the treatment of the abuse of cocaine and methamphetamine. Furthermore, FDA-approved pharmacotherapies to treat the abuse of other psychostimulants, such as nicotine, are not ideal since only about 20% of tobacco smokers sustain long-term (12 months) abstinence, despite the use of available treatment options, that is, bupropion, varenicline, or nicotine replacement.

The lack of progress in the discovery of novel pharmacotherapeutics to treat psychostimulant abuse is, in part, due to a lack of investment by the pharmaceutical industry because of factors associated with the discovery of new therapeutics, in general, and, in particular, the factors associated with the discovery of therapeutics to specifically treat drug abuse. A general impediment is the exorbitant costs associated with the process of discovery and development of a new chemical entity as it progresses from the preclinical laboratory to clinical trials and FDA approval. The process is costly, with estimates of $1–2 billion, and it typically requires 10–15 years to complete. A more specific impediment to the development of new therapeutics to treat drug abuse is the perceived small market size, the risks associated with treating abusers with impaired health, and the expected small return on investment relative to potential returns on other more lucrative treatment indications. Furthermore, there is the perception that the pharmaceutical company's brand will acquire negative associations as a result of being linked to the treatment of drug abuse. An additional consideration is that the hurdle for regulatory approval for therapeutics to treat drug abuse is high, since demonstration of efficacy in clinical trials is defined as a period of abstinence during treatment rather than the reduced use of the abused drug. Another challenge is the limited patient compliance associated with treatment.

The National Institute on Drug Abuse (NIDA) mission is, in part, to provide strategic support of research to significantly improve the treatment of drug abuse, including the discovery and development of therapeutics for this purpose. One strategy to obtain new therapies is to provide support for the repurposing of drugs that are in late-stage development, have been approved by the FDA, or have failed as therapeutics for another indication. An important consideration is that repurposing will be less costly and require less total time for the drug to reach commercialization compared with newly discovered compounds beginning the process at chemical design and synthesis. However, approval of repurposed drugs still requires demonstration of safety and efficacy in double blind, placebo-controlled clinical trials using individuals who are psychostimulant abusers. A number of therapeutics have been approved previously or are in late stages of development to be considered for clinical evaluation as drug abuse treatments. However, in the absence of patent protection, the effectiveness of repurposing is questionable unless economic incentives are adopted.

NIDA also has been a strong proponent of the long-term investment strategy, which supports research focused on the discovery and development of new innovative therapeutics for psychostimulant abuse, most of which has been conceived in the academic arena. It is even more critical at the current time to continue support of the discovery of novel compounds for the treatment of drug abuse to maintain and further develop the pipeline of potential new therapeutics. This support is particularly important since the pharmaceutical industry has reduced their high-risk discovery efforts, severely limiting their pipeline and causing them to pursue new compounds discovered in the academic arena often pursued as academic/industrial alliances. Thus, pursuing both strategies (repurposing and novel compound discovery) likely will provide the best chance of success.

The primary impetus for this volume of *Advances in Pharmacology* is to provide a compilation of some of the important contemporary research discoveries. Not intended to be comprehensive, this volume instead features high-value targets and compounds that have emerged from the efforts of academics pursing drug discovery for the treatment of psychostimulant abuse. The author list constitutes the outstanding investigators from academic and research institutions who are exploiting a variety of targets and pharmacophores in an attempt to provide new efficacious therapeutics to those individuals addicted to psychostimulant drugs. This volume includes reviews of research on novel drugs targeting the classical biogenic amine transporters and receptors, nicotinic receptors, kappa and mu opioid receptors, sigma receptors, and benzodiazepine receptors combined with inhibitors of cortisol synthesis. Also included is a review of innovative work on glia as a drug target. These are complemented by reviews of research on biologic approaches, vaccines, and monoclonal antibodies, aimed at limiting the distribution of the abused drug to brain. Finally, a review of the pharmacology and use of synthetic cathinones is included, as these psychostimulants represent an emerging drug abuse problem.

In closing, I gratefully acknowledge the guidance and assistance of the Series Editor, S.J. Enna, and of the Managing Editor, Lynn LeCount, in the editing of this volume.

LINDA P. DWOSKIN, PH.D.
Department of Pharmaceutical Sciences, College of Pharmacy
University of Kentucky, Lexington, KY, USA

Funding: Work in the Dwoskin laboratory is supported by the National Institute on Drug Abuse (NIDA) U01 DA13519; however, this grant did not play a role in the preparation or contents of this preface.

CONTRIBUTORS

Michael T. Bardo
Department of Psychology, College of Pharmacy, University of Kentucky, Lexington, Kentucky, USA

Patrick M. Beardsley
Virginia Commonwealth University, Richmond, Virginia, USA

Jean M. Bidlack
School of Medicine and Dentistry, University of Rochester, Rochester, New York, USA

Bruce E. Blough
Center for Organic and Medicinal Chemistry, Research Triangle Institute, Research Triangle Park, North Carolina, USA

Caitlin Burzynski
Medicinal Chemistry Section, Molecular Targets and Medications Discovery Branch, National Institute on Drug Abuse—Intramural Research Program, Baltimore, Maryland, USA

F. Ivy Carroll
Center for Organic and Medicinal Chemistry, Research Triangle Institute, Research Triangle Park, North Carolina, USA

Peter A. Crooks
Department of Pharmaceutical Sciences, College of Pharmacy, University of Arkansas for Medical Sciences, Little Rock, Arizona, and College of Pharmacy, University of Kentucky, Lexington, Kentucky, USA

M. Imad Damaj
Pharmacology and Toxicology, Virginia Commonwealth University, Richmond, Virginia, USA

Patricia Di Ciano
Translational Addiction Research Laboratory, Centre for Addiction and Mental Health, University of Toronto, Toronto, Canada

Linda P. Dwoskin
Department of Pharmaceutical Sciences, College of Pharmacy, University of Kentucky, Lexington, Kentucky, USA

Amy W.M. Ewald
School of Biological Sciences, Centre for Biodiscovery, Victoria University of Wellington, Wellington, New Zealand

Helen Fox
Yale Stress Center, Yale University School of Medicine, New Haven Connecticut USA

W. Brooks Gentry
Department of Pharmacology and Toxicology, and Department of Anesthesiology, College of Medicine, University of Arkansas for Medical Sciences, Little Rock, Arkansas, USA

Richard A. Glennon
Department of Medicinal Chemistry, School of Pharmacy, Virginia Commonwealth University, Richmond, Virginia, USA

Nicholas E. Goeders
Department of Pharmacology, Toxicology & Neuroscience, LSU Health Sciences Center, Shreveport, Louisiana, USA

David K. Grandy
Department of Physiology & Pharmacology, School of Medicine, Oregon Health & Science University, Portland, Oregon, USA

Glenn F. Guerin
Department of Pharmacology, Toxicology & Neuroscience, LSU Health Sciences Center, Shreveport, Louisiana, USA

Kurt F. Hauser
Virginia Commonwealth University, Richmond, Virginia, USA

Leonard L. Howell
Yerkes National Primate Research Center, Emory University, Atlanta, Georgia, USA

Nidhi Kaushal
West Virginia University, One Medical Center Drive, Morgantown, West Virginia, USA

Thomas M. Keck
Medicinal Chemistry Section, Molecular Targets and Medications Discovery Branch, National Institute on Drug Abuse—Intramural Research Program, Baltimore, Maryland, USA

Bronwyn M. Kivell
School of Biological Sciences, Centre for Biodiscovery, Victoria University of Wellington, Wellington, New Zealand

Bernard Le Foll
Translational Addiction Research Laboratory, Centre for Addiction and Mental Health; Alcohol Research and Treatment Clinic, Addiction Medicine Services, Ambulatory Care and Structured Treatments; Campbell Family Mental Health Research Institute, Centre for Addiction and Mental Health; Department of Family and Community Medicine; Department of Pharmacology; Department of Psychiatry, Division of Brain and Therapeutics, and Institute of Medical Sciences, University of Toronto, Toronto, Ontario, Canada

Mark G. LeSage
Department of Medicine; Minneapolis Medical Research Foundation, and Department of Psychology, University of Minnesota, Minneapolis, Minnesota, USA

Ronald J. Lukas
Division of Neurobiology, St. Joseph's Hospital and Medical Center, Barrow Neurological Institute, Phoenix, Arizona, USA

S. Wayne Mascarella
Center for Organic and Medicinal Chemistry, Research Triangle Institute, Research Triangle Park, North Carolina, USA

Rae R. Matsumoto
West Virginia University, One Medical Center Drive, Morgantown, West Virginia, USA

Hernán A. Navarro
Discovery Sciences, Research Triangle Institute, Research Triangle Park, North Carolina, USA

S. Stevens Negus
Department of Pharmacology and Toxicology, Virginia Commonwealth University, Richmond, Virginia, USA

Amy Hauck Newman
Medicinal Chemistry Section, Molecular Targets and Medications Discovery Branch, National Institute on Drug Abuse—Intramural Research Program, Baltimore, Maryland, USA

Linda Nguyen
West Virginia University, One Medical Center Drive, Morgantown, West Virginia, USA

Justin R. Nickell
College of Pharmacy, University of Kentucky, Lexington, Kentucky, USA

S. Michael Owens
Department of Pharmacology and Toxicology, College of Medicine, University of Arkansas for Medical Sciences, Little Rock, Arkansas, USA

Paul R. Pentel
Department of Pharmacology; Department of Medicine, University of Minnesota, and Minneapolis Medical Research Foundation, Minneapolis, Minnesota, USA

Eric C. Peterson
Department of Pharmacology and Toxicology, College of Medicine, University of Arkansas for Medical Sciences, Little Rock, Arkansas, USA

Thomas E. Prisinzano
Department of Medicinal Chemistry, University of Kansas, Lawrence, Kansas, USA

Matthew J. Robson
West Virginia University, One Medical Center Drive, Morgantown, West Virginia, USA

Christopher D. Schmoutz
Department of Pharmacology, Toxicology & Neuroscience, LSU Health Sciences Center, Shreveport, Louisiana, USA

Lei Shi
Department of Physiology and Biophysics and Institute for Computational Biomedicine, Weill Cornell Medical College, New York, USA

Rajita Sinha
Yale Stress Center, Yale University School of Medicine, New Haven Connecticut USA

Kiran B. Siripurapu
College of Pharmacy, University of Kentucky, Lexington, Kentucky, USA

Ashish Vartak
College of Pharmacy, University of Kentucky, Lexington, Kentucky, USA

CHAPTER ONE

Glial Modulators as Potential Treatments of Psychostimulant Abuse

Patrick M. Beardsley[1], Kurt F. Hauser
Virginia Commonwealth University, Richmond, Virginia, USA
[1]Corresponding author: e-mail address: pbeardsl@vcu.edu

Contents

Abstract

Glia (including astrocytes, microglia, and oligodendrocytes), which constitute the majority of cells in the brain, have many of the same receptors as neurons, secrete neurotransmitters and neurotrophic and neuroinflammatory factors, control clearance of neurotransmitters from synaptic clefts, and are intimately involved in synaptic plasticity. Despite their prevalence and spectrum of functions, appreciation of their potential general importance has been elusive since their identification in the mid-1800s, and only relatively recently have they been gaining their due respect. This development of appreciation has been nurtured by the growing awareness that drugs of abuse, including the psychostimulants, affect glial activity, and glial activity, in turn, has been found to modulate the effects of the psychostimulants. This developing awareness has begun to

Advances in Pharmacology, Volume 69
ISSN 1054-3589
http://dx.doi.org/10.1016/B978-0-12-420118-7.00001-9

1

illuminate novel pharmacotherapeutic targets for treating psychostimulant abuse, for which targeting more conventional neuronal targets has not yet resulted in a single, approved medication. In this chapter, we discuss the molecular pharmacology, physiology, and functional relationships that the glia have especially in the light in which they present themselves as targets for pharmacotherapeutics intended to treat psychostimulant abuse disorders. We then review a cross section of preclinical studies that have manipulated glial processes whose behavioral effects have been supportive of considering the glia as drug targets for psychostimulant-abuse medications. We then close with comments regarding the current clinical evaluation of relevant compounds for treating psychostimulant abuse, as well as the likelihood of future prospects.

ABBREVIATIONS

AGEs advanced glycation (nonenzymatic glycosylation) end products
BDNF brain-derived neurotrophic factor
CNS central nervous system
Co-REST corepressor of RE1 silencing transcription
CPP conditioned place preference
DAMPs damage-associated molecular patterns
DAT1 dopamine transporter (*SLC6A3* gene)
DC-SIGN dendritic cell-specific intercellular adhesion molecule-3-grabbing nonintegrin
EAAT excitatory amino acid transporter
GABA γ-amino-butyric acid
GDNF glial cell line-derived neurotrophic factor
GSK-3β glycogen synthase kinase-3β
HO-1 heme-oxygenase 1
IL interleukin
LPS lipopolysaccharide
MBP myelin basic protein
MHC-I major histocompatibility complex class I
MHC-II major histocompatibility complex class II
mPFC medial prefrontal cortex
nACC nucleus accumbens
NGF nerve growth factor
NMDA *N*-methyl-D-aspartate
NOD-like receptors nucleotide-binding and oligomerization domain (NOD) receptors
NOS2 nitric oxide synthase 2
PAMPs pathogen-associated molecular patterns
PDE phosphodiesterase
PLP proteolipid protein
PRRs pattern recognition receptors
RAGE receptor for advanced glycation end products
Ret rearranged during transfection (a tyrosine kinase receptor)
RIG-1 retinoic acid-inducible gene 1 protein
TGF-β transforming growth factor-β
TLRs toll-like receptors
TNF-α tumor necrosis factor-α

TrkB tropomyosin receptor kinase B (aka, tropomyosin-related kinase B or neurotrophic tyrosine kinase, receptor, type 2) (*NTRK2* gene)
VMAT2 vesicular monoamine transporter-2 (*SLC18A2* gene)

1. INTRODUCTION

Virchow (1856, 1858) penned the term "neuroglia," specifically, *nervenkitt*, which has been translated as "nerve glue," or perhaps more appropriately as "nerve putty" (Somjen, 1988). The perception that neuroglia were subservient to neurons and were just the "glue" that held them together persisted as a dominant concept for many decades. It was not until the last couple of decades that a more sophisticated vision of some categories of glia became appreciated with greater importance. For instance, it was not until nearly the beginning of this century that the astroglia were viewed as an integral modular component of a "tripartite synapse" in which they were wed as partners with the presynaptic and postsynaptic nerve terminals regulating neuronal activity and synaptic strength (Araque, Parpura, Sanzgiri, & Haydon, 1999).

Glial cells (astrocytes, microglia, and oligodendrocytes) constitute the majority of cells in the brain (Nedergaard, Ransom, & Goldman, 2003; Sherwood et al., 2006). The major subcategories of glial cells include macroglia (most typically defined as astrocytes, oligodendroglia, and ependymal cells) and microglia. Exhaustive reviews on each macroglial cell type and subtype exist and numerous debates on whether additional varieties of macroglia or "stable" populations of oligodendroglial/astroglial progenitors, such as polydendroglia or "NG2" cells (Chan, Hazell, Desjardins, & Butterworth, 2000; Keirstead, Levine, & Blakemore, 1998; Zhu, Bergles, & Nishiyama, 2008), continue. Ependymal cells line the ventricles, are important in brain homeostasis and cerebrospinal fluid transport, and are derived from radial glia during embryonic maturation (Spassky et al., 2005). Of the macroglial types, we will only discuss the role of psychostimulants in astroglia, although emerging findings suggest that cocaine (Feng, 2008; George, Mandyam, Wee, & Koob, 2008; Kristiansen, Bannon, & Meador-Woodruff, 2009; Kovalevich, Corley, Yen, Rawls, & Langford, 2012) disrupts myelin and oligodendrocyte genes and/or their function and it seems likely that other macroglial cell types will be found to facilitate significant aspects of psychostimulant action.

Oligodendroglia remain an understudied glial type that have only been minimally explored in the context of psychostimulant abuse (Miguel-Hidalgo, 2009) and will only be passingly mentioned in this chapter. Oligodendrocyte numbers (George, Mandyam, Wee, & Koob, 2008) and myelin (Kristiansen, Bannon, & Meador-Woodruff, 2009; Kovalevich, Corley, Yen, Rawls, & Langford, 2012) are reduced following cocaine exposure in rats. Cocaine exposure is also known to cause reductions in myelin basic protein (MBP), proteolipid protein (PLP), and other key oligodendroglial transcripts in gene arrays (Albertson et al., 2004; Bannon, Kapatos, & Albertson, 2005). However, unlike the effects of psychostimulants in microglia and astroglia, which have known effects on neuronal function, it is as yet uncertain whether reduced numbers of cells; decreased levels of MBP, PLP, and other transcripts; or hypothetical alterations in oligodendroglia function induced by psychostimulants (Miguel-Hidalgo, 2009) affect neuronal function. Even less is known about the effects of methamphetamine on oligodendrocytes, except that the drug preferentially disrupts the genesis of oligodendroglial precursors in the adult rat medial prefrontal cortex (mPFC) (Mandyam, Wee, Eisch, Richardson, & Koob, 2007). Additional study of psychostimulant action in oligodendrocytes and how the changes in oligodendrocytes affect other neuronal and glial cell types is warranted and overdue. The discussions that follow are limited to astroglia and microglia.

Glia contain receptors (for reviews, see Kimelberg, 1995; Pocock & Kettenmann, 2007) (see in the succeeding text), secrete neurotransmitters and neurotrophic and neuroinflammatory factors (Benz, Grima, & Do, 2004; Bezzi et al., 1998; Kang, Jiang, Goldman, & Nedergaard, 1998; Parpura et al., 1994; Watkins et al., 2007), control clearance of neurotransmitters from synaptic clefts (Camacho & Massieu, 2006), and are involved with synaptic plasticity (e.g., Ullian, Christopherson, & Barres, 2004). Given their prevalence, and their multiple modes of controlling neurological functionality, it is not surprising that glia and their secreted products have been reported to modulate, and be modulated by, the drugs of abuse including the psychostimulants (e.g., Bolanos & Nestler, 2004; Clark, Wiley, & Bradberry, 2013; Cooper, Jones, & Comer, 2012; Ghitza et al., 2010; Haydon, Blendy, Moss, & Jackson, 2009; Narita et al., 2006; Pierce & Bari, 2001).

Astroglia and microglia express a multitude of receptors and drug transporters thought to be directly or indirectly affected by psychostimulants. In fact, there are few examples of G protein-coupled receptors (GPCRs) that are expressed by neurons that are not also expressed by astrocytes (Wilkin, Marriott, & Cholewinski, 1990; Zhang & Barres, 2010). Although this refers to both glial types, astroglia display the greatest phenotypic diversity—rivaled only by neurons in the brain. For this reason, unless the glial type of interest is isolated *in vitro*, it is normally difficult to selectively activate astrocyte (or microglial) receptors without stimulating the same receptor on neurons and vice versa using GPCR agonists or antagonists (Conklin et al., 2008; Fiacco, Agulhon, & McCarthy, 2009). To date, most direct evidence to unambiguously identify a particular drug target or action in microglia or astroglia relies largely on extrapolating findings from *in vitro* studies. Obviously, generalizing any results from cell culture studies to the intact animal has serious limitations. Nevertheless, isolating the response and/or actions of a drug to particular glial type *in vivo* has been exceedingly challenging. Recently, the use of genetic approaches to direct the expression of engineered GPCRs (Coward et al., 1998) into glia, and the utilization of novel ligands to selectively activate these receptors, has been used as a tactic to unambiguously discern glial versus neuronal functions (Conklin et al., 2008). Strategies using designer receptors exclusively activated by designer drugs (DREADDs) (Armbruster, Li, Pausch, Herlitze, & Roth, 2007) or receptors activated solely by a synthetic ligands (RASSLs) (Conklin et al., 2008; Dong, Rogan, & Roth, 2010) hold considerable promise for discriminating the role of a particular glial type such as astroglia or microglia or glial subtype such as dopamine D2 versus non-D2 receptor-expressing astroglia from other cell types. Alternatively, an additional means of differentiating glia from neurons is to examine unique functional markers and their associated responses. Thus, while the "glial" drugs mentioned in this chapter may preferentially act through a single glial cell type, it is extremely tricky to unambiguously assign the actions of a drug to a particular glial cell type or distinguish a drug's action in glia versus neurons using current methodology. Accordingly, even if an action of a drug is preferentially associated with a unique glial function, the glial response may be secondary to the drug's actions in another cell type and likely to be acting preferentially, but not exclusively, in that glial type. Thus, caution is warranted before asserting "glial" action to the most current pharmacotherapeutics.

Manipulating the activity of glia as a target in the development of pharmacotherapeutics for treating psychostimulant disorders is in its infancy, and few mature systematic efforts exist. Thus, this chapter cannot stand as an inventory of current, glial-related strategies in drug development for the treatment of psychostimulant abuse. Instead, we try to introduce the reader to glial physiology presented with a focus on how altering glial processes may provide opportunities for developing psychostimulant medications. We also provide

an overview of key preclinical studies that have reported on drugs that attenuate abuse-related effects of psychostimulants, which likely act through glial
and neuroinflammatory mechanisms. Drugs with the ability to activate or
antagonize receptors that mediate the actions of the psychostimulants have
automatically marked them as potential pharmacotherapeutics. Astroglia
and microglia express most known central nervous system (CNS) receptors
including dopaminergic, opioidergic, glutaminergic, adrenergic, nicotinic,
cannabinergic, serotonergic, ATP/P2X, peptidergic, ionotropic, and GPCRs
such as purinergic, GABAergic, and sigma receptors among others
(Deschepper, 1998; Durand, Carniglia, Caruso, & Lasaga, 2013; Fumagalli
et al., 2003; Hall, Herrera, Ajmo, Cuevas, & Pennypacker, 2009;
Hernandez-Morales & Garcia-Colunga, 2009; ;Hosli & Hosli, 1993 Hosli,
Hosli, Maelicke, & Schroder, 1992; Khan, Koulen, Rubinstein, Grandy, &
Goldman-Rakic, 2001; Kimelberg, 1995; Krisch & Mentlein, 1994;
Morioka, 2011; Pocock & Kettenmann, 2007; Stella, 2010). In fact, cortical
astroglia account for approximately one-third of the total dopamine
D2-receptor binding sites in the cortex (Khan et al., 2001). Although this chapter does address the structure and function of the glia, including their resident
receptors that might modulate psychostimulant effects, it ultimately excludes
discussion of potential pharmacotherapeutics having these conventional receptor targets and instead restricts itself to drugs affecting glia with known anti-
neuroinflammatory consequences. This chapter is consequentially structured
into two major sections. The first section covers microglia and astroglia and
how their molecular pharmacology and neuroinflammatory effects could serve
as provocative targets for psychostimulant pharmacotherapeutic development.
The second section reviews *in vivo* evidence of drugs that affect neuroglia and
have anti-inflammatory consequences that can ameliorate abuse-related effects
of the psychostimulants. This chapter ends with closing comments regarding
the status of glial-drug development for treating psychostimulant abuse and
points to where we think the most interesting targets for future investigation
reside.

2. MOLECULAR BIOLOGY AND PHYSIOLOGY OF THE GLIA

2.1. Glial responses to neuronal injury and stress

2.1.1 Innate immune effectors

Unlike neurons, microglia, and to a lesser extent astroglia, contribute to
innate immunity within the CNS. Microglia, in particular, are the principal

immune effectors in the CNS. Microglia express a wide variety of pattern (or "pathogen," as discussed in the succeeding text) recognition receptors (PRRs) associated with innate immune function, including Toll-like receptors (TLRs); scavenger receptors, such as receptors for advanced glycation end products (RAGEs); nucleotide-binding oligomerization domain receptors (NOD-like receptors or NLRs); and macrophage antigen complex-1 (Mac-1) receptors (see Fig. 1.1). In addition to their role as innate immune effectors, microglia express major histocompatibility complex I (MHC-I) and MHC-II complexes and can thereby recognize both intracellular and extracellular foreign proteins and process these for presentation as antigens to T lymphocytes, hence contributing to adaptive immunity. While it has long been known that astrocytes express MHC-I, cumulative evidence suggests that under duress, astrocytes can also express MHC-II (Jensen, Massie, & De Keyser, 2013).

PRRs were initially characterized for their role in host protection against unique pathogen-associated molecular patterns (PAMPs). It was later realized that many of the same cellular responses that were activated by pathogens could also be triggered by the accompanying damage to the host cell and that in some instances, the damage per se was sufficient to initiate an innate immune response. Consequently, it is not a coincidence that there is considerable overlap in the cellular response to PAMPs and damage (Bianchi, 2007; Srikrishna & Freeze, 2009).

Neuronal damage-associated molecular patterns (DAMPs) can directly activate and, in aberrant or pathologic situations, overactivate microglia (Biber, Neumann, Inoue, & Boddeke, 2007; Block, Zecca, & Hong, 2007). DAMPs are released from stressed or injured cells (Bianchi, 2007; Srikrishna & Freeze, 2009). PRRs are activated by DAMPs and are key regulators of innate immune function. Many classes of PRRs have been purported to be directly or indirectly responsive to substance abuse and especially psychostimulants. Psychostimulants including methamphetamine, cocaine, and ecstasy have been suggested to activate the innate immune system (Clark et al., 2013), which has been proposed to be a necessary neurobiological step in causing some addictions (Crews, Zou, & Qin, 2011). The role of innate immune activation is particularly evident in chronic alcoholism (Crews et al., 2011; Yakovleva, Bazov, Watanabe, Hauser, & Bakalkin, 2011) but is also thought to contribute to cocaine addiction (Crews et al., 2011). The diversity of signals that can act as DAMPs permits the injured cell to communicate sophisticated signals to innate immune effectors, which enables a highly coordinated and measured host response to stress or injury.

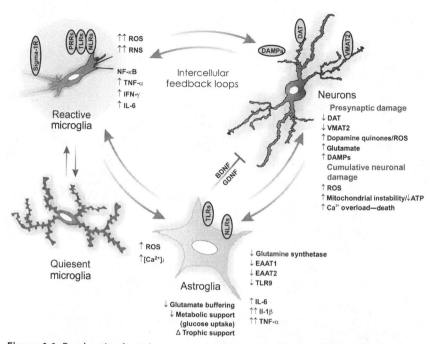

Figure 1.1 Psychostimulants increase synaptic damage through direct actions on neurons and glia including both microglia and astroglia. Psychostimulants damage presynaptic terminals of neurons causing the production of reactive oxygen species (ROS) and nitrogen (species) and the production of damage-associated molecular patterns (DAMPs) that trigger activation of PRRs, including toll-like receptors (TLRs), NOD-like receptors (NLRs), and other PRRs associated with microglia, and to a lesser extent astroglia. Dopaminergic neurons are particularly vulnerable to methamphetamine, which disrupts dopamine transporter (DAT) and vesicular monoamine transporter 1 (VMAT2) function. Importantly, psychostimulants disrupt glial function directly by increasing intracellular Ca^{2+} concentration ($[Ca^{2+}]_i$) and NF-κB transcriptional activity and by activating sigma1 receptors (Sigma-1R) and enzyme systems driving oxidative and nitrosative stress especially in microglia (and other cell types). Increases in NF-κB transcriptional activity result in the increased production of tumor necrosis factor-α (TNF-α), interferon-γ (IFN-γ), and interleukin-6 (IL-6) (among others) and cytokines by microglia and to a lesser degree by astroglia. Psychostimulants also obstruct the buffering of extracellular glutamate by inhibiting excitatory amino acid transporters-1/2 (EAAT1/2) and the conversion of glutamate to glutamine by inhibiting glutamine synthetase, as well as limiting glucose metabolism in astrocytes. Collectively, neuronal damage combined with a heightened state of glial activation promotes positive microglial–astroglial feedback and neuronal–glial feedback that cause spiraling increases in neuroinflammation and neuronal injury. If unchecked, the cumulative insults result in lasting neurodegenerative changes. *Modified and reprinted from Hauser, Fitting, Dever, Podhaizer, and Knapp (2012)—an "open access article distributed under the terms of the Creative Commons Attribution License (http://creativecommons.org/licenses/by/2.5/), which permits unrestrictive use, distribution, and reproduction in any medium, provided the original work is properly cited."* (For color version of this figure, the reader is referred to the online version of this chapter.)

2.1.2 Pattern recognition receptors

2.1.2.1 Toll-like receptors

TLRs are a primitive part of the innate immune system and respond to novel molecular motifs associated with pathogens such as gram-negative and gram-positive bacteria or short lengths of single- and/or double-stranded RNA (dsRNA) or DNA suggestive of viral invasion (Beutler et al., 2006; Kawai & Akira, 2007). Multiple TLRs exist. Each is associated with a distinct pathogen motif or related patterns. Although considerable attention has been given to TLR4 in relation to addiction and neuropathic pain due to its ability to bind opiate agonists and antagonists (Hutchinson et al., 2011; Theberge et al., 2013; Wang, Loram, et al., 2012), emerging evidence suggests that the expression and function of other TLRs may be influenced by psychomotorstimulants. For example, methamphetamine downregulates TLR9, which attenuates the ability of macrophages to recognize and fight intracellular pathogens such as HIV-1 (Cen et al., 2013). Innate immune genes, including TLRs, have been shown to be involved in the sequelae of adaptive neurobiological changes underlying alcohol addiction (Crews et al., 2011) and researchers have speculated that the same mechanisms may be operative for cocaine and perhaps other addictive drugs (Clark et al., 2013; Crews et al., 2011; Frank, Watkins, & Maier, 2011).

2.1.2.2 Receptor for advanced glycation end products

RAGE recognizes a wide variety of advanced glycation end products (AGEs), including S100β, which is released from damaged astrocytes following brain injury (Egea-Guerrero et al., 2012), and high-mobility group box-1, an AGEs-related factor that can be released by neurons and glia during stress or inflammation, which is also recognized by TLR2 and TLR4; Maroso et al., 2010). Methamphetamine produces a number of abnormal immunogenic protein glycation products (Dickerson, Yamamoto, Ruiz, & Janda, 2004; Treweek, Dickerson, & Janda, 2009; Treweek, Wee, Koob, Dickerson, & Janda, 2007).

2.1.2.3 Nucleotide-binding and oligomerization domain receptors

Less is understood about the potential role of nucleotide-binding and oligomerization domain (NOD) receptors (Strober, Murray, Kitani, & Watanabe, 2006) (NOD-like receptors) in psychostimulant actions. Since several of the NOD-like receptor subfamilies contribute to the formation of inflammasomes (Kanneganti, Lamkanfi, & Nunez, 2007; Schroder & Tschopp, 2010), it is likely that they participate in methamphetamine-induced inflammation and neuronal injury. The $NLRP_3$ inflammasome, in particular, is involved in interleukin-1β (IL-1β) processing by macrophages. IL-1β is a key cytokine involved in initiating a variety of inflammatory cascades in microglia.

2.1.2.4 Alternative PRRs

Numerous alternative PRRs exist, including C-type lectin receptors (Geijtenbeek & Gringhuis, 2009), RNA helicases, and retinoic acid-inducible gene 1 (RIG-1 or RIG-I) protein complexes and a wide variety of additional receptor types. Several receptor kinase classes sensing internal homeostatic signals including redox, hyperthermia, and aberrant synaptic function also serve as PRRs. Regarding C-type lectin receptors, a class of receptors that display Ca^{2+}-dependent binding to carbohydrates, the expression and function of dendritic cell-specific intercellular adhesion molecule-3-grabbing nonintegrin (DC-SIGN or CD209) are affected by cocaine (Nair et al., 2004, 2005) and methamphetamine (Nair, Mahajan, Sykes, Bapardekar, & Reynolds, 2006). Disrupting DC-SIGN alters basic immune function and the ability of dendritic cells to present antigens to T lymphocytes. Numerous reviews describe the mechanisms by which psychostimulants cause aberrant intracellular redox potentials (Rubartelli & Lotze, 2007), oxidative and nitrosative stress, hyperthermia (Thomas, Walker, Benjamins, Geddes, & Kuhn, 2004), mitochondrial energetics, and glucose metabolism in neurons and glia (Cadet & Jayanthi, 2013; Cadet & Krasnova, 2009; Coller & Hutchinson, 2012; Davidson, Gow, Lee, & Ellinwood, 2001; Kaushal & Matsumoto, 2011; Kita, Miyazaki, Asanuma, Takeshima, & Wagner, 2009; Krasnova & Cadet, 2009; Quinton & Yamamoto, 2006).

2.2. Microglia

2.2.1 Direct psychostimulant effects on microglia

Methamphetamine and cocaine directly affect microglia through actions at sigma-1 receptors (SIGMA1R). Sigma-1 receptors are associated with the membrane of the endoplasmic reticulum (Hayashi & Su, 2007) and can also serve as intracellular chaperones (Su, Hayashi, Maurice, Buch, & Ruoho, 2010). Sigma-1 receptors are one of several putative molecular targets of methamphetamine (Hayashi et al., 2010; Kaushal & Matsumoto, 2011) and cocaine (Fritz, Klement, El Rawas, Saria, & Zernig, 2011; Katz et al., 2011; Kourrich et al., 2013; Narayanan, Mesangeau, Poupaert, & McCurdy, 2011; Navarro et al., 2010; Robson, Noorbakhsh, Seminerio,

& Matsumoto, 2012; Yao et al., 2011). Despite the emerging importance of sigma-1 receptors in the neurobiology of psychostimulant addiction and some promising lead compounds (Kaushal, Elliott, et al., 2012; Kaushal, Seminerio, Robson, McCurdy, & Matsumoto, 2012; Robson et al., 2013; Xu et al., 2012), as yet, there are no established antagonists highly selective for sigma-1 receptors. Microglia, and potentially astroglia, express sigma-1 receptors and therefore can be directly affected by exposure to methamphetamine and cocaine. Despite some reports that selective sigma-1 receptor activation has been shown to inhibit microglial motility, cytokine release, and intracellular Ca^{2+} in response to lipopolysaccharide (LPS), monocyte chemoattractant protein-1, and ATP (Hall et al., 2009), ligands with agonist properties are more often found to activate proinflammatory microglial responses (Behensky et al., 2013; Cuevas, Rodriguez, Behensky, & Katnik, 2011; Gekker et al., 2006; Yao et al., 2011). The evidence for astroglial expression of sigma-1 receptors is less well established and is based on their expression in a human fetal astroglial SVG cell line (Ben-Ami, Kinor, Perelman, & Yadid, 2006), or ligand binding profiles, or effects in primary astrocytes (Mattson, Rychlik, & Cheng, 1992; Prezzavento et al., 2007) and glioblastoma cell lines (Thomas et al., 1990).

While neurotransmitters tend to be neutral or inhibit the release of proinflammatory cytokines, excess glutamate, extracellular ATP, the tachykinin substance P (Angulo, Angulo, & Yu, 2004), and bradykinin can augment cytokine production by microglia (Farber, Pannasch, & Kettenmann, 2005; Pocock & Kettenmann, 2007). Imbalances in excitatory and inhibitory neurotransmitters have also been proposed to act as DAMPs (Gao & Hong, 2008) and proposed as a mechanism by which methamphetamine activates glia (Pereira et al., 2012). In this regard, microglial glutamate and purine neurotransmitter receptors, specifically AMPA 1 glutamate receptors (GluR1 or GRIA1) (Cadet & Jayanthi, 2013; Hemby, 2004) and P2X4 purinergic receptors (Horvath & Deleo, 2009; Horvath, Romero-Sandoval, & De Leo, 2010), may function as PRRs, thereby distinguishing themselves for their potential involvement in modulating the effects of abused substances directly in microglia. These and other basic steady-state processes are well-established targets of psychostimulants. Thus, by inducing stress and injuring neurons, methamphetamine and cocaine induce the formation of neuronal DAMPs directly, thereby triggering secondary microglial responses. In addition, methamphetamine and cocaine can directly activate the microglia themselves, which may further heighten the innate microglial response to neuronal DAMPs.

2.2.2 Psychostimulant-induced synaptic and neuronal injury result in DAMPs and signals that activate microglia

Many excellent reviews are available that examine the neurotoxic effects of methamphetamine, cocaine, and other psychostimulants in significant detail (Cadet & Jayanthi, 2013; Cadet & Krasnova, 2009; Davidson et al., 2001; Kita et al., 2009; Krasnova & Cadet, 2009) and will only be concisely mentioned. Instead, our goal here is to consider the role of microglia and astroglia in both contributing to and responding to neuronal injury and the extent to which glially directed pharmacotherapies might be advantageous in managing the chronic neuroinflammatory and degenerative effects of these abused substances.

Briefly, methamphetamine can reportedly damage neurons through a variety of mechanisms and the exact sequelae of events resulting in neuronal compromise are not fully understood. Methamphetamine and cocaine are weak bases that restrict intracytoplasmic acidification and reduce the vesicular transmembrane pH gradient necessary for vesicular uptake while prompting excessive release of biogenic amines from presynaptic terminals (Sulzer & Rayport, 1990). While intracytoplasmic dopamine was initially thought to intrinsically promote methamphetamine neurotoxicity (Facchinetti et al., 2004), in reality, the nonenzymatic conversion of dopamine to dopamine quinones (LaVoie & Hastings, 1999a; Sulzer & Zecca, 2000) and the concurrent generation of oxyradicals are believed necessary to elicit a cytotoxic microglial response (Kuhn, Francescutti-Verbeem, & Thomas, 2008; LaVoie & Hastings, 1999b; Sulzer & Zecca, 2000; Thomas, Francescutti-Verbeem, & Kuhn, 2008). Despite this evidence, there remains some skepticism regarding the extent to which methamphetamine-induced intraneuronal dopamine quinone formation is causal in neurodegeneration in addicts (Sulzer & Zecca, 2000). This highly localized response may be exacerbated by excessive peripheral ammonia caused by concurrent methamphetamine-induced hepatotoxicity (Halpin & Yamamoto, 2012). The alterations to pH, nitrogen balance, and redox exact the greatest toll on vesicular trafficking at presynaptic boutons, which results in highly localized increases in oxidative and nitrosative stress that disrupt the dopamine transporter (DAT) (Fleckenstein, Metzger, Wilkins, Gibb, & Hanson, 1997) and vesicular monoamine transporter-2 (VMAT2) function (Larsen, Fon, Hastings, Edwards, & Sulzer, 2002; Miller, Gainetdinov, Levey, & Caron, 1999). Disturbing the transporters promotes the pathologic accumulation of dopamine, a weak oxidant, within the cytoplasmic compartment of presynaptic terminals initiating their damage (Eyerman

& Yamamoto, 2007; Fumagalli et al., 1999; Miller et al., 1999), and VMAT2 reductions are evident in cocaine-addicted individuals (Little, Krolewski, Zhang, & Cassin, 2003). Dopaminergic presynaptic terminal destruction is accompanied by microglial activation, but is thought to be independent of dopamine accumulation in the synaptic cleft or dopamine D1 or D2 receptor blockade (Thomas, Dowgiert, et al., 2004; Thomas, Walker, et al., 2004). Moreover, psychostimulants also disrupt the function of GluN2B subunit-expressing N-methyl-D-aspartate (NMDA) receptors on neurons (Davidson et al., 2007), which are well known to facilitate the excitotoxic effects of excessive and/or extrasynaptic glutamate.

Methamphetamine and other psychostimulants induce atypical increases in extracellular glutamate in the CNS (Cadet, Krasnova, Jayanthi, & Lyles, 2007; Kaushal & Matsumoto, 2011; Miyatake, Narita, Shibasaki, Nakamura, & Suzuki, 2005; Pereira et al., 2012; Quinton & Yamamoto, 2006). Excessive glutamate, especially at extrasynaptic sites (Hardingham, Fukunaga, & Bading, 2002; Sattler, Xiong, Lu, MacDonald, & Tymianski, 2000), induces excitotoxic injury through actions at specific glutamate receptor types and subtypes expressed by neurons (Choi, 1988, 1992; Olney et al., 1991; Rothman & Olney, 1986). Overactivation of extrasynaptic GluN2B NMDA receptors causes synaptodendritic injury and neuron death (Ivanov et al., 2006; Liu et al., 2007). Blockade of NMDA receptors with MK-801 or dextromethorphan prevents methamphetamine-induced neurotoxicity (Thomas & Kuhn, 2005). By contrast, some glutamate receptor types are neuroprotective (Taylor, Diemel, & Pocock, 2003; Venero et al., 2002). For example, GluN2A- (GRIN2A) and GluN2B- (GRIN2B) subunit-containing NMDA receptors typically have opposing roles in synaptic stabilization (Kim, Dunah, Wang, & Sheng, 2005). Not inconsequentially, microglia and astrocytes also express many of these same glutamate receptors, which permit both glial types to respond in coordination with neurons and to assume an immediate defensive posture if necessary. Excitotoxic levels of glutamate can trigger a massive inflammatory response in microglia, including the release of tumor necrosis factor-α (TNF-α) and numerous other proinflammatory cytokines (Hagino et al., 2004; Noda, Nakanishi, Nabekura, & Akaike, 2000). While the presence of TNF-α is often assumed to be problematic, depending on the level and duration of TNF-α exposure, it may alert glia to impending danger and can be cytoprotective to neurons (Bruce et al., 1996; Figiel, 2008; Mattson et al., 1995). Lastly, addictive drugs in general (Robison & Nestler, 2011), including methamphetamine (Cadet & Jayanthi, 2013), cause lasting in gene regulation through epigenetic mechanisms that likely contribute to addiction. Because methamphetamine and cocaine cause fundamental epigenetic changes that dysregulate the normal responses to glutamate, normal responses to glutamate are likely to be distorted and/or inappropriate (Cadet & Jayanthi, 2013; Robison & Nestler, 2011). Chronic (2-week) methamphetamine exposure in rats causes epigenetic changes mediated by a corepressor of RE1 silencing transcription (Co-REST), histone deacetylase 2, methyl-CpG-binding protein 2, and sirtuin 2 complex resulting in the hypoacetylation of histone H4 in the rat striatum (Cadet & Jayanthi, 2013). The epigenetic modification of GluA1 and GluA2 DNA sequences downregulates both AMPA receptor subunit transcripts, and these lasting changes likely contribute to the maladaptive neuroplasticity underlying addiction (Cadet & Jayanthi, 2013).

Besides their potential role in activating microglial PRRs (discussed earlier), AMPA 1 glutaminergic (Bowers, Chen, & Bonci, 2010; Davidson et al., 2007; Palmer et al., 2005; Pierce & Wolf, 2013; Snyder et al., 2000; Yu, Chang, & Gean, 2013) and the P2X4 purinergic receptors (Horvath & Deleo, 2009; Horvath et al., 2010) are further distinguished by their pivotal roles in rewiring the key brain areas that underlie addiction through direct actions in neurons. It is noteworthy that many of the same abnormalities in psychostimulant-induced glutamate and/or ATP neurotransmission contributing to addictive behaviors appear to coordinate increases in neuroinflammation by activating microglial PRRs. Several investigators have proposed that glial involvement in general, and glial inflammation in particular, may be a necessary step in the sequelae of events leading to addiction (Clark et al., 2013; Crews et al., 2011; Frank et al., 2011).

The release of ATP from injured neurons activates microglial receptors, including P2Y12, P2X4, and P2X7 (Zhuo, Wu, & Wu, 2011), as well as the NOD-like receptor NLRP$_3$ (Gombault, Baron, & Couillin, 2012). ATP release from injured cells appears to be highly relevant in the neurotoxicity caused by psychomotor stimulants. As noted, some reports suggest that NLP$_3$ inflammasomes cleave nascent IL-1β into bioactive IL-1β (Costa et al., 2012), a key proinflammatory cytokine released by microglia. The extension of microglial processes in response to neuronal damage in mice is affected by ATP via the P2Y12 receptor (Davalos et al., 2005; Haynes et al., 2006; Ohsawa et al., 2010). Moreover, P2X4 receptor signaling is crucial for the development of neuropathic pain in mice (Tsuda, Inoue, & Salter, 2005; Tsuda et al., 2003). ATP acting via P2X7 receptors is necessary for endotoxin (LPS)-dependent release of IL-1β from microglia (Ferrari, Chiozzi, Falzoni, Hanau, & Di, 1997).

Some neuron-derived signals restrict microglial activation and act as "off" signals. These include CX3CL1 (fractalkine) (Cardona et al., 2006; Fuhrmann et al., 2010; Lee et al., 2010) and γ-amino-butyric acid (GABA) acting via specific GABA$_A$ receptors (Pocock & Kettenmann, 2007) and GABA$_B$ receptors, which restrict LPS-induced release of IL-6 and IL-12p40 (Kuhn et al., 2004). The interest in receptor systems that mediate "off" signals is bolstered by clear evidence implicating them in neurodegenerative processes and the promise of therapeutically switching "off" overactivated microglia. Recent reports suggest that CX3CL1 activation is able to inhibit the dendritic loss and death of striatal neurons induced by the synergistic action of morphine and the pathogenic HIV-1 protein Tat, despite the presence of sustained high levels of TNF-α (Suzuki et al., 2011).

A microglial transcriptional "off" or "inactivation" regulator, with high potential relevance for psychostimulant abuse, is the Nurr1 transcriptional repressor. Nurr1 is essential for the generation and maintenance of dopaminergic neurons and Nurr1 mutations are responsible for familial Parkinson's disease, which was recently discovered to inhibit inflammatory responses in microglia and astroglia (Saijo et al., 2009). Posttranslational modifications of Nurr1 promote the formation of Nurr1/Co-REST corepressor complexes, which trigger the clearance of NF-κB p65 and restore pre-inflammatory transcriptional activity (Saijo et al., 2009). In microglia, Nurr1 expression is upregulated by LPS and downregulated by increased ERK, JNK, and PI3K/Akt pathway activity suggesting ample opportunity for therapeutic manipulation (Fan et al., 2009). Importantly, p65 must be phosphorylated before the NF-κB-p65 complex can be removed by Nurr1/Co-REST, and glycogen synthase kinase-3β (GSK-3β) serves an essential role in this function (Saijo et al., 2009). Interestingly, Nurr1 heterozygote mice display augmented methamphetamine neurotoxicity and greater increases in nNOS activity and 3-nitrosyl adducts (Imam et al., 2005) and show increased neurotoxicity with prolonged methamphetamine exposure (Luo, Wang, Kuang, Chiang, & Hoffer, 2010). Acute methamphetamine exposure (1–3 h following a 4 mg/kg dose) increases Nurr1 transcript levels in several cortical regions and in the ventral tegmental area (VTA) in rats, while chronic exposure (4 mg/kg/day) for 2 weeks attenuates the induction of Nurr1 mRNA levels, suggesting Nurr1 expression becomes blunted with chronic methamphetamine exposure (Akiyama, Isao, Ide, Ishikawa, & Saito, 2008). Thus, in addition to manipulating Nurr1/Co-REST activity, drugs and/or small molecule inhibitors of GSK-3β (Coghlan et al., 2000; Cross et al., 2001) hold additional promise for managing and potentially reversing the deleterious consequences of glial overactivation resulting from psychostimulant abuse.

2.2.3 Consequences of microglial overactivation

As noted earlier in the section on PRRs, many authoritative reviews describe the neurobiological consequences of methamphetamine-induced oxidative, nitrosative damage and neuronal injury and death and need not be repeated here. Microglial activation is triggered to varying degrees by a large number of effectors, which include all the PRRs noted earlier and a combination of key transcriptional regulators. Key aspects of the events triggering microglial activation are briefly summarized in the succeeding text.

The Mac-1, which is also a commonly used macrophage/microglial (and neutrophil) marker (Tang et al., 1997; Zhang, Goncalves, & Mosser, 2008), is essential for microglial-mediated neurotoxicity (Hu et al., 2008). Upon activation, Mac-1 is thought to recruit the p47^{phox} NADPH oxidase subunit to the cell surface, which is requisite for NADPH assembly, superoxide production, and host oxidative defense (Hu et al., 2008). Extracellular reactive oxygen species (ROS) for use in host defense originate from NADPH oxidase, which catalyzes superoxide production from oxygen. NADPH complex activation increases the production of extracellular ROS and can amplify toxic proinflammatory signals through redox signaling, which can be toxic to bystander neurons (Block & Hong, 2007; Block et al., 2007; Halliwell, 1992; Levesque et al., 2010). Methamphetamine and cocaine cause NADPH complex activation in microglia.

A wide variety of PRRs converge on NF-κB to trigger proinflammatory responses. Rel/NF-κB family of transcription factors is central in regulating expression of genes that mediate essential physiological processes, including neuroimmune responses in microglia (Karin, Cao, Greten, & Li, 2002). The family is comprised of five polypeptides (p50, p52, p65/RelA, c-Rel, and RelB) that share a homologous N-terminal Rel homology region (Yakovleva et al., 2011). Rel homology domain polypeptides can interact with different affinities and specificities; each is uniquely regulated by inhibitor IκB proteins and differentially affects nuclear translocation and DNA binding. ROS are implicated as second messengers promoting the activation of NF-κB by TNF-α and IL-1β in microglia (Block et al., 2007) and similarly in astrocytes (El-Hage et al., 2008). The effects of ROS on NF-κB activation are cell-specific and dependent on subcellular localization

(Kabe, Ando, Hirao, Yoshida, & Handa, 2005). NF-κB activity is associated with microglial proinflammatory responses (Guo & Bhat, 2006; Pasparakis, 2009; Pawate, Shen, Fan, & Bhat, 2004), and NF-κB proinflammatory gene expression is directly exacerbated by ROS (Pawate et al., 2004).

2.2.4 Shades of gray: Intermediate states of microglial activation

In reality, the low levels of chronic inflammation that accompany chronic cocaine abuse, and somewhat higher levels of chronic inflammation associated with methamphetamine abuse, are typified by intermediate states of activation/inactivation, rather than all-or-none responses. Colton defines two intermediate states of microglial activation as "alternative activation" and "acquired deactivation" (Colton, 2009).

"Alternative activation" is induced by IL-4 and IL-13 and underscored by reduced levels of proinflammatory cytokine production. This initial state of deactivation is mediated intracellularly by events downstream of STAT6 and highlighted by anti-inflammatory cytokines, the downregulation of nitric oxide synthase 2 (NOS2), and tissue repair and reconstruction. NOS2 is particularly important because it converts arginine into nitric oxide (NO), which is essential in peroxynitrite (ONOO$^-$) production and the generation of reactive nitrogen species. A hallmark of alternative activation is arginine that is primarily used to produce polyamines (via enzymatic conversion by arginase 1), rather than NO, because of the downregulation of NOS2 (Colton, 2009).

"Acquired deactivation" is characterized by a further downregulation of innate immune responses. This "secondary" state of deactivation involves enhanced STAT3/SMAD activity, which is mediated by a downregulation of proinflammatory cytokine production, elevated IL-10 and transforming growth factor-β (TGF-β) anti-inflammatory cytokine release, and upregulation of heme-oxygenase 1 (HO-1) and sphingosine-1-phosphate and typified by heightened "non-immunogenic" phagocytosis of apoptotic cell fragments and immune suppression (Colton, 2009). We propose that chronic psychostimulant abuse, especially cocaine abuse that results in less frank neuropathology than with chronic methamphetamine, results in an "altered" state characterized by "alternative activation" with abortive attempts at "acquired deactivation." The sustained partial switch from an acute to a chronic immune profile is likely to be quite maladaptive and seemingly contributes to the prolonged synaptodendritic instability and a protracted weakening of host defenses via partial immunosuppression that is evident with chronic psychostimulant abuse.

2.2.5 Microglial-induced neuroprotection and restoration of neuronal function

With a long-standing emphasis on cytotoxicity, it is easy to overlook the beneficial role microglia play in supporting normal neuronal function. Microglia serve many beneficial roles by providing trophic support and participate in the repair of damaged neural circuits. For example, during maturation, they are essential for selectively pruning excess synaptic connections required for normal function (Paolicelli et al., 2011). In many instances, such as in an experimental model of amyotrophic lateral sclerosis, the morphologic "activation of microglia and astroglia does not predict [cytotoxic] glial function" (Beers, Henkel, Zhao, Wang, & Appel, 2008). A variety of cues act as microglial "off or inactivation" signals (Block et al., 2007), promoting the release of anti-inflammatory cytokines and trophic factors. These are required for maintaining tissue homeostasis and restricting microglial activation. Anti-inflammatory cytokines include IL-10, while microglial-derived trophic factors include brain-derived neurotrophic factor (BDNF) (Graham et al., 2007; McGinty, Whitfield, & Berglind, 2010) and TGF-β (Ransohoff & Perry, 2009; Streit, 2002). Although microglia can express glial cell line-derived neurotrophic factor (GDNF) and BDNF, astrocytes generate a significant amount of the BDNF and especially GDNF produced in the brain, which is described in the next section. Tropomyosin receptor kinase B (TrkB) and the "rearranged during transfection" (Ret) receptor, the cognate receptors for BDNF and GDNF, respectively, are widely expressed by neurons throughout the brain, including the neostriatum and nucleus accumbens (nACC) (Nosrat, Tomac, Hoffer, & Olson, 1997; Yan et al., 1997). TGF-β receptors are expressed by neurons, astroglia, and microglia. Thus, psychostimulant-induced increases in glial-derived BDNF and GDNF are strategically positioned to maintain and provide trophic support for neighboring neurons, and these glial-neuron signals are critical in promoting neuroplasticity.

2.3. Astroglia

2.3.1 Critical functions

Astroglia form an intimate association with neurons and are involved with fundamental processes including synaptic transmission that were previously thought to be exclusively neuronal (Araque et al., 1999; Haydon & Carmignoto, 2006; Parpura et al., 1994; Volterra & Meldolesi, 2005). As noted earlier, the "tripartite synapse" refers to the intimate structural and functional association between astrocytes and cognate pre- and postsynaptic interconnections. Astrocytes are also critical for interpreting and modifying neuron-to-microglial communication and vice versa—especially during pathologic situations (Maragakis & Rothstein, 2006). Through the selective uptake and/or release (referred to as gliotransmission) of specific neurotransmitters, astroglia play a vital role in synaptic function and can qualitatively and quantitatively affect neurotransmission. Importantly, similar to microglia, astrocytes are also directly affected by psychostimulants. Despite some neuroprotective responses, the net consequences of exposing astroglia to psychostimulants is they are less likely to aid neurons and assuage overactive microglia following drug exposure.

An essential function of astrocytes is in the reuptake and management of glutamate released by neurons during synaptic activity (Boileau et al., 2008; Hertz & Zielke, 2004). Most of the released glutamate undergoes reuptake by astrocytes through glutamate transporters GLT-1 (EAAT2) and GLAST (EAAT1) (Rothstein et al., 1996; Tanaka et al., 1997). The glutamate retrieved by astrocytes is converted to glutamine by glutamine synthetase—an enzyme that is not expressed by neurons or other glial types besides astrocytes. The conversion of glutamate to glutamine is critical because excess extracellular glutamate can be excitotoxic to neurons. Neurons rely exclusively on astrocytes to "detoxify" glutamate and return it as glutamine (via phosphate-activated glutaminase), which is referred to as the glutamate-glutamine shuttle. Importantly, the glutamate transport is coupled to the production of the antioxidant glutathione and GABA biosynthesis.

2.3.2 Psychostimulant effects on astroglia

Glutamate is highly involved in learning behaviors associated with addiction (Hyman, 2005; Kalivas, 2009; Kalivas & Volkow, 2011; Stuber, Britt, & Bonci, 2012), including conditioned place preference (CPP). Because of their essential role in managing glutamate, understanding the neurobiological consequences of psychostimulants in astrocytes is likely to reveal significant mechanisms of action. Indeed, excitatory amino acid transporters-1/2 (EAAT1/2) have been proposed as potential therapeutic targets for methamphetamine and cocaine neurotoxicity (Abulseoud, Miller, Wu, Choi, & Holschneider, 2012; Nakagawa, Fujio, Ozawa, Minami, & Satoh, 2005). The significance of diminished glutamate reuptake in psychostimulant action is revealed by findings demonstrating that a glutamate transport activator, MS-153, given together with methamphetamine or cocaine, significantly decreased CPP without varying locomotor responses in mice (Nakagawa et al., 2005). While few reports of direct actions of methamphetamine or cocaine on EAAT1/2 are reported, Halpin and Yamamoto (2012) suggested that glutamate transporter impairment may result from acute systemic increases in ammonia caused by acute hepatotoxicity. Even slight increases in ammonia decrease EAAT1 expression (Chan et al., 2000; Zhou & Norenberg, 1999) and limit glutamine synthetase activity (Kosenko et al., 2003). Importantly, the deleterious consequences of methamphetamine and/or ammonia were prevented by coadministering the AMPA receptor antagonist, GYKI 52466, implicating extracellular glutamate and its mismanagement in methamphetamine neurotoxicity (Halpin & Yamamoto, 2012).

Astrocytes express DAT and can uptake and metabolize extracellular dopamine (Hertz, 1979; Hertz, Chen, Gibbs, Zang, & Peng, 2004; Miyazaki et al., 2011). Striatal astrocytes exposed to methamphetamine in cell culture display decreased 3,4-dihydroxyphenylacetic acid (DOPAC) formation suggesting that monoamine oxidase is selectively inhibited (Kumari, Hiramatsu, & Ebadi, 1998). Astrocytes isolated from basal ganglia can express dopamine D1, D2, D3, D4, and/or D5 receptors (Miyazaki, Asanuma, Diaz-Corrales, Miyoshi, & Ogawa, 2004; Zanassi, Paolillo, Montecucco, Avvedimento, & Schinelli, 1999). Dopamine upregulates metallothionein expression and secretion by astrocytes (Miyazaki et al., 2011). Metallothionein binds metals, especially Zn^{2+}, and modulates redox potentials affording indirect protection to methamphetamine-exposed neurons (Miyazaki et al., 2011). Recent evidence suggests that stimulating dopamine D2 receptors in astrocytes restricts innate immune activation through αB-crystallin release (Shao et al., 2013). Methamphetamine inhibits glucose uptake by astrocytes and neurons resulting in energetic compromise (Abdel-Salam, 2008).

2.3.3 Astroglial responses to psychostimulant-induced neuronal dysfunction and injury

Besides their role in buffering and managing glutamate, astroglia possess a wide variety of PRRs and respond to DAMPs, and there is an increasing awareness of their key role in innate immune function and its modulation. While astrocytes have long been known to protect neurons from oxidative damage (Desagher, Glowinski, & Premont, 1996; Wilson, 1997), those effects may be overridden by immune signals such as cytokines produced by microglia, other astrocytes, or other immune effector cells (Chao, Hu, & Peterson, 1996; Chao, Hu, Sheng, et al., 1996). Astroglia readily communicate with microglia forming reverberating feedback loops mediating both inflammatory and anti-inflammatory responses—depending on context (Sofroniew & Vinters, 2010). Exposing astrocytes to methamphetamine causes the release of the proinflammatory cytokine IL-6 (Tezuka et al., 2013). The presence or absence of IL-6 coincides with deficits in behavioral correlates of working memory in mice (Tezuka et al., 2013). Moreover, because astrocytes can express numerous classes of neurotransmitter receptors (Glowinski et al., 1994; Hauser. Fitting, Dever, Podhaizer, & Knapp, 2012; Prochiantz & Mallat, 1988; Shao & McCarthy, 1994; Shao, Porter, & McCarthy, 1994), PRRs, and control key neurochemical systems, they are strategically positioned to interpret and convey information regarding neuronal function to microglia and vice versa. In fact, to emphasize the intimate association between neurons, astrocytes, and microglia, especially synaptic remodeling during pathologic processes, it has been suggested that the "tripartite" synapse discussed earlier might be better redefined as "tetrapartite" (De Leo, Tawfik, & Lacroix-Fralish, 2006; Milligan & Watkins, 2009).

Astrocytes are highly plastic and their phenotype can be modified by regional and extrinsic cues within the extracellular environment (Bachoo et al., 2004; El-Hage, Podhaizer, Sturgill, & Hauser, 2011; Theodosis, Poulain, & Oliet, 2008; Zhang & Barres, 2010). For instance, astrocytes isolated from different brain regions display fundamental differences in methamphetamine responsiveness in cell culture (Stadlin, Lau, & Szeto, 1998). The diversity and plasticity of receptor expression by astrocytes are not limited to neurotransmitter receptors. PRRs, which recognize conserved microbial molecular motifs, display considerable diversity in astroglia. Moreover, the appearance and level of expression of individual PRRs appear to be plastic and modifiable by environmental factors and xenobiotics (El-Hage et al., 2011). Psychostimulants themselves or local inflammatory factors from microglia or injured neurons may influence the expression of GPCRs, transporters, or PRRs. PRRs expressed by astrocytes include multiple members of the TLR family including TLR2, TLR3, TLR4, and TLR9 (El-Hage et al., 2011); RAGE (Jones, Minogue, Connor, & Lynch, 2013; Park et al., 2004; Ponath et al., 2007), a novel NOD-like $NLRP_2$ receptor that functions as an inflammasome (Minkiewicz, de Rivero Vaccari, & Keane, 2013) and NOD2 receptors (Jiang, Sun, Kaplan, & Shao, 2012); and "laboratory of genetics and physiology 2" (LGP2), an antiretroviral PRR that recognizes dsRNA (Bruns et al., 2013). Human astrocytes and peripheral blood mononuclear cells can express a novel RAGE splice variant (Δ^8-RAGE) that is likely to have significant functional implications for the subset of psychostimulant abusers who express this allelic variant (Park et al., 2004). The expression of TLR2 and TLR9 is particularly important in the host defense response to viral infections, including human immunodeficiency virus (HIV) (Equils et al., 2003) and herpes simplex virus type-1 (HSV-1) (Villalba et al., 2012; Wang, Bowen, et al., 2012). Methamphetamine exposure has been recently shown to decrease TLR9 expression by macrophages (Cen et al., 2013), but has not yet been explored in astroglia. Based on findings that TLR9 expression by astrocytes is highly plastic and modifiable by other drugs such as opiates or HIV-1 proteins (El-Hage et al., 2011) suggest TLR9 might also be affected by psychostimulants. Collectively, the aforementioned results suggest that psychostimulants can affect the innate immune response by altering one or more TLR signaling pathways.

2.3.4 Neuroprotective astroglial responses

As noted earlier, astrocytes exposed to methamphetamine release metallothionein, a free radical scavenger (Kumari et al., 1998) that protects neurons from the toxic effects of dopamine quinones (Miyazaki et al., 2011). Astrocytes also release HO-1 (Huang, Wu, Lin, & Wang, 2009), which is neuroprotective because it is essential for the production of carbon monoxide, bilirubin, and ferritin (Otterbein, Soares, Yamashita, & Bach, 2003). Pituitary adenylyl cyclase-activating polypeptide 38 (PACAP38) is also released from psychostimulant-exposed astrocytes. PACAP38 (1 mg/kg total administered subcutaneously via Alzet minipump for 7 days) counteracts the effects of four doses of 15 mg/kg methamphetamine at 2 h intervals by increasing the expression of VMAT2 significantly attenuating the neurotoxicity (Guillot et al., 2008).

GDNF is mainly produced by astrocytes, although a few reports suggest that subsets of neurons and microglia may express GDNF at low levels (Appel, Kolman, Kazimirsky, Blumberg, & Brodie, 1997; Sandhu et al., 2009). GDNF first binds to its coreceptor, GDNF family receptor α1, before activating the Ret receptor, which is a member of the tyrosine kinase superfamily (Eketjall, Fainzilber, Murray-Rust, & Ibanez, 1999; Jing et al., 1996; Treanor et al., 1996; Trupp et al., 1996). GDNF is a neurotrophic factor that preferentially protects dopaminergic neurons against methamphetamine neurotoxicity (Boger et al., 2007; Cass, 1996). GDNF is also a potent inhibitor of microglial activation (Rocha, Cristovao, Campos, Fonseca, & Baltazar, 2012). GDNF may be beneficial in treating addiction (Carnicella & Ron, 2009; Gramage & Herradon, 2011), which is discussed in greater detail later in this chapter.

Similar to GDNF, the neurotrophin, BDNF protects neurons against cocaine neurotoxicity (Graham et al., 2007; McGinty et al., 2010). While BDNF can be expressed by subsets of neurons and glia, the proinflammatory cytokine TNF-α uniquely induces the expression and release of BDNF by primary astrocytes (Saha, Liu, & Pahan, 2006). Pahan and colleagues go on to show that, in astrocytes, BDNF expression is regulated through TNF-α-dependent increases in both NF-κB and C/EBPβ transcriptional activity (Saha et al., 2006). Although counterintuitive, the NF-κB-directed concurrent production of both proinflammatory cytokines and BDNF, which may be unique to astrocytes and not shared by microglia, suggests that astrocytes can provide trophic support despite adverse inflammatory conditions. Alternative studies show that the immature, proneurotrophin form of BDNF selectively activates p75 neurotrophin receptors (p75NTR), which can increase NF-κB transcriptional activity; while mature BDNF only stimulates TrkB neurotrophin receptors, which are intrinsically neuroprotective (Reichardt, 2006). Importantly, Nestler and coworkers demonstrate that the selective oblation of the TrkB receptor gene from dopamine D1 or D2 receptor-expressing neurons has diametrically opposing effects on cocaine reward (Lobo et al., 2010). Collectively, these highly provocative findings describe a link between NF-κB-mediated neuroinflammation and BDNF-directed neuroplasticity in the context of psychostimulant addiction.

3. *IN VIVO* EVIDENCE THAT MODULATING GLIA AND NEUROINFLAMMATION PROVIDE PHARMACOTHERAPEUTIC POSSIBILITIES FOR PSYCHOSTIMULANT ABUSE

3.1. Introduction

Considering the multiple functions of glia, and because glia are the most numerous cells in the brain, it is not surprising that psychostimulants affect their activity (see the preceding text). Modulating the activity of the glia has been, in turn, reported to attenuate some of the abuse-related effects of the psychostimulants. Evidence that drugs affecting glial function might emerge as pharmacotherapeutics for treating psychostimulant abuse is reviewed in the next section. Histopathologic and biochemical assessment at autopsy (Büttner, 2011) and positron emission imaging studies (Sekine et al., 2008) in individuals chronically exposed to psychostimulants suggest that cocaine (Little et al., 2009) and methamphetamine (Sekine et al., 2008) can cause astrogliosis and microgliosis with chronic abuse. These findings are not universal, however, since several reports fail to or find intermediate changes following prolonged methamphetamine abuse— suggesting reactive astroglial and microglial responses may markedly differ among individuals (Clark et al., 2013; Kitamura et al., 2010). The disparate results are perhaps not surprising considering the inherent differences in genetics, environment, and drug use patterns among individuals. Moreover, the glial response is likely to be even more dynamic, because astroglia and microglia are highly plastic and modifiable by environmental influences.

Most of the drugs included in this section have multiple effects, some of which do not involve glia, but that nevertheless could participate in their potential effectiveness. We cannot restrict this chapter to drugs with only effects specific to the glia. Instead, the minimally inclusive criteria we apply are drugs that are known to affect the glia and neuroinflammatory processes as a dominant effect and that have consequences for psychostimulant-affected behavior thought to be associated with or predictive of their abuse. With those criteria as a guide, we first discuss drugs affecting glially derived neurotrophic factors and then consider drugs whose actions in glia are unlikely to involve neurotrophic factors.

Two neurotrophic factors widely expressed in glia are GDNF and BDNF. The molecular pharmacology and biochemical mechanisms of BDNF and GDNF are described in detail in Section 2. In summary, GDNF is present in astrocytes and microglia throughout the brain being present in the cortex, basal forebrain, and more particularly nigrostriatal system (Schaar, Sieber, Dreyfus, & Black, 1993). GDNF is secreted by both neuronal (Oo, Ries, Cho, Kholodilov, & Burke, 2005) and glial (astroglial and microglial) cells (Chen et al., 2006; Katoh-Semba et al., 2007; Lin, Doherty, Lile, Bektesh, & Collins, 1993; Ohta et al., 2003; Rocha et al., 2012; Satake et al., 2000) in the CNS. The actions of homodimeric GDNF are mediated through specific binding to the GDNF family receptor alpha 1 coreceptor, leading to activation of the Ret receptor (for review, see Airaksinen & Saarma, 2002). BDNF is distributed widely in the brain including the cortex, cerebellum, hippocampus, and other areas (Zhang et al., 2007) and is contained and secreted by astroglia (Zhang, Lu, Wu, Liu, & Shi, 2012) and microglia (Coull et al., 2005; Keller, Beggs, Salter, & De Koninck, 2007). Activation of the P2X4 purinoceptors

(P2X4Rs) causes the release of BDNF and it subsequently acts via its cognate receptor, TrkB (Trang, Beggs, Wan, & Salter, 2009).

Most of the studies reviewed later that manipulate GDNF and BDNF levels involve their delivery into brain areas or their general up- or down-regulation through pharmacologic, genetic, or other approaches that do not specifically target glia. In fact, most of the reports either lose site or fail to mention that glia, rather than neurons, are the likely source of these neurotrophic factors. Because glia are the major source of these neurotrophic factors, psychostimulant-induced alterations in neurotrophic factors are likely to result from the drugs acting in glia. There have been several, recently published and exhaustive reviews of the importance of GDNF and BDNF in modulating the effects of the drugs of abuse (Bolanos & Nestler, 2004; Carnicella & Ron, 2009; Ghitza et al., 2010; McGinty et al., 2010; Messer et al., 2000; Niwa, Nitta, Yamada, & Nabeshima, 2007; Pierce & Bari, 2001; Ron & Janak, 2005), and it is beyond our objective to follow similarly. Our more limited objective is to attempt provide a selective review of reports sufficiently compelling to seriously consider the use of GDNF and BDNF as pharmacotherapeutic targets for treating psychostimulant abuse.

3.2. Effects of manipulating GDNF and TNF-α levels

One of the earliest demonstrations that GDNF administration into the VTA could attenuate some of the abuse-related effects (biochemical and behavioral) of the psychostimulants was presented by Messer et al. (2000). This group reported that administration of GDNF (2.5 µg/day) via osmotic minipumps into the VTA completely blocked the ability of chronic cocaine (20 mg/kg i.p. for 7 days) to increase levels of tyrosine hydroxylase and the NMDAR1 glutamate receptor subunit. Increasing levels of tyrosine hydroxylase, the enzyme responsible for the rate-limiting conversion of the amino acid L-tyrosine to L-3,4-dihydroxyphenylalanine (Nagatsu, 1995), the precursor of dopamine, and the NMDAR1 glutamate subunit, which is selectively distributed within astrocytic processes and presynaptic axon terminals within the locus coeruleus (Van Bockstaele & Colago, 1996), are typically increased by cocaine exposure (Beitner-Johnson & Nestler, 1991; Fitzgerald, Ortiz, Hamedani, & Nestler, 1996; Sorg, Chen, & Kalivas, 1993). In behavioral studies, they also reported that GDNF-infused rats (2.5 µg/day into the VTA) showed a dose-dependent reduction in the levels of cocaine-induced CPP, although this regimen of GDNF did not abolish place conditioning completely.

In parallel studies, Messer et al. (2000) showed that reducing endogenous levels of GDNF increased the sensitivity to cocaine and opposite to the effects of exogenously administering GDNF. Reducing endogenous GDNF levels by intra-VTA infusion of an anti-GDNF antibody increased the sensitivity of rats to the ability of cocaine to increase tyrosine hydroxylase levels and sensitized them to the ability of a threshold dose of cocaine (2.5 mg/kg) to significantly induce CPP. These latter demonstrations illuminate the importance of normal basal levels of GDNF for controlling the sensitivity to respond, biochemically and behaviorally, to cocaine. Genetically reducing levels of GDNF also sensitized rats to the effects of cocaine. Heterozygous GDNF deficient mice (GDNF (+/−) mice), with diminished levels of GDNF, showed a greater sensitivity for cocaine to establish CPP in that a dose of 5 mg/kg was able to establish CPP in heterozygous but not wild-type mice. GDNF (+/−) mice also showed a greater sensitivity for cocaine to induce locomotor sensitization following its daily injection (10 mg/kg i.p.) for 4 days, relative to wild-type littermates, despite having similar levels of locomotor activation on the first day of treatment. The increased sensitivity of GDNF (+/−) mice versus wild-type controls to cocaine's locomotor-sensitizing effects was, however, not replicated in a subsequent study that used a similar cocaine dosing regimen (Airavaara et al., 2004). Despite this latter ambiguity involving the locomotor-sensitizing effects of cocaine, Messer et al. (2000) firmly documented the importance of GDNF in controlling the biochemical and behavioral responsivity to cocaine exposure, and their results led them to explicitly suggest, for the first time, the possibility that manipulating levels of GDNF might provide a pharmacotherapeutic route to treat drug dependency.

The ability of increased GDNF levels to attenuate even more relevant, abuse-related behaviors was reported by Green-Sadan et al. (2003). These researchers observed that increasing GDNF levels, by augmenting either its endogenous production or its exogenous delivery, reduced levels of lever pressing maintained by 1 mg/kg/inf cocaine under fixed-ratio 1 (FR1) reinforcement schedules during a 12-day access period in Sprague–Dawley rats, relative to untreated or phosphate-buffered saline injection controls. Endogenous generation of GDNF was accomplished by transplanting a human astrocyte-like cell line (simian virus-40 glia (SVG)) into the striatum and nACC; SVG secretes GDNF both tonically and following dopaminergic stimulation. Exogenous delivery of GDNF into the striatal/nACC border at a rate of 2.5 µg/day was accomplished by osmotic minipumps. SVG-induced elevation of GDNF levels significantly attenuated levels of cocaine self-administration evidenced by a slower trajectory and lower obtained level of self-administration by day 12 of cocaine access. This effect on cocaine self-administration appeared not to be due to a general depressant effect, for it did not significantly disrupt rates of lever pressing maintained by water reinforcement in control rats. Exogenous administration of GDNF appeared to completely prevent acquisition of cocaine self-administration, although saline self-administration control groups were not tested to unequivocally make that conclusion.

In other, parallel studies, Green-Sadan et al. (2003) reciprocally found that cocaine self-administration affected GDNF levels. Rats that had self-administered cocaine had a 69% reduction of GDNF mRNA in the striatum, with no changes observed in the nACC, relative to non-cocaine-treated rats.

The hydrophobic dipeptide, Leu-Ile, induces synthesis of GDNF *in vitro* and *in vivo*, and its systemic administration (i.p.) increases the contents of GDNF (and BDNF) in the striatum of mice (Nitta et al., 2004). Leu-Ile (1.5 μmol/kg i.p.) administration with methamphetamine (1 mg/kg s.c.) for 9 days increases levels of GDNF in both neuronal and astroglial cells, relative to the administration of methamphetamine alone (Niwa, Nitta, Yamada, & Nabeshima, 2007; Niwa, Nitta, Yamada, Nakajima, et al., 2007). When mice were pretreated with Leu-Ile (1.5 μmol/kg i.p.) 1 h before administration of methamphetamine (1 mg/kg s.c.), CPP was significantly attenuated relative to treatments with vehicle given prior to methamphetamine administration. Curiously, increasing the dose of Leu-Ile to 15 μmol/kg decreased its effectiveness in attenuating methamphetamine-induced CPP despite inducing similar levels of GDNF (Niwa, Nitta, Yamada, & Nabeshima, 2007; Niwa, Nitta, Yamada, Nakajima, et al., 2007). This latter effect may be due to the bell-shaped dose–effect curve for Leu-Ile-dependent induction of GDNF (Niwa, Nitta, Yamada, & Nabeshima, 2007; Niwa, Nitta, Yamada, Nakajima, et al., 2007). When 1 mg/kg s.c. methamphetamine was administered daily to mice for 9 days, it induced sensitization to its locomotor activity effects. The development of sensitization was significantly attenuated by cotreatment of Leu-Ile (1.5 and 15 μmol/kg) with methamphetamine. Leu-Ile, however, was unable to attenuate the locomotor activity effects induced by methamphetamine's initial administration, as it was unable to inhibit the increase in extracellular dopamine levels induced by a single 1 mg/kg methamphetamine treatment, although it was effective in inhibiting subsequent increases during repeated methamphetamine treatment. This lack of effectiveness of Leu-Ile to blunt the locomotor activity effects of methamphetamine's initial administration while blunting its sensitizing effects (Niwa, Nitta, Yamada, & Nabeshima, 2007; Niwa, Nitta, Yamada, Nakajima, et al., 2007) is reminiscent of the lack of enhanced sensitivity to the locomotor activity effects induced by cocaine's initial administration while displaying enhanced sensitivity to its sensitizing effects in GDNF (+/−) mice (Messer et al., 2000). Surprisingly, when given as five daily injections, Leu-Ile was even effective in attenuating methamphetamine's effects when administered *after* methamphetamine regimens had been completed for inducing CPP and for inducing locomotor sensitizations (Niwa, Nitta, Yamada, & Nabeshima, 2007; Niwa, Nitta, Yamada, Nakajima, et al., 2007).

Leu-Ile also induces TNF-α in cultured neurons as well as *in vivo* under treatment conditions inducing GDNF (Niwa, Nitta, Yamada, & Nabeshima, 2007; Niwa, Nitta, Yamada, Nakajima, et al., 2007). TNF-α and other inflammatory signals can induce GDNF expression in glia (Appel et al., 1997). Accordingly, Niwa, Nitta, Yamada, and Nabeshima (2007) and Niwa, Nitta, Yamada, Nakajima, et al. (2007) suggested that two mechanisms be entertained to explain the ability of Leu-Ile to upregulate GDNF: one is via the expression of TNF-α and another by activating Hsp90/Akt/CREB signaling as reported by Cen (Cen et al., 2006). Observing the lack of effects of Leu-Ile in GDNF (+/−) and TNF-α (−/−) mice in attenuating methamphetamine's CPP effects, these researchers speculated that Leu-Ile's inhibitory effects on methamphetamine-induced CPP and locomotor sensitization were likely attributable to the attenuation of methamphetamine-induced inhibition of dopamine uptake and methamphetamine-dependent increases in extracellular dopamine levels (Niwa, Nitta, Yamada, & Nabeshima, 2007; Niwa, Nitta, Yamada, Nakajima, et al., 2007).

Yan and colleagues from Nabeshima's laboratory (which included Niwa) extended the importance of endogenous GDNF levels as a determinant of methamphetamine abuse-related behaviors in mice in several directions including to its self-administration and relapse (Yan et al., 2007). In these studies, they studied the susceptibility to methamphetamine self-administration in GDNF (+/−) heterozygous mice that had corticolimbic GDNF levels reduced to 54–66% of wild-type littermates. In one study, they implanted indwelling venous catheters and trained mice to nose-poke reinforced with 0.1 mg/kg/inf methamphetamine during 3 h daily experimental sessions. GDNF (+/−) mice required less time to reach stable methamphetamine self-administration than did wild-type controls, although their cumulative intake of methamphetamine during training did not differ. When tested under a dose–response for methamphetamine reinforcement, GDNF (+/−) mice nose-poked more often under all doses of methamphetamine, and significantly so at the intermediate doses of 0.01 and 0.03 mg/kg/inf. When subjected to progressive ratio tests at 0.1 mg/kg/inf methamphetamine, GDNF (+/−) mice demonstrated significantly higher breaking points suggesting a greater "motivation" for methamphetamine. When saline replaced methamphetamine as the infusate, both GDNF (+/−) and wild-type mice extinguished in a similar time course. When tested for the ability of a range of methamphetamine priming doses (0.2–3 mg/kg i.p.) to reinstate extinguished responding, all doses tested between 0.2 and 1.5 mg/kg methamphetamine reinstated greater levels of nose-poking in the GDNF (+/−) mice relative to the wild types. Relative to saline prime tests, 0.4 and 1 mg/kg methamphetamine significantly elevated nose-poking in GDNF (+/−) mice, but methamphetamine did so only at 1 mg/kg in wild-type mice. Representing the methamphetamine infusion-associated cues continued to reinstate extinguished nose-poking in the GDNF (+/−) mice after 6 months of methamphetamine withdrawal, although the effectiveness of these cues had withered in wild-type mice after 3 months. These results suggest that endogenous levels of GDNF can influence the susceptibility to methamphetamine abuse at several points during its abuse cycle, from expanding the range of methamphetamine doses that might come to control behavior and that might precipitate relapse to determining the persistence of the susceptibility to relapse prompted by re-contact with drug-related stimuli. Observing these results, as well as acknowledging other reports indicating the importance of GDNF in determining methamphetamine-associated behaviors, Yan et al. (2007) echoed the suggestion by Messer et al. (2000) that targeting GDNF levels may be a route to developing pharmacotherapies for treating psychostimulant abuse.

Yan and colleagues further extended their earlier studies examining the importance of endogenous GDNF levels as a controller of methamphetamine abuse by comparing mice with elevated GDNF levels induced by bilateral microinjection of adeno-associated viral vectors expressing GDNF (AAV-Gdnf) into their striatum, to control mice similarly injected with adeno-associated virus-mediated enhanced green fluorescent protein (AAV-EGFP) during self-administration and relapse (Yan et al., 2013). Microinjection of AAV-Gdnf vectors increased the density of GDNF in the striatum by nearly threefold relative to AAV-EGFP-injected mice at 2 weeks postinjection. Following intravenous catheterization, the mice were allowed to nose-poke reinforced with 0.1 mg/kg/inf methamphetamine during daily, 3 h experimental sessions. No differences were observed between AAV-Gdnf and AAV-EGFP mice during the initial acquisition (days 1–11) of methamphetamine self-administration. However, once levels stabilized (days 12–16) during the later phase of self-administration, active nose-poking was significantly lower in the AAV-Gdnf-treated mice than in the AAV-EGFP-treated mice. During extinction of nose-poking, there was no significant difference in active nose-poke responses between the two groups. After meeting extinction criteria, the mice were subjected to dose–response (0.2–2.0 mg/kg i.p.) methamphetamine prime-induced reinstatement tests. AAV-EGFP-treated mice showed a dose-dependent induction of reinstatement with nose-poke responding peaking at the 0.4 mg/kg i.p. methamphetamine priming dose. In contrast, the AAV-Gdnf-treated mice failed to show any evidence of reinstatement across all priming doses examined. Because of the variability in responding by the AAV-Gdnf-treated mice, it was unclear whether reinstated responding was statistically greater than extinction levels and results of such tests, if conducted, were not provided. Following an additional extinction phase, the mice were subjected to a cue-induced reinstatement test and then 2 months later were again tested for cue-induced reinstatement. Methamphetamine-associated cues reinstated responding in both groups during both tests in that nose-poking under cue conditions was more frequent than under no-cue conditions. During both tests, however, nose-poking by the AAV-Gdnf group was lower than that by the AAV-EGFP mice. These latter results not only show the effectiveness of elevated GDNF levels for blunting cue-induced precipitated renewal of responding previously reinforced by methamphetamine but also attest to the enduring effectiveness of the adeno-associated viral vector treatment. Observing the effectiveness of AAV-Gdnf striatal treatment in these studies, and the reports of the relatively nontoxic effects of AAV vectors reported by others (Miyazaki et al., 2012), Yan and colleagues speculated, "···that increased expression of exogenous GDNF protein through the microinjection of AAV-Gdnf vectors in the brain may be a gene therapeutic strategy to treat drug dependence and relapse in a clinical setting" (Yan et al., 2013).

3.3. Effects of manipulating BDNF levels

Horger et al. (1999) tested the effects of exogenous administration of BDNF into the NAc and VTA in Sprague–Dawley rats and manipulation of its endogenous levels through the use of BDNF (+/−) heterozygous mice. Chronic infusion via osmotic minipumps of BDNF into the NAc

(1 μg/day/side) resulted in a tripling of the locomotor increasing effects (activity counts) during the 10 min following a 15 mg/kg injection of cocaine relative to control rats. Saline injections also elevated peak locomotor activity by nearly double in BDNF-NAc mice relative to controls that complicated interpretations that the authors attributed to the enhancement of BDNF on mild stress (the injection procedure itself). A subthreshold dose of cocaine (5 mg/kg) in control rats was able to induce locomotor sensitization in BDNF-NAc-injected rats. BDNF-NAc-injected mice also developed sensitization faster to intermediate doses of cocaine (7.5 and 10 mg/kg) than controls. Mice chronically infused with BDNF into the VTA also showed an elevated locomotor activity response to cocaine (15 mg/kg), but the effects were less dramatic than BDNF infusion into the NAc perhaps, as reasoned by the authors, to ceiling effects of this high dose of cocaine. Intra-NAc BDNF infusion not only enhanced the cocaine (10 mg/kg)-induced enhancement of light + tone conditioned reinforcers previously paired with water reinforcement but also enhanced their efficacy in the absence of cocaine. The enhancement of cocaine's effects persisted through repeated (four) tests with cocaine across several days. Although both BDNF (+/−) knockout mice and wild-type mice developed sensitization to cocaine's (10 mg/kg) locomotor activity effects, albeit delayed in BDNF (+/−) mice, wild-type mice showed a significantly greater (60% greater) response to cocaine upon its first administration.

Other studies reported that genetically manipulating BDNF levels controlled the effects of psychostimulants. Hall, Drgonova, Goeb, and Uhl (2003) examined the effects of cocaine on locomotor activity and upon its CPP in heterozygous BDNF (+/−) and wild-type mice. Doses of 5–20 mg/kg s.c. cocaine were tested in each subject during 2 h locomotor activity tests preceded by 1 h habituation periods. BDNF (+/−) mice were less active during wild-type littermates during the first hour of the 3 h test sessions. Although doses of 10 and 20 mg/kg cocaine were able to increase distance traveled in the wild-type mice, only 20 mg/kg cocaine, the highest dose tested, was able to do so in the BDNF (+/−) mice suggesting a reduced sensitivity to cocaine with the assumed reduction of BDNF levels. Similar differential effects of genotype on cocaine dose were observed during the CPP tests in that doses of 10 and 20 mg/kg cocaine were able to induce CPP in the wild-type mice, but only the 20 mg/kg cocaine dose was able to do so in the heterozygous BDNF (+/−) mice. Although Hall and colleagues observed that there had been reports that heterozygous BDNF (+/−) mice demonstrate altered processes determinative of learning and memory, because a higher dose (20 mg/kg) of cocaine established equivalent CPP in both groups, it was unlikely that nonspecific learning deficits could account for the differences in groups at the lower 10 mg/kg cocaine dose. Because CPP involves learning associations between stimuli, and because 10 mg/kg cocaine may represent a more fleeting stimulus than 20 mg/kg if only because of kinetics, dismissing the involvement of learning and memory mechanisms may be premature. Hall and colleagues speculated that because BDNF affects both serotonergic and dopaminergic systems, the effects of partial BDNF deletion on cocaine-induced CPP are largely attributable to the actions of the neurotrophic factor on both of these systems.

Responding previously reinforced by drug delivery can be reinstated during extinction by drug-associated stimuli (de Wit & Stewart, 1981). The level at which responding is reinstated by drug-associated cues may first increase with increases in abstinence and then decrease, and the initial increase in responding with increasing abstinence has been referred by some as an "incubation" effect (Grimm, Hope, Wise, & Shaham, 2001). The "incubation" effect is not special to drug-maintained behavior and can be characteristic of nondrug maintained behavior as well (Grimm et al., 2003). Lu and colleagues trained rats to self-administer 0.75 mg/kg/inf cocaine for 10 days during six 1 h daily sessions and then performed intra-VTA infusions of BDNF (0, 0.075, 0.25, or 0.75 μg) or nerve growth factor (NGF) (0, 0.075, or 0.75 μg) and subsequently tested them for reinstatement on days 3 and 10 of withdrawal (Lu, Dempsey, Liu, Bossert, & Shaham, 2004). Responding was greater after 10 days of withdrawal than after 3 days, consistent with an "incubation" effect. Doses of 0.25 and 0.75 μg BDNF increased responding relative to controls on both withdrawal days. In a subsequent study, these researchers reported that the enhancement of intra-VTA infusion of BDNF persisted for 30 days into withdrawal (Lu et al., 2004). Infusions of NGF were without effect. Neither administering 0.75 μg BDNF into the substantia nigra and testing on days 3 and 10 of withdrawal nor administering it 2 h before the test session on day 3 of withdrawal had an effect. Because intra-VTA infusions of BDNF did not appear to affect the slope of the time-response curve, and given observations that increases of BDNF in the VTA do not always track increases in incubated reward seeking, the authors speculated that BDNF ". . . is probably not directly involved in the basic process underlying the incubation of responsiveness to drug and nondrug reward cues." However, given that BDNF levels were correlated with time-dependent increases in reinstated responding in their previous studies (Grimm et al., 2003), and given the results of the present study, the authors speculated that BDNF-mediated neuroadaptations in mesolimbic areas appear to be involved with persistent cocaine seeking and prolonged withdrawal periods.

Although there have been several other reports in which increasing the presence of BDNF or its receptor, TrkB, in the NAc or VTA (but also including the CA3/dentate gyrus) augments psychostimulant-associated locomotor sensitization, CPP, and self-administration or reinstatement of drug-conditioned behavior (e.g., Bahi, Boyer, Chandrasekar, & Dreyer, 2008; Graham et al., 2007) and decreasing their presence diminishes these psychostimulant effects (e.g., Bahi et al., 2008; Graham et al., 2007, 2009; Shen, Meredith, & Napier, 2006), opposite effects have also been reported when BDNF levels are manipulated in the mPFC (Berglind et al., 2007; McGinty, Berglind, Fuchs, & See, 2006). Berglind and See and colleagues were the first to assess the effects of BDNF infusion into the mPFC on psychostimulant (cocaine) abuse-related behaviors (Berglind et al., 2007; McGinty et al., 2006). Berglind and colleagues trained rats to lever press reinforced with cocaine infusion (0.2 mg/infusion) according to FR1 reinforcement schedules during 2 h daily sessions for 10 consecutive days. In two experiments, BDNF (0.75 µg/side) was infused into the mPFC (anterior cingulate or prelimbic cortex) immediately following the final self-administration session. When rats were tested during a 30 min extinction test (in which lever pressing was without scheduled consequences) preceded by 22 h of cocaine abstinence, intra-mPFC BDNF-infused rats pressed the previously reinforced lever less than vehicle-infused rats. Other BDNF-infused rats tested during extinction preceded by 6 days of abstinence, for cue-reinstatement preceded by 6 days of extinction, and for cocaine prime-induced (10 mg/kg) reinstatement preceded by 6 days of extinction pressed the previously reinforced lever significantly less than controls during each of the three test conditions. Although the first test was identified as an "extinction test," presses of the previously reinforced lever did result in presentations of the light + tone compound stimulus previously associated with cocaine infusion making it, in actuality, also a cue-reinstatement test. Other rats tested during "extinction," but in which lever presses resulted in cocaine-associated cue presentation following 6 days of cocaine abstinence, responded similarly to controls when intra-mPFC infusions occurred 22 h prior to testing indicating a time-sensitive window existed for the ability of BDNF to exert its effects. Other rats given the BDNF infusions following 10 sessions of food-reinforcement training failed to show differences from controls when tested during extinction (when active lever pressing only resulted in presentation of cues previously associated with food delivery) preceded by 6 days of abstinence or during a cue-reinstatement test (whose conditions were little different from the "extinction test") preceded by 6 days of extinction. These results, contrasted with the previously reviewed results that indicate that *decreasing* levels of BDNF may *attenuate* the abuse-related behaviors of BDNF, underscore that globally increasing or decreasing BDNF levels in the CNS with psychostimulant medication may not result in a well-controlled, intended therapeutic effect.

3.4. Sigma-1 receptor effects

As previously described, this chapter was not intended to discuss activity of drugs that bind to conventional neuronal receptors for which there may be similar glial receptors. An exception needs to be made regarding the sigma receptor, which we briefly mention here. As discussed earlier, sigma-1 receptors are one of the several putative molecular targets of methamphetamine (Hayashi et al., 2010; Kaushal & Matsumoto, 2011) and cocaine (Fritz et al., 2011; Katz et al., 2011; Kourrich et al., 2013; Narayanan et al., 2011; Navarro et al., 2010; Robson et al., 2012; Yao et al., 2011). Microglia, and potentially astroglia, express sigma-1 receptors and therefore, can be directly affected by exposure to methamphetamine and cocaine (Gekker et al., 2006; Hall, Cruz, Katnik, Cuevas, & Pennypacker, 2006). There have been previous reviews documenting the importance of sigma receptors in modulating the effects of the drugs of abuse (Banister & Kassiou, 2012; Matsumoto, Liu, Lerner, Howard, & Brackett, 2003; Maurice, Martin-Fardon, Romieu, & Matsumoto, 2002; Maurice & Romieu, 2004; Narayanan et al., 2011; Robson et al., 2012), and their potential as pharmacotherapeutic targets for treating psychostimulant abuse is exhaustively reviewed in this volume by Matsumoto. To the extent that sigma receptor binding agents hold promise as pharmacotherapeutics for treating psychostimulant abuse can be attributed to their interactions with glia, especially the microglia, is not definitively known; however, glia should be kept in mind as possible cellular sites of action contributing to any therapeutic effects of this class of agent.

3.5. Nonspecifically suppressing glial processes

Drugs described as having glial modulating or anti-neuroinflammatory effects as part of their overall profile have been reported to attenuate the abuse-related effects of psychostimulants. Often, the exact mechanism for their anti-psychostimulant effect has not been identified, but their glial/neuroinflammatory-related effects appear to be among the most likely. Some of these drugs include propentofylline, minocycline, and ibudilast.

Propentofylline is a phosphodiesterase (PDE) inhibitor (principally PDF$_{IV}$) that inhibits induced microglial and astroglia TNF-α release, proliferation, and adenosine reuptake (Gregory et al., 2013; Schubert et al., 1997). Methamphetamine-induced (10 μM) activation of purified mouse cortical astrocytes is significantly reduced (~34%) by propentofylline (3 μM) (Narita et al., 2006). Methamphetamine-induced (1 mg/kg) CPP was suppressed by pretreatments with propentofylline (3 mg/kg) (Narita et al., 2006). Supporting the importance of astroglia in mediating the methamphetamine CPP effect, microinjecting astrocyte-conditioned medium (ACM), but not microglia-conditioned medium, into the nACC the day before the CPP preconditioning test that preceded training with methamphetamine (0.0625, 0.125, 0.25, or 0.5 mg/kg s.c.) significantly elevated levels of CPP expression at all doses of methamphetamine at 0.125 and above (Narita et al., 2006). Intracingulate cortex (CG) administration of ACM also enhanced the rewarding effect induced by methamphetamine. Treatment with ACM collected from methamphetamine-treated astrocytes induced an increase in the level of glial fibrillary acidic protein in mouse purified cortical astrocytes suggesting that methamphetamine exposure caused a release of factors from astrocytes promoting activation. Overall, these results indicate that modulating the effects of glial activity with drugs like propentofylline can obtund the rewarding effects of methamphetamine.

Minocycline is a broad-spectrum semisynthetic tetracycline antibiotic that has been in use for over 30 years whose main indication is acne vulgaris and other skin infections (Garrido-Mesa, Zarzuelo, & Galvez, 2013). Minocycline inhibits microglia and their neuroinflammatory processes including the release of cytokines and chemokines (Cui et al., 2008; Sriram, Miller, & O'Callaghan, 2006). Minocycline has other anti-inflammatory effects including the inhibition of phospholipase A2, prostaglandin E2, and Cox-2. It is protectorant against oxidative stress and apoptosis and inhibits glutamate excitotoxicity (for review, see Soczynska et al., 2012). While minocycline clearly acts through microglia, and its actions are often categorically assumed to be acting via this cell type, minocycline also directly affects astroglia (Alvarez, Rama Rao, Brahmbhatt, & Norenberg, 2011; Garwood, Pooler, Atherton, Hanger, & Noble, 2011) and astroglia can also produce cytokines and chemokines and contribute to inflammation. A caveat, noted earlier when discussing DREADDs and RASSLs, is that because astrocytes, microglia, and neurons act in concert and are functionally interdependent, it is not possible to reach unambiguous conclusions regarding the exclusivity of minocycline effects via microglia from *in vivo* studies—without the use of specialized strategies to discriminate among individual neural cell types.

Minocycline readily penetrates the CNS and has been considered for a broad range of CNS disorders including schizophrenia, depression, stroke, Parkinson's disease, and multiple sclerosis (Abdel-Salam, 2008; Blum, Chtarto, Tenenbaum, Brotchi, & Levivier, 2004; Buller, Carty, Reinebrant, & Wixey, 2009; ;Chen et al., 2011 Kim & Suh, 2009; Miyaoka et al., 2007; Soczynska et al., 2012; Stirling, Koochesfahani, Steeves, & Tetzlaff, 2005; Yenari, Kauppinen, & Swanson, 2010). Given minocycline's profile, researchers have begun to investigate its potential application as a pharmacotherapeutic for treating psychostimulant disorders.

Zhang and colleagues reported several *in vivo* and *in vitro* effects of minocycline suggestive of potential in the treatment of methamphetamine abuse. Pretreating mice with minocycline (40 mg/kg) prior to a 3 mg/kg methamphetamine challenge significantly reduced (by ∼50%) the psychostimulant's hyperlocomotor activity effects (Zhang et al., 2006). Doses of 10 and 20 mg/kg of minocycline were without effect. The 40 mg/kg dose of minocycline that was effective did not appear to have locomotor activity effects by itself. Others had reported the ability of a high dose (100 mg/kg s.c.) of minocycline to attenuate the locomotor activity effects (ambulations) of a moderate dose (0.5 mg/kg i.p.) of amphetamine in rats (Kofman et al., 1990). At the 100 mg/kg dose, however, minocycline reduced the number of ambulations relative to vehicle-treated rats making it less clear regarding the specificity of the effect. This dose of minocycline was ineffective in blocking the stereotypy induced by 0.5 and 1 mg/kg apomorphine (Kofman et al., 1990). Administering minocycline at 100 and 150 mg/kg intravenously (but not at 25 mg/kg), however, was able to reduce the total, ambulatory, and vertical activity of rats elevated by 1 mg/kg i.p. of amphetamine (Kofman, van Embden, Alpert, & Fuchs, 1993). Again, however, these doses effective in attenuating amphetamine's effects appeared to reduce activity when given by themselves suggesting a degree of nonspecificity.

Zhang and colleagues also found that daily treatment with 3 mg/kg methamphetamine for 5 days induced sensitization to a 1 mg/kg challenge dose of methamphetamine given 7 days later as inferred from the greater level of activity induced relative to a vehicle-treated group. A group receiving chronic vehicle (i.e., "vehicle" for chronic methamphetamine) followed by a 1 mg/kg methamphetamine challenge was absent to properly infer "sensitization"; however, levels of locomotion elevated by the 1 mg/kg methamphetamine challenge did appear to be at least equal to, if not greater than that induced by the acutely administered 3 mg/kg methamphetamine dose from the earlier study, and this suggested a sensitized effect. Sensitization was significantly attenuated by pretreatment with minocycline (40 mg/kg). Minocycline was unable to attenuate some of methamphetamine's *in vivo* effects, however. For instance, it failed (10–40 mg/kg, b.i.d.) to prevent hyperthermia induced by three injections of 3 mg/kg. Given the same methamphetamine dosing regimen, however, minocycline dose-dependently (10–40 mg/kg, b.i.d.) attenuated the reduction of dopamine and its major metabolite, DOPAC, in the striatum and significantly attenuated the reduction of the density of DAT in the striatum. Surprisingly, even when minocycline was given 2 h after the final treatment with methamphetamine, it attenuated the methamphetamine-induced reductions in dopamine and DAT in the striatum, although its protection was not complete and DOPAC levels were not protected. In *in vivo* microdialysis studies, pretreating mice with 40 mg/kg minocycline prior to a 3 mg/kg methamphetamine challenge significantly inhibited the induced increases in extracellular dopamine levels. Zhang et al. (2006) speculated that minocycline's inhibition of methamphetamine-induced dopamine release was likely, in part, responsible for its mechanism for blunting methamphetamine's *acute* behavioral effects and that its ability to inhibit the activity of p38 mitogen-activated protein kinase (MAPK) could likely be responsible for its inhibition of the induction of methamphetamine-induced sensitization. The neurotoxic effects of methamphetamine, they suggested, were most likely attributable to its striatal inhibition of microglial activation.

Fujita and colleagues examined the effects of 40 mg/kg i.p. minocycline on the establishment of 1 mg/kg s.c. methamphetamine-induced CPP and its elevation of dopamine levels in the nACC in mice (Fujita, Kunitachi, Iyo, & Hashimoto, 2012). When minocycline was administered before methamphetamine and saline injections during CPP training, it resulted in a complete blockade of methamphetamine-induced CPP. Conditioning with minocycline itself resulted in a small, nonsignificant induction of place aversion. Pretreating mice with 40 mg/kg minocycline 30 min before administration of 1 mg/kg methamphetamine significantly reduced extracellular dopamine levels at 30 and 60 min post-methamphetamine administration. Observing their earlier reports that minocycline has neurotrophic effects (Hashimoto & Ishima, 2010), and observing the importance that neuronal plasticity has in drug dependence (Luscher & Malenka, 2011), these researchers speculated that minocycline's role in neuronal plasticity could possibly account for its ability to block methamphetamine-induced CPP. Because minocycline does not alter the pharmacokinetics of methamphetamine in mice (Zhang et al., 2006), it is unlikely that a kinetics explanation could account for its attenuation of methamphetamine's effects. It is also unlikely that the modest level of place aversion induced by minocycline in this study could account for its blockade of methamphetamine's CPP effect, although the lack of a dose–effect curve for minocycline administered by itself leaves the robustness and potential importance of that possible effect unanswered.

Ibudilast (aka, AV411 and MN-166; 3-isobutyryl-2-isopropyl-pyrazolo-[1,5-a]pyridine) is a nonselective PDE inhibitor, glial cell modulator, and anti-inflammatory agent (Gibson et al., 2006; Kishi et al., 2001). Ibudilast attenuates the activation of microglia and astroglia, suppressing the LPS- and interferon-γ (IFN-γ)-induced production of inflammatory TNF-α, interleukins IL-1β and IL-6, and NO while increasing the productions of NGF, GDNF, neurotrophin-4, and anti-inflammatory cytokine IL-10 (Kawanokuchi, Mizuno, Kato, Mitsuma, & Suzumura, 2004; Mizuno et al., 2004; Suzumura, Ito, Yoshikawa, & Sawada, 1999). Ibudilast also inhibits macrophage migration inhibitory factor (MIF) (Cho et al., 2010). Ibudilast is marketed in Japan to treat bronchial asthma and ischemic stroke (Kishi et al., 2001) and is being clinically evaluated for treating neuropathic pain (Ledeboer et al., 2006) and opioid dependency (Hutchinson et al., 2009). Because some inhibitors of glial activation and inhibitors of PDE activity can attenuate methamphetamine's effects (see earlier, e.g., Iyo, Bi, Hashimoto, Inada, & Fukui, 1996; Iyo, Bi, Hashimoto, Tomitaka, et al., 1996; Niwa, Nitta, Shen, Noda, & Nabeshima, 2007; Niwa, Nitta, Yamada, & Nabeshima, 2007; Niwa, Nitta, Yamada, Nakajima, et al., 2007; Yan et al., 2006; Zhang et al., 2006), we examined the ability of ibudilast to attenuate the acute and chronic effects of methamphetamine-induced hyperactivity and sensitization in mice, as well as its ability to reduce ongoing levels of methamphetamine self-administration in rats, and to prevent stress- and prime-induced reinstatement of extinguished lever pressing previously reinforced by methamphetamine in rats (see Fig. 1.2). In some studies, we also tested the amino analog of ibudilast, AV1013, which retains ibudilast's ability to inhibit glial cell activation but has minimal PDE inhibitory effects (Cho et al., 2010), to determine whether PDE inhibition was essential for the initial effects we observed with ibudilast.

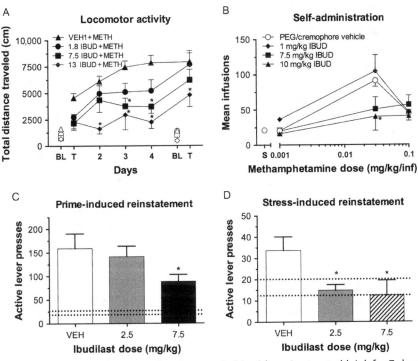

Figure 1.2 Panel A: Results on distance traveled (cm) by mice treated b.i.d. for 7 days with ibudilast (IBUD) or its vehicle (VEH1), beginning 2 days before 5 days of treatment with 3 mg/kg methamphetamine. Ibudilast was administered at 1.8, 7.5, or 13 mg/kg. Data points represent group means (±SEM) obtained during 1 h experimental sessions. Filled data points represent sessions preceded by 3 mg/kg i.p. methamphetamine injections. Unfilled data points represent sessions preceded by i.p. saline injections. $N=8$ for each treatment group. $^*p<0.05$ with respect to mice treated with ibudilast's vehicle. Panel B: Effects of ibudilast or its vehicle on group mean infusions of methamphetamine (0.001, 0.03, and 0.1 mg/kg/inf) obtained during daily 2 h self-administration sessions. Ibudilast was administered at 1, 7.5, or 10 mg/kg i.p. b.i.d. for three consecutive days at each methamphetamine self-administered dose. Data points represent the group means of total infusions obtained during the third day of testing at each ibudilast dose. Bars through symbols indicate ±SEM. Data point above "S" on the abscissa indicates results when saline was self-administered when ibudilast's vehicle was given b.i.d. $N=4$ rats. $^*p<0.05$ with respect to infusions obtained under ibudilast's vehicle condition. Panel C: Mean number of active lever presses during the methamphetamine-prime reinstatement test session as a function of ibudilast dose. Brackets through the bars indicate ±SEM. "VEH," results of the vehicle-treatment group. Dashed horizontal lines indicate the range of the means of active lever presses across test groups occurring during the last session of extinction. Asterisk (*) indicates significantly different from vehicle ($p<0.05$). Panel D: Mean number of active lever presses during the footshock-induced reinstatement test session as a function of ibudilast dose. Other details as in panel C. *(A) Modified and reprinted with permission from Snider et al. (2012). (B) Modified and reprinted with permission from Snider, Hendrick, and Beardsley (2013). (C) Modified and reprinted with permission from Beardsley, Shelton, Hendrick, and Johnson (2010).*

We examined whether ibudilast and AV411 could attenuate methamphetamine-induced locomotor activity and its sensitization in mice (Snider et al., 2012). In these studies, mice were treated b.i.d. with ibudilast (1.8–13 mg/kg), AV1013 (10–56 mg/kg), or their vehicles intraperitoneally for 7 days, beginning 2 days before 5 days of daily 1 h locomotor activity tests. Each test was initiated by either a methamphetamine (3 mg/kg) or a saline injection. Methamphetamine (3 mg/kg) significantly elevated total distance traveled upon its first administration. Each, daily subsequent administration of methamphetamine elevated distance traveled more than the preceding administrations, and distance traveled was significantly greater following its fifth administration compared to its first indicative of sensitization. Neither doses of ibudilast nor AV1013 significantly affected activity when given with methamphetamine's vehicle. Ibudilast reduced distance traveled during all test sessions following methamphetamine administration relative to the vehicle + methamphetamine treatment group and significantly so during test days 2–5 at 13 mg/kg ibudilast and during test days 3 and 4 at 7.5 mg/kg ibudilast (panel A, Fig. 1.2). Ibudilast (13 mg/kg) also significantly prevented the induction of methamphetamine-induced sensitization. AV1013, which lacks ibudilast's potency for inhibiting PDE, but retains its ability to suppress activated glial activity, similarly dose-dependently attenuated methamphetamine's chronic and acute locomotor activity effects, but was ~6–9 fold less potent in doing so. These later observations suggest that the presence of PDE inhibition is not essential for inhibiting methamphetamine's locomotor activity effects, although it likely can contribute if present, and the presence of the other effects of these drugs is sufficient (perhaps including the inhibition of activated glia or upregulation of GDNF).

We also examined whether ibudilast and AV1013, as well as minocycline, could reduce ongoing levels of methamphetamine self-administration in rats (Snider, Hendrick, & Beardsley, 2013). In these studies, we trained Long–Evans hooded rats to press a lever for 0.1 mg/kg/inf methamphetamine according to a FR1 schedule of reinforcement during 2 h daily sessions. Once stable responding was obtained, twice daily ibudilast (1, 7.5, and 10 mg/kg), AV1013 (1, 10, and 30 mg/kg), or once daily minocycline (10, 30, and 60 mg/kg), or their corresponding vehicles, were given i.p. for 3 consecutive days during methamphetamine (0.001, 0.03, and 0.1 mg/kg/inf) self-administration. Under vehicle pretreatment conditions, 0.03 and 0.1 mg/kg methamphetamine was self-administered above saline self-administration indicating that these doses, but not

0.001 mg/kg/inf methamphetamine, were serving as positive reinforcers. The rats self-administered methamphetamine at an average of 3.7–4.5 mg/kg/2 h session when given access to the 0.1 mg/kg/inf dose and an average of 2.74–3.2 mg/kg/2 h session methamphetamine at the 0.03 mg/kg/inf dose. Self-administration of both doses was likely high enough to produce proinflammatory conditions, as it has been shown that a single dose of 1 mg/kg methamphetamine administered subcutaneously produces a significant enhancement of cytokine and chemokine induction in mice (Loftis, Choi, Hoffman, & Huckans, 2011).

Ibudilast (10 mg/kg) (panel B, Fig. 1.2), AV1013 (10 and 30 mg/kg), and minocycline (60 mg/kg) all significantly ($p < 0.05$) reduced responding maintained by 0.03 mg/kg/inf methamphetamine, the methamphetamine dose that had maintained the highest level of infusions under vehicle pre-treatment conditions. These drugs did not significantly reduce levels of 0.1 mg/kg/inf methamphetamine, however, the highest dose self-administered. These latter observations suggested to us that the effects of the test drugs for reducing methamphetamine self-administration could be rate-dependent (Dews, 1955). To test this possibility, we manipulated the fixed-ratio requirement for methamphetamine infusion and matched response rates obtained at 0.03 and 0.1 mg/kg/inf and then retested the effects of 10 mg/kg ibudilast, a dose found previously effective in reducing responding maintained by 0.03 mg/kg/inf methamphetamine. Although 10 mg/kg ibudilast reduced infusion levels of 0.03 mg/kg/inf methamphetamine relative to vehicle control as previously obtained, infusion rates of 0.01 mg/kg/inf methamphetamine in the matched response rate group were again unaffected. These results suggested that the ability of ibudilast to reduce self-administration of the intermediate dose of methamphetamine (0.03 mg/kg/inf), and not at the highest dose (0.1 mg/kg/inf) self-administered, was unlikely attributable to rate-dependent effects and suggested that the highest dose of methamphetamine could insulate reinforced behavior from reductions by these drugs. None of the test drugs increased infusion rates of 0.001 mg/kg/inf, the lowest tested dose of meth-amphetamine, and that was not self-administered under vehicle pre-treatment conditions. This observation suggested that the infusion-rate reducing effects of these drugs at the 0.03 mg/kg/inf dose of methamphet-amine were not attributable to the test drugs "enhancing" the effects 0.03 mg/kg/inf methamphetamine to be functionally experienced as a higher dose (and thus, advancing it along the descending limb of the dose–effect curve).

Bacterial LPS is a gram-negative endotoxin that stimulates inflammation via Toll-like receptor-4 (TLR-4) (Chow, Young, Golenbock, Christ, & Gusovsky, 1999). Methamphetamine and LPS both induce inflammation through the AKT/PI3K pathways and induce NF-κB to translocate to the nucleus and promote transcription of inflammatory cytokines (Ojaniemi et al., 2003; Shah, Silverstein, Singh, & Kumar, 2012). Methamphetamine exacerbates the LPS inflammatory signal (Liu et al., 2012). These effects are likely attributable to both compounds acting via NF-κB, MAPK, and AKT/PI3K pathways (Liu et al., 2012). Ibudilast and AV1013 antagonize macrophage MIF (Cho et al., 2010), a proinflammatory factor essential for TLR-4 function and inflammatory response (Roger, David, Glauser, & Calandra, 2001). If LPS and methamphetamine's inflammatory signals are similar, ibudilast and AV1013's antagonism of the TLR-4 receptor via modulation of MIF may be one mechanism by which these compounds are reducing cytokine production and inflammation. Interestingly, morphine's inflammatory response occurs when the glycoprotein, MD-2, forms a complex with TLR-4 and induces inflammation similar to LPS (Wang, Loram, et al., 2012), thus providing evidence for ibudilast's mechanism of action in reducing opioid-induced inflammation and behavior as well. Minocycline's proposed mechanism also includes interaction with LPS and the NF-κB pathway. Minocycline prevents LPS-induced degradation of IκBα, an inhibitory factor, which ultimately prevents NF-κB translocation to the nucleus and induction of inflammatory cytokine production (Nikodemova, Duncan, & Watters, 2006). Minocycline also decreases binding of NF-κB to DNA that disrupts transcription (Bernardino, Kaushal, & Philipp, 2009). Thus, all three test compounds are hypothesized to inhibit inflammation and methamphetamine-induced behaviors via a similar neurochemical pathway.

We also examined the ability of ibudilast and minocycline to attenuate the reinstatement of extinguished lever pressing previously reinforced with methamphetamine (Beardsley, 2013; Beardsley, Shelton, Hendrick, & Johnson, 2010; Snider, Hendrick, & Beardsley, 2013). Male Long–Evans hooded rats were trained to lever press reinforced with 0.1 mg/kg i.v. methamphetamine infusion according to FR1 reinforcement schedules during daily, 2 h experimental sessions. After performance had stabilized, lever pressing was extinguished for 12 consecutive sessions. During the sessions, doses of 0 (vehicle), 2.5, and 7.5 mg/kg ibudilast were then administered intraperitoneally b.i.d. on the last 2 days of extinction and then once on the test day to separate groups of 12 rats. During testing, the rats were given

15 min of intermittent footshock or a 1 mg/kg i.p. methamphetamine priming dose followed by a 2 h reinstatement test session that effectively reinstated responding above control levels under vehicle pretreatment conditions. Ibudilast (2.5 and 7.5 mg/kg) significantly ($p < 0.05$) reduced response levels of prime- (7.5 mg/kg methamphetamine) and of footshock-induced reinstatement (panels C and D, respectively, Fig. 1.2) of extinguished methamphetamine-maintained responding. Minocycline (15 and 30 mg/kg) was tested under similar methamphetamine prime-induced conditions as described for ibudilast. Minocycline dose-dependently reduced reinstated responding, although the effects did not attain statistical significance. Minocycline (15 and 30 mg/kg) was also tested under cue-induced reinstatement conditions in which the tone–light compound stimulus that had previously accompanied methamphetamine infusions reinstated extinguished lever pressing under vehicle pretreatment conditions. When minocycline was administered as a pretreatment, it dose-dependently reduced cue-induced reinstated responding, significantly so at 30 mg/kg. Overall, these results strengthen interest in ibudilast and minocycline, as well as in other drugs with similar mechanisms of action, as possible candidates for relapse prevention.

4. ONGOING OR PLANNED CLINICAL STUDIES EXAMINING GLIAL MODULATORS IN THE TREATMENT OF PSYCHOSTIMULANT ABUSE

To our knowledge, there are only two drugs reviewed in the aforementioned behavioral studies that are either presently in or proposed for future testing in clinical studies or for which results pertinent to psychostimulant abuse have been reported using human subjects. Those drugs are ibudilast and minocycline. Unfortunately, given ibudilast's multiple actions including its ability to inhibit release of multiple cytokines and chemokines, its inhibition of MIF and PDE, and its promotion of GDNF, the precise mechanism responsible for its success or failure will be difficult to identify. Minocycline also has its own multiplicity of effects including its antibiotic, anti-inflammatory, and neuroprotective effects (Cui et al., 2008; Garrido-Mesa et al., 2013; Soczynska et al., 2012; Sriram et al., 2006), making interpretation regarding its specific mechanism equally challenging.

Reported clinical results with minocycline provided some encouragement that it may eventually have a place in the treatment of d-amphetamine abuse (Sofuoglu, Sato, & Takemori, 1990). In this study, healthy nondependent volunteers were given a 4-day treatment with either minocycline (200 mg/day) or placebo in an outpatient double-blind, placebo-controlled, crossover study. On days 3 and 4, the subjects were challenged with 20 mg/70 kg d-amphetamine and then were given a variety of physiological, subjective effects and behavioral tests. On the fifth test day, the subjects were allowed to self-administer up to four, 5 mg d-amphetamine capsules according to a progressive ratio computer task. Minocycline significantly reduced the rating of "feel good drug effects" and "I feel high" following d-amphetamine challenge, reduced reaction times on a Sustained Attention to Response Test, and reduced cortisol levels. Minocycline, however, did not affect d-amphetamine choice behavior during the progressive ratio task. Although there were limitations of this study, as acknowledged by the authors, including the use of healthy volunteers who chose no drugs for 60% of the options and the fact that dose–effect manipulations were conducted with neither minocycline nor d-amphetamine, the attenuation of the subjective effects of d-amphetamine by minocycline offers some encouragement for its future use in the treatment of psychostimulant abuse.

Recently, the interim results of a phase 1b study involving ibudilast and methamphetamine were reported at the 2013 College on Problems of Drug Dependence Meetings (Shoptaw, 2013). This study was designed to collect safety and tolerability data for ibudilast in the presence of relevant doses of methamphetamine necessary for conducting phase IIa studies. Specific issues addressed were whether 20 or 50 mg b.i.d. ibudilast altered the cardiovascular, pharmacokinetic, and subjective effects of 15 or 30 mg i.v. methamphetamine. The subjects were verified methamphetamine users who were not seeking treatment at the time for their methamphetamine problems. No significant interactions between methamphetamine and dosage regimen of ibudilast on either cardiovascular or subjective effects (Drug Effects Questionnaire) were observed. The high dosage regimen of ibudilast significantly dampened variability and perseveration on a task of sustained attention. Overall, the findings supported safety for evaluating ibudilast efficacy in subsequent outpatient phase IIa studies.

Another clinical study (phase 2) involving ibudilast and methamphetamine is scheduled to begin in the mid-2013 that will involve the recruitment of subjects representing those both positively and negatively presenting with HIV (Heinzerling, 2013). The primary aims of this study will address whether ibudilast reduces methamphetamine use more than placebo and whether it improves treatment retention more than placebo. An additional aim specific to HIV positive subjects involves the effects of ibudilast on CD4 count and HIV viral load, antiretroviral uptake and adherence, neurocognitive function, neuroinflammatory/neurotrophic markers, and serum markers of inflammation.

5. CONCLUSION

This chapter has provided a molecular and pharmacological basis for targeting CNS glia with drugs as potential pharmacotherapeutics for treating psychostimulant abuse disorders. Additionally, the behavioral studies in which manipulating glial activity was reported to modulate behavioral responses to the psychostimulants further strengthen consideration of medications with glial targets for treating psychostimulant abuse. Developing medications for these targets has challenges, some of which may not be practically surmountable in the near term. For instance, elevating GDNF levels might be of benefit for attenuating the behavioral effects of the psychostimulants under some conditions and times; however, GDNF cannot be delivered systemically to penetrate the blood–brain barrier (Lin et al., 1993). Even if one could initiate its elevation through other pharmacological methods, timing would be critical, for a rise in GDNF levels may attenuate the acute reinforcing effects of methamphetamine under low consumption conditions (Niwa, Nitta, Shen, Noda, et al., 2007; Niwa, Nitta, Yamada, & Nabeshima, 2007; Niwa, Nitta, Yamada, Nakajima, et al., 2007), but may actually augment relapse to methamphetamine use following abstinence from higher consumption conditions (Lu et al., 2009). Considering the pervasiveness of the glia throughout the CNS, nonspecifically (anatomically) elevating or depressing either of these glial neurotrophic factors may result in unintended effects. For instance, injecting BDNF into the PFC has desirable effects (as a medication target) on cocaine-seeking behavior (McGinty, 2013; McGinty et al., 2006, 2010) but undesirable effects when injected into the VTA (Lu et al., 2004). How could a systemically administered medication that controlled BDNF levels be expected to have *only* the desirable effect? Other CNS medication candidates, such as the cannabinoid CB1 receptor antagonists, whose targets also have pervasive distribution in the brain (Howlett et al., 2004), have had their development terminated because of untoward effects (Food & Drug Administration, 2007), likely, in part, because of their activity on non-intended targets. Perhaps glial neuroinflammatory factors, as opposed to their neurotrophic factors, would make easier medication targets in the near term. The two drugs currently being examined clinically for their effects on psychostimulant abuse with those principal targets that we have reviewed include minocycline and ibudilast. Both of these drugs have been used safely as medications for other indications for decades, and initial hints of their positive effects with the psychostimulants are encouraging (Shoptaw, 2013; Sofuoglu, Mooney, Kosten, Waters, & Hashimoto, 2011). Perhaps research and development with drugs having similar mechanisms may lead to the earliest approved medications with important glial activity for the treatment of psychostimulant abuse.

CONFLICT OF INTEREST

The authors have no conflicts of interest to declare.

REFERENCES

Abdel-Salam, O. M. E. (2008). Drugs used to treat Parkinson's disease, present status and future directions. *CNS and Neurological Disorders Drug Targets, 7*(4), 321–342. http://dx.doi.org/10.2174/187152708786441867.

Abulseoud, O. A., Miller, J. D., Wu, J., Choi, D. S., & Holschneider, D. P. (2012). Ceftriaxone upregulates the glutamate transporter in medial prefrontal cortex and blocks reinstatement of methamphetamine seeking in a condition place preference paradigm. *Brain Research, 1456*, 14–21. http://dx.doi.org/10.1016/j.brainres.2012.03.045.

Airaksinen, M. S., & Saarma, M. (2002). The GDNF family: Signalling, biological functions and therapeutic value. *Nature Reviews Neuroscience, 3*(5), 383–394. http://dx.doi.org/10.1038/nrn812.

Airavaara, M., Planken, A., Gaddnas, H., Piepponen, T. P., Saarma, M., & Ahtee, L. (2004). Increased extracellular dopamine concentrations and FosB/DeltaFosB expression in striatal brain areas of heterozygous GDNF knockout mice. *The European Journal of Neuroscience, 20*(9), 2336–2344. http://dx.doi.org/10.1111/j.1460-9568.2004.03700.x.

Akiyama, K., Isao, T., Ide, S., Ishikawa, M., & Saito, A. (2008). mRNA expression of the Nurr1 and NGFI-B nuclear receptor families following acute and chronic administration of methamphetamine. *Progress in Neuro-Psychopharmacology & Biological Psychiatry, 32*(8), 1957–1966, Retrieved from PM: 18930103.

Albertson, D. N., Pruetz, B., Schmidt, C. J., Kuhn, D. M., Kapatos, G., & Bannon, M. J. (2004). Gene expression profile of the nucleus accumbens of human cocaine abusers: Evidence for dysregulation of myelin. *Journal of Neurochemistry, 88*(5), 1211–1219. http://dx.doi.org/10.1046/j.1471-4159.2003.02247.x, Retrieved from PM: 15009677.

Alvarez, V. M., Rama Rao, K. V., Brahmbhatt, M., & Norenberg, M. D. (2011). Interaction between cytokines and ammonia in the mitochondrial permeability transition in cultured astrocytes. *Journal of Neuroscience Research, 89*(12), 2028–2040. http://dx.doi.org/10.1002/jnr.22708, Retrieved from PM: 21748779.

Angulo, J. A., Angulo, N., & Yu, J. (2004). Antagonists of the neurokinin-1 or dopamine D1 receptors confer protection from methamphetamine on dopamine terminals of the mouse striatum. *Annals of the New York Academy of Sciences, 1025*, 171–180.

Appel, E., Kolman, O., Kazimirsky, G., Blumberg, P. M., & Brodie, C. (1997). Regulation of GDNF expression in cultured astrocytes by inflammatory stimuli. *Neuroreport, 8*(15), 3309–3312, Retrieved from PM: 9351662.

Araque, A., Parpura, V., Sanzgiri, R. P., & Haydon, P. G. (1999). Tripartite synapses: Glia, the unacknowledged partner. *Trends in Neurosciences, 22*(5), 208–215.

Armbruster, B. N., Li, X., Pausch, M. H., Herlitze, S., & Roth, B. L. (2007). Evolving the lock to fit the key to create a family of G protein-coupled receptors potently activated by an inert ligand. *Proceedings of the National Academy of Sciences of the United States of America, 104*(12), 5163–5168. Retrieved from PM: 17360345.

Bachoo, R. M., Kim, R. S., Ligon, K. L., Maher, E. A., Brennan, C., Billings, N., et al. (2004). Molecular diversity of astrocytes with implications for neurological disorders. *Proceedings of the National Academy of Sciences of the United States of America, 101*(22), 8384–8389, Retrieved from PM: 15155908.

Bahi, A., Boyer, F., Chandrasekar, V., & Dreyer, J. L. (2008). Role of accumbens BDNF and TrkB in cocaine-induced psychomotor sensitization, conditioned-place preference, and reinstatement in rats. *Psychopharmacology, 199*(2), 169–182. http://dx.doi.org/10.1007/s00213-008-1164-1.

Banister, S. D., & Kassiou, M. (2012). The therapeutic potential of sigma (sigma) receptors for the treatment of central nervous system diseases: Evaluation of the evidence. *Current Pharmaceutical Design, 18*(7), 884–901.

Bannon, M., Kapatos, G., & Albertson, D. (2005). Gene expression profiling in the brains of human cocaine abusers. *Addiction Biology, 10*(1), 119–126. http://dx.doi.org/10.1080/13556210412331308921, [pii] N098X4GAP1KET58P. Retrieved from PM: 15849025.

Beardsley, P. M. (2013). Preclinical evidence that chemically modulating glial and neuro-inflammatory activity affects drug-maintained and relapse behavior with a focus on methamphetamine. In *College on problems of drug dependence, San Diego, CA.*

Beardsley, P. M., Shelton, K. L., Hendrick, E., & Johnson, K. W. (2010). The glial cell modulator and phosphodiesterase inhibitor, AV411 (ibudilast), attenuates prime- and stress-induced methamphetamine relapse. *European Journal of Pharmacology, 637*(1–3), 102–108. http://dx.doi.org/10.1016/j.ejphar.2010.04.010.

Beers, D. R., Henkel, J. S., Zhao, W., Wang, J., & Appel, S. H. (2008). CD4 + T cells support glial neuroprotection, slow disease progression, and modify glial morphology in an animal model of inherited ALS. *Proceedings of the National Academy of Sciences of the United States of America, 105*(40), 15558–15563. http://dx.doi.org/10.1073/pnas.0807419105, [pii] 0807419105. Retrieved from PM: 18809917.

Behensky, A. A., Cortes-Salva, M., Seminerio, M. J., Matsumoto, R. R., Antilla, J. C., & Cuevas, J. (2013). In vitro evaluation of guanidine analogs as sigma receptor ligands for potential anti-stroke therapeutics. *The Journal of Pharmacology and Experimental Therapeutics, 344*(1), 155–166. http://dx.doi.org/10.1124/jpet.112.199513, [pii] jpet.112.199513. Retrieved from PM: 23065135.

Beitner-Johnson, D., & Nestler, E. J. (1991). Morphine and cocaine exert common chronic actions on tyrosine hydroxylase in dopaminergic brain reward regions. *Journal of Neurochemistry, 57*(1), 344–347.

Ben-Ami, O., Kinor, N., Perelman, A., & Yadid, G. (2006). Dopamine-1 receptor agonist, but not cocaine, modulates sigma(1) gene expression in SVG cells. *Journal of Molecular Neuroscience, 29*(2), 169–176, doi: JMN:29:2:169 [pii]. Retrieved from PM: 16954606.

Benz, B., Grima, G., & Do, K. Q. (2004). Glutamate-induced homocysteic acid release from astrocytes: Possible implication in glia-neuron signaling. *Neuroscience, 124*(2), 377–386. http://dx.doi.org/10.1016/j.neuroscience.2003.08.067.

Berglind, W. J., See, R. E., Fuchs, R. A., Ghee, S. M., Whitfield, T. W., Miller, S. W., et al. (2007). A BDNF infusion into the medial prefrontal cortex suppresses cocaine seeking in rats. *European Journal of Neuroscience, 26*(3), 757–766. http://dx.doi.org/10.1111/j.1460-9568.2007.05692.x.

Bernardino, A. L., Kaushal, D., & Philipp, M. T. (2009). The antibiotics doxycycline and minocycline inhibit the inflammatory responses to the Lyme disease spirochete Borrelia burgdorferi. *The Journal of Infectious Diseases*, *199*(9), 1379–1388. http://dx.doi.org/10.1086/597807.

Beutler, B., Jiang, Z., Georgel, P., Crozat, K., Croker, B., Rutschmann, S., et al. (2006). Genetic analysis of host resistance: Toll-like receptor signaling and immunity at large. *Annual Review of Immunology*, *24*, 353–389. http://dx.doi.org/10.1146/annurev.immunol.24.021605.090552, Retrieved from PM: 16551253.

Bezzi, P., Carmignoto, G., Pasti, L., Vesce, S., Rossi, D., Rizzini, B. L., et al. (1998). Prostaglandins stimulate calcium-dependent glutamate release in astrocytes. *Nature*, *391*(6664), 281–285. http://dx.doi.org/10.1038/34651.

Bianchi, M. E. (2007). DAMPs, PAMPs and alarmins: All we need to know about danger. *Journal of Leukocyte Biology*, *81*(1), 1–5, Retrieved from PM: 17032697.

Biber, K., Neumann, H., Inoue, K., & Boddeke, H. W. (2007). Neuronal 'On' and 'Off' signals control microglia. *Trends in Neurosciences*, *30*(11), 596–602.

Block, M. L., & Hong, J. S. (2007). Chronic microglial activation and progressive dopaminergic neurotoxicity. *Biochemical Society Transactions*, *35*(Pt. 5), 1127–1132. http://dx.doi.org/10.1042/BST0351127, [pii] BST0351127. Retrieved from PM: 17956294.

Block, M. L., Zecca, L., & Hong, J. S. (2007). Microglia-mediated neurotoxicity: Uncovering the molecular mechanisms. *Nature Reviews Neuroscience*, *8*(1), 57–69, Retrieved from PM: 17180163.

Blum, D., Chtarto, A., Tenenbaum, L., Brotchi, J., & Levivier, M. (2004). Clinical potential of minocycline for neurodegenerative disorders. *Neurobiology of Disease*, *17*(3), 359–366. http://dx.doi.org/10.1016/j.nbd.2004.07.012.

Boger, H. A., Middaugh, L. D., Patrick, K. S., Ramamoorthy, S., Denehy, E. D., Zhu, H., et al. (2007). Long-term consequences of methamphetamine exposure in young adults are exacerbated in glial cell line-derived neurotrophic factor heterozygous mice. *The Journal of Neuroscience*, *27*(33), 8816–8825, Retrieved from PM: 17699663.

Boileau, I., Rusjan, P., Houle, S., Wilkins, D., Tong, J., Selby, P., et al. (2008). Increased vesicular monoamine transporter binding during early abstinence in human methamphetamine users: Is VMAT2 a stable dopamine neuron biomarker? *The Journal of Neuroscience*, *28*(39), 9850–9856. http://dx.doi.org/10.1523/JNEUROSCI.3008-08.2008, [pii] 28/39/9850. Retrieved from PM: 18815269.

Bolanos, C. A., & Nestler, E. J. (2004). Neurotrophic mechanisms in drug addiction. *Neuromolecular Medicine*, *5*(1), 69–83. http://dx.doi.org/10.1385/nmm:5:1:069.

Bowers, M. S., Chen, B. T., & Bonci, A. (2010). AMPA receptor synaptic plasticity induced by psychostimulants: The past, present, and therapeutic future. *Neuron*, *67*(1), 11–24, Retrieved from PM: 20624588.

Bruce, A. J., Boling, W., Kindy, M. S., Peschon, J., Kraemer, P. J., Carpenter, M. K., et al. (1996). Altered neuronal and microglial responses to excitotoxic and ischemic brain injury in mice lacking TNF receptors. *Nature Medicine*, *2*(7), 788–794.

Bruns, A. M., Pollpeter, D., Hadizadeh, N., Myong, S., Marko, J. F., & Horvath, C. M. (2013). ATP hydrolysis enhances RNA recognition and antiviral signal transduction by the innate immune sensor, laboratory of genetics and physiology 2 (LGP2). *The Journal of Biological Chemistry*, *288*(2), 938–946.

Buller, K. M., Carty, M. L., Reinebrant, H. E., & Wixey, J. A. (2009). Minocycline: A neuroprotective agent for hypoxic-ischemic brain injury in the neonate? *Journal of Neuroscience Research*, *87*(3), 599–608. http://dx.doi.org/10.1002/jnr.21890.

Büttner, A. (2011). The neuropathology of drug abuse. *Neuropathology and Applied Neurobiology*, *37*(2), 118–134, Retrieved from PM: 20946118.

Cadet, J. L., & Jayanthi, S. (2013). Epigenetics of methamphetamine-induced changes in glutamate function. *Neuropsychopharmacology*, *38*(1), 248–249, Retrieved from PM: 23147489.

Cadet, J. L., & Krasnova, I. N. (2009). Molecular bases of methamphetamine-induced neurodegeneration. *International Review of Neurobiology*, *88*, 101–119. http://dx.doi.org/10.1016/S0074-7742(09)88005-7, [pii] S0074-7742(09)88005-7. Retrieved from PM: 19897076.

Cadet, J. L., Krasnova, I. N., Jayanthi, S., & Lyles, J. (2007). Neurotoxicity of substituted amphetamines: Molecular and cellular mechanisms. *Neurotoxicity Research*, *11*(3–4), 183–202, Retrieved from PM: 17449459.

Camacho, A., & Massieu, L. (2006). Role of glutamate transporters in the clearance and release of glutamate during ischemia and its relation to neuronal death. *Archives of Medical Research*, *37*(1), 11–18. http://dx.doi.org/10.1016/j.arcmed.2005.05.014.

Cardona, A. E., Pioro, E. P., Sasse, M. E., Kostenko, V., Cardona, S. M., Dijkstra, I. M., et al. (2006). Control of microglial neurotoxicity by the fractalkine receptor. *Nature Neuroscience*, *9*(7), 917–924, Retrieved from PM: 16732273.

Carnicella, S., & Ron, D. (2009). GDNF—A potential target to treat addiction. *Pharmacology & Therapeutics*, *122*(1), 9–18. http://dx.doi.org/10.1016/j.pharmthera.2008.12.001, [pii] S0163-7258(08)00235-0. Retrieved from PM: 19136027.

Cass, W. A. (1996). GDNF selectively protects dopamine neurons over serotonin neurons against the neurotoxic effects of methamphetamine. *The Journal of Neuroscience*, *16*(24), 8132–8139, Retrieved from PM: 8987838.

Cen, X. B., Nitta, A., Ohya, S., Zhao, Y. L., Ozawa, N., Mouri, A., et al. (2006). An analog of a dipeptide-like structure of FK506 increases glial cell line-derived neurotrophic factor expression through cAMP response element-binding protein activated by heat shock protein 90/Akt signaling pathway. *Journal of Neuroscience*, *26*(12), 3335–3344. http://dx.doi.org/10.1523/jneurosci.5010-05.2006.

Cen, P., Ye, L., Su, Q. J., Wang, X., Li, J. L., Lin, X. Q., et al. (2013). Methamphetamine inhibits Toll-like receptor 9-mediated anti-HIV activity in macrophages. *AIDS Research and Human Retroviruses*, *29*(8), 1129–1137. http://dx.doi.org/10.1089/AID.2012.0264, Retrieved from PM: 23751096.

Chan, H., Hazell, A. S., Desjardins, P., & Butterworth, R. F. (2000). Effects of ammonia on glutamate transporter (GLAST) protein and mRNA in cultured rat cortical astrocytes. *Neurochemistry International*, *37*(2–3), 243–248, [pii] S0197-0186(00)00026-7. Retrieved from PM: 10812209.

Chao, C. C., Hu, S., & Peterson, P. K. (1996). Glia: The not so innocent bystanders. *Journal of Neurovirology*, *2*(4), 234–239, Retrieved from PM: 8799214.

Chao, C. C., Hu, S., Sheng, W. S., Bu, D., Bukrinsky, M. I., & Peterson, P. K. (1996). Cytokine-stimulated astrocytes damage human neurons via a nitric oxide mechanism. *Glia*, *16*(3), 276–284. http://dx.doi.org/10.1002/(SICI)1098-1136(199603)16:3<276::AID-GLIA10>3.0.CO;2-X, Retrieved from PM: 8833198.

Chen, X. H., Ma, X. M., Jiang, Y., Pi, R. B., Liu, Y. Y., & Ma, L. L. (2011). The prospects of minocycline in multiple sclerosis. *Journal of Neuroimmunology*, *235*(1–2), 1–8. http://dx.doi.org/10.1016/j.jneuroim.2011.04.006.

Chen, P. S., Peng, G. S., Li, G., Yang, S., Wu, X., Wang, C. C., et al. (2006). Valproate protects dopaminergic neurons in midbrain neuron/glia cultures by stimulating the release of neurotrophic factors from astrocytes. *Molecular Psychiatry*, *11*(12), 1116–1125. http://dx.doi.org/10.1038/sj.mp.4001893.

Cho, Y., Crichlow, G. V., Vermeire, J. J., Leng, L., Du, X., Hodsdon, M. E., et al. (2010). Allosteric inhibition of macrophage migration inhibitory factor revealed by ibudilast. *Proceedings of the National Academy of Sciences of the United States of America*, *107*(25), 11313–11318. http://dx.doi.org/10.1073/pnas.1002716107.

Choi, D. W. (1988). Glutamate neurotoxicity and diseases of the nervous system. *Neuron*, *1*, 623–634.

Choi, D. W. (1992). Excitotoxic cell death. *Journal of Neurobiology*, *23*(9), 1261–1276.

Chow, J. C., Young, D. W., Golenbock, D. T., Christ, W. J., & Gusovsky, F. (1999). Toll-like receptor-4 mediates lipopolysaccharide-induced signal transduction. *The Journal of Biological Chemistry*, *274*(16), 10689–10692.

Clark, K. H., Wiley, C. A., & Bradberry, C. W. (2013). Psychostimulant abuse and neuroinflammation: Emerging evidence of their interconnection. *Neurotoxicity Research*, *23*(2), 174–188. http://dx.doi.org/10.1007/s12640-012-9334-7, Retrieved from PM: 22714667.

Coghlan, M. P., Culbert, A. A., Cross, D. A., Corcoran, S. L., Yates, J. W., Pearce, N. J., et al. (2000). Selective small molecule inhibitors of glycogen synthase kinase-3 modulate glycogen metabolism and gene transcription. *Chemistry & Biology*, *7*(10), 793–803, Retrieved from PM: 11033082.

Coller, J. K., & Hutchinson, M. R. (2012). Implications of central immune signaling caused by drugs of abuse: Mechanisms, mediators and new therapeutic approaches for prediction and treatment of drug dependence. *Pharmacology & Therapeutics*, *134*(2), 219–245.

Colton, C. A. (2009). Heterogeneity of microglial activation in the innate immune response in the brain. *Journal of Neuroimmune Pharmacology*, *4*(4), 399–418, Retrieved from PM: 19655259.

Conklin, B. R., Hsiao, E. C., Claeysen, S., Dumuis, A., Srinivasan, S., Forsayeth, J. R., et al. (2008). Engineering GPCR signaling pathways with RASSLs. *Nature Methods*, *5*(8), 673–678. Retrieved from PM: 18668035.

Cooper, Z. D., Jones, J. D., & Comer, S. D. (2012). Glial modulators: A novel pharmacological approach to altering the behavioral effects of abused substances. *Expert Opinion on Investigational Drugs*, *21*(2), 169–178. http://dx.doi.org/10.1517/13543784.2012.651123.

Costa, A., Gupta, R., Signorino, G., Malara, A., Cardile, F., Biondo, C., et al. (2012). Activation of the NLRP3 inflammasome by group B streptococci. *Journal of Immunology*, *188*(4), 1953–1960.

Coull, J. A., Beggs, S., Boudreau, D., Boivin, D., Tsuda, M., Inoue, K., et al. (2005). BDNF from microglia causes the shift in neuronal anion gradient underlying neuropathic pain. *Nature*, *438*(7070), 1017–1021. http://dx.doi.org/10.1038/nature04223.

Coward, P., Wada, H. G., Falk, M. S., Chan, S. D., Meng, F., Akil, H., et al. (1998). Controlling signaling with a specifically designed Gi-coupled receptor. *Proceedings of the National Academy of Sciences of the United States of America*, *95*(1), 352–357.

Crews, F. T., Zou, J., & Qin, L. (2011). Induction of innate immune genes in brain create the neurobiology of addiction. *Brain, Behavior, and Immunity*, *25*(Suppl. 1), S4–S12. http://dx.doi.org/10.1016/j.bbi.2011.03.003.

Cross, D. A., Culbert, A. A., Chalmers, K. A., Facci, L., Skaper, S. D., & Reith, A. D. (2001). Selective small-molecule inhibitors of glycogen synthase kinase-3 activity protect primary neurones from death. *Journal of Neurochemistry*, *77*(1), 94–102, Retrieved from PM: 11279265.

Cuevas, J., Rodriguez, A., Behensky, A., & Katnik, C. (2011). Afobazole modulates microglial function via activation of both sigma-1 and sigma-2 receptors. *The Journal of Pharmacology and Experimental Therapeutics*, *339*(1), 161–172. http://dx.doi.org/10.1124/jpet.111.182816, [pii] jpet.111.182816. Retrieved from PM: 21715561.

Cui, Y., Liao, X. X., Liu, W., Guo, R. X., Wu, Z. Z., Zhao, C. M., et al. (2008). A novel role of minocycline: Attenuating morphine antinociceptive tolerance by inhibition of p38 MAPK in the activated spinal microglia. *Brain, Behavior, and Immunity*, *22*(1), 114–123. http://dx.doi.org/10.1016/j.bbi.2007.07.014.

Davalos, D., Grutzendler, J., Yang, G., Kim, J. V., Zuo, Y., Jung, S., et al. (2005). ATP mediates rapid microglial response to local brain injury in vivo. *Nature Neuroscience*, *8*(6), 752–758.

Davidson, C., Chen, Q., Zhang, X., Xiong, X., Lazarus, C., Lee, T. H., et al. (2007). Deprenyl treatment attenuates long-term pre- and post-synaptic changes evoked by chronic methamphetamine. *European Journal of Pharmacology*, *573*(1–3), 100–110, Retrieved from PM: 17651730.

Davidson, C., Gow, A. J., Lee, T. H., & Ellinwood, E. H. (2001). Methamphetamine neurotoxicity: Necrotic and apoptotic mechanisms and relevance to human abuse and treatment. *Brain Research Brain Research Reviews*, *36*(1), 1–22.

De Leo, J. A., Tawfik, V. L., & Lacroix-Fralish, M. L. (2006). The tetrapartite synapse: Path to CNS sensitization and chronic pain. *Pain*, *122*(1–2), 17–21.

Desagher, S., Glowinski, J., & Premont, J. (1996). Astrocytes protect neurons from hydrogen peroxide toxicity. *The Journal of Neuroscience*, *16*(8), 2553–2562, Retrieved from PM: 8786431.

Deschepper, C. F. (1998). Peptide receptors on astrocytes. *Frontiers in Neuroendocrinology*, *19*(1), 20–46. http://dx.doi.org/10.1006/frne.1997.0161.

de Wit, H., & Stewart, J. (1981). Reinstatement of cocaine-reinforced responding in the rat. *Psychopharmacology*, *75*(2), 134–143.

Dews, P. B. (1955). Studies on behavior. I. Differential sensitivity to pentobarbital of pecking performance in pigeons depending on the schedule of reward. *The Journal of Pharmacology and Experimental Therapeutics*, *113*(4), 393–401.

Dickerson, T. J., Yamamoto, N., Ruiz, D. I., & Janda, K. D. (2004). Immunological consequences of methamphetamine protein glycation. *Journal of the American Chemical Society*, *126*(37), 11446–11447. http://dx.doi.org/10.1021/ja047690h, Retrieved from PM: 15366884.

Dong, S., Rogan, S. C., & Roth, B. L. (2010). Directed molecular evolution of DREADDs: A generic approach to creating next-generation RASSLs. *Nature Protocols*, *5*(3), 561–573. Retrieved from PM: 20203671.

Durand, D., Carniglia, L., Caruso, C., & Lasaga, M. (2013). mGlu3 receptor and astrocytes: Partners in neuroprotection. *Neuropharmacology*, *66*, 1–11. http://dx.doi.org/10.1016/j.neuropharm.2012.04.009.

Egea-Guerrero, J. J., Revuelto-Rey, J., Murillo-Cabezas, F., Munoz-Sanchez, M. A., Vilches-Arenas, A., Sanchez-Linares, P., et al. (2012). Accuracy of the S100beta protein as a marker of brain damage in traumatic brain injury. *Brain Injury*, *26*(1), 76–82.

Eketjall, S., Fainzilber, M., Murray-Rust, J., & Ibanez, C. F. (1999). Distinct structural elements in GDNF mediate binding to GFRalpha1 and activation of the GFRalpha1-c-Ret receptor complex. *The EMBO Journal*, *18*(21), 5901–5910. http://dx.doi.org/10.1093/emboj/18.21.5901, Retrieved from PM: 10545102.

El-Hage, N., Bruce-Keller, A. J., Yakovleva, T., Bakalkin, G., Knapp, P. E., & Hauser, K. F. (2008). Morphine exacerbates HIV-1 Tat-induced cytokine production in astrocytes through convergent effects on $[Ca^{2+}]_i$, NF-κB trafficking and transcription. *PLoS One*, *3*(12), e4093.

El-Hage, N., Podhaizer, E. M., Sturgill, J., & Hauser, K. F. (2011). Toll-like receptor expression and activation in astroglia: Differential regulation by HIV-1 Tat, gp120, and morphine. *Immunological Investigations*, *40*(5), 498–522, Retrieved from PM: 21425908.

Equils, O., Schito, M. L., Karahashi, H., Madak, Z., Yarali, A., Michelsen, K. S., et al. (2003). Toll-like receptor 2 (TLR2) and TLR9 signaling results in HIV-long terminal repeat trans-activation and HIV replication in HIV-1 transgenic mouse spleen cells: Implications of simultaneous activation of TLRs on HIV replication. *Journal of Immunology*, *170*(10), 5159–5164.

Eyerman, D. J., & Yamamoto, B. K. (2007). A rapid oxidation and persistent decrease in the vesicular monoamine transporter 2 after methamphetamine. *Journal of Neurochemistry*, *103*(3), 1219–1227, Retrieved from PM: 17683483.

Facchinetti, F., Del, G. E., Furegato, S., Passarotto, M., Arcidiacono, D., & Leon, A. (2004). Dopamine inhibits responses of astroglia-enriched cultures to lipopolysaccharide via a β-adrenoreceptor-mediated mechanism. *Journal of Neuroimmunology, 150*(1–2), 29–36, Retrieved from PM: 15081246.

Fan, X., Luo, G., Ming, M., Pu, P., Li, L., Yang, D., et al. (2009). Nurr1 expression and its modulation in microglia. *Neuroimmunomodulation, 16*(3), 162–170, Retrieved from PM: 19246938.

Farber, K., Pannasch, U., & Kettenmann, H. (2005). Dopamine and noradrenaline control distinct functions in rodent microglial cells. *Molecular and Cellular Neurosciences, 29*(1), 128–138.

Feng, Y. (2008). Convergence and divergence in the etiology of myelin impairment in psychiatric disorders and drug addiction. *Neurochemical Research, 33*(10), 1940–1949.

Ferrari, D., Chiozzi, P., Falzoni, S., Hanau, S., & Di, V. F. (1997). Purinergic modulation of interleukin-1 β release from microglial cells stimulated with bacterial endotoxin. *The Journal of Experimental Medicine, 185*(3), 579–582.

Fiacco, T. A., Agulhon, C., & McCarthy, K. D. (2009). Sorting out astrocyte physiology from pharmacology. *Annual Review of Pharmacology and Toxicology, 49*, 151–174. Retrieved from PM: 18834310.

Figiel, I. (2008). Pro-inflammatory cytokine TNF-α as a neuroprotective agent in the brain. *Acta Neurobiologiae Experimentalis (Wars), 68*(4), 526–534, http://www.crossref.org/guestquery/, Retrieved from PM: 19112477.

Fitzgerald, L. W., Ortiz, J., Hamedani, A. G., & Nestler, E. J. (1996). Drugs of abuse and stress increase the expression of GluR1 and NMDAR1 glutamate receptor subunits in the rat ventral tegmental area: Common adaptations among cross-sensitizing agents. *The Journal of Neuroscience, 16*(1), 274–282.

Fleckenstein, A. E., Metzger, R. R., Wilkins, D. G., Gibb, J. W., & Hanson, G. R. (1997). Rapid and reversible effects of methamphetamine on dopamine transporters. *The Journal of Pharmacology and Experimental Therapeutics, 282*(2), 834–838, Retrieved from PM: 9262348.

Food and Drug Administration (2007). Retrieved from http://www.fda.gov/ohrms/dockets/ac/07/briefing/2007-4306b1-00-index.htm.

Frank, M. G., Watkins, L. R., & Maier, S. F. (2011). Stress- and glucocorticoid-induced priming of neuroinflammatory responses: Potential mechanisms of stress-induced vulnerability to drugs of abuse. *Brain, Behavior, and Immunity, 25*(Suppl. 1), S21–S28. http://dx.doi.org/10.1016/j.bbi.2011.01.005, [pii] S0889-1591(11)00010-9. Retrieved from PM: 21256955.

Fritz, M., Klement, S., El Rawas, R., Saria, A., & Zernig, G. (2011). Sigma1 receptor antagonist BD1047 enhances reversal of conditioned place preference from cocaine to social interaction. *Pharmacology, 87*(1–2), 45–48. http://dx.doi.org/10.1159/000322534, [pii] 000322534. Retrieved from PM: 21196793.

Fuhrmann, M., Bittner, T., Jung, C. K., Burgold, S., Page, R. M., Mitteregger, G., et al. (2010). Microglial Cx3cr1 knockout prevents neuron loss in a mouse model of Alzheimer's disease. *Nature Neuroscience, 13*(4), 411–413.

Fujita, Y., Kunitachi, S., Iyo, M., & Hashimoto, K. (2012). The antibiotic minocycline prevents methamphetamine-induced rewarding effects in mice. *Pharmacology, Biochemistry, and Behavior, 101*(2), 303–306. http://dx.doi.org/10.1016/j.pbb.2012.01.005.

Fumagalli, M., Brambilla, R., D'Ambrosi, N., Volonte, C., Matteoli, M., Verderio, C., et al. (2003). Nucleotide-mediated calcium signaling in rat cortical astrocytes: Role of P2X and P2Y receptors. *Glia, 43*(3), 218–230. http://dx.doi.org/10.1002/glia.10248.

Fumagalli, F., Gainetdinov, R. R., Wang, Y. M., Valenzano, K. J., Miller, G. W., & Caron, M. G. (1999). Increased methamphetamine neurotoxicity in heterozygous vesicular monoamine transporter 2 knock-out mice. *The Journal of Neuroscience*, *19*(7), 2424–2431, Retrieved from PM: 10087057.

Gao, H. M., & Hong, J. S. (2008). Why neurodegenerative diseases are progressive: Uncontrolled inflammation drives disease progression. *Trends in Immunology*, *29*(8), 357–365, Retrieved from PM: 18599350.

Garrido-Mesa, N., Zarzuelo, A., & Galvez, J. (2013). Minocycline: Far beyond an antibiotic. *British Journal of Pharmacology*, *169*(2), 337–352. http://dx.doi.org/10.1111/bph.12139.

Garwood, C. J., Pooler, A. M., Atherton, J., Hanger, D. P., & Noble, W. (2011). Astrocytes are important mediators of Aβ-induced neurotoxicity and tau phosphorylation in primary culture. *Cell Death & Disease*, *2*, e167. http://dx.doi.org/10.1038/cddis.2011.50, [pii] cddis201150. Retrieved from PM: 21633390.

Geijtenbeek, T. B., & Gringhuis, S. I. (2009). Signalling through C-type lectin receptors: Shaping immune responses. *Nature Reviews Immunology*, *9*(7), 465–479. http://dx.doi.org/10.1038/nri2569, [pii] nri2569. Retrieved from PM: 19521399.

Gekker, G., Hu, S., Sheng, W. S., Rock, R. B., Lokensgard, J. R., & Peterson, P. K. (2006). Cocaine-induced HIV-1 expression in microglia involves sigma-1 receptors and transforming growth factor-β1. *International Immunopharmacology*, *6*(6), 1029–1033. http://dx.doi.org/10.1016/j.intimp.2005.12.005, [pii] S1567-5769(05)00354-1. Retrieved from PM: 16644490.

George, O., Mandyam, C. D., Wee, S., & Koob, G. F. (2008). Extended access to cocaine self-administration produces long-lasting prefrontal cortex-dependent working memory impairments. *Neuropsychopharmacology*, *33*(10), 2474–2482.

Ghitza, U. E., Zhai, H. F., Wu, P., Airavaara, M., Shaham, Y., & Lu, L. (2010). Role of BDNF and GDNF in drug reward and relapse: A review. *Neuroscience and Biobehavioral Reviews*, *35*(2), 157–171. http://dx.doi.org/10.1016/j.neubiorev.2009.11.009.

Gibson, L. C., Hastings, S. F., McPhee, I., Clayton, R. A., Darroch, C. E., Mackenzie, A., et al. (2006). The inhibitory profile of Ibudilast against the human phosphodiesterase enzyme family. *European Journal of Pharmacology*, *538*(1–3), 39–42. http://dx.doi.org/10.1016/j.ejphar.2006.02.053.

Glowinski, J., Marin, P., Tence, M., Stella, N., Giaume, C., & Premont, J. (1994). Glial receptors and their intervention in astrocyto-astrocytic and astrocyto-neuronal interactions. *Glia*, *11*(2), 201–208. http://dx.doi.org/10.1002/glia.440110214, Retrieved from PM: 7927648.

Gombault, A., Baron, L., & Couillin, I. (2012). ATP release and purinergic signaling in NLRP3 inflammasome activation. *Frontiers in Immunology*, *3*, 414. http://dx.doi.org/10.3389/fimmu.2012.00414.

Graham, D. L., Edwards, S., Bachtell, R. K., DiLeone, R. J., Rios, M., & Self, D. W. (2007). Dynamic BDNF activity in nucleus accumbens with cocaine use increases self-administration and relapse. *Nature Neuroscience*, *10*(8), 1029–1037. http://dx.doi.org/10.1038/nn1929, [pii] nn1929. Retrieved from PM: 17618281.

Graham, D. L., Krishnan, V., Larson, E. B., Graham, A., Edwards, S., Bachtell, R. K., et al. (2009). Tropomyosin-related kinase B in the mesolimbic dopamine system: Region-specific effects on cocaine reward. *Biological Psychiatry*, *65*(8), 696–701. http://dx.doi.org/10.1016/j.biopsych.2008.09.032.

Gramage, E., & Herradon, G. (2011). Connecting Parkinson's disease and drug addiction: Common players reveal unexpected disease connections and novel therapeutic approaches. *Current Pharmaceutical Design*, *17*(5), 449–461, [pii] BSP/CPD/E-Pub/000336. Retrieved from PM: 21375485.

Green-Sadan, T., Kinor, N., Roth-Deri, I., Geffen-Aricha, R., Schindler, C. J., & Yadid, G. (2003). Transplantation of glial cell line-derived neurotrophic factor-expressing cells into the striatum and nucleus accumbens attenuates acquisition of cocaine self-administration in rats. *European Journal of Neuroscience, 18*(7), 2093–2098. http://dx.doi.org/10.1046/j.1460-9568.2003.02943.x.

Gregory, E. N., Delaney, A., AbdelMoaty, S., Bas, D. B., Codeluppi, S., Wigerblad, G., et al. (2013). Pentoxifylline and propentofylline prevent proliferation and activation of the mammalian target of rapamycin and mitogen activated protein kinase in cultured spinal astrocytes. *Journal of Neuroscience Research, 91*(2), 300–312. http://dx.doi.org/10.1002/jnr.23144.

Grimm, J. W., Hope, B. T., Wise, R. A., & Shaham, Y. (2001). Neuroadaptation. Incubation of cocaine craving after withdrawal. *Nature, 412*(6843), 141–142.

Grimm, J. W., Lu, L., Hayashi, T., Hope, B. T., Su, T. P., & Shaham, Y. (2003). Time-dependent increases in brain-derived neurotrophic factor protein levels within the mesolimbic dopamine system after withdrawal from cocaine: Implications for incubation of cocaine craving. *The Journal of Neuroscience, 23*(3), 742–747.

Guillot, T. S., Richardson, J. R., Wang, M. Z., Li, Y. J., Taylor, T. N., Ciliax, B. J., et al. (2008). PACAP38 increases vesicular monoamine transporter 2 (VMAT2) expression and attenuates methamphetamine toxicity. *Neuropeptides, 42*(4), 423–434. http://dx.doi.org/10.1016/j.npep.2008.04.003, [pii] S0143-4179(08)00051-6. Retrieved from PM: 18533255.

Guo, G., & Bhat, N. R. (2006). Hypoxia/reoxygenation differentially modulates NF-κB activation and iNOS expression in astrocytes and microglia. *Antioxidants & Redox Signaling, 8*(5–6), 911–918. http://dx.doi.org/10.1089/ars.2006.8.911, Retrieved from PM: 16771681.

Hagino, Y., Kariura, Y., Manago, Y., Amano, T., Wang, B., Sekiguchi, M., et al. (2004). Heterogeneity and potentiation of AMPA type of glutamate receptors in rat cultured microglia. *Glia, 47*(1), 68–77.

Hall, A., Cruz, Y., Katnik, C., Cuevas, J., & Pennypacker, K. (2006). Sigma receptor agonists suppress the activation of microglia and the subsequent release of cytotoxins. *Experimental Neurology, 198*(2), 570–571. http://dx.doi.org/10.1016/j.expneurol.2006.02.047.

Hall, F. S., Drgonova, J., Goeb, M., & Uhl, G. R. (2003). Reduced behavioral effects of cocaine in heterozygous brain-derived neurotrophic factor (BDNF) knockout mice. *Neuropsychopharmacology, 28*(8), 1485–1490. http://dx.doi.org/10.1038/sj.npp.1300192.

Hall, A. A., Herrera, Y., Ajmo, C. T., Jr., Cuevas, J., & Pennypacker, K. R. (2009). Sigma receptors suppress multiple aspects of microglial activation. *Glia, 57*(7), 744–754. http://dx.doi.org/10.1002/glia.20802.

Halliwell, B. (1992). Reactive oxygen species and the central nervous system. *Journal of Neurochemistry, 59,* 1609–1623.

Halpin, L. E., & Yamamoto, B. K. (2012). Peripheral ammonia as a mediator of methamphetamine neurotoxicity. *The Journal of Neuroscience, 32*(38), 13155–13163. http://dx.doi.org/10.1523/JNEUROSCI.2530-12.2012, [pii] 32/38/13155. Retrieved from PM: 22993432.

Hardingham, G. E., Fukunaga, Y., & Bading, H. (2002). Extrasynaptic NMDARs oppose synaptic NMDARs by triggering CREB shut-off and cell death pathways. *Nature Neuroscience, 5*(5), 405–414. http://dx.doi.org/10.1038/nn835, [pii] nn835. Retrieved from PM: 11953750.

Hashimoto, K., & Ishima, T. (2010). A novel target of action of minocycline in NGF-induced neurite outgrowth in PC12 cells: Translation initiation [corrected] factor eIF4AI. *PLoS One, 5*(11), e15430. http://dx.doi.org/10.1371/journal.pone.0015430.

Hauser, K. F., Fitting, S., Dever, S. M., Podhaizer, E. M., & Knapp, P. E. (2012). Opiate drug use and the pathophysiology of neuroAIDS. *Current HIV Research, 10*(5), 435–452, Retrieved from PM: 22591368.

Hayashi, T., Justinova, Z., Hayashi, E., Cormaci, G., Mori, T., Tsai, S. Y., et al. (2010). Regulation of sigma-1 receptors and endoplasmic reticulum chaperones in the brain of methamphetamine self-administering rats. *The Journal of Pharmacology and Experimental Therapeutics, 332*(3), 1054–1063.

Hayashi, T., & Su, T. P. (2007). Sigma-1 receptor chaperones at the ER-mitochondrion interface regulate Ca^{2+} signaling and cell survival. *Cell, 131*(3), 596–610. http://dx.doi.org/10.1016/j.cell.2007.08.036, [pii] S0092-8674(07)01099-9. Retrieved from PM: 17981125.

Haydon, P. G., Blendy, J., Moss, S. J., & Jackson, F. R. (2009). Astrocytic control of synaptic transmission and plasticity: A target for drugs of abuse? *Neuropharmacology, 56*, 83–90. http://dx.doi.org/10.1016/j.neuropharm.2008.06.050.

Haydon, P. G., & Carmignoto, G. (2006). Astrocyte control of synaptic transmission and neurovascular coupling. *Physiological Reviews, 86*(3), 1009–1031, Retrieved from PM: 16816144.

Haynes, S. E., Hollopeter, G., Yang, G., Kurpius, D., Dailey, M. E., Gan, W. B., et al. (2006). The P2Y12 receptor regulates microglial activation by extracellular nucleotides. *Nature Neuroscience, 9*(12), 1512–1519.

Heinzerling, K. (2013). Brief introduction to current research on glial/neuro-inflammatory processes and drug abuse and summary/discussion of highlights from symposium presentations. In *College on problems of drug dependence, San Diego, CA.*

Hemby, S. E. (2004). Morphine-induced alterations in gene expression of calbindin immunopositive neurons in nucleus accumbens shell and core. *Neuroscience, 126*(3), 689–703.

Hernandez-Morales, M., & Garcia-Colunga, J. (2009). Effects of nicotine on K^+ currents and nicotinic receptors in astrocytes of the hippocampal CA1 region. *Neuropharmacology, 56*(6–7), 975–983. http://dx.doi.org/10.1016/j.neuropharm.2009.01.024.

Hertz, L. (1979). Functional interactions between neurons and astrocytes I. Turnover and metabolism of putative amino acid transmitters. *Progress in Neurobiology, 13*(3), 277–323, [pii] 0301-0082(79)90018-2. Retrieved from PM: 42117.

Hertz, L., Chen, Y., Gibbs, M. E., Zang, P., & Peng, L. (2004). Astrocytic adrenoceptors: A major drug target in neurological and psychiatric disorders? *Current Drug Targets CNS and Neurological Disorders, 3*(3), 239–267.

Hertz, L., & Zielke, H. R. (2004). Astrocytic control of glutamatergic activity: Astrocytes as stars of the show. *Trends in Neurosciences, 27*(12), 735–743.

Horger, B. A., Iyasere, C. A., Berhow, M. T., Messer, C. J., Nestler, E. J., & Taylor, J. R. (1999). Enhancement of locomotor activity and conditioned reward to cocaine by brain-derived neurotrophic factor. *The Journal of Neuroscience, 19*(10), 4110–4122.

Horvath, R. J., & Deleo, J. A. (2009). Morphine enhances microglial migration through modulation of P2X4 receptor signaling. *Journal of Neuroscience, 29*(4), 998–1005, Retrieved from PM: 19176808.

Horvath, R. J., Romero-Sandoval, E. A., & De Leo, J. A. (2010). Inhibition of microglial P2X4 receptors attenuates morphine tolerance, Iba1, GFAP and μ opioid receptor protein expression while enhancing perivascular microglial ED2. *Pain, 150*(3), 401–413, Retrieved from PM: 20573450.

Hosli, E., & Hosli, L. (1993). Receptors for neurotransmitters on astrocytes in the mammalian central-nervous-system. *Progress in Neurobiology, 40*(4), 477–506. http://dx.doi.org/10.1016/0301-0082(93)90019-o.

Hosli, L., Hosli, E., Maelicke, A., & Schroder, H. (1992). Peptidergic and cholinergic receptors on cultured astrocytes of different regions of the rat CNS. *Progress in Brain Research, 94*, 317–329.

Howlett, A. C., Breivogel, C. S., Childers, S. R., Deadwyler, S. A., Hampson, R. E., & Porrino, L. J. (2004). Cannabinoid physiology and pharmacology: 30 years of progress. *Neuropharmacology, 47*, 345–358. http://dx.doi.org/10.1016/j.neuropharm.2004.07.030.

Hu, X., Zhang, D., Pang, H., Caudle, W. M., Li, Y., Gao, H., et al. (2008). Macrophage antigen complex-1 mediates reactive microgliosis and progressive dopaminergic neurodegeneration in the MPTP model of Parkinson's disease. *Journal of Immunology*, *181*(10), 7194–7204, [pii] 181/10/7194. Retrieved from PM: 18981141.

Huang, Y. N., Wu, C. H., Lin, T. C., & Wang, J. Y. (2009). Methamphetamine induces heme oxygenase-1 expression in cortical neurons and glia to prevent its toxicity. *Toxicology and Applied Pharmacology*, *240*(3), 315–326.

Hutchinson, M. R., Lewis, S. S., Coats, B. D., Skyba, D. A., Crysdale, N. Y., Berkelhammer, D. L., et al. (2009). Reduction of opioid withdrawal and potentiation of acute opioid analgesia by systemic AV411 (ibudilast). *Brain, Behavior, and Immunity*, *23*(2), 240–250. http://dx.doi.org/10.1016/j.bbi.2008.09.012.

Hutchinson, M. R., Shavit, Y., Grace, P. M., Rice, K. C., Maier, S. F., & Watkins, L. R. (2011). Exploring the neuroimmunopharmacology of opioids: An integrative review of mechanisms of central immune signaling and their implications for opioid analgesia. *Pharmacological Reviews*, *63*(3), 772–810.

Hyman, S. E. (2005). Addiction: A disease of learning and memory. *The American Journal of Psychiatry*, *162*(8), 1414–1422.

Imam, S. Z., Jankovic, J., Ali, S. F., Skinner, J. T., Xie, W., Conneely, O. M., et al. (2005). Nitric oxide mediates increased susceptibility to dopaminergic damage in Nurr1 heterozygous mice. *The FASEB Journal*, *19*(11), 1441–1450. Retrieved from PM: 16126911.

Ivanov, A., Pellegrino, C., Rama, S., Dumalska, I., Salyha, Y., Ben-Ari, Y., et al. (2006). Opposing role of synaptic and extrasynaptic NMDA receptors in regulation of the extracellular signal-regulated kinases (ERK) activity in cultured rat hippocampal neurons. *The Journal of Physiology*, *572*(Pt. 3), 789–798.

Iyo, M., Bi, Y., Hashimoto, K., Inada, T., & Fukui, S. (1996). Prevention of methamphetamine-induced behavioral sensitization in rats by a cyclic AMP phosphodiesterase inhibitor, rolipram. *European Journal of Pharmacology*, *312*(2), 163–170, [pii] 0014-2999(96)00479-7.

Iyo, M., Bi, Y., Hashimoto, K., Tomitaka, S., Inada, T., & Fukui, S. (1996). Does an increase of cyclic AMP prevent methamphetamine-induced behavioral sensitization in rats? *Annals of the New York Academy of Sciences*, *801*, 377–383.

Jensen, C. J., Massie, A., & De Keyser, J. (2013). Immune players in the CNS: The astrocyte. *Journal of Neuroimmune Pharmacology*, *8*(4), 824–839. http://dx.doi.org/10.1007/s11481-013-9480-6, Retrieved from PM: 23821340.

Jiang, G., Sun, D., Kaplan, H. J., & Shao, H. (2012). Retinal astrocytes pretreated with NOD2 and TLR2 ligands activate uveitogenic T cells. *PLoS One*, *7*(7), e40510.

Jing, S., Wen, D., Yu, Y., Holst, P. L., Luo, Y., Fang, M., et al. (1996). GDNF-induced activation of the ret protein tyrosine kinase is mediated by GDNFR-α, a novel receptor for GDNF. *Cell*, *85*(7), 1113–1124, [pii] S0092-8674(00)81311-2. Retrieved from PM: 8674117.

Jones, R. S., Minogue, A. M., Connor, T. J., & Lynch, M. A. (2013). Amyloid-β-induced astrocytic phagocytosis is mediated by CD36, CD47 and RAGE. *Journal of Neuroimmune Pharmacology*, *8*(1), 301–311.

Kabe, Y., Ando, K., Hirao, S., Yoshida, M., & Handa, H. (2005). Redox regulation of NF-κB activation: Distinct redox regulation between the cytoplasm and the nucleus. *Antioxidants & Redox Signaling*, *7*(3–4), 395–403. http://dx.doi.org/10.1089/ars.2005.7.395, Retrieved from PM: 15706086.

Kalivas, P. W. (2009). The glutamate homeostasis hypothesis of addiction. *Nature Reviews Neuroscience*, *10*(8), 561–572.

Kalivas, P. W., & Volkow, N. D. (2011). New medications for drug addiction hiding in glutamatergic neuroplasticity. *Molecular Psychiatry*, *16*(10), 974–986.

Kang, J., Jiang, L., Goldman, S. A., & Nedergaard, M. (1998). Astrocyte-mediated potentiation of inhibitory synaptic transmission. *Nature Neuroscience*, *1*(8), 683–692. http://dx.doi.org/10.1038/3684.

Kanneganti, T. D., Lamkanfi, M., & Nunez, G. (2007). Intracellular NOD-like receptors in host defense and disease. *Immunity, 27*(4), 549–559.

Karin, M., Cao, Y., Greten, F. R., & Li, Z. W. (2002). NF-κB in cancer: From innocent bystander to major culprit. *Nature Reviews Cancer, 2*(4), 301–310. http://dx.doi.org/10.1038/nrc780, Retrieved from PM: 12001991.

Katoh-Semba, R., Tsuzuki, M., Miyazaki, N., Yoshida, A., Nakajima, H., Nakagawa, C., et al. (2007). Distribution and immunohistochemical localization of GDNF protein in selected neural and non-neural tissues of rats during development and changes in unilateral 6-hydroxydopamine lesions. *Neuroscience Research, 59*(3), 277–287. http://dx.doi.org/10.1016/j.neures.2007.07.007.

Katz, J. L., Su, T. P., Hiranita, T., Hayashi, T., Tanda, G., Kopajtic, T., et al. (2011). A role for sigma receptors in stimulant self administration and addiction. *Pharmaceuticals (Basel), 4*(6), 880–914. http://dx.doi.org/10.3390/ph4060880, Retrieved from PM: 21904468.

Kaushal, N., Elliott, M., Robson, M. J., Iyer, A. K., Rojanasakul, Y., Coop, A., et al. (2012). AC927, a sigma receptor ligand, blocks methamphetamine-induced release of dopamine and generation of reactive oxygen species in NG108-15 cells. *Molecular Pharmacology, 81*(3), 299–308.

Kaushal, N., & Matsumoto, R. R. (2011). Role of sigma receptors in methamphetamine-induced neurotoxicity. *Current Neuropharmacology, 9*(1), 54–57.

Kaushal, N., Seminerio, M. J., Robson, M. J., McCurdy, C. R., & Matsumoto, R. R. (2012). Pharmacological evaluation of SN79, a sigma (σ) receptor ligand, against methamphetamine-induced neurotoxicity in vivo. *European Neuropsychopharmacology, 23*(8), 960–971.

Kawai, T., & Akira, S. (2007). Signaling to NF-κB by Toll-like receptors. *Trends in Molecular Medicine, 13*(11), 460–469.

Kawanokuchi, J., Mizuno, T., Kato, H., Mitsuma, N., & Suzumura, A. (2004). Effects of interferon-β on microglial functions as inflammatory and antigen presenting cells in the central nervous system. *Neuropharmacology, 46*(5), 734–742. http://dx.doi.org/10.1016/j.neuropharm.2003.11.007.

Keirstead, H. S., Levine, J. M., & Blakemore, W. F. (1998). Response of the oligodendrocyte progenitor cell population (defined by NG2 labelling) to demyelination of the adult spinal cord. *Glia, 22*(2), 161–170.

Keller, A. F., Beggs, S., Salter, M. W., & De Koninck, Y. (2007). Transformation of the output of spinal lamina I neurons after nerve injury and microglia stimulation underlying neuropathic pain. *Molecular Pain, 3*, 27. http://dx.doi.org/10.1186/1744-8069-3-27.

Khan, Z. U., Koulen, P., Rubinstein, M., Grandy, D. K., & Goldman-Rakic, P. S. (2001). An astroglia-linked dopamine D2-receptor action in prefrontal cortex. *Proceedings of the National Academy of Sciences of the United States of America, 98*(4), 1964–1969. http://dx.doi.org/10.1073/pnas.98.4.1964.

Kim, M. J., Dunah, A. W., Wang, Y. T., & Sheng, M. (2005). Differential roles of NR2A- and NR2B-containing NMDA receptors in Ras-ERK signaling and AMPA receptor trafficking. *Neuron, 46*(5), 745–760.

Kim, H. S., & Suh, Y. H. (2009). Minocycline and neurodegenerative diseases. *Behavioural Brain Research, 196*(2), 168–179. http://dx.doi.org/10.1016/j.bbr.2008.09.040.

Kimelberg, H. K. (1995). Receptors on astrocytes—What possible functions. *Neurochemistry International, 26*(1), 27–40. http://dx.doi.org/10.1016/0197-0186(94)00118-e.

Kishi, Y., Ohta, S., Kasuya, N., Sakita, S., Ashikaga, T., & Isobe, M. (2001). Ibudilast: A non-selective PDE inhibitor with multiple actions on blood cells and the vascular wall. *Cardiovascular Drug Reviews, 19*(3), 215–225.

Kita, T., Miyazaki, I., Asanuma, M., Takeshima, M., & Wagner, G. C. (2009). Dopamine-induced behavioral changes and oxidative stress in methamphetamine-induced neurotoxicity. *International Review of Neurobiology, 88,* 43–64. http://dx.doi.org/10.1016/ S0074-7742(09)88003-3, [pii] S0074-7742(09)88003-3. Retrieved from PM: 19897074.

Kitamura, O., Takeichi, T., Wang, E. L., Tokunaga, I., Ishigami, A., & Kubo, S. (2010). Microglial and astrocytic changes in the striatum of methamphetamine abusers. *Legal Medicine (Tokyo), 12*(2), 57–62. http://dx.doi.org/10.1016/j.legalmed.2009.11.001, [pii] S1344-6223(09)00360-5. Retrieved from PM: 20110187.

Kofman, O., Klein, E., Newman, M., Hamburger, R., Kimchi, O., Nir, T., et al. (1990). Inhibition by antibiotic tetracyclines of rat cortical noradrenergic adenylate cyclase and amphetamine-induced hyperactivity. *Pharmacology, Biochemistry, and Behavior, 37*(3), 417–424.

Kofman, O., van Embden, S., Alpert, C., & Fuchs, I. (1993). Central and peripheral minocycline suppresses motor activity in rats. *Pharmacology, Biochemistry, and Behavior, 44*(2), 397–402.

Kosenko, E., Llansola, M., Montoliu, C., Monfort, P., Rodrigo, R., Hernandez-Viadel, M., et al. (2003). Glutamine synthetase activity and glutamine content in brain: Modulation by NMDA receptors and nitric oxide. *Neurochemistry International, 43*(4–5), 493–499. http:// dx.doi.org/10.1016/S0197-0186(03)00039-1, [pii]. Retrieved from PM: 12742096.

Kourrich, S., Hayashi, T., Chuang, J. Y., Tsai, S. Y., Su, T. P., & Bonci, A. (2013). Dynamic interaction between sigma-1 receptor and Kv1.2 shapes neuronal and behavioral responses to cocaine. *Cell, 152*(1–2), 236–247. http://dx.doi.org/10.1016/j.cell. 2012.12.004, [pii] S0092-8674(12)01491-2. Retrieved from PM: 23332758.

Kovalevich, J., Corley, G., Yen, W., Rawls, S. M., & Langford, D. (2012). Cocaine-induced loss of white matter proteins in the adult mouse nucleus accumbens is attenuated by administration of a β-lactam antibiotic during cocaine withdrawal. *The American Journal of Pathology, 181*(6), 1921–1927.

Krasnova, I. N., & Cadet, J. L. (2009). Methamphetamine toxicity and messengers of death. *Brain Research Reviews, 60*(2), 379–407. http://dx.doi.org/10.1016/j.brainresrev.2009.03.002, [pii] S0165-0173(09)00034-4. Retrieved from PM: 19328213.

Krisch, B., & Mentlein, R. (1994). Neuropeptide receptors and astrocytes. *International Review of Cytology A Survey of Cell Biology, 148*(148), 119–169.

Kristiansen, L. V., Bannon, M. J., & Meador-Woodruff, J. H. (2009). Expression of transcripts for myelin related genes in postmortem brain from cocaine abusers. *Neurochemical Research, 34*(1), 46–54.

Kuhn, D. M., Francescutti-Verbeem, D. M., & Thomas, D. M. (2008). Dopamine disposition in the presynaptic process regulates the severity of methamphetamine-induced neurotoxicity. *Annals of the New York Academy of Sciences, 1139,* 118–126, Retrieved from PM: 18991856.

Kuhn, S. A., van Landeghem, F. K., Zacharias, R., Farber, K., Rappert, A., Pavlovic, S., et al. (2004). Microglia express GABA$_B$ receptors to modulate interleukin release. *Molecular and Cellular Neurosciences, 25*(2), 312–322. http://dx.doi.org/10.1016/j.mcn.2003.10.023, [pii] S104474310300352X. Retrieved from PM: 15019947.

Kumari, M. V., Hiramatsu, M., & Ebadi, M. (1998). Free radical scavenging actions of metallothionein isoforms I and II. *Free Radical Research, 29*(2), 93–101, Retrieved from PM: 9790511.

Larsen, K. E., Fon, E. A., Hastings, T. G., Edwards, R. H., & Sulzer, D. (2002). Methamphetamine-induced degeneration of dopaminergic neurons involves autophagy and upregulation of dopamine synthesis. *The Journal of Neuroscience, 22*(20), 8951–8960, Retrieved from PM: 12388602.

LaVoie, M. J., & Hastings, T. G. (1999a). Dopamine quinone formation and protein modification associated with the striatal neurotoxicity of methamphetamine: Evidence against a role for extracellular dopamine. *The Journal of Neuroscience, 19*(4), 1484–1491, Retrieved from PM: 9952424.

LaVoie, M. J., & Hastings, T. G. (1999b). Peroxynitrite- and nitrite-induced oxidation of dopamine: Implications for nitric oxide in dopaminergic cell loss. *Journal of Neurochemistry, 73*(6), 2546–2554, Retrieved from PM: 10582617.

Ledeboer, A., Liu, T., Shumilla, J. A., Mahoney, J. H., Vijay, S., Gross, M. I., et al. (2006). The glial modulatory drug AV411 attenuates mechanical allodynia in rat models of neuropathic pain. *Neuron Glia Biology, 2*(4), 279–291. http://dx.doi.org/10.1017/S1740925X0700035X.

Lee, S., Varvel, N. H., Konerth, M. E., Xu, G., Cardona, A. E., Ransohoff, R. M., et al. (2010). CX3CR1 deficiency alters microglial activation and reduces β-amyloid deposition in two Alzheimer's disease mouse models. *The American Journal of Pathology, 177*(5), 2549–2562.

Levesque, S., Wilson, B., Gregoria, V., Thorpe, L. B., Dallas, S., Polikov, V. S., et al. (2010). Reactive microgliosis: Extracellular μ-calpain and microglia-mediated dopaminergic neurotoxicity. *Brain, 133*(Pt. 3), 808–821. http://dx.doi.org/10.1093/brain/awp333, [pii] awp333. Retrieved from PM: 20123724.

Lin, L. F., Doherty, D. H., Lile, J. D., Bektesh, S., & Collins, F. (1993). GDNF: A glial cell line-derived neurotrophic factor for midbrain dopaminergic neurons. *Science, 260*(5111), 1130–1132.

Little, K. Y., Krolewski, D. M., Zhang, L., & Cassin, B. J. (2003). Loss of striatal vesicular monoamine transporter protein (VMAT2) in human cocaine users. *The American Journal of Psychiatry, 160*(1), 47–55.

Little, K. Y., Ramssen, E., Welchko, R., Volberg, V., Roland, C. J., & Cassin, B. (2009). Decreased brain dopamine cell numbers in human cocaine users. *Psychiatry Research, 168*(3), 173–180. http://dx.doi.org/10.1016/j.psychres.2008.10.034, [pii] S0165-1781 (08)00377-6. Retrieved from PM: 19233481.

Liu, X., Silverstein, P. S., Singh, V., Shah, A., Qureshi, N., & Kumar, A. (2012). Methamphetamine increases LPS-mediated expression of IL-8, TNF-α and IL-1β in human macrophages through common signaling pathways. *PLoS One, 7*(3), e33822. http://dx.doi.org/10.1371/journal.pone.0033822.

Liu, Y., Wong, T. P., Aarts, M., Rooyakkers, A., Liu, L., Lai, T. W., et al. (2007). NMDA receptor subunits have differential roles in mediating excitotoxic neuronal death both in vitro and in vivo. *The Journal of Neuroscience, 27*(11), 2846–2857.

Lobo, M. K., Covington, H. E., III, Chaudhury, D., Friedman, A. K., Sun, H., Damez-Werno, D., et al. (2010). Cell type-specific loss of BDNF signaling mimics optogenetic control of cocaine reward. *Science, 330*(6002), 385–390, Retrieved from PM: 20947769.

Loftis, J. M., Choi, D., Hoffman, W., & Huckans, M. S. (2011). Methamphetamine causes persistent immune dysregulation: A cross-species, translational report. *Neurotoxicity Research, 20*(1), 59–68. http://dx.doi.org/10.1007/s12640-010-9223-x.

Lu, L., Dempsey, J., Liu, S. Y., Bossert, J. M., & Shaham, Y. (2004). A single infusion of brain-derived neurotrophic factor into the ventral tegmental area induces long-lasting potentiation of cocaine seeking after withdrawal. *The Journal of Neuroscience, 24*(7), 1604–1611.

Lu, L., Wang, X., Wu, P., Xu, C. M., Zhao, M., Morales, M., et al. (2009). Role of ventral tegmental area glial cell line-derived neurotrophic factor in incubation of cocaine craving. *Biological Psychiatry, 66*(2), 137–145. http://dx.doi.org/10.1016/j.biopsych.2009.02.009.

Luo, Y., Wang, Y., Kuang, S. Y., Chiang, Y. H., & Hoffer, B. (2010). Decreased level of Nurr1 in heterozygous young adult mice leads to exacerbated acute and long-term toxicity after repeated methamphetamine exposure. *PLoS One, 5*(12), e15193, Retrieved from PM: 21151937.

Luscher, C., & Malenka, R. C. (2011). Drug-evoked synaptic plasticity in addiction: From molecular changes to circuit remodeling. *Neuron, 69*(4), 650–663. http://dx.doi.org/10.1016/j.neuron.2011.01.017.

Mandyam, C. D., Wee, S., Eisch, A. J., Richardson, H. N., & Koob, G. F. (2007). Meth-amphetamine self-administration and voluntary exercise have opposing effects on medial prefrontal cortex gliogenesis. *The Journal of Neuroscience, 27*(42), 11442–11450. http://dx. doi.org/10.1523/JNEUROSCI.2505-07.2007, [pii] 27/42/11442. Retrieved from PM: 17942739.

Maragakis, N. J., & Rothstein, J. D. (2006). Mechanisms of disease: Astrocytes in neurode-generative disease. *Nature Clinical Practice Neurology, 2*(12), 679–689. http://dx.doi.org/ 10.1038/ncpneuro0355, [pii] ncpneuro0355. Retrieved from PM: 17117171.

Maroso, M., Balosso, S., Ravizza, T., Liu, J., Aronica, E., Iyer, A. M., et al. (2010). Toll-like receptor 4 and high-mobility group box-1 are involved in ictogenesis and can be targeted to reduce seizures. *Nature Medicine, 16*(4), 413–419, Retrieved from PM: 20348922.

Matsumoto, R. R., Liu, Y., Lerner, M., Howard, E. W., & Brackett, D. J. (2003). σ Receptors: Potential medications development target for anti-cocaine agents. *European Journal of Pharmacology, 469*(1–3), 1–12. http://dx.doi.org/10.1016/s0014-2999(03) 01723-0.

Mattson, M. P., Cheng, B., Baldwin, S. A., Smith-Swintosky, V. L., Keller, J., Geddes, J. W., et al. (1995). Brain injury and tumor necrosis factors induce calbindin D-28k in astro-cytes: Evidence for a cytoprotective response. *Journal of Neuroscience Research, 42,* 357–370.

Mattson, M. P., Rychlik, B., & Cheng, B. (1992). Degenerative and axon outgrowth-altering effects of phencyclidine in human fetal cerebral cortical cells. *Neuropharmacology, 31,* 279–291.

Maurice, T., Martin-Fardon, W., Romieu, P., & Matsumoto, R. R. (2002). Sigma$_1$ (σ_1) receptor antagonists represent a new strategy against cocaine addiction and toxicity. *Neuroscience and Biobehavioral Reviews, 26*(4), 499–527. http://dx.doi.org/10.1016/ s0149-7634(02)00017-9.

Maurice, T., & Romieu, P. (2004). Involvement of the sigma$_1$ receptor in the appetitive effects of cocaine. *Pharmacopsychiatry, 37,* S198–S207. http://dx.doi.org/10.1055/ s-2004-832678.

McGinty, J. F. (2013). Intra-PFC BDNF suppresses cocaine-seeking by rescuing ERK MAPK and CREB signaling. *Journal of Neurochemistry, 125,* 19.

McGinty, J. F., Berglind, W. J., Fuchs, R. L., & See, R. E. (2006). A single BDNF infusion into the medial prefrontal cortex suppresses contextual-, cue-, and cocaine-induced rein-statement of cocaine-seeking behavior. *Neuropsychopharmacology, 31,* S4.

McGinty, J. F., Whitfield, T. W., Jr., & Berglind, W. J. (2010). Brain-derived neurotrophic factor and cocaine addiction. *Brain Research, 1314,* 183–193. http://dx.doi.org/10.1016/ j.brainres.2009.08.078.

Messer, C. J., Eisch, A. J., Carlezon, W. A., Jr., Whisler, K., Shen, L., Wolf, D. H., et al. (2000). Role for GDNF in biochemical and behavioral adaptations to drugs of abuse. *Neuron, 26*(1), 247–257.

Miguel-Hidalgo, J. J. (2009). The role of glial cells in drug abuse. *Current Drug Abuse Reviews, 2*(1), 76–82, Retrieved from PM: 19606280.

Miller, G. W., Gainetdinov, R. R., Levey, A. I., & Caron, M. G. (1999). Dopamine trans-porters and neuronal injury. *Trends in Pharmacological Sciences, 20*(10), 424–429.

Milligan, E. D., & Watkins, L. R. (2009). Pathological and protective roles of glia in chronic pain. *Nature Reviews Neuroscience, 10*(1), 23–36, Retrieved from PM: 19096368.

Minkiewicz, J., de Rivero Vaccari, J. P., & Keane, R. W. (2013). Human astrocytes express a novel NLRP2 inflammasome. *Glia, 61*(7), 1113–1121.

Miyaoka, T., Yasukawa, R., Yasuda, H., Hayashida, M., Inagaki, T., & Horiguchi, J. (2007). Possible antipsychotic effects of minocycline in patients with schizophrenia. *Progress in Neuro-Psychopharmacology & Biological Psychiatry, 31*(1), 304–307. http://dx.doi.org/ 10.1016/j.pnpbp.2006.08.013.

Miyatake, M., Narita, M., Shibasaki, M., Nakamura, A., & Suzuki, T. (2005). Glutamatergic neurotransmission and protein kinase C play a role in neuron-glia communication during the development of methamphetamine-induced psychological dependence. *European Journal of Neuroscience, 22*(6), 1476–1488.

Miyazaki, Y., Adachi, H., Katsuno, M., Minamiyama, M., Jiang, Y. M., Huang, Z., et al. (2012). Viral delivery of miR-196a ameliorates the SBMA phenotype via the silencing of CELF2. *Nature Medicine, 18*(7), 1136–1141. http://dx.doi.org/10.1038/nm.2791.

Miyazaki, I., Asanuma, M., Diaz-Corrales, F. J., Miyoshi, K., & Ogawa, N. (2004). Direct evidence for expression of dopamine receptors in astrocytes from basal ganglia. *Brain Research, 1029*(1), 120–123. http://dx.doi.org/10.1016/j.brainres.2004.09.014, [pii] S0006-8993(04)01539-2. Retrieved from PM: 15533323.

Miyazaki, I., Asanuma, M., Kikkawa, Y., Takeshima, M., Murakami, S., Miyoshi, K., et al. (2011). Astrocyte-derived metallothionein protects dopaminergic neurons from dopamine quinone toxicity. *Glia, 59*(3), 435–451.

Mizuno, T., Kurotani, T., Komatsu, Y., Kawanokuchi, J., Kato, H., Mitsuma, N., et al. (2004). Neuroprotective role of phosphodiesterase inhibitor ibudilast on neuronal cell death induced by activated microglia. *Neuropharmacology, 46*(3), 404–411. http://dx.doi.org/10.1016/j.neuropharm.2003.09.009.

Morioka, N. (2011). The roles of ATP receptors in the regulation of various functions in spinal microglia. *Yakugaku Zasshi: Journal of the Pharmaceutical Society of Japan, 131*(7), 1047–1052.

Nagatsu, T. (1995). Tyrosine hydroxylase: Human isoforms, structure and regulation in physiology and pathology. *Essays in Biochemistry, 30*, 15–35.

Nair, M. P., Mahajan, S. D., Schwartz, S. A., Reynolds, J., Whitney, R., Bernstein, Z., et al. (2005). Cocaine modulates dendritic cell-specific C type intercellular adhesion molecule-3-grabbing nonintegrin expression by dendritic cells in HIV-1 patients. *Journal of Immunology, 174*(11), 6617–6626, Retrieved from PM: 15905500.

Nair, M. P., Mahajan, S., Sykes, D., Bapardekar, M. V., & Reynolds, J. L. (2006). Methamphetamine modulates DC-SIGN expression by mature dendritic cells. *Journal of Neuroimmune Pharmacology, 1*(3), 296–304. http://dx.doi.org/10.1007/s11481-006-9027-1, Retrieved from PM: 18040806.

Nair, M. P., Schwartz, S. A., Mahajan, S. D., Tsiao, C., Chawda, R. P., Whitney, R., et al. (2004). Drug abuse and neuropathogenesis of HIV infection: Role of DC-SIGN and IDO. *Journal of Neuroimmunology, 157*(1–2), 56–60.

Nakagawa, T., Fujio, M., Ozawa, T., Minami, M., & Satoh, M. (2005). Effect of MS-153, a glutamate transporter activator, on the conditioned rewarding effects of morphine, methamphetamine and cocaine in mice. *Behavioural Brain Research, 156*(2), 233–239.

Narayanan, S., Mesangeau, C., Poupaert, J. H., & McCurdy, C. R. (2011). Sigma receptors and cocaine abuse. *Current Topics in Medicinal Chemistry, 11*(9), 1128–1150, [pii] BSP/CTMC/E-Pub/-00016-11-3. Retrieved from PM: 21050176.

Narita, M., Miyatake, M., Shibasaki, M., Shindo, K., Nakamura, A., Kuzumaki, N., et al. (2006). Direct evidence of astrocytic modulation in the development of rewarding effects induced by drugs of abuse. *Neuropsychopharmacology, 31*(11), 2476–2488. http://dx.doi.org/10.1038/sj.npp.1301007.

Navarro, G., Moreno, E., Aymerich, M., Marcellino, D., McCormick, P. J., Mallol, J., et al. (2010). Direct involvement of sigma-1 receptors in the dopamine D1 receptor-mediated effects of cocaine. *Proceedings of the National Academy of Sciences of the United States of America, 107*(43), 18676–18681. http://dx.doi.org/10.1073/pnas.1008911107, [pii] 1008911107. Retrieved from PM: 20956312.

Nedergaard, M., Ransom, B., & Goldman, S. A. (2003). New roles for astrocytes: Redefining the functional architecture of the brain. *Trends in Neurosciences, 26*(10), 523–530. http://dx.doi.org/10.1016/j.tins.2003.08.008.

Nikodemova, M., Duncan, I. D., & Watters, J. J. (2006). Minocycline exerts inhibitory effects on multiple mitogen-activated protein kinases and IκBα degradation in a stimulus-specific manner in microglia. *Journal of Neurochemistry, 96*(2), 314–323. http://dx.doi.org/10.1111/j.1471-4159.2005.03520.x.

Nitta, A., Nishioka, H., Fukumitsu, H., Furukawa, Y., Sugiura, H., Shen, L., et al. (2004). Hydrophobic dipeptide Leu-Ile protects against neuronal death by inducing brain-derived neurotrophic factor and glial cell line-derived neurotrophic factor synthesis. *Journal of Neuroscience Research, 78*(2), 250–258. http://dx.doi.org/10.1002/jnr.20258.

Niwa, M., Nitta, A., Shen, L., Noda, Y., & Nabeshima, T. (2007). Involvement of glial cell line-derived neurotrophic factor in inhibitory effects of a hydrophobic dipeptide Leu-Ile on morphine-induced sensitization and rewarding effects. *Behavioural Brain Research, 179*(1), 167–171. http://dx.doi.org/10.1016/j.bbr.2007.01.026.

Niwa, M., Nitta, A., Yamada, K., & Nabeshima, T. (2007). The roles of glial cell line-derived neurotrophic factor, tumor necrosis factor-α, and an inducer of these factors in drug dependence. *Journal of Pharmacological Sciences, 104*(2), 116–121. http://dx.doi.org/10.1254/jphs.CP0070017.

Niwa, M., Nitta, A., Yamada, Y., Nakajima, A., Saito, K., Seishima, M., et al. (2007). An inducer for glial cell line-derived neurotrophic factor and tumor necrosis factor-alpha protects against methamphetamine-induced rewarding effects and sensitization. *Biological Psychiatry, 61*(7), 890–901. http://dx.doi.org/10.1016/j.biopsych.2006.06.016.

Noda, M., Nakanishi, H., Nabekura, J., & Akaike, N. (2000). AMPA-kainate subtypes of glutamate receptor in rat cerebral microglia. *The Journal of Neuroscience, 20*(1), 251–258.

Nosrat, C. A., Tomac, A., Hoffer, B. J., & Olson, L. (1997). Cellular and developmental patterns of expression of Ret and glial cell line-derived neurotrophic factor receptor alpha mRNAs. *Experimental Brain Research, 115*(3), 410–422.

Ohsawa, K., Irino, Y., Sanagi, T., Nakamura, Y., Suzuki, E., Inoue, K., et al. (2010). P2Y12 receptor-mediated integrin-β1 activation regulates microglial process extension induced by ATP. *Glia, 58*(7), 790–801.

Ohta, K., Kuno, S., Mizuta, I., Fujinami, A., Matsui, H., & Ohta, M. (2003). Effects of dopamine agonists bromocriptine, pergolide, cabergoline, and SKF-38393 on GDNF, NGF, and BDNF synthesis in cultured mouse astrocytes. *Life Sciences, 73*(5), 617–626.

Ojaniemi, M., Glumoff, V., Harju, K., Liljeroos, M., Vuori, K., & Hallman, M. (2003). Phosphatidylinositol 3-kinase is involved in Toll-like receptor 4-mediated cytokine expression in mouse macrophages. *European Journal of Immunology, 33*(3), 597–605. http://dx.doi.org/10.1002/eji.200323376.

Olney, J. W., Labruyere, J., Wang, G., Wozniak, D. F., Price, M. T., & Sesma, M. A. (1991). NMDA antagonist neurotoxicity: Mechanism and prevention. *Science, 254*(5037), 1515–1518.

Oo, T. F., Ries, V., Cho, J. W., Kholodilov, N., & Burke, R. E. (2005). Anatomical basis of glial cell line-derived neurotrophic factor expression in the striatum and related basal ganglia during postnatal development of the rat. *The Journal of Comparative Neurology, 484*(1), 57–67. http://dx.doi.org/10.1002/cne.20463.

Otterbein, L. E., Soares, M. P., Yamashita, K., & Bach, F. H. (2003). Heme oxygenase-1: Unleashing the protective properties of heme. *Trends in Immunology, 24*(8), 449–455, [pii] S1471490603001819. Retrieved from PM: 12909459.

Palmer, A. A., Verbitsky, M., Suresh, R., Kamens, H. M., Reed, C. L., Li, N., et al. (2005). Gene expression differences in mice divergently selected for methamphetamine sensitivity. *Mammalian Genome, 16*(5), 291–305, Retrieved from PM: 16104378.

Paolicelli, R. C., Bolasco, G., Pagani, F., Maggi, L., Scianni, M., Panzanelli, P., et al. (2011). Synaptic pruning by microglia is necessary for normal brain development. *Science, 333*(6048), 1456–1458.

Park, I. H., Yeon, S. I., Youn, J. H., Choi, J. E., Sasaki, N., Choi, I. H., et al. (2004). Expression of a novel secreted splice variant of the receptor for advanced glycation end products (RAGE) in human brain astrocytes and peripheral blood mononuclear cells. *Molecular Immunology, 40*(16), 1203–1211.

Parpura, V., Basarsky, T. A., Liu, F., Jeftinija, K., Jeftinija, S., & Haydon, P. G. (1994). Glutamate-mediated astrocyte-neuron signalling. *Nature, 369*(6483), 744–747. http://dx.doi.org/10.1038/369744a0.

Pasparakis, M. (2009). Regulation of tissue homeostasis by NF-κB signalling: Implications for inflammatory diseases. *Nature Reviews Immunology, 9*(11), 778–788. http://dx.doi.org/10.1038/nri2655, [pii] nri2655. Retrieved from PM: 19855404.

Pawate, S., Shen, Q., Fan, F., & Bhat, N. R. (2004). Redox regulation of glial inflammatory response to lipopolysaccharide and interferon-γ. *Journal of Neuroscience Research, 77*(4), 540–551. http://dx.doi.org/10.1002/jnr.20180, Retrieved from PM: 15264224.

Pereira, F. C., Cunha-Oliveira, T., Viana, S. D., Travassos, A. S., Nunes, S., Silva, C., et al. (2012). Disruption of striatal glutamatergic/GABAergic homeostasis following acute methamphetamine in mice. *Neurotoxicology and Teratology, 34*(5), 522–529.

Pierce, R. C., & Bari, A. A. (2001). The role of neurotrophic factors in psychostimulant-induced behavioral and neuronal plasticity. *Reviews in the Neurosciences, 12*(2), 95–110.

Pierce, R. C., & Wolf, M. E. (2013). Psychostimulant-induced neuroadaptations in nucleus accumbens AMPA receptor transmission. *Cold Spring Harbor Perspectives in Medicine, 3*(2), a012021, Retrieved from PM: 23232118.

Pocock, J. M., & Kettenmann, H. (2007). Neurotransmitter receptors on microglia. *Trends in Neurosciences, 30*(10), 527–535.

Ponath, G., Schettler, C., Kaestner, F., Voigt, B., Wentker, D., Arolt, V., et al. (2007). Autocrine S100B effects on astrocytes are mediated via RAGE. *Journal of Neuroimmunology, 184*(1–2), 214–222.

Prezzavento, O., Campisi, A., Ronsisvalle, S., Li, V. G., Marrazzo, A., Bramanti, V., et al. (2007). Novel sigma receptor ligands: Synthesis and biological profile. *Journal of Medicinal Chemistry, 50*(5), 951–961. http://dx.doi.org/10.1021/jm0611197, Retrieved from PM: 17328523.

Prochiantz, A., & Mallat, M. (1988). Astrocyte diversity. *Annals of the New York Academy of Sciences, 540*, 52–63, Retrieved from PM: 2462828.

Quinton, M. S., & Yamamoto, B. K. (2006). Causes and consequences of methamphetamine and MDMA toxicity. *The AAPS Journal, 8*(2), E337–E347. http://dx.doi.org/10.1208/aapsj080238, Retrieved from PM: 16796384.

Ransohoff, R. M., & Perry, V. H. (2009). Microglial physiology: Unique stimuli, specialized responses. *Annual Review of Immunology, 27*, 119–145. http://dx.doi.org/10.1146/annurev.immunol.021908.132528.

Reichardt, L. F. (2006). Neurotrophin-regulated signalling pathways. *Philosophical Transactions of the Royal Society of London Series B, Biological Sciences, 361*(1473), 1545–1564. http://dx.doi.org/10.1098/rstb.2006.1894, [pii] G280147415872711. Retrieved from PM: 16939974.

Robison, A. J., & Nestler, E. J. (2011). Transcriptional and epigenetic mechanisms of addiction. *Nature Reviews Neuroscience, 12*(11), 623–637.

Robson, M. J., Noorbakhsh, B., Seminerio, M. J., & Matsumoto, R. R. (2012). Sigma-1 receptors: Potential targets for the treatment of substance abuse. *Current Pharmaceutical Design, 18*(7), 902–919.

Robson, M. J., Turner, R. C., Naser, Z. J., McCurdy, C. R., Huber, J. D., & Matsumoto, R. R. (2013). SN79, a sigma receptor ligand, blocks methamphetamine-induced microglial activation and cytokine upregulation. *Experimental Neurology, 247C*, 134–142. http://dx.doi.org/10.1016/j.expneurol.2013.04.009.

Rocha, S. M., Cristovao, A. C., Campos, F. L., Fonseca, C. P., & Baltazar, G. (2012). Astrocyte-derived GDNF is a potent inhibitor of microglial activation. *Neurobiology of Disease, 47*(3), 407–415. http://dx.doi.org/10.1016/j.nbd.2012.04.014.

Roger, T., David, J., Glauser, M. P., & Calandra, T. (2001). MIF regulates innate immune responses through modulation of Toll-like receptor 4. *Nature, 414*(6866), 920–924. http://dx.doi.org/10.1038/414920a.

Ron, D., & Janak, P. H. (2005). GDNF and addiction. *Reviews in the Neurosciences, 16*(4), 277–285.

Rothman, S. M., & Olney, J. W. (1986). Glutamate and the pathophysiology of hypoxic—Ischemic brain damage. *Annals of Neurology, 19*, 105–111.

Rothstein, J. D., Dykes-Hoberg, M., Pardo, C. A., Bristol, L. A., Jin, L., Kuncl, R. W., et al. (1996). Knockout of glutamate transporters reveals a major role for astroglial transport in excitotoxicity and clearance of glutamate. *Neuron, 16*(3), 675–686, Retrieved from PM: 8785064.

Rubartelli, A., & Lotze, M. T. (2007). Inside, outside, upside down: Damage-associated molecular-pattern molecules (DAMPs) and redox. *Trends in Immunology, 28*(10), 429–436.

Saha, R. N., Liu, X., & Pahan, K. (2006). Up-regulation of BDNF in astrocytes by TNF-α: A case for the neuroprotective role of cytokine. *Journal of Neuroimmune Pharmacology, 1*(3), 212–222. http://dx.doi.org/10.1007/s11481-006-9020-8, Retrieved from PM: 18040799.

Saijo, K., Winner, B., Carson, C. T., Collier, J. G., Boyer, L., Rosenfeld, M. G., et al. (2009). A Nurr1/CoREST pathway in microglia and astrocytes protects dopaminergic neurons from inflammation-induced death. *Cell, 137*(1), 47–59, Retrieved from PM: 19345186.

Sandhu, J. K., Gardaneh, M., Iwasiow, R., Lanthier, P., Gangaraju, S., Ribecco-Lutkiewicz, M., et al. (2009). Astrocyte-secreted GDNF and glutathione antioxidant system protect neurons against 6OHDA cytotoxicity. *Neurobiology of Disease, 33*(3), 405–414. http://dx.doi.org/10.1016/j.nbd.2008.11.016, [pii] S0969-9961(08)00286-6. Retrieved from PM: 19118631.

Satake, K., Matsuyama, Y., Kamiya, M., Kawakami, H., Iwata, H., Adachi, K., et al. (2000). Up-regulation of glial cell line-derived neurotrophic factor (GDNF) following traumatic spinal cord injury. *NeuroReport, 11*(17), 3877–3881.

Sattler, R., Xiong, Z., Lu, W. Y., MacDonald, J. F., & Tymianski, M. (2000). Distinct roles of synaptic and extrasynaptic NMDA receptors in excitotoxicity. *The Journal of Neuroscience, 20*(1), 22–33, Retrieved from PM: 10627577.

Schaar, D. G., Sieber, B. A., Dreyfus, C. F., & Black, I. B. (1993). Regional and cell-specific expression of GDNF in rat brain. *Experimental Neurology, 124*(2), 368–371.

Schroder, K., & Tschopp, J. (2010). The inflammasomes. *Cell, 140*(6), 821–832.

Schubert, P., Ogata, T., Rudolphi, K., Marchini, C., McRae, A., & Ferroni, S. (1997). Support of homeostatic glial cell signaling: A novel therapeutic approach by propentofylline. *Annals of the New York Academy of Sciences, 826*, 337–347.

Sekine, Y., Ouchi, Y., Sugihara, G., Takei, N., Yoshikawa, E., Nakamura, K., et al. (2008). Methamphetamine causes microglial activation in the brains of human abusers. *The Journal of Neuroscience, 28*(22), 5756–5761. http://dx.doi.org/10.1523/JNEUROSCI.1179-08.2008, [pii] 28/22/5756. Retrieved from PM: 18509037.

Shah, A., Silverstein, P. S., Singh, D. P., & Kumar, A. (2012). Involvement of metabotropic glutamate receptor 5, AKT/PI3K signaling and NF-κB pathway in methamphetamine-mediated increase in IL-6 and IL-8 expression in astrocytes. *Journal of Neuroinflammation, 9*, 52. http://dx.doi.org/10.1186/1742-2094-9-52.

Shao, Y., & McCarthy, K. D. (1994). Plasticity of astrocytes. *Glia, 11*, 147–155.

Shao, Y., Porter, J. T., & McCarthy, K. D. (1994). Neuroligand receptor heterogeneity among astroglia. *Perspectives on Developmental Neurobiology, 2*(3), 205–215, Retrieved from PM: 7850353.

Shao, W., Zhang, S. Z., Tang, M., Zhang, X. H., Zhou, Z., Yin, Y. Q., et al. (2013). Suppression of neuroinflammation by astrocytic dopamine D2 receptors via αB-crystallin. *Nature, 494*(7435), 90–94. http://dx.doi.org/10.1038/nature11748, [pii] nature11748. Retrieved from PM: 23242137.

Shen, F., Meredith, G. E., & Napier, T. C. (2006). Amphetamine-induced place preference and conditioned motor sensitization requires activation of tyrosine kinase receptors in the hippocampus. *The Journal of Neuroscience, 26*(43), 11041–11051. http://dx.doi.org/10.1523/JNEUROSCI.2898-06.2006.

Sherwood, C. C., Stimpson, C. D., Raghanti, M. A., Wildman, D. E., Uddin, M., Grossman, L. I., et al. (2006). Evolution of increased glia-neuron ratios in the human frontal cortex. *Proceedings of the National Academy of Sciences of the United States of America, 103*(37), 13606–13611. http://dx.doi.org/10.1073/pnas.0605843103.

Shoptaw, S. (2013). Safety and subjective effects of ibudilast for methamphetamine dependence. In *College on problems of drug dependence, San Diego, CA.*

Snider, S. E., Hendrick, E. S., & Beardsley, P. M. (2013). Glial cell modulators attenuate methamphetamine self-administration in the rat. *European Journal of Pharmacology, 701*(1–3), 124–130. http://dx.doi.org/10.1016/j.ejphar.2013.01.016.

Snider, S. E., Vunck, S. A., van den Oord, E., Adkins, D. E., McClay, J. L., & Beardsley, P. M. (2012). The glial cell modulators, ibudilast and its amino analog, AV1013, attenuate methamphetamine locomotor activity and its sensitization in mice. *European Journal of Pharmacology, 679*(1–3), 75–80. http://dx.doi.org/10.1016/j.ejphar.2012.01.013.

Snyder, G. L., Allen, P. B., Fienberg, A. A., Valle, C. G., Huganir, R. L., Nairn, A. C., et al. (2000). Regulation of phosphorylation of the GluR1 AMPA receptor in the neostriatum by dopamine and psychostimulants in vivo. *The Journal of Neuroscience, 20*(12), 4480–4488, Retrieved from PM: 10844017.

Soczynska, J. K., Mansur, R. B., Brietzke, E., Swardfager, W., Kennedy, S. H., Woldeyohannes, H. O., et al. (2012). Novel therapeutic targets in depression: Minocycline as a candidate treatment. *Behavioural Brain Research, 235*(2), 302–317. http://dx.doi.org/10.1016/j.bbr.2012.07.026.

Sofroniew, M. V., & Vinters, H. V. (2010). Astrocytes: Biology and pathology. *Acta Neuropathologica, 119*(1), 7–35.

Sofuoglu, M., Mooney, M., Kosten, T., Waters, A., & Hashimoto, K. (2011). Minocycline attenuates subjective rewarding effects of dextroamphetamine in humans. *Psychopharmacology, 213*(1), 61–68. http://dx.doi.org/10.1007/s00213-010-2014-5.

Sofuoglu, M., Sato, J., & Takemori, A. E. (1990). Maintenance of morphine dependence by naloxone in acutely dependent mice. *The Journal of Pharmacology and Experimental Therapeutics, 254*(3), 841–846.

Somjen, G. G. (1988). Nervenkitt: Notes on the history of the concept of neuroglia. *Glia, 1*, 2–9.

Sorg, B. A., Chen, S. Y., & Kalivas, P. W. (1993). Time course of tyrosine hydroxylase expression after behavioral sensitization to cocaine. *The Journal of Pharmacology and Experimental Therapeutics, 266*(1), 424–430.

Spassky, N., Merkle, F. T., Flames, N., Tramontin, A. D., Garcia-Verdugo, J. M., & Alvarez-Buylla, A. (2005). Adult ependymal cells are postmitotic and are derived from radial glial cells during embryogenesis. *The Journal of Neuroscience, 25*(1), 10–18. http://dx. doi.org/10.1523/JNEUROSCI.1108-04.2005, [pii] 25/1/10. Retrieved from PM: 15634762.

Srikrishna, G., & Freeze, H. H. (2009). Endogenous damage-associated molecular pattern molecules at the crossroads of inflammation and cancer. *Neoplasia, 11*(7), 615–628, Retrieved from PM: 19568407.

Sriram, K., Miller, D. B., & O'Callaghan, J. P. (2006). Minocycline attenuates microglial activation but fails to mitigate striatal dopaminergic neurotoxicity: Role of tumor necrosis factor-α. *Journal of Neurochemistry, 96*(3), 706–718. http://dx.doi.org/10.1111/j.1471-4159.2005.03566.x.

Stadlin, A., Lau, J. W., & Szeto, Y. K. (1998). A selective regional response of cultured astrocytes to methamphetamine. *Annals of the New York Academy of Sciences, 844,* 108–121.

Stella, N. (2010). Cannabinoid and cannabinoid-like receptors in microglia, astrocytes, and astrocytomas. *Glia, 58*(9), 1017–1030. http://dx.doi.org/10.1002/glia.20983.

Stirling, D. P., Koochesfahani, K. M., Steeves, J. D., & Tetzlaff, W. (2005). Minocycline as a neuroprotective agent. *The Neuroscientist, 11*(4), 308–322. http://dx.doi.org/10.1177/1073858405275175.

Streit, W. J. (2002). Microglia as neuroprotective, immunocompetent cells of the CNS. *Glia, 40*(2), 133–139, Retrieved from PM: 12379901.

Strober, W., Murray, P. J., Kitani, A., & Watanabe, T. (2006). Signalling pathways and molecular interactions of NOD1 and NOD2. *Nature Reviews Immunology, 6*(1), 9–20. http://dx.doi.org/10.1038/nri1747, [pii] nri1747. Retrieved from PM: 16493424.

Stuber, G. D., Britt, J. P., & Bonci, A. (2012). Optogenetic modulation of neural circuits that underlie reward seeking. *Biological Psychiatry, 71*(12), 1061–1067.

Su, T. P., Hayashi, T., Maurice, T., Buch, S., & Ruoho, A. E. (2010). The sigma-1 receptor chaperone as an inter-organelle signaling modulator. *Trends in Pharmacological Sciences, 31*(12), 557–566.

Sulzer, D., & Rayport, S. (1990). Amphetamine and other psychostimulants reduce pH gradients in midbrain dopaminergic neurons and chromaffin granules: A mechanism of action. *Neuron, 5*(6), 797–808, [pii] 0896-6273(90)90339-H. Retrieved from PM: 2268433.

Sulzer, D., & Zecca, L. (2000). Intraneuronal dopamine-quinone synthesis: A review. *Neurotoxicity Research, 1*(3), 181–195, Retrieved from PM: 12835101.

Suzuki, M., El-Hage, N., Zou, S., Hahn, Y. K., Sorrell, M. E., Sturgill, J. L., et al. (2011). Fractalkine/CX3CL1 protects striatal neurons from synergistic morphine and HIV-1 Tat-induced dendritic losses and death. *Molecular Neurodegeneration, 6*(1), 78, Retrieved from PM: 22093090.

Suzumura, A., Ito, A., Yoshikawa, M., & Sawada, M. (1999). Ibudilast suppresses TNFα production by glial cells functioning mainly as type III phosphodiesterase inhibitor in the CNS. *Brain Research, 837*(1–2), 203–212.

Tanaka, K., Watase, K., Manabe, T., Yamada, K., Watanabe, M., Takahashi, K., et al. (1997). Epilepsy and exacerbation of brain injury in mice lacking the glutamate transporter GLT-1. *Science, 276*(5319), 1699–1702.

Tang, T., Rosenkranz, A., Assmann, K. J., Goodman, M. J., Gutierrez-Ramos, J. C., Carroll, M. C., et al. (1997). A role for Mac-1 (CDIIb/CD18) in immune complex-stimulated neutrophil function in vivo: Mac-1 deficiency abrogates sustained Fcγ receptor-dependent neutrophil adhesion and complement-dependent proteinuria in acute glomerulonephritis. *The Journal of Experimental Medicine, 186*(11), 1853–1863, Retrieved from PM: 9382884.

Taylor, D. L., Diemel, L. T., & Pocock, J. M. (2003). Activation of microglial group III metabotropic glutamate receptors protects neurons against microglial neurotoxicity. *The Journal of Neuroscience, 23*(6), 2150–2160.

Tezuka, T., Tamura, M., Kondo, M. A., Sakaue, M., Okada, K., Takemoto, K., et al. (2013). Cuprizone short-term exposure: Astrocytic IL-6 activation and behavioral changes relevant to psychosis. *Neurobiology of Disease, 59C,* 63–68. http://dx.doi.org/10.1016/j.ncbrbd.2013.07.003, Retrieved from PM: 23867234.

Theberge, F. R., Li, X., Kambhampati, S., Pickens, C. L., St. Laurent, R., Bossert, J. M., et al. (2013). Effect of chronic delivery of the Toll-like receptor 4 antagonist (+)-naltrexone on incubation of heroin craving. *Biological Psychiatry, 73*(8), 729–737.

Theodosis, D. T., Poulain, D. A., & Oliet, S. H. (2008). Activity-dependent structural and functional plasticity of astrocyte-neuron interactions. *Physiological Reviews*, *88*(3), 983–1008, Retrieved from PM: 18626065.

Thomas, D. M., Dowgiert, J., Geddes, T. J., Francescutti-Verbeem, D., Liu, X., & Kuhn, D. M. (2004). Microglial activation is a pharmacologically specific marker for the neurotoxic amphetamines. *Neuroscience Letters*, *367*(3), 349–354, Retrieved from PM: 15337264.

Thomas, D. M., Francescutti-Verbeem, D. M., & Kuhn, D. M. (2008). The newly synthesized pool of dopamine determines the severity of methamphetamine-induced neurotoxicity. *Journal of Neurochemistry*, *105*(3), 605–616, Retrieved from PM: 18088364.

Thomas, D. M., & Kuhn, D. M. (2005). MK-801 and dextromethorphan block microglial activation and protect against methamphetamine-induced neurotoxicity. *Brain Research*, *1050*(1–2), 190–198.

Thomas, G. E., Szücs, M., Mamone, J. Y., Bem, W. T., Rush, M. D., Johnson, F. E., et al. (1990). Sigma and opioid receptors in human brain tumors. *Life Sciences*, *46*, 1279–1286.

Thomas, D. M., Walker, P. D., Benjamins, J. A., Geddes, T. J., & Kuhn, D. M. (2004). Methamphetamine neurotoxicity in dopamine nerve endings of the striatum is associated with microglial activation. *Journal of Pharmacology and Experimental Therapeutics*, *311*(1), 1–7.

Trang, T., Beggs, S., Wan, X., & Salter, M. W. (2009). P2X4-receptor-mediated synthesis and release of brain-derived neurotrophic factor in microglia is dependent on calcium and p38-mitogen-activated protein kinase activation. *The Journal of Neuroscience*, *29*(11), 3518–3528. http://dx.doi.org/10.1523/JNEUROSCI.5714-08.2009.

Treanor, J. J., Goodman, L., de Sauvage, F., Stone, D. M., Poulsen, K. T., Beck, C. D., et al. (1996). Characterization of a multicomponent receptor for GDNF. *Nature*, *382*(6586), 80–83. http://dx.doi.org/10.1038/382080a0, Retrieved from PM: 8657309.

Treweek, J. B., Dickerson, T. J., & Janda, K. D. (2009). Drugs of abuse that mediate advanced glycation end product formation: A chemical link to disease pathology. *Accounts of Chemical Research*, *42*(5), 659–669. http://dx.doi.org/10.1021/ar800247d, Retrieved from PM: 19275211.

Treweek, J., Wee, S., Koob, G. F., Dickerson, T. J., & Janda, K. D. (2007). Self-vaccination by methamphetamine glycation products chemically links chronic drug abuse and cardiovascular disease. *Proceedings of the National Academy of Sciences of the United States of America*, *104*(28), 11580–11584. http://dx.doi.org/10.1073/pnas.0701328104, [pii] 0701328104. Retrieved from PM: 17592122.

Trupp, M., Arenas, E., Fainzilber, M., Nilsson, A. S., Sieber, B. A., Grigoriou, M., et al. (1996). Functional receptor for GDNF encoded by the c-ret proto-oncogene. *Nature*, *381*(6585), 785–789. http://dx.doi.org/10.1038/381785a0, Retrieved from PM: 8657281.

Tsuda, M., Inoue, K., & Salter, M. W. (2005). Neuropathic pain and spinal microglia: A big problem from molecules in "small" glia. *Trends in Neurosciences*, *28*(2), 101–107.

Tsuda, M., Shigemoto-Mogami, Y., Koizumi, S., Mizokoshi, A., Kohsaka, S., Salter, M. W., et al. (2003). P2X4 receptors induced in spinal microglia gate tactile allodynia after nerve injury. *Nature*, *424*(6950), 778–783.

Ullian, E. M., Christopherson, K. S., & Barres, B. A. (2004). Role for glia in synaptogenesis. *Glia*, *47*(3), 209–216. http://dx.doi.org/10.1002/glia.20082.

Van Bockstaele, E. J., & Colago, E. E. (1996). Selective distribution of the NMDA-R1 glutamate receptor in astrocytes and presynaptic axon terminals in the nucleus locus coeruleus of the rat brain: An immunoelectron microscopic study. *The Journal of Comparative Neurology*, *369*(4), 483–496. http://dx.doi.org/10.1002/(SICI)1096-9861(19960610)369:4<483::AID-CNE1>3.0.CO;2-0.

Venero, J. L., Santiago, M., Tomas-Camardiel, M., Matarredona, E. R., Cano, J., & Machado, A. (2002). DCG-IV but not other group-II metabotropic receptor agonists induces microglial BDNF mRNA expression in the rat striatum. Correlation with neuronal injury. *Neuroscience, 113*(4), 857–869.

Villalba, M., Hott, M., Martin, C., Aguila, B., Valdivia, S., Quezada, C., et al. (2012). Herpes simplex virus type 1 induces simultaneous activation of Toll-like receptors 2 and 4 and expression of the endogenous ligand serum amyloid A in astrocytes. *Medical Microbiology and Immunology, 201*(3), 371–379.

Virchow, R. (1856). *Gesammelte Abhandlungen zur Wissenschaftlichen Medicin.* Frankfurt: Hamm.

Virchow, R. (1858). *Cellularpathologie in ihre Begründung auf Physiogische und Pathologische Gewebelehre.* Berlin: A. Hirschwald, F.C. (1863), Trans.

Volterra, A., & Meldolesi, J. (2005). Astrocytes, from brain glue to communication elements: The revolution continues. *Nature Reviews Neuroscience, 6*(8), 626–640.

Wang, J. P., Bowen, G. N., Zhou, S., Cerny, A., Zacharia, A., Knipe, D. M., et al. (2012). Role of specific innate immune responses in herpes simplex virus infection of the central nervous system. *Journal of Virology, 86*(4), 2273–2281.

Wang, X., Loram, L. C., Ramos, K., de Jesus, A. J., Thomas, J., Cheng, K., et al. (2012). Morphine activates neuroinflammation in a manner parallel to endotoxin. *Proceedings of the National Academy of Sciences of the United States of America, 109*(16), 6325–6330. http://dx.doi.org/10.1073/pnas.1200130109.

Watkins, L. R., Hutchinson, M. R., Ledeboer, A., Wieseler-Frank, J., Milligan, E. D., & Maier, S. F. (2007). Norman Cousins Lecture. Glia as the "bad guys": Implications for improving clinical pain control and the clinical utility of opioids. *Brain, Behavior, and Immunity, 21*(2), 131–146. http://dx.doi.org/10.1016/j.bbi.2006.10.011.

Wilkin, G. P., Marriott, D. R., & Cholewinski, A. J. (1990). Astrocyte heterogeneity. *Trends in Neurosciences, 13*, 43–46.

Wilson, J. X. (1997). Antioxidant defense of the brain: A role for astrocytes. *Canadian Journal of Physiology and Pharmacology, 75*(10–11), 1149–1163, Retrieved from PM: 9431439.

Xu, Y. T., Robson, M. J., Szeszel-Fedorowicz, W., Patel, D., Rooney, R., McCurdy, C. R., et al. (2012). CM156, a sigma receptor ligand, reverses cocaine-induced place conditioning and transcriptional responses in the brain. *Pharmacology, Biochemistry, and Behavior, 101*(1), 174–180.

Yakovleva, T., Bazov, I., Watanabe, H., Hauser, K. F., & Bakalkin, G. (2011). Transcriptional control of maladaptive and protective responses in alcoholics: A role of the NF-κB system. *Brain, Behavior, and Immunity, 25*(Suppl. 1), S29–S38. http://dx.doi.org/10.1016/j.bbi.2010.12.019.

Yan, Y., Miyamoto, Y., Nitta, A., Muramatsu, S.-I., Ozawa, K., Yamada, K., et al. (2013). Intrastriatal gene delivery of GDNF persistently attenuates methamphetamine self-administration and relapse in mice. *The International Journal of Neuropsychopharmacology/ Official Scientific Journal of the Collegium Internationale Neuropsychopharmacologicum (CINP), 16*(7), 1559–1567. http://dx.doi.org/10.1017/s1461145712001575.

Yan, Y., Nitta, A., Mizuno, T., Nakajima, A., Yamada, K., & Nabeshima, T. (2006). Discriminative-stimulus effects of methamphetamine and morphine in rats are attenuated by cAMP-related compounds. *Behavioural Brain Research, 173*(1), 39–46. http://dx.doi.org/10.1016/j.bbr.2006.05.029.

Yan, Q., Radeke, M. J., Matheson, C. R., Talvenheimo, J., Welcher, A. A., & Feinstein, S. C. (1997). Immunocytochemical localization of TrkB in the central nervous system of the adult rat. *The Journal of Comparative Neurology, 378*(1), 135–157.

Yan, Y., Yamada, K., Niwa, M., Nagai, T., Nitta, A., & Nabeshima, T. (2007). Enduring vulnerability to reinstatement of methamphetamine-seeking behavior in glial-cell-line-derived neurotrophic factor mutant mice. *FASEB Journal, 21*(9), 1994–2004. http://dx.doi.org/10.1096/fj.06-7772com.

Yao, H., Kim, K., Duan, M., Hayashi, T., Guo, M., Morgello, S., et al. (2011). Cocaine hijacks sigma1 receptor to initiate induction of activated leukocyte cell adhesion molecule: Implication for increased monocyte adhesion and migration in the CNS. *The Journal of Neuroscience*, *31*(16), 5942–5955. http://dx.doi.org/10.1523/JNEUROSCI.5618-10.2011, [pii] 31/16/5942. Retrieved from PM: 21508219.

Yenari, M. A., Kauppinen, T. M., & Swanson, R. A. (2010). Microglial activation in stroke: Therapeutic targets. *Neurotherapeutics*, *7*(4), 378–391.

Yu, Y. J., Chang, C. H., & Gean, P. W. (2013). AMPA receptor endocytosis in the amygdala is involved in the disrupted reconsolidation of Methamphetamine-associated contextual memory. *Neurobiology of Learning and Memory*, *103*, 72–81, Retrieved from PM: 23603364.

Zanassi, P., Paolillo, M., Montecucco, A., Avvedimento, E. V., & Schinelli, S. (1999). Pharmacological and molecular evidence for dopamine D(1) receptor expression by striatal astrocytes in culture. *Journal of Neuroscience Research*, *58*(4), 544–552. http://dx.doi.org/10.1002/(SICI)1097-4547(19991115)58:4<544::AID-JNR7>3.0.CO;2-9, [pii]. Retrieved from PM: 10533046.

Zhang, Y., & Barres, B. A. (2010). Astrocyte heterogeneity: An underappreciated topic in neurobiology. *Current Opinion in Neurobiology*, *20*(5), 588–594, Retrieved from PM: 20655735.

Zhang, X., Goncalves, R., & Mosser, D. M. (2008). The isolation and characterization of murine macrophages. *Current Protocols in Immunology*, (Suppl. 83). http://dx.doi.org/10.1002/0471142735.im1401s83, Chapter 14, Unit 14.1. Retrieved from PM:19016445.

Zhang, L., Kitaichi, K., Fujimoto, Y., Nakayama, H., Shimizu, E., Iyo, M., et al. (2006). Protective effects of minocycline on behavioral changes and neurotoxicity in mice after administration of methamphetamine. *Progress in Neuro-Psychopharmacology & Biological Psychiatry*, *30*(8), 1381–1393. http://dx.doi.org/10.1016/j.pnpbp.2006.05.015.

Zhang, H. T., Li, L. Y., Zou, X. L., Song, X. B., Hu, Y. L., Feng, Z. T., et al. (2007). Immunohistochemical distribution of NGF, BDNF, NT-3, and NT-4 in adult rhesus monkey brains. *The Journal of Histochemistry & Cytochemistry*, *55*(1), 1–19. http://dx.doi.org/10.1369/jhc.6A6952.2006.

Zhang, F., Lu, Y. F., Wu, Q., Liu, J., & Shi, J. S. (2012). Resveratrol promotes neurotrophic factor release from astroglia. *Experimental Biology and Medicine (Maywood, NJ)*, *237*(8), 943–948. http://dx.doi.org/10.1258/ebm.2012.012044.

Zhou, B. G., & Norenberg, M. D. (1999). Ammonia downregulates GLAST mRNA glutamate transporter in rat astrocyte cultures. *Neuroscience Letters*, *276*(3), 145–148, [pii] S0304394099008162. Retrieved from PM:10612626.

Zhu, X., Bergles, D. E., & Nishiyama, A. (2008). NG2 cells generate both oligodendrocytes and gray matter astrocytes. *Development*, *135*(1), 145–157.

Zhuo, M., Wu, G., & Wu, L. J. (2011). Neuronal and microglial mechanisms of neuropathic pain. *Molecular Brain*, *4*, 31–34. http://dx.doi.org/10.1186/1756-6606-4-31.

CHAPTER TWO

The Vesicular Monoamine Transporter-2: An Important Pharmacological Target for the Discovery of Novel Therapeutics to Treat Methamphetamine Abuse

Justin R. Nickell[*], **Kiran B. Siripurapu**[*], **Ashish Vartak**[*],
Peter A. Crooks[*], **Linda P. Dwoskin**[†,1]

[*]College of Pharmacy, University of Kentucky, Lexington, Kentucky, USA
[†]Department of Pharmaceutical Sciences, College of Pharmacy, University of Kentucky, Lexington, Kentucky, USA
[1]Corresponding author: e-mail address: ldwoskin@email.uky.edu

Contents

Abstract

Methamphetamine abuse escalates, but no approved therapeutics are available to treat addicted individuals. Methamphetamine increases extracellular dopamine in reward-relevant pathways by interacting at vesicular monoamine transporter-2 (VMAT2) to inhibit dopamine uptake and promote dopamine release from synaptic vesicles, increasing cytosolic dopamine available for reverse transport by the dopamine transporter (DAT). VMAT2 is the target of our iterative drug discovery efforts to identify pharmacotherapeutics for methamphetamine addiction. Lobeline, the major alkaloid

Advances in Pharmacology, Volume 69
ISSN 1054-3589
http://dx.doi.org/10.1016/B978-0-12-420118-7.00002-0

in *Lobelia inflata*, potently inhibited VMAT2, methamphetamine-evoked striatal dopamine release, and methamphetamine self-administration in rats but exhibited high affinity for nicotinic acetylcholine receptors (nAChRs). Defunctionalized, unsaturated lobeline analog, *meso*-transdiene (MTD), exhibited lobeline-like *in vitro* pharmacology, lacked nAChR affinity, but exhibited high affinity for DAT, suggesting potential abuse liability. The 2,4-dichlorophenyl MTD analog, UKMH-106, exhibited selectivity for VMAT2 over DAT, inhibited methamphetamine-evoked dopamine release, but required a difficult synthetic approach. Lobelane, a saturated, defunctionalized lobeline analog, inhibited the neurochemical and behavioral effects of methamphetamine; tolerance developed to the lobelane-induced decrease in methamphetamine self-administration. Improved druglikeness was afforded by the incorporation of a chiral N-1,2-dihydroxypropyl moiety into lobelane to afford GZ-793A, which inhibited the neurochemical and behavioral effects of methamphetamine, without tolerance. From a series of 2,5-disubstituted pyrrolidine analogs, AV-2-192 emerged as a lead, exhibiting high affinity for VMAT2 and inhibiting methamphetamine-evoked dopamine release. Current results support the hypothesis that potent, selective VMAT2 inhibitors provide the requisite preclinical behavioral profile for evaluation as pharmacotherapeutics for methamphetamine abuse and emphasize selectivity for VMAT2 relative to DAT as a criterion for reducing abuse liability of the therapeutic.

ABBREVIATIONS

AV-2-192 *cis*-2,5-di(2-benzyl)-pyrrolidine
AV-2-197 1-methyl-*cis*-2,5-di(2-benzyl)-pyrrolidine
CNS central nervous system
CHO Chinese hamster ovary
CPP conditioned place preference
DA dopamine
DAT dopamine transporter
DTBZ dihydrotetrabenazine
DOPAC dihydroxyphenylacetic acid
GZ-793A (*R*)-3-[2,6-*cis*-di(4-methoxyphenethyl)piperidin-1-yl]propane-1,2-diol
METH methamphetamine
MTD *meso*-transdiene
MLA methyllycaconitine
MAO monoamine oxidase
MPP$^+$ 1-methyl-4-phenylpyridinium
MPTP *N*-methyl-1,2,3,6-tetrahydropyridine
NIC nicotine
nAChR nicotinic acetylcholine receptor
SERT serotonin transporter
TBZ tetrabenazine
UKMH-105 (3*Z*,5*E*)-3,5-bis(2,4-dichlorobenzylidene)-1-methylpiperidine
UKMH-106 (3*Z*,5*Z*)-3,5-bis(2,4-dichlorobenzylidene)-1-methylpiperidine
VMAT vesicular monoamine transporter
VMAT2 vesicular monoamine transporter-2

1. METHAMPHETAMINE ADDICTION

Psychostimulant abuse is an escalating problem, with 100,000 new methamphetamine (METH) users in the United States each year (Drug and Alcohol Services Information System (DASIS, 2008)). Methamphetamine use poses significant health risks, including long-term neuronal damage and concomitant deleterious effects on cognitive processes, such as memory and attention (Nordahl, Salo, & Leamon, 2003). The problem is complicated by the fact that treatment centers lack an effective means to combat its abuse (DASIS, 2008). Despite the serious consequences of METH use, there are currently no approved therapeutics available for those individuals suffering from METH addiction. Increasing emphasis has been placed on identifying the underlying mechanisms of METH action and relevant pharmacological targets for the development of novel therapeutic agents to treat METH addiction.

2. METHAMPHETAMINE: MECHANISM OF ACTION

Methamphetamine (Fig. 2.1), a powerful central nervous system (CNS) stimulant, exerts its pharmacological and behavioral effects through alterations in the brain dopaminergic reward circuitry, which is generally accepted as responsible for the rewarding effects of drugs of abuse (Di Chiara et al., 2004; Koob, 1992; Wise & Bozarth, 1987; Wise & Hoffman, 1992). Methamphetamine self-administration and conditioned place preference (CPP) in rodents are gold-standard assays used to demonstrate the reinforcing and rewarding effects of this drug (Hart, Ward, Haney, Foltin, & Fischman, 2001; Xu, Mo, Yung, Yang, & Leung, 2008; Yokel & Pickens, 1973). Amphetamines (including METH) enter dopaminergic presynaptic terminals by acting as substrates for the plasmalemma dopamine transporter (DAT) and by diffusion through the plasmalemma (Fig. 2.2; Johnson, Eshleman, Meyers, Neve, & Janowsky, 1998; Sulzer et al., 1995). Once inside the presynaptic terminal, amphetamines elicit the release of vesicular dopamine (DA) stores into the cytosol through an interaction with reserpine sites on the vesicular monoamine transporter-2 (VMAT2) protein (Ary & Komiskey, 1980; Liang & Rutledge, 1982; Peter, Jimenez, Liu, Kim, & Edwards, 1994; Philippu & Beyer, 1973; Pifl,

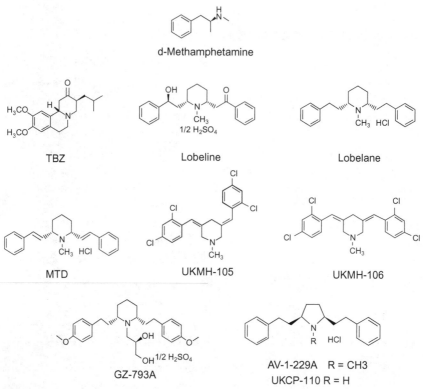

Figure 2.1 *Chemical structures.* Tetrabenazine (TBZ) is a benzoquinolizine compound that reversibly inhibits VMAT2 function. Lobeline is a lipophilic, nonpyridino alkaloid present in *Lobelia inflata.* Lobelane is a defunctionalized, saturated *meso*-analog of lobeline. MTD is a lobelane analog bearing unsaturated phenethyl side chain linkers. GZ-793A is a lobelane analog bearing a dihydroxypropyl moiety on the central nitrogen atom and methoxy substituents in the *para*-position on the phenyl rings. AV-1-229 bears a high degree of structural similarity to lobelane, with substitution of a pyrrolidine ring for the piperidine ring. UKCP-110, also known as AV-1-228, is the demethylated *nor*-analog of AV-1-229.

Drobny, Reither, Hornykiewicz, & Singer, 1995) and via disruption of the vesicular proton gradient as a consequence of its weak basicity and high lipophilicity (Barlow & Johnson, 1989). Amphetamines promote DA release from synaptic vesicles into the cytosol of the dopaminergic presynaptic terminal, redistributing DA stores and increasing cytosolic DA concentrations (Pifl et al., 1995; Sulzer et al., 1995), and inhibit DA uptake from the cytosol by VMAT2 (Brown, Hanson, & Fleckenstein, 2000, 2001; Fleckenstein, Volz, Riddle, Gibb, & Hanson, 2007). As amphetamines also inhibit the

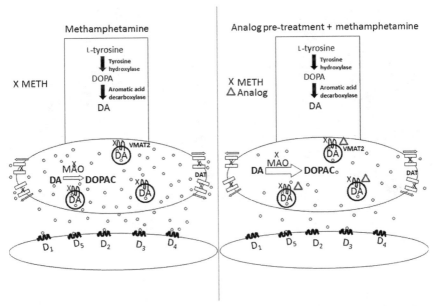

Figure 2.2 Model of the DA presynaptic terminal in the presence of methamphetamine (left) and in the presence of lobeline analog plus methamphetamine. (For color version of this figure, the reader is referred to the online version of this chapter.)

activity of the mitochondrial enzyme monoamine oxidase (MAO), the elevated concentrations of cytosolic DA are not subjected to metabolism (Mantle, Tipton, & Garrett, 1976). With increased cytosolic DA concentrations, DA is available for release into the synaptic cleft via reversal of DAT (Ary & Komiskey, 1980; Fischer & Cho, 1979; Liang & Rutledge, 1982; Sulzer et al., 1995). Enhanced DA release and increased stimulation of postsynaptic DA receptors that follows lead to the rewarding effects and high degree of abuse liability associated with these psychostimulant drugs (Carr & White, 1983; Hiroi & White, 1991; Hoebel et al., 1983; Lyness, Friedle, & Moore, 1979; Wise & Bozarth, 1987). Furthermore, the demonstration that heterologous VMAT2 knockout mice exhibit reduced amphetamine conditioned reward, enhanced amphetamine locomotion, and enhanced sensitivity to amphetamine also indicates that VMAT2 plays a critical role in mediating the behavioral effects of this drug of abuse (Takahashi et al., 1997; Wang et al., 1997). Although the effects of METH on VMAT2 are not the only mechanism responsible for its behavioral effects, we have considered VMAT2 as a key pharmacological target for developing pharmacotherapies to treat psychostimulant abuse (Dwoskin & Crooks, 2002), because this protein is an essential cellular component contributing to the increased extracellular DA concentrations produced by the actions of METH.

Furthermore, studies evaluating VMAT2 expression levels and function in both rodents and humans, together with results from imaging studies, led to the conclusion that VMAT2 protein levels and function are not changed by acute or chronic psychostimulant administration (Eiden & Weihe, 2011; Kilbourn et al., 2010). However, other investigators provide evidence that VMAT2 function and expression are altered by psychostimulant drugs of abuse (Riddle, Fleckenstein, & Hanson, 2005). Methamphetamine administration to rats reduced VMAT2 expression and clearance rates of DA in purified striatal vesicle preparations (Brown et al., 2000; Hogan, Staal, & Sonsalla, 2000), while cocaine increased V_{max} of DA uptake in these preparations (Brown et al., 2001). Corroborating evidence revealed that administration of monoamine releasers, such as amphetamine or METH, resulted in a redistribution of vesicular pools in the presynaptic terminal, leading to a reduction in VMAT2 available to clear DA from the cytosol (Fleckenstein et al., 2007). Taken together, these findings implicate VMAT2 as a dynamic presynaptic target for psychostimulant drugs of abuse, specifically amphetamines, and that VMAT2 may be a viable target for the discovery of pharmacotherapeutics to treat psychostimulant abuse.

3. IDENTIFICATION AND CLASSIFICATION OF VESICULAR MONOAMINE TRANSPORTERS

The discovery of secretory vesicles (Hillarp, 1958) led to the subsequent discovery of the vesicular monoamine transporter (VMAT) and the characterization of the structure and function of this protein. Early research revealed several distinguishing features of this class of transporters, including a preference to transport monoamines (e.g., serotonin, DA, and norepinephrine), the dependence of substrate transport on an electrochemical gradient across the vesicular lipid bilayer membrane, and the inhibition of substrate transport by both reserpine and tetrabenazine (TBZ) (Fig. 2.1; Henry, Gasnier, Roisin, Isamber, & Scherman, 1987; Johnson, 1988; Kanner & Schuldiner, 1987; Njus, Kelley, & Harnadek, 1986). The molecular structure of VMAT was first elucidated using Chinese hamster ovary (CHO) cells via expression cloning from rat pheochromocytoma PC12 cells (Liu, Peter, et al., 1992). Successful expression of the transporter in CHO cells provided protection against the neurotoxic effects of 1-methyl-4-phenylpyridinium (MPP$^+$), the active metabolite of N-methyl-1,2,3,6-tetrahydropyridine (MPTP), demonstrating that intracellular sequestration of MPP^+ via VMAT was responsible for the resistance to toxicity observed in PC12 cells (Liu, Peter, et al., 1992; Liu, Roghani, & Edwards, 1992). Gene transfer followed by plasmid rescue identified a cDNA clone for the VMAT isoform, designated VMAT1, which was predicted to be a 70-kDa protein having 12 transmembrane-spanning domains, internal carboxy and amino termini, and a large hydrophilic loop between transmembrane regions 1 and 2 (Liu, Peter, et al., 1992; Liu, Roghani, et al., 1992). Overall, the molecular structure for VMAT1 expressed in CHO cells was determined to be remarkably similar to the plasmalemma neurotransmitter transporters, yet its amino acid sequence showed homology to a multitude of bacterial resistance transporters (e.g., transporters encoded by tetracycline and methylenomycin resistance genes). An alternate isoform of VMAT was discovered contemporaneously by employing an expression cloning strategy using a mammalian cell line (CV-1), such that the expression of the protein by CV-1 cells resulted in transport of serotonin, DA, and norepinephrine (Erickson, Eiden, & Hoffman, 1992). The predicted molecular structure of this transporter, designated VMAT2, also suggested 12 transmembrane domains and internal carboxy and amino termini.

While having similar molecular structures, the development of polyclonal antibodies specific for each isoform revealed important differences between VMAT1 and VMAT2. Immunohistochemistry studies showed that VMAT1 is located primarily within the lipid bilayer membrane of large dense-core vesicles within chromaffin granule cells in the medulla of the adrenal, whereas scant expression of VMAT1 was found in the peripheral sympathetic neurons and blood platelets. In contrast, VMAT2 had a more ubiquitous expression pattern. VMAT2 is expressed widely by monoaminergic neurons of the CNS, histaminergic mast cells, peripheral sympathetic neurons, and β-cells of the pancreas (Erickson, Schafer, Bonner, Eiden, & Weihe, 1996; Peter et al., 1995; Weihe, Schafer, Erickson, & Eiden, 1995; Wimalasena, 2010). Isolation of VMAT1 to the peripheral nervous system and a likely minimal role in processes underlying psychostimulant abuse reduce the importance of this protein as a target for the discovery of pharmacotherapeutics for psychostimulant abuse.

4. VMAT2 FUNCTION

VMAT2 is critical as a functional component of monoaminergic neurotransmission. Within presynaptic terminals of monoaminergic neurons,

VMAT2 translocates monoamines from the cytosol across the vesicle membrane into the vesicle lumen following neurotransmitter biosynthesis and/or clearance from the extracellular space. Intravesicular sequestration of monoamines by VMAT2 occurs despite the high concentrations ($\sim$0.5 M) of monoamines within the vesicle. Transport is driven by the transmembrane proton gradient, generated by a vesicular H^+-ATPase, which shuttles protons into the vesicle by active transport. With respect to VMAT2, initial binding and movement of a hydrogen atom to the luminal face of VMAT2 induces a conformational change in the cytosolic face of the protein, exposing a high-affinity substrate binding site to which monoamines located in the cytosol bind. Following binding of substrate to the high-affinity site on VMAT2, a second proton binds to its luminal face, signaling a return to its original conformational state, which is accompanied by antiport of the hydrogen atom and monoamine molecule (Chaudhry, Edwards, & Fonnum, 2008; Wimalasena, 2010). Thus, intravesicular transport of a single monoamine molecule from the cytosol into the vesicle requires efflux of two protons from inside the vesicle to the cytosol.

5. VMAT2 BINDING SITES

Classically speaking, two distinct ligand binding sites have been identified on VMAT2: a reserpine binding site and a high-affinity TBZ binding site. Reserpine is obtained from *Rauwolfia serpentina* and was utilized originally to treat hypertension. Reserpine produces a long-lasting depletion of monoaminergic content from vesicles that express VMAT2. The use of reserpine as a first-line antihypertensive was discontinued due to its inhibition of VMAT2 on vesicles in monoaminergic neurons in the CNS and to the untoward side effect of depression resulting from vesicular monoamine depletion (Frize, 1954). Nonetheless, reserpine continues to be an important tool to evaluate the binding of novel compounds to and their subsequent functional inhibition of VMAT2. Reserpine binds in an irreversible manner to the substrate recognition site on VMAT2 following translocation of the initial proton from the vesicle lumen to the cytosol (Schuldiner, Liu, & Edwards, 1993). As such, reserpine is classified as a competitive monoamine uptake inhibitor at VMAT1 and VMAT2. In contrast, TBZ binding to VMAT2 is not affected by pH and is inhibited by high concentrations of monoamines (Darchen, Scherman, & Henry, 1989), suggesting a site of interaction different from that of reserpine. A single injection of reserpine *in vivo* inhibits TBZ binding to VMAT2 in rat striatal slices (Naudon et al., 1996). Furthermore, TBZ also inhibits reserpine binding to VMAT2 (Darchen et al., 1989; Schuldiner et al., 1993), suggesting either that reserpine and TBZ binding sites are overlapping or that each drug interacts with a functionally distinct conformation of the transporter (Liu & Edwards, 1997).

Several studies identified amino acid sequences in VMAT2 critical to protein function and that constitute the ligand binding sites. Photolabeling of purified VMAT2 revealed that the TBZ binding site is localized to the N-terminus of the protein (Sagne, Isambert, Vandekerckhove, Henry, & Gasnier, 1997; Sievert & Ruoho, 1997). Furthermore, mutagenesis of cysteine-439 resulted in >80% inhibition of dihydrotetrabenazine (DTBZ) binding, revealing a critical role of this amino acid in binding to the TBZ site (Thiriot & Ruoho, 2001). Mutation of aspartate-33 in the first transmembrane domain and of the serines 180–182 in the third transmembrane domain impaired substrate recognition by the transporter, suggesting that these amino acid residues are critical for interaction with the cationic amino groups and hydroxyl groups, respectively, of the monoamine substrate (Merickel, Rosandich, Peter, & Edwards, 1995). Additionally, mutation of transmembrane regions 9 through 12 revealed that tyrosine-434 and aspartate-461 are responsible for VMAT2 having greater affinity for TBZ, histamine, and serotonin compared with VMAT1 (Finn & Edwards, 1997).

6. ABERRANT VMAT2 EXPRESSION AND FUNCTION

Generation of VMAT2 knockout mice in 1997 allowed investigation of the role that VMAT2 plays in the physiological function of a number of different systems. Elimination of VMAT2 protein results in hypolocomotion in comparison with wild-type and heterozygous littermates and, moreover, is lethal within 2 weeks following birth due to the failure to gain weight (Fon et al., 1997; Takahashi et al., 1997; Wang et al., 1997). Morphological abnormalities were not observed in VMAT2 knockout mice (Takahashi et al., 1997; Wang et al., 1997), and monoaminergic neurons exhibited normal dendritic processes and axonal projections, despite having decreased whole-brain levels of monoamines (Fon et al., 1997; Takahashi et al., 1997; Wang et al., 1997). VMAT2 heterozygotes exhibited physiological and behavioral similarities to wild-type littermates, including viability into adulthood, normal weight gain, expression of conditioned passive avoidance behavior and stress responses emitted upon exposure to a novel environment, and unchanged monoamine receptor densities and affinities (Takahashi et al., 1997). Presynaptic vesicles within monoaminergic neurons from heterozygote mice express VMAT2 protein at 50% of the expression levels found in wild-type mice, as evidenced by the amount of [^{3}H]DTBZ binding to vesicle membranes (Takahashi et al., 1997). Cultures of midbrain neurons from heterozygote mice released ~50% less DA when depolarized compared to cultures from wild-type mice (Fon et al., 1997), revealing the necessity for VMAT2 expression and function for proper distribution and storage of monoamines for exocytotic release. VMAT2 heterozygotes administered amphetamine exhibited enhanced locomotor activity and a reduction in amphetamine reward in comparison with wild-type littermates in CPP assays (Takahashi et al., 1997). Following MPTP administration, the substantia nigra of heterozygotes exhibited twice the dopaminergic neuronal loss compared to wild-type mice (Takahashi et al., 1997), indicating enhanced sensitivity to its neurotoxic effects when VMAT2 protein levels were reduced. Collectively, these data indicate that appropriate VMAT2 expression is required for viability of the organism and that VMAT2 provides neuroprotection against some CNS toxins. Furthermore, VMAT2 appears to play a role in a variety of amphetamine-induced behaviors, which leads to the hypothesis that reversible inhibition of VMAT2 function may attenuate the behavioral effects of METH.

The role of VMAT2 in the protection of monoaminergic neurons from toxic insult gained attention in the clinical arena. VMAT2 sequesters MPP$^+$ from the cytosol in cell lines expressing VMAT2 (Liu, Roghani, & Edwards, 1992), thus limiting MPP$^+$ exposure and damage to the mitochondria and cellular respiration processes and the development of Parkinson's-like behavioral symptoms. Furthermore, elevated cytosolic DA concentrations are of particular concern, as DA inhibits mitochondrial respiration and DA auto-oxidation generates harmful free radicals (Ben-Shachar, Zuk, & Glinka, 1995; Hastings, Lewis, & Zigmond, 1996). Parkinson's disease is characterized by reduced motor coordination with an underlying etiology of loss of dopaminergic neurons in the substantia nigra pars compacta, which innervates the striatum. Given that VMAT2 provides neuroprotection from MPP$^+$-induced Parkinson's-like symptoms, clinicians employed a variety of neuroimaging and genetic screens to evaluate VMAT2 expression levels in Parkinson's patients to determine the role of this transporter in the disease. Results indicated that polymorphisms in the coding sequence of VMAT2 are extremely rare and, thus, likely did not account for the incidence of Parkinson's disease (Glatt et al., 2001). However, investigators found numerous gain-of-function haplotypes present in the genetic sequence responsible for the transcription of VMAT2 that seemed to confer a neuro-protective effect, specifically in women (Glatt, Wahner, White, Ruiz-Linares, & Ritz, 2006). Results from clinical studies employing positron emission tomography and photon emission computed tomography imaging techniques led to the speculation that the ratio of DAT to VMAT2 expression may be a critical parameter in predicting vulnerability of monoaminergic neurons to neurotoxic insult (Frey et al., 1996; Kazumata et al., 1998; Madras et al., 1998; Miller, Gainetdinov, Levey, & Caron, 1999; Uhl, 1998). Toxins gain rapid access to the presynaptic terminal through DAT and are removed from the cytosol by VMAT2 at a slower rate. Thus, toxins have increased access to vital intracellular organelles in individuals with a high DAT to VMAT2 expression ratio. Taken together, results from VMAT2 heterozygous mouse studies and from clinical studies suggest that inhibition of VMAT2 may attenuate the behavioral effects of METH. Further, a criterion for VMAT2 inhibitors developed as therapeutics to treat METH abuse is selectivity at VMAT2 relative to DAT in order to minimize abuse liability of the therapeutic.

7. CONCLUSION

7.1. Lobeline

This review focuses on the discovery of novel compounds that interact with VMAT2 and inhibit the pharmacological effect of METH. Lobeline, the major lipophilic, nonpyridino alkaloidal constituent of *Lobelia inflata* (also known as Indian tobacco), inhibits DA uptake by VMAT2 (Teng, Crooks, & Dwoskin, 1998; Teng, Crooks, Sonsalla, & Dwoskin, 1997). Lobeline also has high affinity for the [^{3}H]DTBZ binding site on VMAT2 protein (Fig. 2.2; Kilbourn, Lee, Vander Borght, Jewett, & Frey, 1995; Miller et al., 2004). Importantly, lobeline decreases amphetamine-evoked DA release from superfused rat striatal slices, but did not inhibit field stimulation-evoked DA release, indicating a selective inhibition of the effect of amphetamine (Miller et al., 2001).

Lobeline also decreases METH-induced hyperactivity, behavioral sensitization, and self-administration in rats (Harrod, Dwoskin, Crooks,

Klebaur, & Bardo, 2001; Miller, Green, et al., 2000; Miller et al., 2001). The development of locomotor sensitization has been suggested to result from neuroadaptations in response to repeated METH administration and may play a role in the development of dependence (Kalivas & Stewart, 1991; Vezina, 1996). In Miller, Green, et al. (2000), adult male rats were pretreated with lobeline (3 mg/kg) 10 min prior to METH (1 mg/kg) for 10 consecutive days. Lobeline significantly reduced locomotor activity in response to METH relative to saline-pretreated rats on each day. Thus, lobeline attenuates the induction of METH behavioral sensitization, leading to the prediction that lobeline may attenuate METH dependence. Lobeline decreased responding for food reinforcers; however, tolerance developed to this effect of lobeline (Harrod et al., 2001). Moreover, the lobeline-induced decrease in responding for METH persisted, revealing specificity upon repeated administration. Furthermore, this effect of lobeline was not surmountable upon increasing the unit dose of METH. Importantly, lobeline is not self-administered and does not produce CPP (Harrod, Dwoskin, Green, Gehrke, & Bardo, 2003). Lobeline did not substitute for METH and did not reinstate responding for METH following extinction, suggesting that the alkaloid does not act as a substitute reinforcer and that it lacks abuse liability (Harrod et al., 2001, 2003). Based on these preclinical findings, lobeline has been evaluated as a treatment for METH abuse and has completed phase 1b clinical trials, which determined that lobeline was safe in METH addicts (http://www.clinicaltrials.gov/ct2/show/NCT00439504?term=NCT00439504&rank=1).

The interaction of lobeline with VMAT2 was hypothesized to be the mechanism underlying the ability of lobeline to decrease the neurochemical and behavioral effects of METH (Dwoskin & Crooks, 2002; Miller et al., 2001; Teng et al., 1997). Lobeline, in a manner comparable to METH, inhibits the transport of cytosolic DA into synaptic vesicles via potent inhibition of VMAT2 function; however, lobeline does not inhibit MAO. Moreover, lobeline is more potent in inhibiting DA uptake at VMAT2 than it is in releasing DA from the vesicles, whereas amphetamine is more potent in releasing DA from the vesicles than it is in inhibiting DA uptake into the vesicles. Importantly, lobeline reduces METH-evoked DA release *in vitro* while concurrently increasing extracellular dihydroxyphenylacetic acid (DOPAC) concentrations (Miller et al., 2001; Wilhelm, Johnson, Eshleman, & Janowsky, 2008). Collectively, these results suggest that the decreased reinforcing effects of METH are the result of lobeline decreasing the cytosolic pool of DA available for METH-induced reverse transport by

DAT (Dwoskin & Crooks, 2002). However, lobeline is not selective for VMAT2, acting as an inhibitor of DAT and the serotonin transporter (SERT; Miller et al., 2004) and as a potent inhibitor of [^{3}H]nicotine (NIC) and [^{3}H]methyllycaconitine (MLA) binding to rat brain membranes. Additionally, lobeline decreases NIC-evoked ^{86}Rb$^+$ efflux from rat thalamic synaptosomes, suggesting that it acts as an alpha4beta2* and alpha7* nicotinic acetylcholine receptor (nAChR) antagonist (Damaj, Patrick, Creasy, & Martin, 1997; Flammia, Dukat, Damaj, Martin, & Glennon, 1999; Miller, Crooks, & Dwoskin, 2000; Miller et al., 2004).

7.2. *meso*-Transdiene

To enhance selectivity, a number of analogs similar in structure to lobeline were synthesized and evaluated for selectivity for VMAT2 and affinity for the DA uptake site on VMAT2. Lobeline consists of a central piperidine ring with phenyl rings attached at C-2 and C-6 of the piperidine ring by ethylene linkers containing hydroxyl and keto functionalities at the C8 and C10 positions on the linkers, respectively (Fig. 2.1). Both affinity at and selectivity for VMAT2 were improved as a result of alterations in structure, with the emergence of two new lead compounds, N-methyl-2,6-bis(*cis*-phenylethenyl) piperidine (*meso*-transdiene, MTD; Fig. 2.1) and N-methyl-2,6-bis(*cis*-phenylethyl)piperidine (lobelane; Fig. 2.1; Miller et al., 2004; Nickell et al., 2010; Zheng, Dwoskin, Deaciuc, Norrholm, & Crooks, 2005). MTD is a lobeline analog with defunctionalized and unsaturated (double bonds) linker units. Compared with lobeline, MTD exhibited similar affinity for the [^{3}H]DTBZ binding site on VMAT2 and dramatically decreased affinity for alpha4beta2* and alpha7* nAChRs, thus revealing increased selectivity for VMAT2 (Miller et al., 2004; Zheng, Dwoskin, Deaciuc, Norrholm, et al., 2005). Importantly, MTD inhibited METH-evoked DA release from superfused rat striatal slices (Nickell et al., 2010). Furthermore, MTD specifically decreased METH self-administration in rats, but only at the highest dose (17 mg/kg) evaluated (Horton, Siripurapu, Norrholm, et al., 2011). However, MTD exhibited a 100-fold higher affinity for DAT and a 6.5-fold lower affinity for SERT, compared with lobeline (Miller et al., 2004). The affinity of MTD at DAT was similar to that for cocaine and methylphenidate ($K_i = 300$ and 100 nM, respectively; Han & Gu, 2006), suggesting the potential for abuse liability. Due to the observation that MTD inhibited DAT more potently than VMAT2, suggesting the potential for abuse liability, and given that MTD had limited solubility, its potential was diminished for development as a pharmacotherapy for METH abuse. As such, mechanistic studies evaluating the effect of MTD on depolarization-stimulated DA release were not pursued and other more promising analogs were evaluated.

Nevertheless, taking into account these encouraging findings, but tempered by the limitations associated with the potential for abuse liability, modifications to the MTD molecule were evaluated in the search for preclinical candidates for the treatment of METH abuse (Horton, Siripurapu, Norrholm, et al., 2011). Structural modifications of MTD were made, including lengthening the linkers and either introducing substituents (4-methoxy, 4-methyl, or 2,4-dichloro) into the phenyl rings or replacing the phenyl rings with furan or thiophene rings. The effects of altering the geometry of the C5 double bond of the piperidine ring were evaluated in analogs with longer linkers or an aromatic 2,4-dicholor-substituted phenyl ring. In this series of analogs, affinity for VMAT2 was retained and affinity for DAT was reduced by 50- to 1000-fold, importantly increasing selectivity for VMAT2 over DAT, compared with MTD. UKMH-105 and UKMH-106, 2,4-dicholorophenyl analogs (Fig. 2.1), exhibiting 20- to 30-fold higher potency at VMAT2 over DAT, were evaluated for inhibition of METH-evoked DA release. Interestingly, the effect of METH was inhibited by UKMH-106, but not by UKMH-105, revealing an important geometric specificity of inhibition and suggesting that these isomers may interact with different sites on VMAT2 to inhibit DA uptake and METH-evoked DA release (Horton, Siripurapu, Norrholm, et al., 2011). Although UKMH-106 and UKMH-105 exhibit no differences in selectivity for the substrate uptake site on VMAT2, differences in affinity for the DTBZ binding site on VMAT2 have been noted. Thus, incorporation of the phenylethylene moiety of MTD into the piperidine ring and the addition of the dichloro groups resulted in a novel compound, UKMH-106, which had improved water solubility, reduced affinity for DAT and nAChRs, increased selectivity for VMAT2, and, importantly, inhibited the effect of METH to increase the extracellular concentration of DA.

7.3. Lobelane

Defunctionalization of lobeline afforded lobelane, with the hydroxyl and keto groups of lobeline eliminated from the saturated linkers. Lobelane is also a minor alkaloid of *L. inflata*. Preclinical evaluation of lobelane, as well as analogs based on the lobelane structural scaffold, revealed that this structural modification was sufficient to eliminate affinity for nAChRs, to provide a 10-fold increase in affinity for the DA uptake site on VMAT2 and a two-fold enhancement in the affinity for the DTBZ binding site on VMAT2, compared with lobeline (Beckmann et al., 2010; Nickell et al., 2010; Zheng, Dwoskin, Deaciuc, Zhu, et al., 2005). Kinetic analysis revealed that lobelane inhibited DA uptake at VMAT2 via a competitive mechanism. Furthermore, lobelane exhibited 35-fold greater potency for VMAT2 than for DAT (i.e., reduced affinity for DAT). Moreover, lobelane potently and nearly completely inhibited METH-evoked DA release from superfused rat striatal slices (Nickell et al., 2010). Taking into account these *in vitro* results, considerable enthusiasm was generated for the potential for lobelane as a lead compound.

Preclinical assessment of the ability of lobelane to decrease the behavioral effects of METH revealed that lobelane dose-dependently decreased METH self-administration while having no effect on sucrose-maintained responding (Neugebauer et al., 2007). However, lobelane appeared to have a shorter duration of action than lobeline in the self-administration assay. Furthermore, only the highest dose (10 mg/kg) of lobelane decreased locomotor activity. Unfortunately, tolerance developed to the effect of lobelane to decrease METH self-administration, revealing a transient effect of this alkaloid across seven consecutive sessions. The development of tolerance with repeated lobelane administration was in contrast with results obtained with lobeline using similar behavioral procedures. Lobelane appears to be a better substrate for hepatic metabolic oxidation compared to lobeline, which is consistent with the shorter duration of action of lobelane and metabolic issues being a factor in the development of tolerance to the effects of lobelane. Furthermore, lobelane exhibited decreased water solubility and as such reduced drug-likeness due to its decreased polarity as a result of the elimination of the keto and hydroxyl functionalities in lobeline.

Further structural modification of lobelane revealed that the most potent ($K_i = 13-16$ nM) and selective analogs included *para*-methoxyphenyl *nor*-lobelane, *para*-methoxyphenyl lobelane, and 2,4-dichlorphentyl lobelane (Nickell, Zheng, Deaciuc, Crooks, & Dwoskin, 2011; Zheng, Dwoskin, Deaciuc, Zhu, et al., 2005). Kinetic analyses revealed a competitive mechanism of inhibition of VMAT2 function. Also, these analogs had >100-fold higher affinity for VMAT2 than DAT, predicting low abuse liability.

7.4. GZ-793A

To improve water solubility and enhance drug-likeness properties of the lobelane scaffold, the *N*-methyl moiety of the central piperidine ring of lobelane was replaced with a chiral N-1,2-dihydroxypropyl (N-1,2-diol) moiety, which was predicted to enhance water solubility based on computational modeling. As such, a new series of lobelane analogs was synthesized by incorporating the chiral N-1,2-diol, altering the configuration of this moiety, and incorporating phenyl ring substituents (2-methoxy, 3-methoxy, 4-methoxy, 3-flouro, 2,4-flouro, and 3,4-methylenedioxy) into both phenyl rings or replacing the phenyl rings with naphthalene or biphenyl rings. Emerging from the *in vitro* pharmacological evaluation of this series of analogs was (R)-3-[2,6-*cis*-di(4-methoxyphenethyl)piperidin-1-yl]propane-1,2-diol (GZ-793A; Fig. 2.1), a potent, VMAT2-selective, drug-like lead (Horton, Siripurapu, Zheng, Crooks, & Dwoskin, 2011). GZ-793A was a potent competitive inhibitor of DA uptake at VMAT2, exhibiting a K_i value of 29 nM and an I_{max} of 86%. Thus, the pharmacophore for inhibiting VMAT2 function accommodates the N-1,2-diol moiety, which not only improved water solubility and drug-likeness but also enhanced the pharmacological characteristics of the molecule. For example, GZ-793A was 50-fold selective for inhibiting VMAT2 function over DAT or SERT, suggesting that GZ-793A would have low abuse liability at relevant doses. Importantly, GZ-793A inhibited METH-evoked DA release from superfused striatal slices (Horton, Siripurapu, Zheng, et al., 2011), and GZ-793A reduced the duration of the METH-induced increase in extracellular DA in nucleus accumbens in microdialysis studies (Meyer et al., 2013). Taking a more molecular approach, GZ-793A was found recently to inhibit METH-evoked DA release from isolated striatal synaptic vesicles via a surmountable allosteric inhibition and to interact with VMAT2 at several distinct sites on the protein, both extravesicular and intravesicular (Horton, Nickell, Zheng, Crooks, & Dwoskin, 2013). These results from the neurochemical assays support VMAT2 as an important pharmacological target and GZ-793A as a lead compound for reducing the neurochemical effects of METH.

Moreover, GZ-793A, administered peripherally across a reasonable dose range (3–30 mg/kg), decreased METH self-administration in rats, without altering responding for food reinforcers (Beckmann et al., 2012). Similar doses of GZ-793A blocked METH CPP, and GZ-793A itself did not induce place preference. Importantly, tolerance did not develop to the GZ-793A-induced decrease in responding for METH in the self-administration assay (Beckmann et al., 2012). Furthermore, the results of this study showed that increasing the unit dose of self-administered METH did not surmount the GZ-793A-induced decrease in responding for METH. GZ-793A was evaluated also for its ability to attenuate cue- and

METH-induced reinstatement of METH-seeking after a period of extinction (Alvers et al., 2012). GZ-793A (15 mg/kg) was found to decrease reinstatement following exposure to conditioned cue or METH administration. GZ-793A did not produce response suppressive effects in the absence of the conditioned cue stimuli; however, this lead compound did produce response suppressive effects in the METH reinstatement experiments. Thus, GZ-793A specifically blocks the primary and conditioned rewarding effects of METH and also decreases reinstatement of METH-seeking following presentation of conditioned cues and is predicted to have low abuse liability. In a subsequent investigation, oral dosing of GZ-793A (240 mg/kg) was shown to attenuate METH self-administration 85% relative to the control baseline responding rate while producing no alteration in responding for food (Wilmouth, Zheng, Crooks, Dwoskin, & Bardo, 2013). Thus, GZ-793A is orally bioavailable. Together, these results support the hypothesis that analogs that exhibit potent and selective inhibition of VMAT2 function translate to the requisite behavioral profile in preclinical studies, supporting their clinical evaluation as a pharmacotherapies for METH abuse.

7.5. 2,5-Disubstituted pyrrolidine analogs

To further generate the pharmacophore, a recent approach with respect to structural modification of the lobelane molecule was the introduction of a smaller, more conformationally constrained pyrrolidine ring in place of the central piperidine ring in the lobelane scaffold, which afforded a novel series of 2,5-disubstituted pyrrolidine analogs. Changes in the chemical structure also incorporated various linker lengths of the phenylethyl side chain and the addition of various substituents to the phenyl rings (Fig. 2.3). The pyrrolidine analogs were synthesized in the Department of Pharmaceutical Sciences in the College of Pharmacy at the University of Kentucky. The chemical structures were verified by ^{1}H and ^{13}C NMR spectroscopy, mass spectrometry, and X-ray crystallography.

These 2,5-disubstituted pyrrolidine analogs were evaluated first for inhibition of [^{3}H]DTBZ binding to VMAT2 using modifications of a previously published method (Teng et al., 1998). Briefly, vesicular suspension (15 μg protein/100 μl) from whole rat brain was added to each well of a 96-well plate, containing 5 nM [^{3}H]DTBZ, 50 μl of analog (1 nM–1 mM), and 50 μl of assay buffer. Samples were incubated at room temperature for 30 min. Nonspecific binding was determined in the presence of (2R,3S,11bS)-2-ethyl-3-isobutyl-9,10-dimethoxy-2,2,4,6,7,11b-hexahydro-1H-pyrido[2,1a]

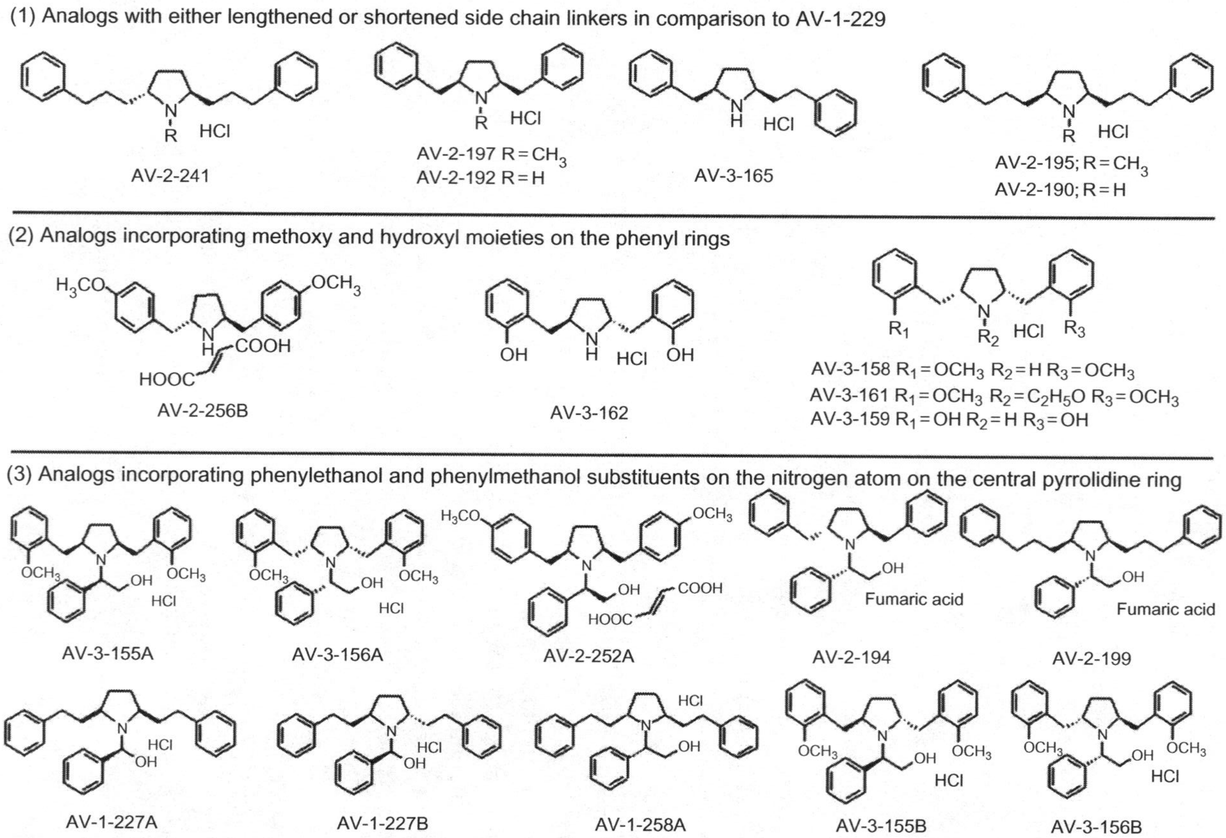

Figure 2.3 *Chemical structures of the novel 2,5-disubstituted pyrrolidine analogs.* Analogs are grouped according to structural similarity: Group 1: analogs with either lengthened or shortened side chain linkers in comparison with AV-1-229; Group 2: analogs incorporating methoxy and hydroxyl moieties on the phenyl rings; and Group 3: analogs incorporating phenylethanol and phenylmethanol substituents on the nitrogen atom on the central pyrrolidine ring.

isoquinolin-2-ol (Ro4-1284; 10 µM). Following incubation, plates were filtered, filters washed with 350 µl of ice-cold buffer (25 mM HEPES, 100 mM potassium tartrate, 5 mM MgSO$_4$, and 10 mM NaCl, pH 7.5), dried, sealed, and 40 µl of scintillation cocktail added to each well, and radioactivity determined by liquid scintillation spectrometry.

All of the pyrrolidine analogs inhibited [^{3}H]DTBZ binding (Table 2.1), although only AV-2-190 ($K_i = 0.27$ µM) exhibited greater affinity for VMAT2 than lobelane ($K_i = 0.97$ µM). Thus, AV-2-190, a *nor*-analog incorporating an additional methylene in each of its methylene linker units, exhibited the highest affinity at the DTBZ binding site in this series of analogs. The majority of analogs inhibited [^{3}H]DTBZ binding at concentrations of 1–10 µM, although several exceptions with low affinity were noted, including AV-3-156B ($K_i = 96.6$ µM), AV-3-158 ($K_i = 74.7$ µM), AV-3-159 ($K_i = 89.9$ µM), and AV-3-162 ($K_i = 82.6$ µM). Low-affinity analogs had methoxy groups in the *ortho*-position on the phenyl rings. Interestingly, analogs bearing methoxy groups in the *para*-position on the phenyl rings, including AV-1-252B and AV-2-256B, exhibited relatively high affinity ($K_i = 1.23$ and 1.39 µM, respectively) for the DTBZ binding site on VMAT2. Generally, *nor*-pyrrolidine analogs inhibited [^{3}H]DTBZ binding with higher affinity than their respective pyrrolidine *N*-methylated analogs.

The ability of the pyrrolidine analogs to inhibit vesicular [^{3}H]DA uptake was determined using our reported method employing synaptic vesicle preparations (Teng et al., 1997). Briefly, rat striatal vesicular suspension (100 µl) was added to assay tubes containing buffer, various concentrations of analog (0.1 nM–10 mM), and 0.1 µM [^{3}H]DA in a final volume of 500 µl. Samples were incubated at 37 °C for 8 min and filtered, and radioactivity remaining on the filter determined. Pyrrolidine analogs exhibited >90% inhibition of VMAT2 function (Table 2.1). Many of these analogs exhibited greater affinity for the DA uptake site on VMAT2 compared to lobelane ($K_i = 0.045$ µM). The *nor*-pyrrolidine analog AV-2-192, with a reduced number of methylene linker units having *cis* geometry, had an affinity of <10 nM. The *nor*-pyrrolidine analog AV-1-228 (Fig. 2.1; also known as UKCP-110) with the greatest structural resemblance to lobelane also inhibited VMAT2 function with high affinity ($K_i = 28$ nM). AV-2-252A and AV-2-252B, incorporating methoxy moieties in the *para*-position on the phenyl rings, exhibited high affinity ($K_i = 5.3$ and 50 nM, respectively) for the DA uptake site on VMAT2. In all cases, the *nor*-pyrrolidine analogs exhibited higher affinity for the DA uptake site than the respective pyrrolidine *N*-methylated analogs.

Table 2.1 K_i and I_{max} values for 2,5-disubstituted lobelane analog inhibition of [^{3}H]DTBZ binding and [^{3}H]DA uptake at VMAT2

Compound	[^{3}H]DTBZ binding K_i (μM)	I_{max} (%)	VMAT2 [^{3}H]DA uptake K_i (μM)	I_{max} (%)
Standards				
TBZ	0.013 ± 0.001^a	100	0.054 ± 0.015	92 ± 3
Lobelane	0.97 ± 0.19	90 ± 3	0.045 ± 0.002	100
AV-1-229A	8.80 ± 2.30	97 ± 2	0.27 ± 0.035	100
AV-1-228	2.66 ± 0.37	100	0.028 ± 0.0010	100
Group 1				
AV-2-192	1.64 ± 0.12	100	0.0093 ± 0.00075	100
AV-2-197	2.46 ± 0.42	96 ± 1	0.019 ± 0.00091	100
AV-2-190	0.27 ± 0.0067	100	0.014 ± 0.0011	100
AV-2-195	2.78 ± 0.63	100	0.12 ± 0.011	100
AV-3-165	5.18 ± 0.47	100	0.042 ± 0.0035	100
AV-2-241	11.2 ± 1.17	97 ± 2	0.21 ± 0.019	98 ± 1
Group 2				
AV-2-256B	1.39 ± 0.062	100	0.16 ± 0.0071	100
AV-3-161	25.6 ± 7.31	64 ± 1	2.23 ± 0.29	100
AV-3-158	74.7 ± 14.4	47 ± 2	3.38 ± 0.27	100
AV-3-159	89.9 ± 5.14	50 ± 2	2.39 ± 0.53	100
AV-3-162	82.6 ± 11.9	57 ± 6	1.78 ± 0.47	100
Group 3				
AV-3-155A	1.49 ± 0.77	58 ± 1	0.38 ± 0.066	99 ± 1
AV-3-156A	7.55 ± 1.45	60 ± 2	0.69 ± 0.19	100
AV-3-156B	96.6 ± 21.9	56 ± 2	2.42 ± 0.20	98 ± 1
AV-3-155B	3.94 ± 2.29	55 ± 2	0.43 ± 0.052	100
AV-2-252A	1.06 ± 0.047	100	0.0053 ± 0.00045	100
AV-2-199	2.23 ± 0.58	85 ± 2	0.40 ± 0.087	99 ± 1
AV-2-194	1.84 ± 0.35	91 ± 1	0.51 ± 0.024	100
AV-1-227A	4.34 ± 0.71	85 ± 2	1.29 ± 0.24	100
AV-1-227B	5.05 ± 1.05	97 ± 2	1.94 ± 0.47	99 ± 1
AV-1-258A	2.75 ± 0.63	74 ± 8	0.14 ± 0.049	97 ± 3

[a]Data represent mean $\pm$ SEM; $n =$ three to four rats per compound.

In an effort to further generate the pharmacophore via a thorough analysis of structure–activity relationship on this series of compounds, analogs were divided into three groups (Fig. 2.3; Table 2.1) based upon similarities in chemical structure. The pyrrolidine analog most structurally similar to lobelane was AV-1-229A (Fig. 2.1), with one less methylene group in the central heterocyclic ring. AV-1-229A exhibited a K_i of 270 nM at the DA uptake site on VMAT2, which had six-fold lower affinity compared with lobelane. The N-methylated analog AV-2-195, with an increased number of methylene linker units (Fig. 2.3, Group 1), exhibited a two-fold higher affinity for the DA uptake site on VMAT2, relative to AV-1-229A. Interestingly, the N-methylated analog AV-2-197, with only one methylene linker unit, exhibited 14 orders-of-magnitude increased affinity for the DA uptake site on VMAT2 compared with AV-1-229A. Demethylation of the central pyrrolidine N-atom to afford *nor*-pyrrolidines AV-2-192 and AV-2-190 resulted in increased affinity at both the DTBZ binding and DA uptake sites on VMAT2. The greatest impact of N-demethylation occurred with analogs incorporating three methylene linker units, for example, AV-2-190, which exhibited an order-of-magnitude higher affinity than AV-2-195. Thus, the loss of one methylene moiety from each linker unit in AV-1-229A produced the greatest increase in affinity for the DA uptake site.

Pyrrolidine analogs incorporating either a methoxy or hydroxyl moiety at various positions of the phenyl rings (Fig. 2.3, Group 2) had reduced affinity at both the [^{3}H]DTBZ binding and DA uptake sites on VMAT2 in comparison with AV-1-229A. Furthermore, a final group of pyrrolidine analogs consisting of various structural modifications was evaluated. These analogs (Fig. 2.3, Group 3) had altered linker lengths, methoxy substituents in the phenyl rings or N-phenethanol or N-phenmethanol groups in place of the N-methyl of AV-1-229A. Generally, these analogs had reduced affinity at both uptake and binding sites compared to AV-1-229A.

Most analogs exhibited affinities for the DA uptake site at least 10-fold higher than their respective affinities for the [^{3}H]DTBZ binding site on VMAT2, and a positive correlation between uptake and binding affinity was found (Spearman $r = 0.72$; $p < 0.001$; Fig. 2.4). These results are in contrast with previous results evaluating this relationship for a different series of lobelane analogs with phenyl ring substituents (Nickell et al., 2011). At least for the pyrrolidine analog series, the high-throughput binding assay serves as a predictive screen for inhibition of DA uptake by VMAT2. While a positive correlation was found, affinity for the majority of analogs at the DTBZ binding site was within a relatively restricted range of 1–10 μM, whereas a greater

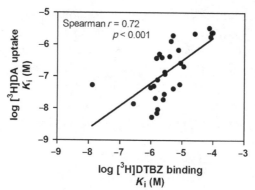

Figure 2.4 *Positive correlation between 2,5-disubstituted pyrrolidine analog affinity for the DTBZ binding site and the DA uptake site.* Data are K_i values obtained from concentration–response curves for analog-induced inhibition of [^{3}H]DTBZ binding and [^{3}H]DA uptake (data not shown). Spearman analysis revealed a positive correlation (Spearman $r = 0.72$; $p < 0.001$) between pyrrolidine analog affinity for the DTBZ binding site and the DA uptake site on VMAT2.

range of 0.005–0.7 µM was obtained for affinity at the DA uptake site. Thus, structural modification did not alter interactions with the binding site to as great a degree as interactions with the DA uptake site.

Furthermore, the current results support previous findings of alternative recognition sites on VMAT2, including a ketanserine binding site near the N-terminal of the VMAT2 protein and a TBZ site located near the C-terminus of the VMAT2 protein (Sievert & Ruoho, 1997; Weaver & Deupree, 1982). Interestingly, studies investigating interactions of novel compounds at VMAT2 and DAT reveal that compounds exhibiting large differences in affinity between binding and uptake sites act as transporter substrates, while compounds equipotent inhibiting binding and uptake act purely as uptake inhibitors (Andersen, 1987; Matecka et al., 1997; Partilla et al., 2006; Rothman, Ayestas, Dersch, & Baumann, 1999). If allowed to extrapolate from these previous studies, all of the pyrrolidine analogs evaluated herein, with the exception of AV-1-227A and AV-1-227B, would be predicted to act as substrates for VMAT2 and to inhibit DA uptake in a competitive manner.

To determine the mechanism of inhibition of [^{3}H]DA uptake (i.e., competitive vs. noncompetitive) for the lead pyrrolidine analogs, kinetic analyses were performed. The methylated pyrrolidine AV-2-192 and its *nor*-counterpart AV-2-197 (Fig. 2.3, Group 1) were selected for evaluation of mechanism of inhibition of DA uptake at VMAT2, as both compounds displayed high affinity for the DA uptake site and moderate affinity for the [^{3}H]DTBZ binding site. Concentrations of these lead compounds, AV-2-192 and AV-2-197 (9.3 and 19 nM, respectively), were chosen based on K_i values obtained from the [^{3}H]DA uptake assays. Incubations were initiated by the addition of 50 µl of vesicular suspension to 150 µl assay buffer, 25 µl of inhibitor or assay buffer (control), and 25 µl of a range of concentrations of [^{3}H]DA (0.001–5.0 µM). Nonspecific uptake was determined in the presence of Ro4-1284 (10 µM). Following an 8 min incubation, [^{3}H]DA uptake was terminated by filtration, and radioactivity retained by the filters determined as previously described. Both AV-2-192 and AV-2-197 increased ($p < 0.05$) the K_m value relative to control, without altering V_{max} (Fig. 2.5; Table 2.2), indicating that the analogs competitively inhibit [^{3}H]DA uptake by VMAT2, in agreement with the earlier-mentioned prediction and indicating that methylation of the pyrrolidine N-atom was not an important factor in the interaction of these analogs with VMAT2.

The ability of the leads, AV-2-192 and AV-2-197, to inhibit [^{3}H]DA uptake at DAT in synaptosomal preparations was determined according to previous methods (Teng et al., 1997). Synaptosomal suspension (25 µl) was added to assay tubes containing assay buffer and various concentrations

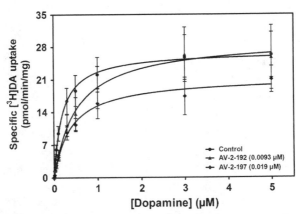

Figure 2.5 *Kinetic analysis of the inhibition of [^{3}H]DA uptake at VMAT2 by AV-2-192 and AV-2-197.* The *nor*-pyrrolidine analog (AV-2-192) containing single methylene unit side chain linkers in the *cis* conformation and its *N*-methyl counterpart (AV-2-197) were evaluated to determine mechanism of inhibition of [^{3}H]DA uptake. Concentrations of analog utilized (in parentheses) for the kinetic analysis were the respective K_i concentrations from the inhibition curves (data not shown). V_{max} and K_m values (±SEM) are provided in Table 2.2 ($n = 4$–6 rats/analog).

Table 2.2 K_m and V_{max} values for AV-2-192 and AV-2-197 from kinetic analysis of [³H]DA uptake at VMAT2

Compound[a]	K_m (µM)	V_{max} (pmol/min/mg)
Control[b]	0.19 ± 0.021[c]	29.9 ± 4.30
AV-2-192	0.51 ± 0.025[d]	29.6 ± 7.28
AV-2-197	0.43 ± 0.13[d]	22.0 ± 4.36

[a]Concentrations of analogs utilized for kinetic analyses were the K_i concentrations from the inhibition curves (AV-2-192, 0.0093 µM; AV-2-197, 0.019 µM).
[b]Control represents the absence of analog.
[c]Data are mean ± SEM for K_m and V_{max} values.
[d]$p < 0.05$ different from control, two-tailed t test ($n = 4$–6 rats/analog).

of analog (100 µM–1 nM) and incubated at 34 °C for 5 min. Nonspecific uptake was determined in the presence of nomifensine (10 µM). Samples were placed on ice, and 50 µl of 0.1 µM [³H]DA was added, and then, incubation proceeded for 10 min at 34 °C. Samples were filtered and radioactivity retained by the filters determined. No difference was found between AV-2-192 and AV-2-197 affinities for DAT ($K_i = 2.63 \pm 0.35$ and 5.40 ± 0.53 µM, respectively). Both analogs were 1- to 2-orders-of-magnitude more potent inhibiting DA uptake at VMAT2 relative to inhibiting DA uptake at DAT; thus, these leads are not likely to possess abuse liability.

The ability of AV-2-192 and AV-2-197 to inhibit METH-evoked DA release from striatal slices was determined as previously reported (Teng et al., 1997). Coronal striatal slices were incubated in Krebs buffer at 34 °C in a metabolic shaker for 60 min. Slices were superfused (1 ml/min) for 60 min with Krebs buffer. Then, two 5 min basal samples (1 ml into 100 µl of 0.1 M perchloric acid) were collected. Superfusion continued for 30 min in the absence or presence of a single concentration (0.3–30 µM) of AV-2-192 or AV-2-197. Then, METH (5 µM) was added to the buffer and superfusion continued for 15 min. Slices were superfused for another 20 min with analog in the absence of METH. In each experiment, a striatal slice was superfused for 90 min in the absence of analog or METH, serving as the buffer control. Duplicate slices were superfused with METH in the absence of analog, serving as the METH control. Samples (500 µl) were processed immediately by adding 20 µl of ascorbate oxidase (81 U/1 ml), vortexing for 30 s, followed by injection of 100 µl onto the HPLC with electrochemical detection (Table 2.3).

Analysis of the effect of AV-2-192 and AV-2-197 on fractional DOPAC release during the 30 min period prior to addition of METH to the

Table 2.3 Summary of data for lead compounds: Affinity for nAChRs, DTBZ site on VMAT2 affinity, substrate site on VMAT2 and DAT, mechanism of VMAT2 inhibition, potency for inhibition of METH-evoked DA release, and inhibition of the behavioral effects of METH

Compound	nAChR K_i value (μM)	DTBZ site K_i value (μM)	VMAT2 substrate site K_i value (μM)	Mechanism of VMAT2 inhibition	DAT K_i value (μM)	IC_{50} and I_{max} values for analog inhibition of METH-evoked DA release (μM)	Inhibition of METH behavioral effects
Lobeline	[^{3}H] NIC $= 0.016$ [^{3}H] MLA $= 11.6$	2.04	0.47	Competitive	31.6	$IC_{50} = 0.42$ $I_{max} = 56\%$	Hyperactivity Self-administration CPP Discrimination Reinstatement
Lobelane	[^{3}H] NIC $= 77.3$ [^{3}H] MLA $= 43.1$	0.97	0.045	Competitive	1.57	$IC_{50} = 0.65$ $I_{max} = 73\%$	Hyperactivity Self-administration
MTD	[^{3}H] NIC $= >100$ [^{3}H] MLA $= >100$	9.88	0.46	Competitive	0.039	$IC_{50} = 0.44$ $I_{max} = 76\%$	Self-administration
UKMH-105	[^{3}H] NIC $= >100$ [^{3}H] MLA $= >100$	4.60	0.22	Competitive	6.27	No inhibition	Not evaluated

Continued

Table 2.3 Summary of data for lead compounds: Affinity for nAChRs, DTBZ site on VMAT2 affinity, substrate site on VMAT2 and DAT, mechanism of VMAT2 inhibition, potency for inhibition of METH-evoked DA release, and inhibition of the behavioral effects of METH—cont'd

Compound	nAChR K_i value (μM)	DTBZ site K_i value (μM)	VMAT2 substrate site K_i value (μM)	Mechanism of VMAT2 inhibition	DAT K_i value (μM)	IC_{50} and I_{max} values for analog inhibition of METH-evoked DA release (μM)	Inhibition of METH behavioral effects
UKMH-106	[³H]NIC = >100 [³H]MLA = >100	41.3	0.32	Competitive	6.90	$IC_{50} = 0.38$ $I_{max} = 50\%$	Not evaluated
GZ-793A	[³H]NIC = >100 [³H]MLA = >100	8.29	0.029	Competitive	1.44	$IC_{50} = 10.6$ $I_{max} = 85\%$	Self-administration CPP Reinstatement
AV-2-192	[³H]NIC = Not evaluated [³H]MLA = Not evaluated	1.64	0.0093	Competitive	2.63	$IC_{50} = 5.2$ $I_{max} = 55\%$	Not evaluated
AV-2-197	[³H]NIC = Not evaluated [³H]MLA = Not evaluated	2.46	0.019	Competitive	5.40	$IC_{50} = 4.2$ $I_{max} = 63\%$	Not evaluated

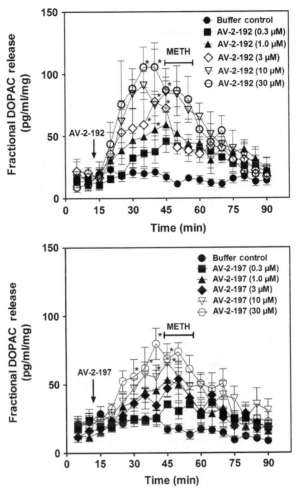

Figure 2.6 *AV-2-192 and AV-2-197 stimulate fractional DOPAC release from rat striatal slice preparations.* Top and bottom panels illustrate the time course for AV-2-192 and AV-2-197, respectively, to stimulate fractional DOPAC release. Each striatal slice was superfused with either a single concentration (0.3–30 μM) of AV-2-192 or AV-2-197 alone during the 30 min time period prior to the inclusion of 5 μM methamphetamine (METH) in the buffer. Arrow denotes time point at which analog was added to the buffer. METH was added to the buffer after 30 min and remained in the buffer for 15 min. Buffer control represents slices superfused in the absence of analog and METH. Data are mean (±SEM) pg/min/ml slice weight. $^{*}p < 0.05$ different from buffer control condition.

superfusion buffer revealed a concentration–dependent increase in DOPAC (Fig. 2.6). The increase in extracellular DOPAC levels was observed consistent with findings using lobeline and lobelane (Nickell et al., 2010). The lowest concentration of AV-2-192 and AV-2-197 to increase

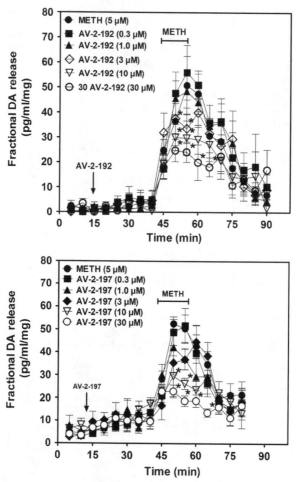

Figure 2.7 *Time course of AV-2-192 and AV-2-197 inhibition of methamphetamine (METH)-evoked fractional DA release.* Top and bottom panels illustrate the time course for AV-2-192 and AV-2-197, respectively, to inhibit METH-evoked fractional DA release. Each striatal slice was superfused with either a single concentration (0.3–30 μM) of AV-2-192 or AV-2-197 alone during the 30-min time period prior to the inclusion of 5 μM METH in the buffer. Arrow denotes time point at which analog was added to the buffer. METH was added to the buffer after 30 min and remained in the buffer for 15 min. METH control represents slices superfused with METH in the absence of analog. Data are mean (±SEM) pg/min/ml slice weight. *$p < 0.05$ different from the METH control condition.

extracellular DOPAC was 3 and 10 μM, respectively. Across the concentration range, addition of either AV-2-192 or AV-2-197 to the superfusion buffer (15–45 min) alone did not alter fractional DA release (Fig. 2.7), indicating that the lead compounds lacked intrinsic activity with respect to

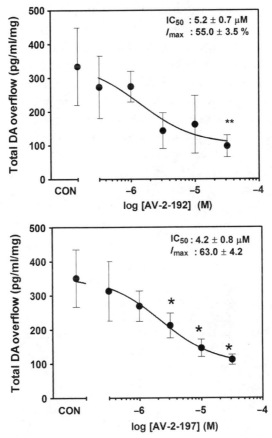

Figure 2.8 *AV-2-192 and AV-2-197 inhibit methamphetamine-evoked total DA overflow from rat striatal slices.* Data are total DA overflow following methamphetamine administration as a function of concentration of AV-2-192 (top panel) and AV-2-197 (bottom panel). CON denotes slice superfused with 5 μM methamphetamine in absence of analog. Data are mean (±SEM) pg/ml/mg slice weight. *$p < 0.05$ and **$p < 0.01$ different from the methamphetamine control condition.

releasing DA. METH (5 μM) increased fractional DA release compared to the buffer control condition. Both AV-2-192 and AV-2-197 attenuated METH-evoked DA release. When the data were expressed as total DA overflow (Fig. 2.8), the IC_{50} value for AV-2-192 to inhibit this effect of METH was 5.2 ± 0.7 μM and the I_{max} was $55.0 \pm 3.5\%$, and similarly, the IC_{50} value for AV-2-197 was 4.2 ± 0.8 μM and the I_{max} was $63.0 \pm 4.2\%$. Thus, AV-2-192 and AV-2-197 were equipotent but incompletely inhibited METH-evoked DA release.

The current results obtained with superfusion of striatal slices with AV-2-192 and AV-2-197 alone (Figs. 2.6 and 2.7) are consistent with our previous findings when employing the parent compounds lobeline and lobelane. This family of compounds inhibits DA uptake at VMAT2 and promotes DA release from the synaptic vesicles via an interaction with VMAT2, presumably increasing the cytosolic concentration of DA. The increase in cytosolic DA is then exposed to intracellular MAO, an avid enzyme that metabolizes the cytosolic DA to DOPAC, and the observed outcome is an increase in DOPAC, but not DA, in superfusate (the extracellular compartment). Thus, this family of compounds clearly does not inhibit MAO activity. The increased DOPAC concentrations in superfusate, in combination with the lack of change in DA concentration, are the result of MAO metabolizing the increased cyotosolic DA as a component of the analog effect. Furthermore, consistent with the interaction of these lead analogs at the DA uptake site on VMAT2, methylation of the pyrrolidine N-atom was not a factor in the inhibition of METH-evoked DA release from intact striatal slices.

The results presented herein show that 2,5-disubstituted pyrrolidine analogs constitute a promising series of analogs for further preclinical evaluation as potential pharmacotherapeutics for METH addiction. Specifically, the pyrrolidine analogs with a short linker length (AV-2-192 and AV-2-197) afforded modest affinity at the DTBZ binding site on VMAT2, high affinity at DA uptake site, and competitive inhibition at the DA uptake site on VMAT2; were not potent inhibitors of DAT function; and, moreover, inhibited the effect of METH to release DA from intact striatal slices. Future studies will determine the ability of these lead analogs in the 2,5-disubstituted pyrrolidine series to decrease reinforcement produced by METH in behavioral studies.

CONFLICT OF INTEREST

The University of Kentucky holds patents on the compounds described in the current work, some of which have been licensed by Yaupon Therapeutics/Ceptaris Inc. A potential royalty stream to LPD and PAC may occur consistent with the University of Kentucky policy. Both LPD and PAC are founders of, and have financial interest in, Yaupon Therapeutics/Ceptaris Inc.

ACKNOWLEDGMENTS

This research was supported by NIH grants U01 DA013519, UL1TR000117, and T32 DA016176.

REFERENCES

Alvers, K. M., Beckmann, J. S., Zheng, G., Crooks, P. A., Dwoskin, L. P., & Bardo, M. T. (2012). The effect of VMAT2 inhibitor GZ-793A on the reinstatement of methamphetamine-seeking in rats. *Psychopharmacology, 224*, 255–262.

Andersen, P. H. (1987). Biochemical and pharmacological characterization of [³H]GBR 12935 binding in vitro to rat striatal membranes: Labeling of the dopamine uptake complex. *Journal of Neurochemistry, 48*, 1887–1896.

Ary, T. E., & Komiskey, H. L. (1980). Phencyclidine: Effect on the accumulation of ³H-dopamine in synaptic vesicles. *Life Sciences, 26*, 575–578.

Barlow, R. B., & Johnson, O. (1989). Relations between structure and nicotine-like activity: X-ray crystal structure analysis of (−)-cytisine and (−)-lobeline hydrochloride and a comparison with (−)-nicotine and other nicotine-like compounds. *British Journal of Pharmacology, 98*, 799–808.

Beckmann, J. S., Denehy, E. D., Zheng, G., Crooks, P. A., Dwoskin, L. P., & Bardo, M. T. (2012). The effect of a novel VMAT2 inhibitor, GZ-793A, on methamphetamine reward in rats. *Psychopharmacology, 220*, 295–403.

Beckmann, J. S., Siripurapu, K. B., Nickell, J. R., Horton, D. B., Denehy, E. D., Vartak, A., et al. (2010). The novel pyrrolidine nor-lobelane analog UKCP-110 [cis-2,5-di-(2-phenethyl)-pyrrolidine hydrochloride] inhibits VMAT2 function, methamphetamine-evoked dopamine release, and methamphetamine self-administration in rats. *The Journal of Pharmacology and Experimental Therapeutics, 335*, 841–851.

Ben-Shachar, D., Zuk, R., & Glinka, Y. (1995). Dopamine neurotoxicity: Inhibition of mitochondrial respiration. *Journal of Neurochemistry, 64*, 718–723.

Brown, J. M., Hanson, G. R., & Fleckenstein, A. E. (2000). Methamphetamine rapidly decreases vesicular dopamine uptake. *Journal of Neurochemistry, 74*, 2221–2223.

Brown, J. M., Hanson, G. R., & Fleckenstein, A. E. (2001). Regulation of the vesicular monoamine transporter-2: A novel mechanism for cocaine and other psychostimulants. *The Journal of Pharmacology and Experimental Therapeutics, 296*, 762–767.

Carr, G. D., & White, N. M. (1983). Conditioned place preference from intra-accumbens but not intra-caudate amphetamine injections. *Life Sciences, 33*, 2551–2557.

Chaudhry, F. A., Edwards, R. H., & Fonnum, F. (2008). Vesicular neurotransmitter transporters as targets for endogenous and exogenous toxic substances. *Annual Review of Pharmacology and Toxicology, 48*, 277–301.

Damaj, M. I., Patrick, G. S., Creasy, K. R., & Martin, B. R. (1997). Pharmacology of lobeline, a nicotinic receptor ligand. *The Journal of Pharmacology and Experimental Therapeutics, 282*, 410–419.

Darchen, F., Scherman, D., & Henry, J. P. (1989). Reserpine binding to chromaffin granules suggests the existence of two conformations of the monoamine transporter. *Biochemistry, 28*, 1692–1697.

DASIS, Drug and Alcohol Services Information System (DASIS) (2008). The DASIS Report. Primary methamphetamine/amphetamine admissions to substance abuse treatment: 2005. http://www.oas.samhsa.gov/2k8/methamphetamineTx/meth.htm.

Di Chiara, G., Bassareo, V., Fenu, S., De Luca, M. A., Spina, L., Cadoni, C., et al. (2004). Dopamine and drug addiction: The nucleus accumbens shell connection. *Neuropharmacology, 47*, 227–241.

Dwoskin, L. P., & Crooks, P. A. (2002). A novel mechanism and potential use for lobeline as a treatment for psychostimulant abuse. *Biochemical Pharmacology, 63,* 89–98.

Eiden, L. E., & Weihe, E. (2011). VMAT2: A dynamic regulator of brain monoaminergic neuronal function interacting with drugs of abuse. *Annals of the New York Academy of Sciences, 1216,* 86–98.

Erickson, J. D., Eiden, L. E., & Hoffman, B. J. (1992). Expression cloning of a reserpine-sensitive vesicular monoamine transporter. *Proceedings of the National Academy of Sciences of the United States of America, 89,* 10993–10997.

Erickson, J. D., Schafer, M. K., Bonner, T. I., Eiden, L. E., & Weihe, E. (1996). Distinct pharmacological properties and distribution in neurons and endocrine cells of two isoforms of the human vesicular monoamine transporter. *Proceedings of the National Academy of Sciences of the United States of America, 93,* 5166–5171.

Finn, J. P., III, & Edwards, R. H. (1997). Individual residues contribute to multiple differences in ligand recognition between vesicular monoamine transporters 1 and 2. *The Journal of Biological Chemistry, 272,* 16301–16307.

Fischer, J. F., & Cho, A. K. (1979). Chemical release of dopamine from striatal homogenates: Evidence for an exchange diffusion model. *The Journal of Pharmacology and Experimental Therapeutics, 208,* 203–209.

Flammia, D., Dukat, M., Damaj, M. I., Martin, B., & Glennon, R. A. (1999). Lobeline: Structure-affinity investigation of nicotinic acetylcholinergic receptor binding. *Journal of Medicinal Chemistry, 42,* 3726–3731.

Fleckenstein, A. E., Volz, T. J., Riddle, E. L., Gibb, J. W., & Hanson, G. R. (2007). New insights into the mechanism of action of amphetamines. *Annual Review of Pharmacology and Toxicology, 47,* 681–698.

Fon, E. A., Pothos, E. N., Sun, B., Killeen, N., Sulzer, D., & Edwards, R. H. (1997). Vesicular transport regulates monoamine storage and release but is not essential for amphetamine action. *Neuron, 19,* 1271–1283.

Frey, K. A., Koeppe, R. A., Kilbourn, M. R., Vander Borght, T. M., Albin, R. L., Gilman, S., et al. (1996). Presynaptic monoaminergic vesicles in Parkinson's disease and normal aging. *Annals of Neurology, 40,* 873–884.

Frize, E. D. (1954). Mental depression in hypertensive patients treated for long periods with high doses of reserpine. *The New England Journal of Medicine, 251,* 1006–1008.

Glatt, C. E., DeYoung, J. A., Delgado, S., Service, S. K., Giacomini, K. M., Edwards, R. H., et al. (2001). Screening a large reference sample to identify very low frequency sequence variants: Comparison between two genes. *Nature Genetics, 27,* 435–438.

Glatt, C. E., Wahner, A. D., White, D. J., Ruiz-Linares, A., & Ritz, B. (2006). Gain-of-function haplotypes in the vesicular monoamine transporter promoter are protective for Parkinson disease in women. *Human Molecular Genetics, 15,* 299–305.

Han, D. D., & Gu, H. H. (2006). Comparison of the monoamine transporters from human and mouse in their sensitivities to psychostimulant drugs. *BMC Pharmacology, 6,* 6.

Hart, C. L., Ward, A. S., Haney, M., Foltin, R. W., & Fischman, M. W. (2001). Methamphetamine self-administration by humans. *Psychopharmacology, 157,* 75–81.

Harrod, S. B., Dwoskin, L. P., Crooks, P. A., Klebaur, J. E., & Bardo, M. T. (2001). Lobeline attenuates d-methamphetamine self-administration in rats. *The Journal of Pharmacology and Experimental Therapeutics, 298,* 172–179.

Harrod, S. B., Dwoskin, L. P., Green, T. A., Gehrke, B. J., & Bardo, M. T. (2003). Lobeline does not serve as a reinforcer in rats. *Psychopharmacology, 165,* 397–404.

Hastings, T. G., Lewis, D. A., & Zigmond, M. F. (1996). Reactive dopamine metabolites and neurotoxicity: Implications for Parkinson's disease. *Advances in Experimental Medicine and Biology, 387,* 97–106.

Henry, J. P., Gasnier, B., Roisin, M. P., Isamber, M. F., & Scherman, D. (1987). Molecular pharmacology of the monoamine transporter of the chromaffin granule membrane. *Annals of the New York Academy of Sciences, 493*, 194–206.

Hillarp, N. A. (1958). The release of catechol amines from the amine containing granules of the adrenal medulla. *Acta Physiologica Scandinavica, 43*, 292–302.

Hiroi, N., & White, N. M. (1991). The lateral nucleus of the amygdala mediates expression of the amphetamine produced conditioned place preference. *The Journal of Neuroscience, 11*, 2107–2116.

Hoebel, B. G., Monaco, A. P., Hernandez, L., Aulisi, E. F., Stanley, B. G., & Lenard, L. (1983). Self-injection of amphetamine directly into the brain. *Psychopharmacology, 81*, 158–163.

Hogan, K. A., Staal, R. G., & Sonsalla, P. K. (2000). Analysis of VMAT2 binding after methamphetamine or MPTP treatment: Disparity between homogenates and vesicle preparations. *Journal of Neurochemistry, 74*, 2217–2220.

Horton, D. B., Nickell, J. R., Zheng, G., Crooks, P. A., & Dwoskin, L. P. (2013). GZ-793A, a lobelane analog, interacts with the vesicular monoamine transporter-2 to inhibit the effect of methamphetamine. *Journal of Neurochemistry, 127*, 177–186.

Horton, D. B., Siripurapu, K. B., Norrholm, S. D., Culver, J. P., Hojahmat, M., Beckmann, J. S., et al. (2011). meso-Transdiene analogs inhibit vesicular monoamine transporter-2 function and methamphetamine-evoked dopamine release. *The Journal of Pharmacology and Experimental Therapeutics, 336*(3), 940–951.

Horton, D. B., Siripurapu, K. B., Zheng, G., Crooks, P. A., & Dwoskin, L. P. (2011). Novel N-1,2-dihydroxypropyl analogs of lobelane inhibit vesicular monoamine transporter-2 function and methamphetamine-evoked dopamine release. *The Journal of Pharmacology and Experimental Therapeutics, 339*, 286–297.

Johnson, R. G. (1988). Accumulation of biological amines into chromaffin granules: A model for hormone and neurotransmitter transport. *Physiological Reviews, 68*, 232–307.

Johnson, R. A., Eshleman, A. J., Meyers, T., Neve, K. A., & Janowsky, A. (1998). Substrate- and cell-specific effects of uptake inhibitors on human dopamine and serotonin transporter-mediated efflux. *Synapse, 30*, 97–106.

Kalivas, P. W., & Stewart, J. (1991). Dopamine transmission in the initiation and expression of drug- and stress-induced sensitization of motor activity. *Brain Research. Brain Research Reviews, 16*, 223–244.

Kanner, B. I., & Schuldiner, S. (1987). Mechanism of transport and storage of neurotransmitters. *CRC Critical Reviews in Biochemistry, 22*, 1–38.

Kazumata, K., Dhawan, V., Chaly, T., Antonini, A., Marqouleff, C., Belakhlef, A., et al. (1998). Dopamine transporter imaging with fluorine-18-FPCIT and PET. *Journal of Nuclear Medicine, 39*, 1521–1530.

Kilbourn, M. R., Butch, E. R., Desmond, T., Sherman, P., Harris, P. E., & Frey, K. A. (2010). In vivo [^{11}H]dihydrotetrabenazine binding in rat striatum: Sensitivity to dopamine concentrations. *Nuclear Medicine and Biology, 37*, 3–8.

Kilbourn, M., Lee, L., Vander Borght, T., Jewett, D., & Frey, K. (1995). Binding of alpha-dihydrotetrabenazine to the vesicular monoamine transporter is stereospecific. *European Journal of Pharmacology, 278*, 249–252.

Koob, G. F. (1992). Neural mechanisms of drug reinforcement. *Annals of the New York Academy of Sciences, 654*, 171–191.

Liang, N. Y., & Rutledge, C. O. (1982). Comparison of the release of [^{3}H]dopamine from isolated corpus striatum by amphetamine, fenfluramine and unlabelled dopamine. *Biochemical Pharmacology, 31*, 983–992.

Liu, Y., & Edwards, R. H. (1997). The role of vesicular transport proteins in synaptic transmission and neural degeneration. *Annual Review of Neuroscience, 20*, 125–156.

Liu, Y., Peter, D., Roghani, A., Schuldiner, S., Prive, G. G., Eisenberg, D., et al. (1992). A cDNA that suppresses MPP$^+$ toxicity encodes a vesicular amine transporter. *Cell, 70*, 539–551.

Liu, Y., Roghani, A., & Edwards, R. H. (1992). Gene transfer of a reserpine-sensitive mechanism of resistance to N-methyl-4-phenylpyridinium. *Proceedings of the National Academy of Sciences of the United States of America, 89*, 9074–9078.

Lyness, W. H., Friedle, N. M., & Moore, K. E. (1979). Destruction of dopaminergic nerve terminals in nucleus accumbens: Effect on d-amphetamine self-administration. *Pharmacology, Biochemistry, and Behavior, 11*, 553–556.

Madras, B. K., Meltzer, P. C., Liang, A. Y., Elmaleh, D. R., Babich, J., & Fischman, A. J. (1998). Altropane, a SPECT or PET imaging probe for dopamine neurons: I. Dopamine transporter binding in primate brain. *Synapse, 29*, 93–104.

Mantle, T. J., Tipton, K. F., & Garrett, N. J. (1976). Inhibition of monoamine oxidase by amphetamine and related compounds. *Biochemical Pharmacology, 25*, 2073–2077.

Matecka, D., Lewis, D., Rothman, R. B., Dersch, M., Wojnicki, F. H., Glowa, J. R., et al. (1997). Heteroaromatic analogs of 1-[2-(diphenylmethoxy)ethyl]- and 1-[2-[bis(4-fluorophenyl)-methoxy]ethyl]-4-(3-phenylpropyl)piperazines (GBR 12935 and GBR 12909) as high-affinity dopamine reuptake inhibitors. *Journal of Medicinal Chemistry, 40*, 705–716.

Merickel, A., Rosandich, P., Peter, D., & Edwards, R. H. (1995). Identification of residues involved in substrate recognition by a vesicular monoamine transporter. *The Journal of Biological Chemistry, 270*, 25798–25804.

Meyer, A. C., Neugebauer, N. M., Zheng, G., Crooks, P. A., Dwoskin, L. P., & Bardo, M. T. (2013). Effects of VMAT2 inhibitors lobeline and GZ-793A on methamphetamine-induced changes in dopamine release, metabolism and synthesis in vivo. *Journal of Neurochemistry, 127*, 187–198.

Miller, D. K., Crooks, P. A., & Dwoskin, L. P. (2000). Lobeline inhibits nicotine-evoked [^{3}H]dopamine overflow from rat striatal slices and nicotine-evoked ^{86}RB$^+$ efflux from thalamic synaptosomes. *Neuropharmacology, 39*, 2654–2662.

Miller, D. K., Crooks, P. A., Teng, L. H., Witkin, J. M., Munzar, P., Goldberg, S. R., et al. (2001). Lobeline inhibits the neuronal and behavioral effects of amphetamine. *The Journal of Pharmacology and Experimental Therapeutics, 296*, 1023–1034.

Miller, D. K., Crooks, P. A., Zheng, G., Grinevich, V. P., Norrholm, S. D., & Dwoskin, L. P. (2004). Lobeline analogs with enhanced affinity and selectivity for plasmalemma and vesicular monoamine transporters and diminished affinity at $\alpha 4 \beta 2^*$ and $\alpha 7^*$ nicotinic receptors. *The Journal of Pharmacology and Experimental Therapeutics, 310*, 1035–1045.

Miller, G. W., Gainetdinov, R. R., Levey, A. I., & Caron, M. G. (1999). Dopamine transporter and neuronal injury. *Trends in Pharmacological Sciences, 20*, 424–429.

Miller, D. K., Green, T. A., Harrod, S. B., Bardo, M. T., Crooks, P. A., & Dwoskin, L. P. (2000). Effects of lobeline on methamphetamine and nicotine-induced hyperactivity and sensitization. *Drug and Alcohol Dependence, 60*, 151.

Naudon, L., Raisman-Vozari, R., Edwards, R. H., Leroux-Nicollet, I., Peter, D., Liu, Y., et al. (1996). Reserpine affects differentially the density of the vesicular monoamine transporter and dihydrotetrabenazine binding sites. *The European Journal of Neuroscience, 8*, 842–846.

Neugebauer, N. M., Harrod, S. B., Stairs, D. J., Crooks, P. A., Dwoskin, L. P., & Bardo, M. T. (2007). Lobelane decreases methamphetamine self-administration in rats. *European Journal of Pharmacology, 571*, 33–38.

Nickell, J. R., Krishnamurthy, S., Norrholm, S., Deaciuc, G., Siripurapu, K. B., Zheng, G., et al. (2010). Lobelane inhibits methamphetamine-evoked dopamine release via inhibition of the vesicular monoamine transporter-2. *The Journal of Pharmacology and Experimental Therapeutics, 332*, 612–621.

Nickell, J. R., Zheng, G., Deaciuc, A. G., Crooks, P. A., & Dwoskin, L. P. (2011). Phenyl ring-substituted lobelane analogs: Inhibition of [³H]dopamine uptake at the vesicular monoamine transporter-2. *The Journal of Pharmacology and Experimental Therapeutics, 336*(3), 724–733.

Njus, D., Kelley, P. M., & Harnadek, G. J. (1986). Bioenergetics of secretory vesicles. *Biochimica et Biophysica Acta, 853*, 237–265.

Nordahl, T. E., Salo, R., & Leamon, M. (2003). Neuropsychological effects of chronic methamphetamine use on neurotransmitters and cognition: A review. *The Journal of Neuropsychiatry and Clinical Neurosciences, 15*, 317–325.

Partilla, J. S., Dempsey, A. G., Nagpal, A. S., Blough, B. E., Baumann, M. H., & Rothman, R. B. (2006). Interaction of amphetamines and related compounds at the vesicular monoamine transporter. *The Journal of Pharmacology and Experimental Therapeutics, 319*, 237–246.

Peter, D., Jimenez, J., Liu, Y., Kim, J., & Edwards, R. H. (1994). The chromaffin granule and synaptic vesicle amine transporters differ in substrate recognition and sensitivity to inhibitors. *The Journal of Biological Chemistry, 269*, 7231–7237.

Peter, D., Liu, Y., Sternini, C., de Giorgio, R., Brecha, N., & Edwards, R. H. (1995). Differential expression of two vesicular monoamine transporters. *The Journal of Neuroscience, 15*, 6179–6188.

Philippu, A., & Beyer, J. (1973). Dopamine and noradrenaline transport into subcellular vesicles of the striatum. *Naunyn-Schmiedeberg's Archives of Pharmacology, 278*, 387–402.

Pifl, C., Drobny, H., Reither, H., Hornykiewicz, O., & Singer, E. A. (1995). Mechanism of the dopamine-releasing actions of amphetamine and cocaine: Plasmalemmal dopamine transporter versus vesicular monoamine transporter. *Molecular Pharmacology, 47*, 368–373.

Riddle, E. L., Fleckenstein, A. E., & Hanson, G. R. (2005). Role of monoamine transporters in mediating psychostimulant effects. *The AAPS Journal, 7*, 847–851.

Rothman, R. B., Ayestas, M. A., Dersch, C. M., & Baumann, M. H. (1999). Aminorex, fenfluramine, and chlorphentermine are serotonin transporter substrates: Implications for primary pulmonary hypertension. *Circulation, 100*, 869–875.

Sagne, C., Isambert, M. F., Vandekerckhove, J., Henry, J. P., & Gasnier, B. (1997). The photoactivatable inhibitor 7-azido-8-iodoketanserin labels the N terminus of the vesicular monoamine transporter from bovine chromaffin granules. *Biochemistry, 36*, 3345–3352.

Schuldiner, S., Liu, Y., & Edwards, R. H. (1993). Reserpine binding to a vesicular amine transporter expressed in Chinese hamster ovary fibroblasts. *The Journal of Biological Chemistry, 268*, 29–34.

Sievert, M. K., & Ruoho, A. E. (1997). Peptide mapping of the [125I]Iodoazidoketanserin and [125I]2-N-[(3'-iodo-4'-azidophenyl)propionyl]tetrabenazine binding sites for the synaptic vesicle monoamine transporter. *The Journal of Biological Chemistry, 272*, 26049–26055.

Sulzer, D., Chen, T. K., Lau, Y. Y., Kristensen, H., Rayport, S., & Ewing, A. (1995). Amphetamine redistributes dopamine from synaptic vesicles to the cytosol and promotes reverse transport. *The Journal of Neuroscience, 15*, 4102–4108.

Takahashi, N., Miner, L. L., Sora, I., Ujike, H., Revay, R. S., Kostic, V., et al. (1997). VMAT2 knockout mice: Heterozygotes display reduced locomotion, and enhanced MPTP toxicity. *Proceedings of the National Academy of Sciences of the United States of America, 94*, 9938–9943.

Teng, L. H., Crooks, P. A., & Dwoskin, L. P. (1998). Lobeline displaces [³H] dihydrotetrabenazine binding and releases [³H]dopamine from rat striatal synaptic vesicles: Comparison with d-amphetamine. *Journal of Neurochemistry, 71*, 258–265.

Teng, L., Crooks, P. A., Sonsalla, P. K., & Dwoskin, L. P. (1997). Lobeline and nicotine evoke [3H]overflow from rat striatal slices preloaded with [3H]dopamine: Differential inhibition of synaptosomal and vesicular [3H]dopamine uptake. *The Journal of Pharmacology and Experimental Therapeutics, 280,* 1432–1444.

Thiriot, D. S., & Ruoho, A. E. (2001). Mutagenesis and derivatization of human monoamine vesicle transporter-2 (VMAT2) cysteines identifies transporter domains involved in tetrabenazine binding and substrate transport. *The Journal of Biological Chemistry, 276,* 27304–27315.

Uhl, G. R. (1998). Hypothesis: The role of dopaminergic transporters in selective vulnerability of cells in Parkinson's disease. *Annals of Neurology, 43,* 555–560.

Vezina, P. (1996). D1 dopamine receptor activation is necessary for the induction of sensitization by amphetamine in the ventral tegmental area. *The Journal of Neuroscience, 16,* 2411–2420.

Wang, Y., Gainetdinov, R. R., Fumagalli, F., Xu, F., Jones, S. R., Bock, C. B., et al. (1997). Knockout of the vesicular monoamine transporter 2 gene results in neonatal death and supersensitivity to cocaine and amphetamine. *Neuron, 19,* 1285–1296.

Weaver, J. A., & Deupree, J. D. (1982). Conditions required for reserpine binding to the catecholamine transporter on chromaffin granule ghosts. *European Journal of Pharmacology, 80,* 437–438.

Weihe, E., Schafer, M. K., Erickson, J. D., & Eiden, L. E. (1995). Localization of vesicular monoamine transporter isoforms (VMAT1 and VMAT2) to endocrine cells and neurons in rat. *Journal of Molecular Neuroscience, 5,* 149–164.

Wilhelm, C. J., Johnson, R. A., Eshleman, A. J., & Janowsky, A. (2008). Lobeline effects on tonic and methamphetamine-induced dopamine release. *Biochemical Pharmacology, 75,* 1411–1415.

Wilmouth, C. E., Zheng, G., Crooks, P. A., Dwoskin, L. P., & Bardo, M. T. (2013). Oral administration of GZ-793A, a VMAT2 inhibitor, decreases methamphetamine self-administration in rats. *Pharmacology, Biochemistry, and Behavior, 112,* 29–33.

Wimalasena, K. (2010). Vesicular monoamine transporters: Structure-function, pharmacology and medicinal chemistry. *Medicinal Research Reviews, 31,* 483–519.

Wise, R. A., & Bozarth, M. A. (1987). A psychomotor stimulant theory of addiction. *Psychological Review, 94,* 469–492.

Wise, R. A., & Hoffman, D. C. (1992). Localization of drug reward mechanisms by intracranial injections. *Synapse, 10,* 247–263.

Xu, D. D., Mo, Z. X., Yung, K. K., Yang, Y., & Leung, A. W. (2008). Individual and combined effects of methamphetamine and ketamine on conditioned place preference and NR1 receptor phosphorylation in rats. *Neurosignals, 15,* 322–331.

Yokel, R. A., & Pickens, R. (1973). Self-administration of optical isomers of amphetamine and methylamphetamine by rats. *The Journal of Pharmacology and Experimental Therapeutics, 187,* 27–33.

Zheng, G., Dwoskin, L. P., Deaciuc, A. G., Norrholm, S. D., & Crooks, P. A. (2005). Defunctionalized lobeline analogues: Structure-activity of novel ligands for the vesicular monoamine transporter. *Journal of Medicinal Chemistry, 48,* 5551–5560.

Zheng, G., Dwoskin, L. P., Deaciuc, A. G., Zhu, J., Jones, M. D., & Crooks, P. A. (2005). Lobelane analogues as novel ligands for the vesicular monoamine transporter-2. *Bioorganic & Medicinal Chemistry Letters, 13,* 3899–3909.

CHAPTER THREE

Customizing Monoclonal Antibodies for the Treatment of Methamphetamine Abuse: Current and Future Applications

Eric C. Peterson[*], W. Brooks Gentry[*,†], S. Michael Owens[*,1]

[*]Department of Pharmacology and Toxicology, College of Medicine, University of Arkansas for Medical Sciences, Little Rock, Arkansas, USA
[†]Department of Anesthesiology, College of Medicine, University of Arkansas for Medical Sciences, Little Rock, Arkansas, USA
[1]Corresponding author: e-mail address: mowens@uams.edu

Contents

Abstract

Monoclonal antibody-based medications designed to bind (+)-methamphetamine (METH) with high affinity are among the newest approaches to the treatment of METH abuse and the associated medical complications. The potential clinical indications for these medications include treatment of overdose, reduction of drug dependence, and protection of vulnerable populations from METH-related complications. Research designed to discover and conduct preclinical and clinical testing of these antibodies suggests a scientific vision for how intact monoclonal antibody (mAb) (singular and plural) or small antigen-binding fragments of mAb could be engineered to optimize the proteins for specific therapeutic applications. In this review, we discuss keys to success in this development process including choosing predictors of specificity, efficacy, duration of action, and safety of the medications in disease models of acute and chronic drug abuse. We consider important aspects of METH-like hapten design and how hapten structural features influence specificity and affinity, with an example of a high-resolution X-ray crystal structure of a high-affinity antibody to demonstrate this structural relationship. Additionally, several prototype anti-METH mAb forms such as antigen-binding fragments and single-chain variable fragments are under development. Unique, customizable aspects of these fragments are presented with specific possible clinical indications. Finally, we discuss clinical trial progress of the first in kind anti-METH mAb, for which METH is the disease target instead of vulnerable central nervous system networks of receptors, binding sites, and neuronal connections.

ABBREVIATIONS

AMP (+)-amphetamine
CDR complementarity determining region
Cls systemic clearance
CNS central nervous system
DA dopamine
Fab antigen-binding fragment
FcRn neonatal Fc receptor
IgG immunoglobulin gamma
i.v. intravenous
K_d equilibrium dissociation rate constant
mAb monoclonal antibody
(+/−)-MDMA (+/−) 3,4-methylenedioxymethamphetamine
METH (+)-methamphetamine
PCKN pharmacokinetics
PCP phencyclidine
scFv single-chain variable fragment
$t_{1/2\lambda n}$ terminal elimination half-life
V_d apparent volume of distribution
V_H variable heavy chain
V_L variable light chain

1. INTRODUCTION

Methamphetamine (METH) addiction causes serious medical conditions (Table 3.1). The positive and motivating effects that promote its continued use include a sense of increased energy and euphoria, heightened awareness, self-confidence, increased sexual drive and performance, and

Table 3.1 Acute and chronic medical problems caused by methamphetamine abuse[a]
Acute medical problems[b]

Neuropsychiatric	Aggression, acute psychosis, violence
CNS	Cerebral hemorrhage, hyperthermia, stroke, and seizures leading to brain injury
Cardiovascular	Dysrhythmias, hypertension, myocardial infarction, vasoconstriction
Renal	Acute renal failure caused by rhabdomyolysis
General health	Death

Chronic medical problems[c]

Neuropsychiatric	Addiction, delirium, paranoia, hallucinations, psychosis
CNS	Neurological changes including short-term memory loss, neurotoxicity, cerebral hemorrhage, hyperthermia, stroke, and seizures
Cardiovascular	Dysrhythmias, hypertension, myocardial infarction
Hepatic	Liver toxicity
Renal	Electrolyte imbalance
General health	Malnutrition, significant weight loss, increased risk of infectious diseases (i.e., hepatitis and HIV/AIDS)

[a]These medical effects of METH abuse are adapted from the report of Gentry, Rüedi-Bettschen, and Owens (2009) and compiled from the following references.
[b]Acute effects: Albertson, Derlet, and Van Hoozen (1999), Callaway and Clark (1994), Mendelson, Jones, Upton, and Jacob (1995), Richards et al. (1999).
[c]Chronic effects: Albertson et al. (1999), Hong, Matsuyama, and Nur (1991), Nordahl, Salo, and Leamon (2003), Richards et al. (1999), Sato (1992), Urbina and Jones (2004), Yu, Larson, and Watson (2003).

reduced appetite (Cho, 1990; Rawson, Washton, Domier, & Reiber, 2002). Unfortunately, these initial positive effects are reinforcers of METH use and likely play a role in the establishment of METH addiction. When METH users attempt to continue the pleasurable effects through more frequent use, tolerance develops (Cho, 1990; Cook et al., 1993). To maintain their "high," users often increase the METH dose and shorten the interval between self-administrations. They accomplish this with a so-called speed run, which usually includes rapid input of the drug by smoking, snorting, or intravenous (i.v.) delivery. While initial doses of 10 mg of METH are common, 150 mg to 1 g doses of METH are sometimes consumed during a binge period (Cho, 1990). METH is the chief among a class of dangerous

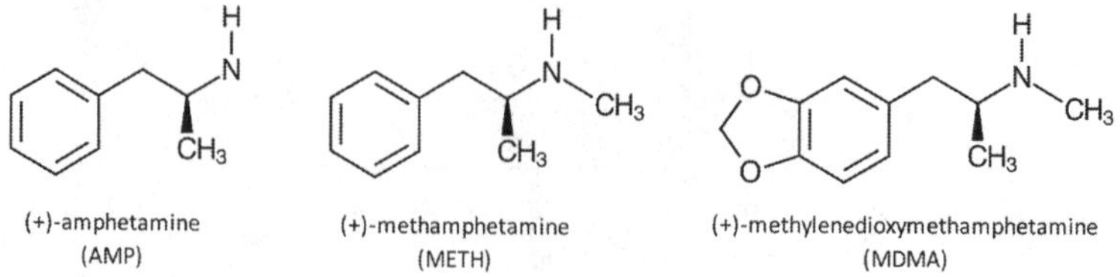

Figure 3.1 Chemical structures of (+)-methamphetamine, (+)-amphetamine, and (+)-3,4-methylenedioxymethamphetamine.

stimulants that include amphetamine (AMP, also a metabolite of METH) and the structurally related stimulant (+/−) 3,4-methylenedioxymethamphetamine (MDMA, or ecstasy) (Fig. 3.1, note that MDMA is shown as the (+)-isomer and not as a racemic mixture).

Binge use may lead to adverse complications that require medical intervention. As indicated by the most recent reports from 2011, METH/AMP-related problems accounted for 159,840 emergency department visits, which were 12.8% of the visits resulting from all illicit drugs (DAWN, 2013). This represents a 71% increase over 2009 statistics. When METH users come to emergency departments, many need treatment for acute toxicity or psychiatric symptoms. The number of METH/AMP users that sought chronic detoxification and longer-term treatment for their drug use increased nearly 50% between 2009 and 2011.

When METH is used at high binge doses, the medical effects can be very prolonged, especially since METH's half-life is about 12 h in humans (Cook et al., 1982, 1993; Mendelson et al., 2006). To recover, users might sleep for days (Kramer, 1967). This abusive cycle of METH use causes severe depression and sometimes a psychosis that is similar to paranoid schizophrenia (Derlet & Heischober, 1990; Lee, Boehm, Chester, Begent, & Perkins, 2002). Abusive and violent behaviors often occur (Kramer, 1967). Serious or medically harmful effects are so significant at higher METH doses (see Table 3.1) that studies of these effects are not safe in humans; thus, alternative animal models are required.

2. METH MECHANISMS OF ACTION, TOXICITY, AND CURRENT THERAPIES

The actions of METH in the central nervous system (CNS) result from complex interactions with a diverse set of neurotransmitters, ion channels, and presynaptic catecholamine uptake systems (Seger, 2010).

The effects on the CNS dopaminergic system are particularly profound because METH is a substrate for the dopamine (DA) transporter, leading to extraneural DA transport. METH can also increase neuronal release of DA through processes not controlled by the DA transporter. Together, these increased levels of presynaptic DA cause increased postsynaptic transmission (Cho, 1990). Other important METH-induced brain changes lead to excitation, excessive motor movements, mood changes, and a suppressed appetite. The CNS clinical syndromes resulting from METH's diverse mechanisms at multiple CNS sites emphasize the difficulty in discovering a single small molecule agonist or antagonist that could safely treat METH effects without addiction liability.

Effective medications are needed for the treatment of a plethora of medical problems related to METH abuse, which range from drug overdose to long-term neurotoxicity. Current therapies for METH medical effects are largely supportive. For instance, in overdose situations, patients are treated with hydration, anticonvulsants/sedatives, antihypertensives, or surface cooling while medical personnel wait for the most severe effects to dissipate (Beebe & Walley, 1995; Derlet & Heischober, 1990). While behavioral therapies for METH abuse exist, effective pharmacotherapies for drug abuse and addiction are missing. According to the National Institute on Drug Abuse (NIDA), the optimal characteristics of an effective addiction treatment program would combine counseling and therapeutic medicines, along with support services to meet individual patient needs.

3. THERAPEUTIC MONOCLONAL ANTIBODIES TO COUNTERACT METH EFFECTS

Immunopharmacological treatments fall into one of two broad categories (Gentry et al., 2009; Kosten & Owens, 2005). The first is active immunization, which requires 2–3 months of immunizations with a drug–protein conjugate before a long-lasting immunologic memory against the drug of abuse is established. This therapeutic strategy will not be discussed in this chapter. The second potential treatment is administration of monoclonal antibody (mAb) (singular and plural). This involves the infusion of a high-quality, pharmaceutical-grade antibody for immediate and long-term protection against the drug of abuse, without creating an immunologic memory. The mAb dose and frequency of dosing can be easily controlled, unlike the variable patient-to-patient response sometimes found with active immunization (Roskos, Davis, & Schwab, 2004). In addition, the beneficial response from infusion of a mAb can be immediate and long lasting. This makes it feasible to treat both the immediate urgency of a drug overdose and chronic drug addiction. The major disadvantages are cost of the medication and the possibility of allergic reaction to the protein.

Therapeutic mAb represent a rapidly growing area of clinical drug development, with more than 30 mAb medications already approved by the US Food and Drug Administration. These therapeutic mAb have diverse mechanisms of action including (1) neutralizing toxins or drugs, (2) delivering drugs to targeted sites, and (3) altering cellular function (Lobo, Hansen, & Balthasar, 2004). The first of these mechanisms best describes the mode of action for mAb treatment of drug abuse. To summarize their actions, anti-METH mAb changes both the amount and the rate of METH entry into medically critical site(s) of action in the CNS and cardiovascular system (Gentry, Rüedi-Bettschen, & Owens, 2010).

Three important and unique properties of mAb are as follows: IgG mAb has a long duration of action, the disease target for the mAb medications is the METH molecule, and the mAb medications modulate METH effect without leaving the blood stream. This medication profile is profoundly different from most small molecule agonist and antagonist that are short-acting, target the binding sites within the CNS, and must cross the blood–brain barrier to be effective (Camí & Farré, 2003).

Table 3.2 summarizes some of the most important prototype antibodies and antibody-binding fragments (Fabs) that could be used for treating medical problems caused by METH abuse. mAb medications are classified as pharmacokinetic antagonists because they bind to the target molecule (METH) and alter its distribution, metabolism, and elimination. There is no abuse liability, which is a negative characteristic of many small molecule agonist therapies. Because the mAb rapidly binds METH in the blood stream and prevents it from reaching its sites of action, the mAb or antibody fragment can reverse or prevent acute toxicities (Gentry et al., 2010; Hardin, Wessinger, Proksch, & Owens, 1998). The mAb dose and frequency of dosing can be easily controlled to achieve the desired level of effect, unlike active immunization. Finally, mAb have a long elimination half-life (~7 days in rats and ~21 days in humans; Bazin-Redureau, Renard, & Scherrmann, 1997; Joos et al., 2006), which limits the need for frequent repetitive dosing and improves the likelihood of patient compliance. This makes IgG mAb a very novel prototype for treating the chronic effects of addiction.

Table 3.2 Anti-METH mAb forms designed for customization of duration of action and specific clinical treatment scenarios

mAb medication (molecular size) $t_{1/2\lambda n}$	Possible human medical indication	Immunochemical selection criteria	Pharmacological testing and expected mAb-induced changes in rats
IgG (150,000 Da) weeks	• Overdose • Detoxification • Reduced harmful health effects from binge use	• K_d for METH <20 nM • K_d for AMP and/or and MDMA of <20 nM • No significant cross-reactivity with other medications or neurotransmitters	• Favorable pharmacokinetic profile • Long-acting METH binding in rodents (i.e., minimum of 2 weeks) • Reduction of METH-induced locomotor activity • Reduction of adverse medical effects
Fab (50,000 Da) hours	• Overdose • Detoxification	Above plus: • Ease of production • Lower protein dose required for drug binding	• Short-acting METH binding in rodents (i.e., 8 h) • Short-term reduction of adverse medical effects
scFv (25,000 Da) minutes to hours	• Overdose • Detoxification	Above plus: • Easily modified through molecular engineering • Can be modified to improve the duration of action or function (e.g., PEGylation and nanoparticles)	• Very short-acting METH binding in rodents (i.e., 2–3 h) • Short-term reduction of adverse medical effects

4. PREDICTING THERAPEUTIC EFFECTIVENESS

The complex pharmacokinetic relationship between mAb and a target ligand(s) makes it difficult to predict therapeutic effectiveness without an integrated program of mAb design and preclinical testing. Optimizing the mAb medications requires a multidisciplinary approach including chemistry, immunology, behavioral science, and clinical pharmacology. Important factors mediating mAb efficacy include mAb affinity and specificity, molar ratio of the mAb/drug, time of mAb administration in relation to METH use, dose of mAb, and disposition of mAb *in vivo* (Lobo et al., 2004; Peterson, Laurenzana, Atchley, Hendrickson, & Owens, 2008).

While the focus of this chapter is not on behavioral models of addiction, we use several important behavioral models to discover the best anti-METH mAb for treating METH abuse. These include measures of changes in locomotor activity (Byrnes-Blake et al., 2003; Gentry et al., 2006) and mAb effects on drug discrimination (McMillan, Hardwick, Li, & Owens, 2002), on METH self-administration (McMillan et al., 2004), and on the cardiovascular system (Gentry et al., 2006). While it is essential to use these types of preclinical testing, there are no rodent models that are proven to predict human clinical efficacy.

5. METH METABOLISM AND PHARMACOKINETICS: CHOOSING THE APPROPRIATE ANIMAL TESTING MODEL

In addition to understanding how these antibody-related factors contribute to the pharmacokinetic mechanisms of mAb effects, it is also important to understand how METH metabolism and pharmacokinetics impact mAb effects. Because AMP is a major psychoactive metabolite of METH, it is necessary to consider the pharmacokinetic properties of METH and AMP in humans and how they relate to the values in rats (our primary preclinical animal model). The METH pharmacokinetic values for the male rat (Rivière, Byrnes, Gentry, & Owens, 1999) and man (Cook et al., 1993) after i.v. administration are as follows: volume of distribution (V_d), 9.0 l/kg versus 3.7 l/kg; systemic clearance (Cls), 126 ml/min/kg versus 3.2 ml/min/kg; and terminal elimination half-life ($t_{1/2\lambda z}$), 63 min versus 13.1 h, respectively. While the pharmacokinetic values for V_d for the two species differ only by a factor of 2.4, the Cls is 39-fold greater in the rat. Metabolism of METH is the major route of elimination in the rat, with renal elimination constituting only a minor route of the total clearance (9–13% of the dose). In contrast, renal elimination is a significant component of human Cls, with 37–45% of the METH dose appearing in the urine (Cook et al., 1993). These data suggest physiological and treatment factors that could increase urinary elimination of METH could be an effective treatment in humans. Possible candidates for this therapeutic strategy are anti-METH antigen-binding fragments and single-chain variable fragments (Fab or scFv, respectively; Table 3.2), which can be cleared by kidney passive filtration. For example, the use of a monoclonal anti-PCP Fab can significantly increase renal passive filtration of PCP in rats (Proksch, Gentry, & Owens, 1998). Although an anti-METH scFv can rapidly change the apparent volume of distribution of METH in serum, the scFv's specific effects on METH clearance by individual organs like the kidney and liver have not been determined (Peterson et al., 2008).

The short $t_{1/2\lambda_z}$ of METH in rats (about 1 h), compared with that in humans (about 12 h), appears mostly due to a significantly greater capacity for metabolic elimination in the male rat (Milesi-Hallé, Hendrickson, Laurenzana, Gentry, & Owens, 2005). Because METH is partially cleared by the CYP2D6 enzymatic pathway in humans (Lin et al., 1997) and approximately 5–10% of the Caucasian North American population are deficient in this enzymatic pathway (KImura, Umeno, Skoda, Meyer, & Gonzalez, 1989), many METH users will be poor metabolizers of the drug. These patients may be more profoundly affected for longer periods of time and more vulnerable to adverse effects.

Because of some limitations with the male rat as an animal model of human METH use, we explored the possible advantages of using the female rat as a preclinical model (Milesi-Hallé et al., 2005). We find sex-dependent differences in METH pharmacokinetics, metabolism, and locomotor response between male and female rats, with females (but not males) showing dose dependency in the pharmacokinetic parameters at the highest dose tested (3 mg/kg). Dose-dependent METH (Cook et al., 1993) and $(+/-)-$MDMA (de la Torre et al., 2000) pharmacokinetics are reported in male humans. There are no reports in females. We also find the female rat has a significantly slower METH Cls and nonrenal clearance, lower AMP formation, and greater METH urinary excretion compared to the male rat. Based on these parameters, the female rat pharmacokinetic profile is more consistent with METH pharmacokinetics in male humans. However, the differences are not great enough to prefer the use of female to the male rat.

Rather, we view the female and male rats as representative models of human patients with different levels of METH vulnerability.

6. THE ROLE OF AFFINITY, BINDING CAPACITY, AND *In Vivo* MODIFICATIONS IN mAb FUNCTION

Optimizing and maximizing *in vivo* affinity of the mAb for METH is a critical first step (Byrnes-Blake, Laurenzana, Landes, Gentry, & Owens, 2005; Peterson et al., 2007). For instance, high-affinity anti-METH mAb6H4 ($K_d = 4$ nM) is much more effective at antagonizing METH locomotor effects than the lower affinity anti-METH mAb6H8 ($K_d = 250$ nM). Other studies from our laboratory with an antiphencyclidine mAb (anti-PCP mAb6B5, $K_d = 1$ nM) show that binding capacity for the PCP does not limit therapeutic effectiveness as much as was initially predicted based solely on the number of binding sites (Hardin et al., 1998; Laurenzana, Gunnell, Gentry, & Owens, 2003; Proksch, Gentry, & Owens, 2000). In these studies, a mAb dose of only 1/100th the PCP body burden significantly decreased brain PCP concentrations, reversed PCP-induced behavioral effects, prevented adverse PCP-induced health effects, and even prevented death.

We think the mechanism of these favorable effects results from synergy among several following factors: (1) the blood–brain barrier restricts the antibody to the plasma in the blood stream of the brain but METH freely crosses the blood–brain barrier, (2) there is an extremely small volume of the vascular cerebral space relative to the general circulation, and (3) the amount of METH in the brain is an extremely small fraction of the total METH dose (0.1% of the total dose) (Laurenzana, Byrnes-Blake, et al., 2003). These factors, along with the mAb's high affinity and rapid association with the PCP, act synergistically to allow temporary greater drug–mAb occupancy with each pass through the brain. This is an important discovery indicating that mAb pharmacokinetic antagonism of PCP (and perhaps METH) actions might not be as easily "surmounted" as previously thought.

In vivo changes that alter mAb affinity, binding capacity, or pharmacokinetics have an impact on mAb effectiveness. Studies from our laboratory indicate that our high-affinity anti-METH mAb6H4 may be at least partially inactivated *in vivo* (Byrnes-Blake et al., 2003). Although anti-METH mAb6H4 protected against METH-induced locomotor activity acutely over the first several hours, the effectiveness is reduced for METH challenges given 3 days later and significantly diminished after 7 days. This contrasts with other studies showing a single dose of anti-PCP mAb6B5 protects against PCP-induced effects for at least 2 weeks (Hardin et al., 2002; Laurenzana, Gunnell, et al., 2003) and can still reduce PCP brain concentrations 1 month later in rats (Proksch et al., 2000).

The greatly reduced effectiveness of our anti-METH mAb6H4 after 24 h suggests that the mAb is somehow altered *in vivo* to affect affinity and/or binding capacity. The experimental data show there are no changes in the pharmacokinetic properties, such as increased clearance (Laurenzana et al., 2009). Thus, binding function, such as changes in K_d or capacity, appears to be the reason for the unexpected loss of the mAb6H4 binding function. Fortunately, a redesign of the METH-like hapten solved the problem (Carroll et al., 2009; Owens, Atchley, Hambuchen, Peterson, & Gentry, 2011).

7. HAPTEN DESIGN FOR IMPROVED TARGET SPECIFICITY AND mAb FUNCTIONALITY

The hapten design and (IgG) immunoglobulin gamma DNA sequencing described in this section have been ongoing in our laboratory group over the past decade (Carroll et al., 2009, 2011; Peterson et al., 2007; Peterson, Owens, & Henry, 2006). Through experience in molecular modeling and sequence analysis, we were able to analyze a library of mAb function and sequence data and then elucidate important IgG sequence and structural features involved in antibody–METH interactions. This work revealed key hapten features that are important for shaping critical molecular interactions during immunization (Peterson et al., 2006).

Because the chemical composition and molecular orientation of the drug-like haptens on the antigen are crucial determinants in generating antibodies against small molecules (Landsteiner & Van der Scheer, 1931), the goal of these long-term studies was to discover design criteria needed to produce long-acting anti-METH, anti-AMP, and anti-MDMA mAb medications. This led to the discovery of mAb medications with the potential specificity needed to treat overdose and addiction indications resulting from METH, AMP, and/or MDMA abuse. Although high affinity for METH was always our foremost goal, we wanted to generate a single mAb with high affinity for the metabolite AMP and a related compound, (+)-MDMA.

Molecular orientation of the hapten on the protein carrier is critical to the control of antibody specificity for its target ligand. This is because antibodies generated against hapten–protein conjugates primarily react to the portion of the hapten antigenic epitope that is distal to the point of chemical attachment on the carrier protein. Our goal was to generate antibodies against the (+)-isomers of METH-like compounds. (+)-Isomers produce significantly more psychomimetic effects, locomotor activity, stereotyped behavior, monoamine oxidase inhibition, and addiction liability than (−)-isomers (Cho, 1990; Marquardt, DiStefano, & Ling, 1978). From a chemical synthesis point of view, this meant the hapten linker needed to be attached to the phenyl ring structure of (+)-METH, to increase the distance from the chiral center. This maximized the immune system's potential to select for antibodies with high affinity and specificity for (+)-isomers (Peterson et al., 2007).

Using these criteria, we progressively generated haptens with changes in linker length (e.g., 4, 6, and 10 molecules), molecular modification to the linker constituents (e.g., addition of an oxygen molecule to mimic the oxygen in MDMA), and attachment to the METH phenyl ring at the para, ortho, and meta positions. The longer (+)-METH MO10 spacer was created to allow more flexibility of the hapten when attached to the carrier protein, in the hopes of discovering mAb(s) with broader recognition of (+)-METH-like structures (Carroll et al., 2009; Peterson et al., 2007). Using these haptens, we generated the groups of antibodies with different affinities for METH (from 4 to 250 nM) and specificities (METH, AMP, and (+)-MDMA). While we hypothesized that mAb affinity is the primary driving force for therapeutic efficacy, we learned that the duration of action and function of our anti-(+)METH mAb *in vivo* cannot be predicted from simple *in vitro* characterization or from the pharmacokinetic properties of the antibodies (Laurenzana et al., 2009), as discussed in an earlier section.

Our first generation of mAbs was produced from short-chain haptens linked to the phenyl ring structure of METH. The linker chains had 4 and 6 molecule spacer groups bound at the para and meta positions of the phenyl ring of the hapten. The other end of the spacer was designed for easy covalent attachment to amino acids of the protein carrier (Peterson et al., 2007). The resulting mAbs had virtually no cross-reactivity with AMP, but high affinity for METH and (+)-MDMA. When we produced our second generation of haptens with a 10 molecule spacer, including an oxygen attached directly to the METH component of the hapten, we began to discover mAb with specificity for METH, AMP, and (+)-MDMA. One mAb in particular (mAb4G9) had the additional advantages of increased duration of action of METH binding *in vivo* and improved efficacy (Carroll et al., 2009; Owens et al., 2011). mAb4G9 also had a very long duration of *in vivo* function

(Laurenzana et al., 2009). We now know this is related to the important chemical properties of the MO10 hapten, since we have recently identified other long-acting mAb from immunization with MO10 hapten. One of these mAb is mAb7F9 (METH $K_d = 9$ nM), which is our lead candidate medication and a human chimeric version is currently in phase I clinical trials for treating METH abuse.

8. RELATIONSHIP BETWEEN HAPTEN STRUCTURE AND mAb FUNCTION: APPLICATION TO OTHER ANTIBODY FORMS

Numerous studies have attempted to elucidate structural features of antibodies that lead to high affinity and specificity binding. The structural classifications of antibody-binding sites for ligands are generally grouped into four classes: concave, moderately concave, rigid, and planar (MacCallum, Martin, & Thornton, 1996). The crucial interactions for mAb binding are mediated primarily by the amino acids within the complementarity determining regions (CDR) of the antibody heavy and light chains. CDR contacts for domains on protein antigens generally involve the side chains of 15–20 amino acids (Poljak, 1973). Very small molecule drugs like METH (149 Da) interact with a limited number of these amino acids due to the small surface area and low number of charged atoms. This likely limits the potential for discovery of extremely high-affinity mAb binding (e.g., 200 pM) and is a major factor in why even our highest affinity antibodies are only in the low nanomolar range of K_d values (i.e., 4–9 nM).

Information derived from X-ray crystallography studies help to elucidate antibody mechanisms of binding and provide the foundation for customizing affinity and specificity. We first determined the crystal structures of a Fab derived from murine anti-PCP mAb6B5 (Lim, Owens, Arnold, Sacchettini, & Linthicum, 1998) and later the structure of Fab fragments from anti-METH mAb (Celikel, Peterson, Owens, & Varughese, 2009) in complex with their target drugs of abuse. Both of these antibodies have a deep pocket mode of binding (as demonstrated for METH in Fig. 3.2). A unique feature of the binding site of anti-PCP mAb6B5 is a tryptophan at position 97H (H-chain). The side chain of this residue acts as a hydrophobic umbrella over the ligand in the antigen-binding pocket, which appears to significantly contribute to its high affinity for PCP (Lim et al., 1998).

Since IgG molecules of anti-METH mAb are difficult to crystallize due to their flexible nature, antibody structure is studied by examinations of

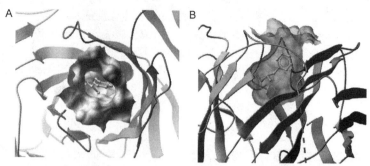

Figure 3.2 X-ray crystal structure of high-affinity anti-METH scFv6H4 reveals METH-binding configuration is influenced by hapten design. Top (A) and side (B) views of anti-METH scFv6H4 crystal structure showing that METH is bound in a deep cavity, which tightly fits the shape of METH. The position of the para-carbon of the METH aromatic ring, the attachment point of the 6-carbon linker of the hapten, is nearest the entrance to the binding pocket. This structure strongly supports that the binding pocket shaping is dictated by hapten design. Binding pocket surface representations are colored by binding property. Molecular interactions are a balance of neutral (white), hydrophobic (green), hydrogen bonding acceptor (red), and hydrogen bonding donor (blue) potentials. Two water molecules in the pocket also form key hydrogen bonds with METH (not shown for clarity). (For interpretation of the references to color in this figure legend, the reader is referred to the online version of this chapter.)

other, smaller customized forms (Table 3.2). Specifically, we use the antigen-binding fragments Fab and scFv. Anti-METH scFv6H4 binds METH with high affinity and the crystal structure of this complex shows that the METH molecule is encased almost completely in a deep binding pocket. In fact, only 3% of the surface area of METH is solvent accessible in the structure of the complex (Fig. 3.2). The METH ligand is oriented in the binding site with the aromatic ring towards the entrance and the side chain pointing to the interior. This is not surprising since the hapten used to discover mAb6H4 contains a linkage of the aromatic ring to the para position of the METH aromatic ring structure (Peterson et al., 2007).

Both hydrophobic interactions and hydrophilic interactions appear to stabilize METH binding. The entrance of the binding site is lined with six aromatic residues. These combine to form a hydrophobic barrel around the aromatic portion of METH that covers 68% of the METH surface area. This forms the majority of interaction surface for the METH/scFv6H4 configuration. Although the binding is mediated mostly by hydrophobic interactions, the secondary amine of METH plays an important role because it is the only charged atom in METH (as well as AMP and MDMA). A salt bridge exists between this nitrogen and the carboxyl oxygen of a key glutamate from the heavy chain and a second hydrogen bond to a histidine of the light chain. Thus, it appears that the para-position orientation of the original METH-like hapten linker favored the formation of this crucial hydrogen bond. If the linker were at another position, the charged nitrogen might not be exposed and available for interaction with amino acid residues so deep in the pocket. While this binding configuration generated very high-affinity anti-METH antibodies, this mAb proved ineffective for chronic treatment with the intact mAb6H4. Fortunately, other high-affinity antibodies against METH have been discovered, which are very long acting *in vivo* (Owens et al., 2011).

9. ANTIBODY FORM AND DURATION OF ACTION

With a half-life of about 3 weeks in humans (Joos et al., 2006), IgG isotype mAb exhibits one of the longest durations of action of any small molecule- or biological-based medications. This long half-life is due in part to the ability of the antibody to be repeatedly salvaged from catabolism pathways by the neonatal Fc receptor (FcRn) through interactions with the Fc portion of the IgG (Lobo et al., 2004; Roskos et al., 2004). Under normal conditions, IgG circulates in the vasculature where it is internalized via pinocytosis into epithelial cells. In the next step of the process, IgG is recycled in a pH-dependent manner (Ghetie & Ward, 2002). If this recycling occurs, the antibody is protected from degradation and released back into the vasculature. While FcRn-mediated recycling of IgG dramatically increases the mAb half-life in the circulation, the process exposes the protein to microenvironment pH changes. This can potentially alter the protonation states of amino acid side chains and affect the binding pocket charge and protein conformation (Sinha, Mohan, Lipschultz, & Smith-Gill, 2002).

Small antibody-binding fragments such as Fab and scFv lack the IgG domains required for FcRn binding and thus are not subject to recycling and the associated pH-dependent change. Their clearance is predominately dependent on renal elimination (Proksch et al., 1998). Thus, their half-life is much shorter. In clinical situations like METH overdose or other acute treatment scenarios, this short half-life could be advantageous. For instance, a short-acting Fab or scFv could be used to rapidly clear the body of high doses of METH and other stimulants (Peterson & Owens, 2009). Treatment of rats with an anti-METH scFv6H4 monomer shows the scFv6H4 monomer is quickly converted to multivalent forms or cleared. This results in an apparent $t_{1/2\lambda n}$ of 5.8 min for the monomer (Peterson et al., 2008). In contrast, the larger scFv6H4 multivalent forms (e.g., trimers) that spontaneously associate *in vivo* show a $t_{1/2\lambda n}$ of 3.8 h. scFv6H4 binding to METH directly correlates with scFv6H4 serum molar concentrations. These data suggest the scFv6H4 binding sites are (nearly) fully occupied in the serum and high-affinity METH binding is the cause of the significant increases in METH serum concentrations.

These data also suggest that the scFv6H4 multimers (and not the monomer) are responsible for the increase in duration of action. *In vitro* multimer formation is often found with scFv proteins; the relative amounts of each form depend upon linker length, pH, ionic strength, and the presence or absence of antigen (Arndt, Müller, & Pluckthun, 1998). This dimerization between the V_L and the V_H domains can occur through two proposed mechanisms (Hudson & Souriau, 2003). In the first scenario, the domains "open" or separate around the linker and bind to the domains of another unhinged scFv. This scenario results in an intermediate that is unable to bind to antigen since the binding site requires the coordination of both domains. The second mechanism is a simpler "back to back" conformation. In this scenario, the regions of the V_L and the V_H domains associate with those of another scFv, instead of forming interactions with globular domains of the constant region. This conformation does not require temporary loss of activity, and we think this is the mechanism through which anti-METH scFv6H4 form multimers, especially since it is able to bind to METH in equimolar ratios during the entire time in the serum.

Because multimerization can extend half-life, it has been explored as a method to customize the pharmacokinetic properties of antibodies. Unfortunately, because multimerization is not always predictable, it is unlikely that modification of the scFv solely through molecular engineering would produce reliable products. The main weakness in this approach is that the scFv molecules tend to self-associate in unpredictable mixtures of dimers and trimers and larger molecular weight multimers (Dolezal et al., 2000). This leads to large-scale production problems and less than optimal formulations.

While scFv has potential advantages over IgG in terms of cost, ease of production, and amount of protein needed for treatment, the variability of scFv multimer formation needs to be addressed. Fortunately, the conversion of the IgG to the single-gene scFv format makes molecular reengineering easier. For instance, the cysteine codon can be incorporated into the DNA coding sequence as a potential conjugation site on the protein for addition of polyethylene glycol (Chapman, 2002; Lobo et al., 2004) or nanoparticles (Nanaware-Kharade, Gonzalez, Lay, Hendrickson, & Peterson, 2012). These customizable fragments present many opportunities for tailoring individual therapies for specific clinical indications in the next generation of immunotherapies for treatment of drug abuse.

10. CONCLUSION

From our anti-METH mAb discovery process, we have chosen the murine anti-METH mAb7F9 (Carroll et al., 2009; Owens et al., 2011) to develop as a human treatment for METH addiction. mAb7F9 was converted to a mouse–human chimeric antibody by reengineering the protein to include the METH-binding variable regions from the original murine antibody (i.e., mAb7F9, $K_d = 9$ nM) and the constant domains from a human IgG2κ mAb. This form of the antibody has been administered to humans as part of a phase 1 clinical trial. Preliminary analysis of the data from this study suggests it will be safe for administration to humans. In the future, we think it will be possible to further customize our anti-METH mAbs to significantly improve on the affinity constants or to shorten or prolong the half-life of the antibodies to improve their utility for treatment of overdose and detoxification.

CONFLICT OF INTEREST

S. M. O. and W. B. G. have financial interests in and serve as chief scientific officer and chief medical officer of InterveXion Therapeutics LLC (Little Rock, AR), a pharmaceutical biotechnology company focused on treating human drug addiction with antibody-based therapy.

ACKNOWLEDGMENTS

The National Institute on Drug Abuse (DA11560, DA026423, DA031944), Arkansas Biosciences Institute (the major research component of the Arkansas Tobacco Settlement Proceeds Act of 2000), and the National Center for Advancing Translational Sciences (UL1TR000039) supported this work.

REFERENCES

Albertson, T. E., Derlet, R. W., & Van Hoozen, B. E. (1999). Methamphetamine and the expanding complications of amphetamines. *Western Journal of Medicine, 170*(4), 214–219.

Arndt, K. M., Müller, K. M., & Pluckthun, A. (1998). Factors influencing the dimer to monomer transition of an antibody single-chain Fv fragment. *Biochemistry, 37*(37), 12918–12926.

Bazin-Redureau, M. I., Renard, C. B., & Scherrmann, J. M. (1997). Pharmacokinetics of heterologous and homologous immunoglobulin G, F(ab')2 and Fab after intravenous administration in the rat. *The Journal of Pharmacy and Pharmacology, 49*(3), 277–281.

Beebe, D. K., & Walley, E. (1995). Smokable methamphetamine ("ice"): An old drug in a different form. *American Family Physician, 51*(2), 449–453.

Byrnes-Blake, K. A., Laurenzana, E. M., Carroll, F. I., Abraham, P., Gentry, W. B., Landes, R. D., et al. (2003). Pharmacodynamic mechanisms of monoclonal antibody-based antagonism of (+)-methamphetamine in rats. *European Journal of Pharmacology*, *461*(2–3), 119–128.

Byrnes-Blake, K. A., Laurenzana, E. M., Landes, R. D., Gentry, W. B., & Owens, S. M. (2005). Monoclonal IgG affinity and treatment time alters antagonism of (+)-methamphetamine effects in rats. *European Journal of Pharmacology*, *521*(1–3), 86–94.

Callaway, C. W., & Clark, R. F. (1994). Hyperthermia in psychostimulant overdose. *Annals of Emergency Medicine*, *24*(1), 68–76.

Camí, J., & Farré, M. (2003). Drug addiction. *New England Journal of Medicine*, *349*(10), 975–986.

Carroll, F. I., Abraham, P., Gong, P. K., Pidaparthi, R. R., Blough, B. E., Che, Y., et al. (2009). The synthesis of haptens and their use for the development of monoclonal antibodies for treating methamphetamine abuse. *Journal of Medicinal Chemistry*, *52*(22), 7301–7309.

Carroll, F. I., Blough, B. E., Pidaparthi, R. R., Abraham, P., Gong, P. K., Deng, L., et al. (2011). Synthesis of mercapto-(+)-methamphetamine haptens and their use for obtaining improved epitope density on (+)-methamphetamine conjugate vaccines. *Journal of Medicinal Chemistry*, *54*(14), 5221–5228.

Celikel, R., Peterson, E. C., Owens, S. M., & Varughese, K. I. (2009). Crystal structures of a therapeutic single chain antibody in complex with two drugs of abuse-methamphetamine and 3,4-methylenedioxymethamphetamine. *Protein Science*, *18*(11), 2336–2345.

Chapman, A. P. (2002). PEGylated antibodies and antibody fragments for improved therapy: A review. *Advanced Drug Delivery Reviews*, *54*(4), 531–545.

Cho, A. K. (1990). Ice: A new dosage form of an old drug. *Science*, *249*(4969), 631–634.

Cook, C. E., Brine, D. R., Jeffcoat, A. R., Hill, J. M., Wall, M. E., Perez-Reyes, M., et al. (1982). Phencyclidine disposition after intravenous and oral doses. *Clinical Pharmacology and Therapeutics*, *31*(5), 625–634.

Cook, C. E., Jeffcoat, A. R., Hill, J. M., Pugh, D. E., Patetta, P. K., Sadler, B. M., et al. (1993). Pharmacokinetics of methamphetamine self-administered to human subjects by smoking S-(+)-methamphetamine hydrochloride. *Drug Metabolism and Disposition*, *21*(4), 717–723.

DAWN (2013). *Substance Abuse and Mental Health Services Administration, Drug Abuse Warning Network, 2011: National Estimates of Drug-Related Emergency Department Visits* (No. HHS Publication No. (SMA) 13-4760). *samhsa.gov* (39 ed. pp. 1–93). Rockville, MD: Substance Abuse and Mental Health Services Administration, 2013. Retrieved from http://www.samhsa.gov/data/2k13/DAWN2k11ED/DAWN2k11ED.pdf.

de la Torre, R., Farré, M., Ortuño, J., Mas, M., Brenneisen, R., Roset, P. N., et al. (2000). Non-linear pharmacokinetics of MDMA ("ecstasy") in humans. *British Journal of Clinical Pharmacology*, *49*(2), 104–109.

Derlet, R. W., & Heischober, B. (1990). Methamphetamine. Stimulant of the 1990s? *Western Journal of Medicine*, *153*(6), 625–628.

Dolezal, O., Pearce, L., Lawrence, L., McCoy, A., Hudson, P., & Kortt, A. (2000). ScFv multimers of the anti-neuraminidase antibody NC10: Shortening of the linker in single-chain Fv fragment assembled in V(L) to V(H) orientation drives the formation of dimers, trimers, tetramers and higher molecular mass multimers. *Protein Engineering*, *13*(8), 565–574.

Gentry, W. B., Laurenzana, E. M., Williams, D. K., West, J. R., Berg, R. J., Terlea, T., et al. (2006). Safety and efficiency of an anti-(+)-methamphetamine monoclonal antibody in the protection against cardiovascular and central nervous system effects of (+)-methamphetamine in rats. *International Immunopharmacology*, *6*(6), 968–977.

Gentry, W. B., Rüedi-Bettschen, D., & Owens, S. M. (2009). Development of active and passive human vaccines to treat methamphetamine addiction. *Human Vaccines*, *5*(4), 206–213.

Gentry, W. B., Rüedi-Bettschen, D., & Owens, S. M. (2010). Anti-(+)-methamphetamine monoclonal antibody antagonists designed to prevent the progression of human diseases of addiction. *Clinical Pharmacology and Therapeutics*, *88*(3), 390–393.

Ghetie, V., & Ward, E. (2002). Transcytosis and catabolism of antibody. *Immunological Research*, *25*(2), 97–113.

Hardin, J. S., Wessinger, W. D., Proksch, J. W., & Owens, S. M. (1998). Pharmacodynamics of a monoclonal antiphencyclidine Fab with broad selectivity for phencyclidine-like drugs. *Journal of Pharmacology and Experimental Therapeutics*, *285*(3), 1113–1122.

Hardin, J. S., Wessinger, W. D., Wenger, G. R., Proksch, J. W., Laurenzana, E. M., & Owens, S. M. (2002). A single dose of monoclonal anti-phencyclidine IgG offers long-term reductions in phencyclidine behavioral effects in rats. *Journal of Pharmacology and Experimental Therapeutics*, *302*(1), 119–126.

Hong, R., Matsuyama, E., & Nur, K. (1991). Cardiomyopathy associated with the smoking of crystal methamphetamine. *Journal of the American Medical Association*, *265*(9), 1152–1154.

Hudson, P. J., & Souriau, C. (2003). Engineered antibodies. *Nature Medicine*, *9*(1), 129–134.

Joos, B., Trkola, A., Kuster, H., Aceto, L., Fischer, M., Stiegler, G., et al. (2006). Long-term multiple-dose pharmacokinetics of human monoclonal antibodies (MAbs) against human immunodeficiency virus type 1 envelope gp120 (MAb 2G12) and gp41 (MAbs 4E10 and 2F5). *Antimicrobial Agents and Chemotherapy*, *50*(5), 1773–1779.

KImura, S., Umeno, M., Skoda, R. C., Meyer, U. A., & Gonzalez, F. J. (1989). The human debrisoquine 4-hydroxylase (CYP2D) locus: Sequence and identification of the polymorphic CYP2D6 gene, a related gene, and a pseudogene. *American Journal of Human Genetics*, *45*(6), 889–904.

Kosten, T., & Owens, S. M. (2005). Immunotherapy for the treatment of drug abuse. *Pharmacology and Therapeutics*, *108*(1), 76–85.

Kramer, J. C. (1967). Amphetamine abuse: Pattern and effects of high doses taken intravenously. *Journal of the American Medical Association*, *201*(5), 305.

Landsteiner, K., & Van der Scheer, J. (1931). On the specificity of serological reactions with simple chemical compounds (inhibition reactions). *The Journal of Experimental Medicine*, *54*(3), 295–305.

Laurenzana, E. M., Byrnes-Blake, K. A., Milesi-Hallé, A., Gentry, W. B., Williams, D. K., & Owens, S. M. (2003). Use of anti-(+)-methamphetamine monoclonal antibody to significantly alter (+)-methamphetamine and (+)-amphetamine disposition in rats. *Drug Metabolism and Disposition*, *31*(11), 1320–1326.

Laurenzana, E. M., Gunnell, M. G., Gentry, W. B., & Owens, S. M. (2003). Treatment of adverse effects of excessive phencyclidine exposure in rats with a minimal dose of monoclonal antibody. *Journal of Pharmacology and Experimental Therapeutics*, *306*(3), 1092–1098.

Laurenzana, E. M., Hendrickson, H. P., Carpenter, D., Peterson, E. C., Gentry, W. B., West, M., et al. (2009). Functional and biological determinants affecting the duration of action and efficacy of anti-(+)-methamphetamine monoclonal antibodies in rats. *Vaccine*, *27*(50), 7011–7020.

Lee, Y. C., Boehm, M. K., Chester, K. A., Begent, R. H. J., & Perkins, S. J. (2002). Reversible dimer formation and stability of the anti-tumour single-chain Fv antibody MFE-23 by neutron scattering, analytical ultracentrifugation, and NMR and FT-IR spectroscopy. *Journal of Molecular Biology*, *320*(1), 107–127.

Lim, K., Owens, S. M., Arnold, L., Sacchettini, J. C., & Linthicum, D. S. (1998). Crystal structure of monoclonal 6B5 Fab complexed with phencyclidine. *The Journal of Biological Chemistry*, *273*(44), 28576–28582.

Lin, L. Y., Di Stefano, E. W., Schmitz, D. A., Hsu, L., Ellis, S. W., Lennard, M. S., et al. (1997). Oxidation of methamphetamine and methylenedioxymethamphetamine by CYP2D6. *Drug Metabolism and Disposition, 25*(9), 1059–1064.

Lobo, E. D., Hansen, R. J., & Balthasar, J. P. (2004). Antibody pharmacokinetics and pharmacodynamics. *Journal of Pharmacological Sciences, 93*(11), 2645–2668.

MacCallum, R., Martin, A., & Thornton, J. (1996). Antibody-antigen interactions: Contact analysis and binding site topography. *Journal of Molecular Biology, 262*(5), 732–745.

Marquardt, G., DiStefano, V., & Ling, L. (1978). Effects of racemic, (S)- and (R)-methylenedioxyamphetamine on synaptosomal uptake and release of tritiated norepinephrine. *Biochemical Pharmacology, 27*(10), 1497–1501.

McMillan, D. E., Hardwick, W. C., Li, M., Gunnell, M. G., Carroll, F. I., Abraham, P., et al. (2004). Effects of murine-derived anti-methamphetamine monoclonal antibodies on (+)-methamphetamine self-administration in the rat. *Journal of Pharmacology and Experimental Therapeutics, 309*(3), 1248–1255.

McMillan, D. E., Hardwick, W. C., Li, M., & Owens, S. M. (2002). Pharmacokinetic antagonism of (+)-methamphetamine discrimination by a low-affinity monoclonal anti-methamphetamine antibody. *Behavioural Pharmacology, 13*(5–6), 465–473.

Mendelson, J., Jones, R. T., Upton, R., & Jacob, P. (1995). Methamphetamine and ethanol interactions in humans. *Clinical Pharmacology and Therapeutics, 57*(5), 559–568.

Mendelson, J., Uemura, N., Harris, D., Nath, R. P., Fernandez, E., Jacob, P., et al. (2006). Human pharmacology of the methamphetamine stereoisomers. *Clinical Pharmacology and Therapeutics, 80*(4), 403–420.

Milesi-Hallé, A., Hendrickson, H. P., Laurenzana, E. M., Gentry, W. B., & Owens, S. M. (2005). Sex- and dose-dependency in the pharmacokinetics and pharmacodynamics of (+)-methamphetamine and its metabolite (+)-amphetamine in rats. *Toxicology and Applied Pharmacology, 209*(3), 203–213.

Nanaware-Kharade, N., Gonzalez, G. A., Lay, J. O., Hendrickson, H. P., & Peterson, E. C. (2012). Therapeutic anti-methamphetamine antibody fragment-nanoparticle conjugates: Synthesis and in vitro characterization. *Bioconjugate Chemistry, 23*(9), 1864–1872.

Nordahl, T. E., Salo, R., & Leamon, M. (2003). Neuropsychological effects of chronic methamphetamine use on neurotransmitters and cognition: A review. *The Journal of Neuropsychiatry and Clinical Neurosciences, 15*(3), 317–325.

Owens, S. M., Atchley, W. T., Hambuchen, M. D., Peterson, E. C., & Gentry, W. B. (2011). Monoclonal antibodies as pharmacokinetic antagonists for the treatment of (+)-methamphetamine addiction. *CNS & Neurological Disorders—Drug Targets, 10*(8), 892–898.

Peterson, E. C., Gunnell, M., Che, Y., Goforth, R. L., Carroll, F. I., Henry, R., et al. (2007). Using hapten design to discover therapeutic monoclonal antibodies for treating methamphetamine abuse. *Journal of Pharmacology and Experimental Therapeutics, 322*(1), 30–39.

Peterson, E. C., Laurenzana, E. M., Atchley, W. T., Hendrickson, H. P., & Owens, S. M. (2008). Development and preclinical testing of a high-affinity single-chain antibody against (+)-methamphetamine. *Journal of Pharmacology and Experimental Therapeutics, 325*(1), 124–133.

Peterson, E. C., & Owens, S. M. (2009). Designing immunotherapies to thwart drug abuse. *Molecular Interventions, 9*(3), 119–124.

Peterson, E., Owens, S. M., & Henry, R. L. (2006). Monoclonal antibody form and function: Manufacturing the right antibodies for treating drug abuse. *The AAPS Journal, 8*(2), E383–E390.

Poljak, R. (1973). X-ray crystallographic studies of immunoglobulins. *Contemporary Topics in Molecular Immunology, 2*, 1–26.

Proksch, J., Gentry, W., & Owens, S. (1998). Pharmacokinetic mechanisms for obtaining high renal coelimination of phencyclidine and a monoclonal antiphencyclidine antigen-binding fragment of immunoglobulin G in the rat. *Journal of Pharmacology and Experimental Therapeutics, 287*(2), 616–624.

Proksch, J. W., Gentry, W. B., & Owens, S. M. (2000). Anti-phencyclidine monoclonal antibodies provide long-term reductions in brain phencyclidine concentrations during chronic phencyclidine administration in rats. *Journal of Pharmacology and Experimental Therapeutics, 292*(3), 831–837.

Rawson, R. A., Washton, A., Domier, C. P., & Reiber, C. (2002). Drugs and sexual effects: Role of drug type and gender. *Journal of Substance Abuse Treatment, 22*(2), 103–108.

Richards, J. R., Bretz, S. W., Johnson, E. B., Turnipseed, S. D., Brofeldt, B. T., & Derlet, R. W. (1999). Methamphetamine abuse and emergency department utilization. *Western Journal of Medicine, 170*(4), 198–202.

Rivière, G. J., Byrnes, K. A., Gentry, W. B., & Owens, S. M. (1999). Spontaneous locomotor activity and pharmacokinetics of intravenous methamphetamine and its metabolite amphetamine in the rat. *Journal of Pharmacology and Experimental Therapeutics, 291*(3), 1220–1226.

Roskos, L. K., Davis, C. G., & Schwab, G. M. (2004). The clinical pharmacology of therapeutic monoclonal antibodies. *Drug Development Research, 61*(3), 108–120.

Sato, M. (1992). A lasting vulnerability to psychosis in patients with previous methamphetamine psychosis. *Annals of the New York Academy of Sciences, 654*, 160–170.

Seger, D. (2010). Cocaine, metamfetamine, and MDMA abuse: The role and clinical importance of neuroadaptation. *Clinical Toxicology, 48*(7), 695–708, Informa Healthcare New York.

Sinha, N., Mohan, S., Lipschultz, C., & Smith-Gill, S. (2002). Differences in electrostatic properties at antibody-antigen binding sites: Implications for specificity and cross-reactivity. *Biophysical Journal, 83*(6), 2946–2968.

Urbina, A., & Jones, K. (2004). Crystal methamphetamine, its analogues, and HIV infection: Medical and psychiatric aspects of a new epidemic. *Clinical Infectious Diseases: An Official Publication of the Infectious Diseases Society of America, 38*(6), 890–894.

Yu, Q., Larson, D. F., & Watson, R. R. (2003). Heart disease, methamphetamine and AIDS. *Life Sciences, 73*(2), 129–140.

CHAPTER FOUR

Monoamine Transporter Inhibitors and Substrates as Treatments for Stimulant Abuse

Leonard L. Howell[*,1], S. Stevens Negus[†]

[*]Yerkes National Primate Research Center, Emory University, Atlanta, Georgia, USA
[†]Department of Pharmacology and Toxicology, Virginia Commonwealth University, Richmond, Virginia, USA
[1]Corresponding author: e-mail address: lhowell@emory.edu

Contents

Abstract

The acute and chronic effects of abused psychostimulants on monoamine transporters and associated neurobiology have encouraged development of candidate medications that target these transporters. Monoamine transporters, in general, and dopamine transporters, in particular, are critical molecular targets that mediate abuse-related effects of psychostimulants such as cocaine and amphetamine. Moreover, chronic administration of psychostimulants can cause enduring changes in neurobiology reflected in dysregulation of monoamine neurochemistry and behavior. The current review will

Advances in Pharmacology, Volume 69
ISSN 1054-3589
http://dx.doi.org/10.1016/B978-0-12-420118-7.00004-4
129

evaluate evidence for the efficacy of monoamine transporter inhibitors and substrates to reduce abuse-related effects of stimulants in preclinical assays of stimulant self-administration, drug discrimination, and reinstatement. In considering deployment of monoamine transport inhibitors and substrates as agonist-type medications to treat stimulant abuse, the safety and abuse liability of the medications are an obvious concern, and this will also be addressed. Future directions in drug discovery should identify novel medications that retain efficacy to decrease stimulant use but possess lower abuse liability and evaluate the degree to which efficacious medications can attenuate or reverse neurobiological effects of chronic stimulant use.

ABBREVIATIONS

ADHD attention deficit hyperactivity disorder
DAT dopamine transporter
FDG fluorodeoxyglucose
GBR 12909 1-[2-[bis-(4-fluorophenyl)methoxy]ethyl]-4-(3-phenylpropyl)piperazine
NET norepinephrine transporter
PAL-287 1-naphthyl-2-aminopropane
PET positron emission tomography
PTT 2β-propanoyl-3β-(4-tolyl)-tropane
RTI-112 (1R,2S,3S)-methyl3-(4-chloro-3-methylphenyl)-8-methyl-8-azabicyclo[3.2.1]octane-2-carboxylate
RTI-113 phenyl 3-(4-chlorophenyl)-8-methyl-8-azabicyclo[3.2.1]octane-2-carboxylate
RTI-177 5-[(1R,2S,3S,5S)-3-(4-chlorophenyl)-8-methyl-8-azabicyclo[3.2.1]octan-2-yl]-3-(4-methylphenyl)-1,2-oxazole
RTI-336 3β-(4-chlorophenyl)-2β-[3-(4β-methylphenyl)isoxazol-5-yl]tropane hydrochloride
SERT serotonin transporter

1. INTRODUCTION

Preclinical assessment of candidate medications to treat drug addiction relies on a two-step process that involves (1) detection of abuse-related effects produced by the target drug of abuse, followed by (2) evaluation of the efficacy and safety of candidate medications to reduce those abuse-related effects. Drug addiction is an operant behavior in which maladaptive patterns of drug use are maintained by drug delivery, and as a result, preclinical operant conditioning procedures have played a key role in medication development. This review will focus on use of preclinical operant procedures to evaluate inhibitors and substrates of monoamine transporters as candidate medications to treat psychostimulant addiction. The review will be divided into three sections. First, principles of operant behavior will be reviewed to illustrate their use in characterizing abuse-related effects of psychostimulants and evaluating efficacy of candidate medications to treat psychostimulant addiction. Second, we will discuss evidence from these and related procedures that implicates monoamine transporters as molecular targets of psychostimulants that mediate abuse liability and adapt to chronic stimulant exposure. Lastly, we will review evidence that regimens of treatment with monoamine transporter inhibitors and substrates can reduce abuse-related effects of psychostimulants in these preclinical procedures and in human laboratory studies and clinical trials. Taken together, the data to be discussed will show that monoamine transporter inhibitors and releasers can reduce abuse-related effects of psychostimulants and warrant further consideration as candidate medications for the treatment of psychostimulant addiction. Figure 4.1 illustrates categories of research on abuse-related behavior and neurobiological effects of abused stimulants.

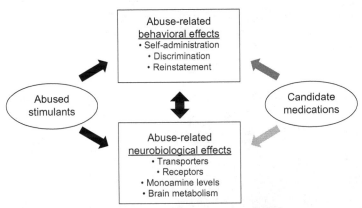

Figure 4.1 Categories of research on abuse-related behavioral and neurobiological effects of abused stimulants in the absence or presence of treatment with candidate medications. A large database now exists on behavioral and neurobiological effects of abused stimulants, and this work provides insight on mechanisms of stimulant addiction. This database also provides a foundation for research to examine effects of candidate medications on abuse-related behavioral and neurobiological effects of abused stimulants. At present, a substantial and growing body of data has examined effects of monoamine transporter inhibitors and substrates on abuse-related behavioral effects of stimulants, whereas a much smaller body of work has addressed effects of these compounds on abuse-related neurobiological effects of stimulants. Optimal candidate medications will reduce expression of abuse-related behavioral effects and reverse abuse-related neurobiological effects of abused stimulants.

2. OPERANT BEHAVIOR IN MEDICATION DEVELOPMENT

Drug addiction is a maladaptive pattern of drug use leading to clinically significant impairment or distress (American_Psychiatric_Association, 2013). The development of medications to treat addiction is founded on the premise that addiction is caused in part by effects of the abused drug that can be blocked or reversed by medications. However, all drugs of abuse produce multiple effects, only some of which are likely to promote abuse. Cocaine, for example, produces local anesthetic, cardiovascular, and neurobiological effects, but only a subset of neurobiological effects is thought to contribute to addiction (Biebuyck, 1990; Catterall & Mackie, 2005; Johanson & Fischman, 1989; O'Brien, 2006). One challenge in preclinical research on medication development is to identify those "abuse-related" effects that contribute to a drug's abuse potential and that might serve as reasonable targets for intervention with medications.

One fruitful approach to this challenge has conceptualized drug addiction as an example of operant behavior, which can be defined as behavior shaped by its consequences in the framework of a 3-term contingency. This 3-term contingency can be diagrammed as follows:

$$S^D \rightarrow R \rightarrow S^C$$

where S^D signifies a *discriminative stimulus*, R designates a *response* on the part of the organism, and S^C designates a *consequent stimulus* (Ferster & Skinner, 1957; Skinner, 1938). The arrows specify the contingency that, in the presence of the discriminative stimulus S^D, performance of the response R will result in delivery of the consequent stimulus S^C. Consequent stimuli that increase responding leading to their delivery are operationally defined as *reinforcers*. The contingencies that relate discriminative stimuli, responses, and consequent stimuli are defined by the *schedule of reinforcement*. For example, under a fixed-ratio (FR) schedule, a fixed number of responses in the presence of the S^D are required to produce delivery of the S^C (e.g., an FR 10 schedule would require 10 responses). Far more complex schedules of reinforcement are also possible. Drugs can function as either the discriminative or consequent stimulus in the 3-term contingency, and procedures that use drugs in these capacities play a key role in research to evaluate both the abuse liability of drugs and the efficacy of medications to treat drug abuse. Three commonly used families of procedures are briefly reviewed later.

2.1. Drug self-administration

In drug self-administration procedures, drug delivery serves as the consequent stimulus (Katz, 1989; Negus & Banks, 2011; Young & Herling, 1986). More specifically, conditions are established such that, in the presence of some discriminative stimulus (e.g., a stimulus light), emission of a response (e.g., pressing a response lever) produces delivery of a drug dose (e.g., i.v. delivery via a chronic i.v. catheter). A drug is considered to function as a reinforcer if some drug dose maintains higher response rates than vehicle, and many drugs of abuse including psychostimulants function as reinforcers in drug self-administration procedures. The high concordance between preclinical measures of drug reinforcement and clinical measures of abuse liability has encouraged use of drug self-administration for practical applications such as abuse liability assessment by regulatory agencies like the U.S. Drug Enforcement Agency (Ator & Griffiths, 2003; Carter & Griffiths, 2009). Moreover, drug self-administration by laboratory animals has clear parallels to human patterns of drug abuse that also involve sequences of behavior culminating in drug consumption. For all these reasons, drug reinforcement in assays of drug self-administration is often viewed as the most significant "abuse-related" effect amenable to preclinical study, and candidate medications can be evaluated for the degree to which they reduce self-administration of a target drug of abuse such as cocaine (Comer et al., 2008; Haney & Spealman, 2008; Mello & Negus, 1996).

Experiments to examine medication effects on drug self-administration can include many nuances (Mello & Negus, 1996). Three of those will be mentioned here. First, to be clinically efficacious, medication effects should be sustained rather than transient, because drug addiction is a chronic disorder that often demands chronic treatment. Assessment of the persistence of medication effects requires experimental designs that use chronic medication delivery. Second, to be clinically safe, medications should reduce consumption of the abused drug without producing undesirable effects. Although toxicology screens play a key role in safety assessment, useful insights to safety can also be provided by comparing medication effects on drug self-administration with effects on responding maintained by a nondrug reinforcer such as food. Some level of safety is implied by a profile of medication effects that includes selective reduction in drug self-administration with lesser effects on responding maintained by another reinforcer. Finally, medication effects on drug self-administration may vary as a function of the schedule of reinforcement used to maintain drug self-administration. This issue has been discussed in detail elsewhere (e.g., Negus & Banks, 2011) and is beyond the scope of this review. However, as a general rule, the strength of preclinical evidence for medication efficacy depends in part on the breadth of conditions across which a medication reduces drug self-administration.

2.2. Drug discrimination

In drug discrimination procedures, the drug serves as the discriminative stimulus of the 3-term contingency (Colpaert, 1999; Glennon & Young, 2011). In a common example, subjects have access to two response levers, and responding on these levers produces food reinforcement contingent on the presence or absence of a training dose of a training drug. Specifically, responding on only one lever (the drug-appropriate lever) produces food reinforcement after drug delivery, and responding on only the other lever (the vehicle-appropriate lever) produces food after vehicle delivery. A drug is considered to function as a discriminative stimulus if subjects can be trained to respond differentially to its presence or absence. Both abused and nonabused drugs can produce discriminative-stimulus effects, so the mere ability of a drug to function as a discriminative stimulus is not sufficient to signify abuse liability; however, all drugs of abuse can function as discriminative stimuli, and abuse liability of a test drug is indicated if it shares discriminative-stimulus effects with a known drug of abuse (e.g., if the test drug produces drug-appropriate responding in a subject trained to discriminate a known drug of abuse such as cocaine) (Ator & Griffiths, 2003; Overton, 1987). In addition, discriminative-stimulus effects of drugs in animals are homologous to subjective drug effects in humans, where discrimination is evidenced by different patterns of verbal behavior rather than by differential lever-pressing behavior (Carter & Griffiths, 2009; Schuster & Johanson, 1988). In view of these considerations, discriminative-stimulus effects can also be considered as a category of abuse-related drug effects. Drug discrimination is used in medication development to assess the degree to which candidate medications mimic or modify discriminative-stimulus effects of the target drug of abuse.

2.3. Reinstatement

Reinstatement procedures constitute a subtype of drug self-administration that adds a focus on the function of nondrug stimuli (Shaham, Shalev, Lu, De Wit, & Stewart, 2003). In a common example, a nondrug stimulus (e.g., a stimulus light) functions as a discriminative stimulus in a drug self-administration procedure. Additional nondrug stimuli (e.g., additional stimulus lights or sounds) may also be paired with drug delivery such that, by classical conditioning mechanisms, they come to function as conditioned reinforcers. Once drug self-administration is established, some period of drug abstinence is imposed when self-administration sessions as a whole are omitted, or more commonly, when modified sessions are conducted during which the operant manipulandum is present but drug and some or all nondrug stimuli are omitted. This abstinence period produces not only withdrawal from the self-administered drug but also a decline in rates of the operant behavior that produced drug, either because whole sessions are omitted and the operant behavior is not possible or because drug and nondrug stimuli have been omitted and operant behavior extinguishes. At the conclusion of the abstinence period, test stimuli are introduced and rates of operant responding are reevaluated, usually with continued omission of drug reinforcement. In general, three types of test stimuli are used: (a) non-contingent treatments with the self-administered drug, (b) reintroduction of omitted nondrug discriminative stimuli and/or conditioned reinforcers (often collectively referred to as "cues"), and (c) stimuli such as foot shock intended to induce "stress." Each of these drug, cue, and stress stimuli can increase (or "reinstate") rates of operant responding, and candidate medications can be evaluated for the degree to which they reduce stimulus-induced reinstatement.

One goal in the use of reinstatement procedures is to model the phenomenon of relapse in drug addiction, and by extension, medication effects on reinstatement are often interpreted as predictive of their utility to treat relapse (Epstein, Preston, Stewart, & Shaham, 2006; Martin-Fardon & Weiss, 2013). However, the relationship between experimental reinstatement and clinical relapse is controversial (Katz & Higgins, 2003), and medication effects on reinstatement might be more profitably interpreted in terms of their effects on the stimulus functions of test stimuli. For example, drug-induced reinstatement likely involves multiple behavioral mechanisms that include discriminative-stimulus effects (Gerber & Stretch, 1975). During a drug self-administration session, each self-administered drug dose can function not only as a reinforcing stimulus that increases the probability of preceding behaviors but also as a discriminative stimulus associated with access to contingencies of drug availability. Consequently, noncontingent administration of drug can be expected to produce discriminative-stimulus effects associated with drug availability and conducive to operant responding, and medication effects on drug reinstatement can be expected to resemble medication effects on discriminative-stimulus effects of the drug under other circumstances (e.g., in conventional drug discrimination assays).

3. MONOAMINE TRANSPORTERS AS MOLECULAR TARGETS FOR MEDICATION DEVELOPMENT

3.1. Monoamine transporter function

Monoamine transporters are transmembrane proteins located in plasma membranes of monoaminergic neurons and include the dopamine transporter (DAT), serotonin transporter (SERT), and norepinephrine transporter (NET) (Amara & Kuhar, 1993; Langer & Galzin, 1988) (see Lin et al., 2011). Their main function is to terminate monoamine transmission by inward transport of released neurotransmitter. Within the cell, vesicular monoamine transporters (VMAT) concentrate neurotransmitter molecules in synaptic vesicles for additional cycles of release (Erickson, Eiden, & Hoffman, 1992; Schuldiner, Shirvan, & Linial, 1995). VMAT1 is preferentially expressed in neuroendocrine cells and VMAT2 is primarily expressed in the CNS (see Wimalasena, 2011).

Monoamines play important roles in normal brain function and are implicated in various neuropsychiatric disorders. Accordingly, the regulation of monoamines is critically important. Dopamine is implicated in many physiological processes such as movement, cognition, memory, and reward (Greengard, 2001). Cell bodies that produce dopamine are localized to the substantia nigra, the ventral tegmental area, and the hypothalamus. Dopamine neurons project to the caudate nucleus, putamen, nucleus accumbens, and prefrontal cortex (Westerink, 2006). Serotonin is also implicated in many functions, including mood, sleep, appetite, anxiety, fear, reward, and aggression (Barnes & Sharp, 1999; Hoyer, Hannon, & Martin, 2002). Serotonin neurons are restricted to the raphe nuclei in the brain stem and project to the cortex, thalamus, basal ganglia, hippocampus, and amygdala (Jacobs & Azmitia, 1992). Norepinephrine plays a critical role in arousal (Astier, Van Bockstaele, Aston-Jones, & Pieribone, 1990), attention, memory, and mood (Grant, Aston-Jones, & Redmond, 1988) and is synthesized primarily in the locus coeruleus and surrounding nuclei in mammals, including humans (Carpenter & Sutin, 1983). Anatomical studies have shown consistently that monoaminergic neurons each express a specific plasma membrane transporter (Hoffman, Hansson, Mezey, & Palkovits, 1998). Alteration of cell-surface expression of transporters is a critical mechanism for regulating monoamine transport. Trafficking of plasma membrane transporters has been shown to occur under basal conditions (Loder & Melikian, 2003) and can also be induced by transporter substrates (Chi & Reith, 2003; Furman et al., 2009) and inhibitors (Daws et al., 2002; Little, Elmer, Zhong, Scheys, & Zhang, 2002; Rothman, Blough, & Baumann, 2007).

Psychostimulants enhance monoaminergic signaling by interfering with transporter function. However, psychostimulants differ in their relative affinity for DAT, SERT, and NET. For example, cocaine has approximately equal affinity for these three transporters, whereas amphetamine, methamphetamine, and methylphenidate all have relatively lower affinity for SERT compared to their affinity for DAT and NET (see Howell & Kimmel, 2008). In addition, psychostimulants differ in their actions as reuptake inhibitors versus substrate-type releasers (Fleckenstein, Gibb, & Hanson, 2000; Rothman et al., 2007). Transporter inhibitors, including cocaine, interfere with transporter function but are not transported into the nerve terminal. In contrast, substrate-type releasers, including amphetamine and methamphetamine, are transported into the cytoplasm of the nerve terminal. Transporter substrates elevate extracellular monoamine levels by reversing the process of transporter-mediated exchange. They also increase cytoplasmic levels of monoamines by interfering with vesicular storage (Rudnick, 1997; Rudnick & Clark, 1993). Typically, substrates are more effective than inhibitors in increasing extracellular monoamines because the former increase the pool of neurotransmitters available for release by transporter-mediated exchange. Moreover, the effectiveness of substrates in increasing extracellular monoamines is not dependent upon the basal rate of neurotransmitter release. In contrast, the effectiveness of inhibitors is impulse-dependent and, therefore, limited by the tone of presynaptic activity.

3.2. Role of monoamine transporters in acute behavioral effects of psychostimulants

Abundant evidence implicates monoamine transporters, in general, and DATs, in particular, as molecular targets that mediate abuse-related effects of psychostimulants such as cocaine and amphetamine (Koob, 1992; Lile & Nader, 2003; Natarajan & Yamamoto, 2011; Rothman & Glowa, 1995; Woolverton & Johnson, 1992). For example, the potency and efficacy of cocaine and a series of related drugs to maintain drug self-administration correlated with their potency to inhibit uptake of dopamine but not serotonin or norepinephrine (Ritz, Lamb, Goldberg, & Kuhar, 1987). Similarly, cocaine-like reinforcing effects (Bergman, Madras,

Johnson, & Spealman, 1989; Hiranita, Soto, Newman, & Katz, 2009; Howell & Byrd, 1995; Woolverton, 1987) and discriminative-stimulus effects (Katz, Izenwasser, & Terry, 2000; Kleven, Anthony, & Woolverton, 1990; Schama, Howell, & Byrd, 1997; Spealman, 1993, 1995) are produced by dopamine-selective uptake inhibitors, but generally not by serotonin- or norepinephrine-selective uptake inhibitors. With amphetamine and other monoamine releasers, it has been more difficult to identify compounds that dissociate effects mediated by dopamine and norepinephrine release, and abused releasers like amphetamine generally display similar to slightly higher (~threefold) potency to promote release of norepinephrine versus dopamine in *in vitro* assays (Rothman et al., 2001). However, potency and efficacy of a series of releasers to maintain self-administration or produce cocaine-like discriminative-stimulus effects were correlated with potency to release dopamine/norepinephrine (Negus, Mello, Blough, Baumann, & Rothman, 2007; Wee et al., 2005). Lastly, disruption of dopaminergic signaling disrupts expression of abuse-related effects by abused psychostimulants. For example, the reinforcing and/or discriminative-stimulus effects of cocaine can be blocked by lesions to the mesolimbic dopamine system (Caine & Koob, 1994), by genetic modification of DATs (Thomsen, Hall, Uhl, & Caine, 2009; Thomsen, Han, Gu, & Caine, 2009), or by pharmacological antagonists of dopamine receptors (Bergman, Kamien, & Spealman, 1990; Caine & Koob, 1994; Caine, Negus, Mello, & Bergman, 2000; Negus, Mello, Lamas, & Mendelson, 1996).

The dopaminergic system is clearly an important site of action for abused stimulants, but preclinical studies have also indicated that the serotonergic system can effectively modulate the behavioral effects of cocaine and amphetamine. Although compounds that selectively increase serotonin neurotransmission lack behavioral-stimulant effects and do not reliably maintain self-administration behavior (Howell & Byrd, 1995; Vanover, Nader, & Woolverton, 1992), a negative relationship was observed between the potencies of several cocaine- and amphetamine-like drugs in self-administration studies and their binding affinities for serotonin-uptake sites (Ritz & Kuhar, 1989; Ritz et al., 1987). Coadministration of agents that induce robust increases in both dopamine and serotonin produces minimal behavioral-stimulant effects (Bauer, Banks, Blough, & Negus, 2013; Baumann et al., 2000) and does not maintain self-administration behavior (Glatz et al., 2002) in rodents. Similarly, monoamine-releasing agents have decreased reinforcing efficacy in rhesus monkeys when serotonin-releasing potency is increased relative to dopamine (Negus et al., 2007; Wee et al.,

2005). The behavioral and neurochemical profile of DAT inhibitors is also influenced by their actions at multiple monoamine transporters in squirrel monkeys (Ginsburg, Kimmel, Carroll, Goodman, & Howell, 2005).

Studies in nonhuman primates also support a significant but subordinate role for norepinephrine uptake in the discriminative-stimulus effects of cocaine (Spealman, 1995). More recent studies in squirrel monkeys have also documented that NET inhibition can play a significant role in cocaine-induced reinstatement (Platt, Rowlett, & Spealman, 2007). There is also a significant positive correlation between potency of drug-induced norepinephrine release and the drug dose that produces stimulant-like subjective effects in humans following oral administration (Rothman et al., 2001). However, it should be noted that there is little evidence that norepinephrine plays a primary role in the reinforcing properties of psychomotor stimulants in rodents (Tella, 1995) or nonhuman primates (Kleven & Woolverton, 1990; Mello, Lukas, Bree, & Mendelson, 1990; Woolverton, 1987).

This evidence implicating monoamine transporters, and especially DATs, as molecular targets of abused psychostimulants provides a sound rationale for development of transporter inhibitors and substrates as medications that also target monoamine transporters. A second line of evidence derives from studies showing that chronic exposure to abused psychostimulants can modulate monoamine transporters, associated monoaminergic systems, and indices of cortical function.

3.3. Neurobiological effects of chronic psychostimulant administration

Chronic administration of psychostimulants can cause enduring changes in neurobiology and corresponding changes in sensitivity to acute drug effects on neurochemistry and behavior. Both sensitization and tolerance have been reported to develop during repeated administration of stimulants in animal studies (Woolverton & Weiss, 1998). However, the outcome can depend upon a variety of procedural variables including the drug effect under investigation, the dosing regimen, the environmental context associated with drug administration, and the animal species. The vast majority of studies have focused on sensitization to locomotor-stimulant effects in rodent models. Stimulants including cocaine and amphetamines can produce robust sensitization in rodents, usually identified as a progressive increase in locomotor activity or stereotyped behavior with drug dosing (Robinson & Berridge, 2000). There is substantial evidence that the mesocorticolimbic dopamine system and its excitatory glutamatergic inputs are critical for the development of sensitization to the behavioral effects of psychostimulants in rodents (Carlezon & Nestler, 2002; Wolf, Sun, Mangiavacchi, & Chao, 2004). In contrast, tolerance to the neurochemical effects of cocaine has been reported in nonhuman primates. Rhesus monkeys trained to self-administer cocaine showed a significant increase in striatal extracellular dopamine following the first injection of a session, but the response to cocaine was attenuated following the second injection, indicative of acute tolerance (Bradberry, 2000). In a related study initiated in drug-naive rhesus monkeys, subjects were trained to self-administer cocaine under limited-access conditions (1 h/day) for 10 weeks, followed by extended-access conditions (4 h/day) for 10 weeks, and micro-dialysis studies were conducted at the end of each phase (Kirkland Henry, Davis, & Howell, 2009). Under both self-administration conditions, cocaine-induced increases in extracellular dopamine were blunted compared to drug-naive conditions, indicating that cocaine self-administration resulted in a hypofunctional dopamine system.

Efforts to define the long-term neurobiological consequences of psychostimulant administration in rodents have focused primarily on the dopaminergic system and have yielded inconsistent results. For example, cocaine exposure has been reported to increase, decrease, or have no effect on DAT density in rodents (Boulay, Duterte-Boucher, Leroux-Nicollet, Naudon, & Costentin, 1996; Claye, Akunne, Davis, DeMattos, & Soliman, 1995; Letchworth, Daunais, Hedgecock, & Porrino, 1997; Letchworth et al., 1999; Pilotte, Sharpe, & Kuhar, 1994; Tella, Ladenheim, Andrews, Goldberg, & Cadet, 1996; Wilson et al., 1994). Similarly, chronic cocaine administration in rodents has been reported to increase, decrease, or have no effect on dopamine D1- or D2-receptor density (Dwoskin, Peris, Yasuda, Philpott, & Zahniser, 1988; Goeders & Kuhar, 1987; Kleven, Perry, Woolverton, & Seiden, 1990; Kuhar & Pilotte, 1996). The equivocal results likely reflect different dosing regimens and withdrawal periods, as well as the use of noncontingent drug administration protocols that do not model voluntary drug use. Active drug self-administration protocols and periods of drug abstinence can have profound influences on the neurobiology of dopamine systems (Mateo, Lack, Morgan, Roberts, & Jones, 2005). Accordingly, a more consistent picture has emerged from nonhuman primate studies of cocaine self-administration (Table 4.1). For example, in rhesus monkeys trained to self-administer i.v. cocaine, initial exposure led to moderate decreases in DAT density in the striatum as determined postmortem with quantitative autoradiography (Letchworth et al., 2001). However, longer

Table 4.1 Neurobiological effects of chronic cocaine administration in nonhuman primates and humans

Effect	Nonhuman primates	Humans
Dopamine transporter	↑ Letchworth, Nader, Smith, Friedman, and Porrino (2001)	↑ Little, Kirkman, Carroll, Clark, and Duncan (1993)
	= Czoty, Reboussin, Calhoun, Nader, and Nader (2007)	↑ Staley, Hearn, Ruttenber, Wetli, and Mash (1994)
Dopamine D1 receptor	↓ Moore, Vinsant, Nader, Porrino, and Friedman (1998a)	= Martinez et al. (2009)
	↓ Nader et al. (2002)	
Dopamine D2 receptor	↓ Moore, Vinsant, Nader, Porrino, and Friedman (1998b)	↓ Volkow and Fowler (2000)
	↓ Nader et al. (2002)	↓ Volkow, Chang, Wang, Fowler, Ding, et al. (2001)
	↓ Czoty, Morgan, Shannon, Gage, and Nader (2004)	
Dopamine release	↓ Kirkland Henry et al. (2009)	↓ Martinez et al. (2007)
		↓ Volkow et al. (1997a, 1997b)
Serotonin transporter	↑ Banks et al. (2008)	↑ Jacobsen et al. (2000)
	↑ Gould et al. (2011)	↑ Mash, Staley, Izenwasser, Basile, and Ruttenber (2000)
Serotonin 5HT2A receptor	↑ Sawyer et al. (2012)	
Norepinephrine transporter		↑ Ding et al. (2010)
Distribution of cerebral activation	↑ Henry, Murnane, Votaw, and Howell (2010)	
Cerebral perfusion		↓ Volkow et al. (1988)
Cerebral metabolism		↓ Reivich et al. (1985)
		↓ Volkow, Chang, Wang, Fowler, Ding, et al. (2001)

exposure resulted in increased striatal DAT density that was most pronounced in the ventral striatum at the level of the nucleus accumbens. Importantly, the increases in DAT binding observed after long-term cocaine self-administration in nonhuman primates corresponded closely to increases observed in postmortem tissue of human cocaine addicts (Little et al., 1993; Staley et al., 1994). In related studies, rhesus monkeys trained to self-administer cocaine on a daily basis over 18–22 months showed lower dopamine D1 binding density as determined postmortem with quantitative autoradiography (Moore et al., 1998a; Nader et al., 2002). In parallel studies using the same self-administration schedule and quantitative autoradiography, dopamine D2 binding density was lower in all regions of the striatum rostral to the anterior commissure (Moore et al., 1998b; Nader et al., 2002). Collectively, these drug-induced changes provide additional evidence of a hypofunctional dopamine system that may contribute to the development of dependence associated with long-term psychostimulant use.

Chronic exposure to cocaine also induces changes in the serotonin system. Increases in SERT density following chronic cocaine exposure have been reported in cells (Kittler, Lau, & Schloss, 2010), rodents (Cunningham, Paris, & Goeders, 1992), nonhuman primates (Banks et al., 2008; Gould et al., 2011), and humans (Jacobsen et al., 2000; Mash et al., 2000). Cocaine exposure has also been reported to affect density and/or function of postsynaptic 5HT receptors, ranging from decreases in 5HT3 receptors in the nucleus accumbens shell of rats sensitized to cocaine (Ricci, Stellar, & Todtenkopf, 2004) to reduced sensitivity of 5HT1A receptors (Baumann & Rothman, 1998). Cocaine exposure and withdrawal also have been reported to affect 5HT2A receptor expression and function, although no consensus has been reached as to the exact nature of these effects (Carrasco & Battaglia, 2007; Carrasco et al., 2006; Huang, Liang, Lee, Wu, & Hsu, 2009). Overall, chronic cocaine clearly results in an altered state of the serotonin system, which could contribute to the development of cocaine dependence.

Functional neuroimaging permits longitudinal evaluation of drug effects on neurochemistry using designs that involve repeated measures over extended periods of time. This approach has been used effectively in nonhuman primates to characterize both transient and long-lasting changes in brain chemistry that are associated with drug history. For example, positron emission tomography (PET) imaging studies conducted in socially housed cynomolgus monkeys characterized the effects of chronic cocaine exposure in dominant and subordinate subjects. Although dominant male monkeys initially exhibited higher D2 receptor availability and lower rates of cocaine self-administration (Morgan et al., 2002), chronic exposure to self-administered cocaine resulted in reductions in D2 receptor availability and enhanced cocaine self-administration to levels comparable with subordinate monkeys (Czoty et al., 2004). A subsequent study examined D2 receptor availability during extended cocaine abstinence (Nader et al., 2006). In subjects with short-term exposure over 1 week, D2 receptor availability returned to predrug levels within 3 weeks. In subjects with long-term exposure over 1 year, some showed complete recovery within 3 months, whereas others did not recover after 1 year of abstinence. It is interesting to note that individual differences in the rate of recovery of D2 receptor availability have also been observed following drug-induced increases by the D2 receptor antagonist raclopride (Czoty, Gage, & Nader, 2005). Baseline DAT availability as determined by PET imaging was negatively correlated with sensitivity to cocaine reinforcement in female cynomolgus monkeys (Nader et al., 2012). However, self-administration of a low dose of cocaine over 9 weeks did not significantly affect DAT availability in any brain region (Czoty et al., 2007). Likewise, rhesus monkeys employed in a within-subject, longitudinal design showed increased 5HT2A receptor availability following a 3-month period of cocaine self-administration (Sawyer et al., 2012). Collectively, these studies demonstrate substantial but yet to be fully elucidated plasticity of monoamine systems in response to exposure to stimulants.

Human studies that have used functional imaging to characterize the effects of psychostimulant use on neurobiology have focused primarily on long-term changes in individuals with a complex history of multidrug use. Similar to nonhuman primates, chronic exposure to stimulant drugs in humans may also lead to significant changes in neuronal markers of dopaminergic function. PET studies characterizing dopamine D2 receptors have reliably documented long-lasting decreases in D2 receptor density in stimulant abusers (Volkow & Fowler, 2000). The reduction in D2 receptor function may further decrease the sensitivity of reward circuits to stimulation by natural rewards and increase the risk for drug taking (Volkow, Fowler, Wang, & Swanson, 2004). Interestingly, no difference in D1 receptor density was observed between cocaine-dependent subjects and matched controls (Martinez et al., 2009). In cocaine abusers, DAT density appears to be elevated shortly after cocaine abstinence but then to normalize with long-term detoxification (Malison et al., 1998). Methamphetamine also induces changes in the density of brain dopamine markers in human users

(Johanson et al., 2006; McCann, Szabo, Scheffel, Dannals, & Ricaurte, 1998; Sekine et al., 2001; Volkow, Chang, Wang, Fowler, Ding, et al., 2001; Volkow, Chang, Wang, Fowler, Franceschi et al., 2001a, 2001b). Interestingly, reduced DAT availability correlated with the duration of drug use, and impaired memory function was associated with a reduction in DAT availability (Volkow, Chang, Wang, Fowler, Leonido-Yee, et al., 2001). PET imaging to quantify DAT availability identified partial recovery of DAT binding in methamphetamine abusers during protracted abstinence (Volkow, Chang, Wang, Fowler, Franceschi, et al., 2001a). A subsequent study found that memory deficits in abstinent methamphetamine users were associated with decreases in striatal DAT binding potentials (McCann et al., 2008). Lastly, NET availability in humans (Ding et al., 2010) was greater in subjects with a cocaine self-administration history compared to control groups.

PET imaging measures of protein binding *in vivo* are complemented by studies that have documented cocaine-induced changes in brain metabolic activity as a function of cocaine self-administration history (Henry et al., 2010). Experimentally, naive rhesus monkeys were given increasing access to cocaine self-administration, and PET imaging with fluorodeoxyglucose (FDG) was used to measure acute cocaine-induced changes in brain metabolism in the cocaine-naive state and during limited- and extended-access conditions. In the cocaine-naive state, cocaine-induced increases in brain metabolism were restricted to the anterior cingulate and medial prefrontal cortex, consistent with other studies reporting acute activation of the anterior cingulate by cocaine (Howell, Votaw, Goodman, & Lindsey, 2010; Murnane & Howell, 2010). Others have reported deficits in basal brain metabolic activity determined with PET imaging that were closely linked to cocaine-induced cognitive impairments in rhesus monkeys (Gould, Duke, & Nader, 2013; Gould, Gage, & Nader, 2012). Interestingly, increased cocaine exposure from limited through extended access, reported by Henry et al. (2010), recruited cocaine-induced metabolic effects in frontal cortical areas and within the striatum. In apparent contrast, tolerance to cocaine- and amphetamine-induced synaptic release of dopamine in the striatum was observed in these same animals under both access conditions (Kirkland Henry et al., 2009). It is noteworthy that blunting of dopamine release has also been recorded in cocaine-dependent humans, in experiments using PET imaging (Martinez et al., 2007). Accordingly, further investigation of the relationship between drug self-administration, tolerance to the dopaminergic effects of cocaine, and recruitment of cortical activation may be highly relevant toward efforts to develop treatments for cocaine addiction.

PET imaging has documented drug-induced brain metabolic effects in chronic cocaine users (Volkow, Mullani, Gould, Adler, & Krajewski, 1988). Measures of brain glucose metabolism with FDG in chronic users documented transient increases in metabolic activity in dopamine-associated brain regions during cocaine withdrawal (Volkow et al., 1991), whereas decreases in frontal brain metabolism persisted after months of detoxification. The same pattern of decreased glucose metabolism (Reivich et al., 1985) and perfusion deficits (Volkow et al., 1988) was observed in the prefrontal cortex of cocaine users who were imaged on multiple occasions. Moreover, detoxified cocaine abusers had a marked decrease in dopamine release as measured by PET imaging (Volkow et al., 1997a, 1997b). Self-reports of "high" induced by methylphenidate were also less intense in cocaine abusers. A recent study using fMRI during a working memory task in cocaine-dependent subjects showed impaired activation in frontal, striatal, and thalamic brain regions (Moeller et al., 2010). Importantly, thalamic activation significantly correlated with response to cognitive behavioral therapy in combination with pharmacotherapy that included amphetamine and modafinil. Lastly, regional brain glucose metabolism has been characterized in conjunction with dopamine D2 receptor availability (Volkow, Chang, Wang, Fowler, Ding, et al., 2001). Reductions in striatal D2 receptors were associated with decreased metabolic activity in the orbital frontal cortex and anterior cingulate cortex in detoxified individuals. In contrast, the orbital frontal cortex was hypermetabolic in active cocaine abusers (Volkow et al., 1991). In addition, chronic methamphetamine users showed reduced striatal D2 receptors, the loss of which was related to the function of the orbitofrontal cortex (Volkow, Chang, Wang, Fowler, Ding, et al., 2001), a region important for executive functions. Collectively, these findings observed in stimulant abusers document the significant dysregulation of dopamine systems that are reflected in brain metabolic changes in areas involved in reward circuitry.

4. EVALUATION OF MONOAMINE TRANSPORTER INHIBITORS AND SUBSTRATES ON ABUSE-RELATED EFFECTS OF PSYCHOSTIMULANTS

The acute and chronic effects of abused psychostimulants on monoamine transporters and associated neurobiology have encouraged development of candidate medications that target these transporters. It is theoretically possible to develop medications that might block psychostimulant effects at monoamine transporters without affecting normal transporter function to mediate uptake of endogenous monoamines. For example, DAT mutants have been identified that have low affinity for cocaine but transport dopamine normally (Thomsen, Han, et al., 2009), and one theme in medication development has focused on compounds that might function as stimulant antagonists with lesser effects on dopamine transport (Meltzer, Liu, Blanchette, Blundell, & Madras, 2002; Rothman, Dersch, Ananthan, & Partilla, 2009; Rothman et al., 1993). To date, though, these efforts have not yielded promising compounds, and research has focused instead on compounds that function as monoamine transporter inhibitors or substrates. In the broader context of medication development for drug abuse, this constitutes an example of an "agonist" approach to drug abuse treatment (Grabowski, Shearer, Merrill, & Negus, 2004; Lile & Nader, 2003; Rothman, Blough, & Baumann, 2002; Rothman et al., 2007). Agonist approaches are typified by the use of opioid agonists like methadone or buprenorphine to treat opioid dependence or the use of nicotine formulations to treat tobacco dependence. In both cases, treatment is accomplished by chronic delivery of a medication that shares pharmacodynamic effects with the abused drug, and utility as an antiaddiction medication is associated with four attributes. First, agonist medications can be expected to produce some level of reinforcing effect similar to that produced by the abused drug, and this reinforcing effect can be leveraged by clinicians to promote medication compliance and reinforce therapeutically desirable behaviors. Second, agonist medications also mitigate withdrawal from the abused drug by replacing effects of the abused drug at the molecular target. Third, ideal agonist medications have a relatively slow onset of action and long duration of action relative to the abused drug. The slow onset of action is thought to reduce abuse liability, and the long duration of action facilitates maintenance of stable drug levels to minimize cycling of drug effects and associated biological adaptations. In a last and related point, agonist medications are administered via routes of administration (e.g., oral, sublingual, or transdermal) that contribute to slow onset and long duration while also being safer than intravenous or smoked routes of administration common in addiction.

The remainder of this review will focus on evidence for the efficacy of chronic treatment with monoamine transporter inhibitors and substrates to reduce abuse-related effects of stimulants in preclinical assays of stimulant self-administration, drug discrimination, and reinstatement. Most of this work has evaluated modulation of abuse-related effects of cocaine, but, where available, data on modulation of abuse-related effects of other stimulants will also be considered. Effects of monoamine transporter inhibitors will be discussed first, followed by review of data with transporter substrates. In considering deployment of monoamine transporter inhibitors and substrates as agonist-type medications to treat stimulant abuse, the safety and abuse liability of the medications are an obvious concern, and this will also be addressed.

4.1. Effects of monoamine transporter inhibitors

Preclinical studies in nonhuman primates provide convincing evidence that selective inhibitors of dopamine uptake may be useful pharmacotherapies in the treatment of cocaine abuse. Several cocaine analogs and other DAT inhibitors have been developed and characterized for their ability to reduce cocaine self-administration. Perhaps the largest class of compounds studied is the 3-phenyltropane analogs (Carroll, Howell, & Kuhar, 1999). The phenyltropane analog phenyl 3-(4-chlorophenyl)-8-methyl-8-azabicyclo [3.2.1]octane-2-carboxylate (RTI-113) effectively decreased cocaine self-administration in squirrel monkeys (Howell, Czoty, Kuhar, & Carrol, 2000) and rhesus monkeys (Negus, Mello, Kimmel, Howell, & Carroll, 2009) trained under second-order schedules of i.v. cocaine delivery. Moreover, RTI-113 maintained its effectiveness when the unit dose of cocaine was increased from 0.1 to 0.3 mg/kg/injection, indicating that the ability of RTI-113 to suppress cocaine self-administration could not be surmounted by a higher dose of cocaine (Howell et al., 2000). However, doses of RTI-113 that suppressed cocaine self-administration also caused a general disruption of operant behavior maintained by a comparable schedule of stimulus termination (Howell et al., 2000) or food delivery (Negus, Baumann, Rothman, Mello, & Blough, 2009). Similar results have been obtained with the cocaine analog 2β-propanoyl-3β-(4-tolyl)-tropane (PTT) in rhesus monkeys trained under a fixed-interval schedule of i.v. cocaine delivery (Nader, Grant, Davies, Mach, & Childers, 1997). Presession administration of PTT decreased response rates and total session intake at multiple unit doses of cocaine (0.03 and 0.1 mg/kg/injection). The effectiveness of selective DAT inhibitors to decrease cocaine self-administration extends to phenylpiperazine derivatives. 1-[2-[bis-(4-fluorophenyl)methoxy]ethyl]-4-(3-phenylpropyl)piperazine (GBR 12909) dose-dependently decreased cocaine self-administration in rhesus monkeys trained under multiple FR schedules of i.v. cocaine and food delivery (Glowa, Wojnicki, Matecka, & Bacher, 1995). Although GBR 12909 decreased rates of responding maintained by cocaine and food, large decreases in cocaine-maintained responding could be obtained at doses of GBR 12909 that had little effect on food-maintained responding. Hence, there was evidence for a selective decrease in cocaine-maintained responding at a low unit dose of cocaine (0.01 mg/kg/injection). However, the selectivity was not evident at a higher unit dose of cocaine (0.056 mg/kg/injection). When GBR 12909 was administered chronically as a decanoate derivative, selective reductions in cocaine self-administration were sustained over a 4-week period (Glowa et al., 1996).

A subsequent series of studies was conducted in nonhuman primates that evaluated the effectiveness of DAT inhibitors in reducing cocaine self-administration, and PET neuroimaging quantified DAT occupancy at behaviorally relevant doses. Selective DAT inhibitors were effective in reducing cocaine self-administration but only at high levels of DAT occupancy. For example, effective doses of the DAT-selective inhibitor RTI-113, which dose-dependently reduced cocaine-maintained responding, produced DAT occupancies between 72% and 84% (Wilcox et al., 2002). Similar results were observed with other DAT-selective inhibitors, including the phenyltropane RTI-177 and the phenylpiperazine GBR 12909 (Lindsey et al., 2004). At doses that decreased rates of cocaine self-administration by 50%, DAT occupancy was approximately 70% for both compounds. Clearly, DAT inhibitors can be effective in reducing cocaine self-administration. However, high levels of DAT occupancy may be required.

A possible limitation to the use of selective DAT inhibitors as medications for treatment of cocaine addiction is their potential for abuse, given their documented reinforcing effects (Howell & Wilcox, 2001). Selective DAT inhibitors, including phenyltropanes (Howell, Carroll, Votaw, Goodman, & Kimmel, 2007; Howell et al., 2000; Lindsey et al., 2004; Wilcox et al., 2002) and phenylpiperazines (Bergman et al., 1989; Howell & Byrd, 1991; Lindsey et al., 2004), reliably maintain self-administration behavior in nonhuman primates. However, several selective DAT inhibitors maintained lower rates of responding compared with cocaine across a broad range of doses, even though DAT occupancy was equal to or greater than that observed for cocaine (Howell et al., 2007; Lindsey et al., 2004; Wilcox et al., 2002). In behavioral studies in rodents and nonhuman primates, these compounds had a slower onset and a longer duration of action compared with cocaine (Howell et al., 2000; Kimmel, Joyce, Carroll, & Kuhar, 2001). Moreover, in PET neuroimaging studies that characterized the time course of drug uptake in the brain, there was a clear trend toward an inverse relationship between the time to peak uptake of drugs in the striatum and the peak number of infusions received under a progressive-ratio schedule of i.v. self-administration, such that the faster-onset drugs produced greater levels of responding relative to the slower-onset drugs (Kimmel et al., 2008). There also was a close correspondence between the time course of drug uptake in the brain and drug-induced increases in extracellular dopamine in the striatum (Ginsburg et al., 2005; Kimmel, O'Connor, Carroll, & Howell, 2007; Kimmel et al., 2008). Hence, the reinforcing effects and pattern of drug self-administration are likely influenced by pharmacokinetics in addition to steady-state levels of DAT occupancy. Accordingly, pharmacokinetic considerations should play an important role in medication development.

A number of clinical studies suggest that the wake-promoting drug modafinil may improve the clinical outcomes for treatment of cocaine dependence (Anderson et al., 2009; Dackis, Kampman, Lynch, Pettinati, & O'Brien, 2005; Dackis et al., 2003; Hart, Haney, Vosburg, Rubin, & Foltin, 2008), although a recent study did not find a significant main effect of modafinil on the rate or duration of cocaine use in cocaine-dependent patients (Dackis et al., 2012). The potential therapeutic effects of modafinil for the treatment of cocaine dependence may involve a DAT-mediated mechanism (Volkow et al., 2009; Zolkowska et al., 2009). To this end, recent studies in rhesus monkeys demonstrated that the *in vivo* effects of modafinil at the DAT are similar to other stimulants, such as cocaine (Andersen et al., 2010; Newman, Negus, Lozama, Prisinzano, & Mello, 2010). Modafinil induced nocturnal locomotor-stimulant effects, reinstated extinguished responding previously maintained by cocaine and exhibited cocaine-like discriminative-stimulus effects. An effective dose of modafinil resulted in approximately 60% DAT occupancy in the striatum and significantly increased extracellular dopamine levels, comparable to effects observed following cocaine doses that reliably maintain self-administration (Votaw et al., 2002; Wilcox et al., 2005). Importantly, chronic treatment with modafinil selectively reduced cocaine self-administration compared to food-maintained behavior (Newman et al., 2010). Collectively, these results document low-potency DAT-related effects in nonhuman primates that may be relevant for its therapeutic effectiveness in humans. Regarding its abuse potential, low potency at the DAT appears to limit modafinil self-administration in nonhuman primates

(Gold & Balster, 1996) and its abuse liability in humans (Jasinski, 2000; Vosburg, Hart, Haney, Rubin, & Foltin, 2010).

Preclinical studies have clearly indicated that serotonin plays an important role in the behavioral effects of cocaine. Acute administration of SERT inhibitors attenuates the behavioral-stimulant effects of cocaine in squirrel monkeys (Howell & Byrd, 1995; Howell, Czoty, & Byrd, 1997) and decreases cocaine self-administration in rodents (Carroll, Lac, Asencio, & Kragh, 1990) and nonhuman primates (Czoty, Ginsburg, & Howell, 2002; Kleven & Woolverton, 1993). The SERT inhibitor alaproclate also attenuated cocaine-induced increases in extracellular dopamine in squirrel monkeys (Czoty et al., 2002) and cocaine-induced activation of prefrontal cortex in rhesus monkeys (Howell et al., 2002). Moreover, the SERT inhibitor fluoxetine attenuated cue-induced reinstatement of cocaine self-administration in rodents (Baker, Tran-Nguyen, Fuchs, & Neisewander, 2001; Burmeister, Lungren, & Neisewander, 2003) and decreased ratings of cocaine's positive subjective effects in a human laboratory setting (Walsh, Preston, Sullivan, Fromme, & Bigelow, 1994). Consistent with these findings, acute administration of the SERT inhibitors fluoxetine and citalopram attenuated cocaine-induced reinstatement in rhesus monkeys (Fig. 4.2; unpublished data). Fluoxetine also attenuated reinstatement by the psychostimulants MDMA and benzylpiperazine (McClung, Fantegrossi, & Howell, 2010). Despite the overwhelming evidence suggesting that SERT inhibitors can reduce abuse-related effects of cocaine, fluoxetine has typically failed to show reductions in cocaine abuse in clinical trials (Grabowski et al., 1995; Lima, Reisser, Soares, & Farrell, 2003; Schmitz et al., 2001; Winstanley, Bigelow, Silverman, Johnson, & Strain, 2011). This may be due in part to the different dosing regimens employed by the preclinical and clinical studies; preclinical studies generally employ single-dose treatments, whereas clinical studies administer the drug chronically. However, clinical studies with more selective SERT inhibitors have shown more promise. For example, citalopram reduced cocaine use in cocaine-dependent patients (Moeller et al., 2007) and sertraline delayed relapse in recently abstinent cocaine-dependent patients (Oliveto et al., 2012).

A recent study was the first to examine the effects of chronic fluoxetine treatment at clinically relevant concentrations in a nonhuman primate model of cocaine abuse (Sawyer et al., 2012). Chronic fluoxetine treatment attenuated cocaine-induced reinstatement and dopamine overflow. Furthermore, these effects persist up to 6 weeks after the conclusion of

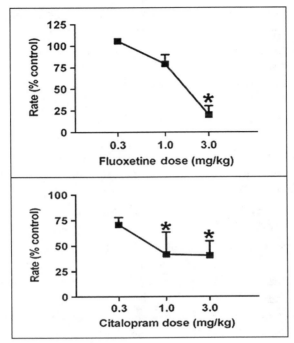

Figure 4.2 Effects of acute IM pretreatments with the SERT inhibitors fluoxetine or citalopram on cocaine-induced reinstatement of extinguished cocaine self-administration in rhesus monkeys ($N = 3$). Subjects were trained to self-administer cocaine under a second-order schedule and could take a maximum of 0.5 mg/kg per session 5 days per week. Subsequently, saline was substituted for cocaine, and once extinction criteria were met (response rates <20% of cocaine-maintained rates), response-independent cocaine (0.1 mg/kg) was administered i.v. prior to extinction sessions. Both fluoxetine and citalopram significantly attenuated cocaine-induced reinstatement (*$p < 0.05$ with respect to control).

fluoxetine treatment. It is also noteworthy that RTI-112, a mixed-action inhibitor of DAT and SERT, significantly reduced cocaine self-administration by rhesus monkeys at doses producing levels of DAT occupancy below the limit of detection (Lindsey et al., 2004). Furthermore, coadministration of the selective SERT inhibitors fluoxetine or citalopram and the selective DAT inhibitor 3β-(4-chlorophenyl)-2β-[3-(4β-methylphenyl)isoxazol-5-yl]tropane hydrochloride (RTI-336) produced more robust reductions in cocaine self-administration than RTI-336 alone, even at comparable levels of DAT occupancy by RTI-336 (Howell et al., 2007). Collectively, there is convincing evidence that SERT inhibition can enhance suppression of cocaine self-administration by DAT inhibitors, indicating that dual DAT/SERT inhibitors warrant consideration as viable medications for cocaine addiction.

NET inhibitors appear less promising as therapeutics for psychostimulant abuse. Studies in squirrel monkeys indicate that NET inhibition may contribute to the discriminative-stimulus effects of cocaine (Spealman, 1995) and cocaine-induced reinstatement (Platt et al., 2007). However, pretreatment with desipramine in rhesus monkeys trained under a second-order schedule of i.v. cocaine delivery had inconsistent effects and actually increased cocaine self-administration in some animals (Mello et al., 1990). In addition, food-maintained behavior was affected by pretreatment doses that influenced drug self-administration, demonstrating a lack of selectivity. In another study, pretreatment with desipramine in rhesus monkeys trained under multiple FR schedules of i.v. cocaine and food delivery had no effect on cocaine self-administration (Kleven & Woolverton, 1990). Desipramine was one of the first medications reported to be effective in an outpatient, controlled clinical trial. An initial meta-analysis found desipramine to be effective in reducing relapse to cocaine use (Levin & Lehman, 1991), but subsequent clinical trials did not confirm its effectiveness (Arndt, Dorozynsky, Woody, McLellan, & O'Brien, 1992; Campbell, Thomas, Gabrielli, Liskow, & Powell, 1994). A recent study with atomoxetine, a NET inhibitor used in the treatment of attention deficit hyperactivity disorder (ADHD), provided no support for its utility in the treatment of cocaine dependence (Walsh et al., 2013).

A recent study in rhesus monkeys evaluated the effects of chronic methylphenidate, a DAT and NET inhibitor used in the treatment of ADHD, and found that methylphenidate treatment either disrupted food-maintained behavior or increased cocaine self-administration (Czoty, Martelle, Gould, & Nader, 2013). Indatraline is an example of a nonselective monoamine transporter inhibitor with similar potencies at DAT, SERT, and NET. Pretreatment with indatraline in rhesus monkeys trained under alternating daily sessions of cocaine and food availability produced dose-dependent decreases in cocaine self-administration over a broad range of cocaine doses (Negus, Brandt, & Mello, 1999). Moreover, reductions in cocaine self-administration were sustained during 7 consecutive days of indatraline pretreatment. When substituted for cocaine in self-administration sessions, indatraline maintained lower rates of responding compared with cocaine. However, indatraline had undesirable side effects, including behavioral stereotypies and trends toward weight loss that limit its clinical utility. In clinical studies, mazindol, a DAT and NET inhibitor used in the treatment of obesity, did not alter the subjective effects of cocaine in a human laboratory study (Preston, Sullivan, Berger, & Bigelow, 1993). Moreover, in a 6-week, placebo-controlled study in cocaine-dependent subjects, mazindol did not differ from placebo in reducing cocaine use and mazindol treatment was not well tolerated (Stine, Krystal, Kosten, & Charney, 1995).

4.2. Effects of monoamine transporter substrates

Studies with amphetamine have provided the most compelling evidence to date for efficacy of monoamine transporter substrates to treat cocaine addiction. Clinical trials (Grabowski et al., 2001; Mariani et al., 2012) and drug self-administration studies in humans (Greenwald, Lundahl, & Steinmiller, 2010; Rush, Stoops, Sevak, & Hays, 2010), nonhuman primates (Czoty, Martelle, Garrett, & Nader, 2008; Negus, 2003; Negus & Mello, 2003a, 2003b), and rats (Chiodo, Lack, & Roberts, 2008; Thomsen, Barrett, Negus, & Caine, 2013) agree in showing that amphetamine maintenance reduces cocaine-taking behavior. An example of this effect is shown in Fig. 4.3 (Negus & Mello, 2003b). In this study, rhesus monkeys were equipped with chronic double-lumen i.v. catheters and trained to respond for food or cocaine during alternating daily components of food and cocaine availability. Self-administered cocaine injections (0.001–0.1 mg/kg/injection) were delivered through one lumen of the double-lumen catheter and the second lumen was used to chronically infuse saline or various amphetamine doses (0.01–0.1 mg/kg/h; 23 h/day) for periods of 7–28 consecutive days. Amphetamine produced a dose-dependent decrease in both cocaine- and food-maintained responding; however, tolerance developed to amphetamine effects on food-maintained responding, and for most of the treatment period, monkeys responded at saline control levels for food pellets. Moreover, all monkeys maintained their body weights during amphetamine treatment. Conversely, cocaine self-administration was nearly eliminated by the fifth day of treatment, remained suppressed for the remainder of treatment, and gradually recovered only after termination of treatment.

Five additional points also warrant mention. First, the experiment in Fig. 4.3 shows similar amphetamine-induced reductions in cocaine- and food-maintained responding during the first 7 days of treatment, and behavioral selectivity of amphetamine effects did not emerge until after the first week. However, other experiments with amphetamine have shown that,

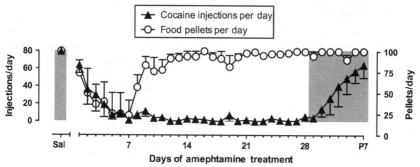

Figure 4.3 Effects of continuous treatment with D-amphetamine (0.1 mg/kg/h, IV) for 28 days on responding maintained by cocaine (0.01 mg/kg/injection, IV) and food pellets (1 g banana-flavored pellets) in rhesus monkeys ($N = 4$). Monkeys could earn a maximum of 80 cocaine injections and 100 food pellets each during alternating components of cocaine and food availability. Points above "Sal" show rates of cocaine- and food-maintained responding during saline treatment. Amphetamine treatment produced an initial decrease in cocaine- and food-maintained responding, but tolerance developed to effects on food-maintained responding, while cocaine self-administration was depressed throughout the 28-day treatment period. *Adapted from Negus and Mello (2003b).*

even at these early time points, amphetamine can selectively decrease cocaine self-administration more than food-maintained responding, and this effect is apparent across a broad range of self-administered cocaine doses (Negus & Mello, 2003b). Second, amphetamine reduced cocaine self-administration at daily amphetamine doses of 0.74–2.3 mg/kg/day (0.032–0.1 mg/kg/h × 23 h/day). This dose range overlaps with the range of amphetamine doses that decreased cocaine use in clinical trials (Grabowski et al., 2004; Mariani et al., 2012) and with recommended amphetamine doses for treating disorders such as narcolepsy and attention deficit hyperactivity disorder. Third, amphetamine maintenance also reduced cocaine self-administration under other schedules of reinforcement, including progressive-ratio schedules (Chiodo et al., 2008; Czoty et al., 2008; Negus & Mello, 2003a) and concurrent schedules of cocaine versus food choice (Banks, Blough, & Negus, 2013; Negus & Mello, 2003b; Thomsen et al., 2013). Fourth, selective reduction in cocaine self-administration by amphetamine or related medications depends on sustained maintenance of treatment and is not apparent with acute treatment. Indeed, acute treatment with amphetamine or related medications can increase self-administration of low cocaine doses or of saline (Thomsen et al., 2013), a phenomenon that may be related to cocaine-like discriminative-stimulus effects of these medications (see later). Lastly, the profile of amphetamine effects on cocaine- and food-maintained responding under this procedure is unusual relative to effects of other candidate medications. For example, dopamine receptor antagonists or opioid receptors agonists/antagonists may also decrease cocaine self-administration in this procedure, but those effects are often transient, and rates of food-maintained responding are often reduced as much or more than rates of cocaine self-administration (Do Carmo, Mello, Rice, Folk, & Negus, 2006; Negus & Banks, 2011; Negus & Mello, 2002, 2004; Negus, Mello, Portoghese, & Lin, 1997; Negus et al., 1996).

Amphetamine has also been evaluated in assays of cocaine discrimination and reinstatement of cocaine self-administration. When administered acutely, amphetamine substitutes fully for the discriminative-stimulus effects of cocaine (D'Mello & Stolerman, 1977; Negus, Baumann, et al., 2009), which is consistent with its related mechanism of action, its cocaine-like subjective effects in humans (Fischman et al., 1976), and its putative potential to function as an agonist medication for treatment of cocaine addiction. As might be expected from its similar discriminative-stimulus effects, acute amphetamine also reinstates extinguished cocaine self-administration (Gerber & Stretch, 1975; Schenk & Partridge, 1999). However, chronic amphetamine administration produces cross-tolerance to both the discriminative-stimulus effects and reinstating effects of cocaine (Norman, Norman, Hall, & Tsibulsky, 1999; Peltier, Li, Lytle, Taylor, & Emmett-Oglesby, 1996). Taken as a whole, these findings converge in suggesting that amphetamine maintenance reduces expression of the abuse-related effects of cocaine.

In contrast to the growing literature describing effects of amphetamine maintenance on abuse-related reinforcing, discriminative stimulus, and reinstating effects of cocaine, far fewer studies have examined effects of amphetamine maintenance on abuse-related effects of other stimulants. Amphetamine treatment produces tolerance to its own discriminative-stimulus effects (Barrett, Caul, & Smith, 2005) and cross-tolerance to the amphetamine-like discriminative-stimulus effects of the weak transporter substrate cathine (Schechter, 1990). However, it has been suggested that transporter substrates may function more effectively as medications to treat abuse of transporter inhibitor stimulants like cocaine, and conversely, transporter inhibitors may function as more effective medications for treatment of addiction to transporter substrate stimulants like amphetamine (Stoops & Rush, 2013).

Many transporter substrates other than amphetamine have been identified, and one important dimension along which they vary is relative selectivity to promote release of dopamine/norepinephrine versus serotonin.
Amphetamine has relatively high selectivity as a substrate for DAT/NET
versus SERT, and it occupies one end of this spectrum, whereas the
serotonin-selective releaser fenfluramine occupies the other end of this spectrum (higher relative potency as a substrate for SERT vs. DAT/NET).
Other compounds have been identified with DAT/NET versus SERT
selectivities intermediate between those of amphetamine and fenfluramine
(Baumann et al., 2012; Rothman, Clark, Partilla, & Baumann, 2003;
Rothman, Katsnelson, et al., 2002). Preclinical metrics of abuse liability correlate positively with DAT/NET selectivity, such that DAT/NET-selective
substrates like amphetamine reliably maintain drug self-administration and
produce other abuse-related effects such as cocaine-like discriminative-
stimulus effects; however, expression of these effects declines as DAT/NET
versus SERT selectivity declines (Bauer et al., 2013; Wee et al., 2005). Consequently, manipulation of DAT/NET versus SERT selectivity has offered
one potential strategy to reduce abuse liability of transporter substrates as
candidate medications. Moreover, as noted earlier, chronic stimulant exposure associated with abuse can disrupt both dopaminergic and serotonergic
signaling, and this has led to the hypothesis that stimulant abuse may produce
a "dual-deficit" in dopaminergic and serotonergic systems that can be mitigated by medications with dual action at DAT and SERT (Rothman,
Blough, & Baumann, 2008).

In view of these considerations, recent studies have compared changes
in cocaine self-administration produced by a series of transporter substrates
that varied in their selectivity for DAT/NET versus SERT (Banks,
Blough, & Negus, 2011; Kohut, Fivel, Blough, Rothman, & Mello, 2013;
Negus, Baumann, et al., 2009; Negus et al., 2007; Rothman et al., 2005).
Illustrative results are shown in Fig. 4.4 from an experimental procedure
similar to that shown earlier with amphetamine (Negus et al., 2007). Specifically, responding maintained in rhesus monkeys by food and cocaine
(0.01 mg/kg/injection) was evaluated during continuous infusion for 7
consecutive days with saline or with various compounds including methamphetamine (DAT/NET > SERT), 1-naphthyl-2-aminopropane (PAL-287)
(DAT/NET = SERT), and fenfluramine (DAT/NET < SERT). These three
transporter substrates all produced dose-dependent and sustained decreases in
cocaine self-administration, but they differed in their relative effects on
food-maintained responding. Like amphetamine, methamphetamine

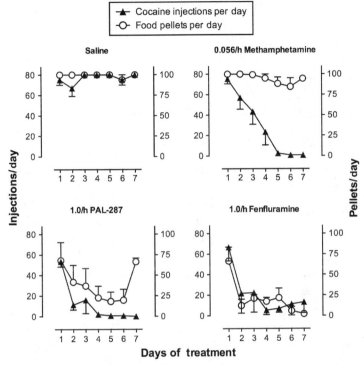

Figure 4.4 Effects of 7-day treatment with saline or transporter substrates on responding maintained by cocaine (0.01 mg/kg/injection) or food pellets by rhesus monkeys. Monkeys could earn a maximum of 80 cocaine injections and 100 food pellets each day during alternating components of cocaine and food availability. Treatment consisted of continuous infusion with saline (upper left) or optimal treatment doses of the DAT/NET > SERT-selective substrate methamphetamine (0.056 mg/kg/h), the nonselective DAT/NET/SERT substrate PAL-287 (1.0 mg/kg/h), or the SERT > DAT/NET-selective substrate fenfluramine (1.0 mg/kg/h). All substrates produced sustained decreases in cocaine self-administration, and behavioral selectivity to decrease cocaine-maintained responding corresponded to pharmacological selectivity for DAT/NET versus SERT. *Adapted from Negus et al. (2007).*

selectively decreased cocaine self-administration at a dose that produced little effect on food-maintained responding, and in this experiment, the selective reduction in cocaine self-administration was evident during the first days of treatment. Similar results have been obtained in this or similar procedures with other transporter substrates selective for DAT/NET versus SERT including phenmetrazine and phentermine (Negus, Baumann, et al., 2009; Negus et al., 2007; Wojnicki, Rothman, Rice, & Glowa, 1999), and these results with methamphetamine also agree with a clinical trial that showed efficacy of methamphetamine maintenance to decrease cocaine use by cocaine-dependent patients (Mooney et al., 2009). Conversely, the doses of PAL-287 and fenfluramine that reduced cocaine self-administration also produced concurrent decreases in food-maintained responding. Similar results were also found with these and other compounds in a different procedure that assessed concurrent choice between cocaine and food in rhesus monkeys (Banks et al., 2011). Specifically, chronic infusion with DAT/NET-selective compounds reduced cocaine choice and promoted reallocation of behavior to food choice, but nonselective or SERT-selective compounds only reduced overall responding without affecting cocaine versus food choice. Taken together, these results suggest that decreasing pharmacological selectivity for DAT/NET versus SERT correlated with decreased behavioral selectivity to reduce cocaine- versus food-maintained responding. The implication for medications development is that SERT activity may reduce abuse liability of transporter substrates but it is also associated with recruitment of other undesirable effects likely to impede use of these compounds as medications.

Selectivity for DAT/NET versus SERT also influences the discriminative stimulus and reinstating effects of transporter substrates. For example, the cocaine-like discriminative-stimulus effects (Negus et al., 2007) and reinstatement effects (Burmeister et al., 2003; Schenk, Hely, Gittings, Lake, & Daniela, 2008; Spealman, Barrett-Larimore, Rowlett, Platt, & Khroyan, 1999) of transporter substrates decline as selectivity for DAT/NET versus SERT declines. Acute fenfluramine treatment attenuated cue-induced reinstatement and partially reduced cocaine-induced reinstatement of cocaine self-administration (Burmeister et al., 2003); however, effects of chronic treatment with transporter substrates other than amphetamine have not been examined in studies of cocaine discrimination or cocaine reinstatement.

Little work has been done to examine effects of transporter substrates other than amphetamine on abuse-related effects of stimulants other than cocaine. In one study, acute pretreatment with the DAT/NET > SERT substrate phentermine decreased self-administration of the DAT-selective uptake inhibitor GBR12909, suggesting that substrates may be effective to reduce abuse liability of transporter inhibitors other than cocaine (Wojnicki et al., 1999). Alternatively, a regimen of chronic methamphetamine administration increased subsequent self-administration of methamphetamine (Woolverton, Cervo, & Johanson, 1984), a finding potentially consistent with the hypothesis that transporter inhibitors will be more effective than substrates for treating abuse of substrates (Stoops & Rush, 2013).

However, this study used high methamphetamine doses (up to 40 mg/kg/day) relative to doses that effectively decreased cocaine self-administration, and methamphetamine self-administration was evaluated 1–1.5 months after methamphetamine treatment rather than during treatment.

Although increases in SERT activity reduce abuse liability of transporter substrates, increased SERT activity is also associated with other undesirable effects that are likely to limit clinical utility. Consequently, other approaches are also being explored to reduce abuse liability of substrate medications while retaining both DAT/NET selectivity and behavioral selectivity to reduce cocaine-maintained responding. One alternative approach is to use prodrugs that generate DAT/NET-selective substrates as active metabolites. Use of prodrugs has the potential to reduce abuse liability by delaying onset of drug action after drug administration (Schindler, Panlilio, & Thorndike, 2009). As one example, lisdexamfetamine is a schedule II drug approved for treatment of ADHD, and it is a prodrug for amphetamine that has a slower onset of action and functions as a less reliable reinforcer than amphetamine (Heal et al., 2013). As another example, phendimetrazine is a weak transporter inhibitor that also functions as a prodrug for the DAT/NET-selective substrate phenmetrazine (Banks, Blough, Fennel, Snyder, & Negus, 2013; Banks, Blough, & Negus, 2013; Rothman, Katsnelson, et al., 2002). Phendimetrazine is a clinically available schedule III anorectic agent, and preclinical studies suggest it has lower abuse liability than its metabolite phenmetrazine or other DAT/NET-selective substrates like amphetamine (Corwin, Woolverton, Schuster, & Johanson, 1987). Despite being a weak transporter inhibitor with low abuse liability, Fig. 4.5 shows that maintenance on phendimetrazine produces a reduction in cocaine versus food choice by rhesus monkeys that is similar to the effect produced by amphetamine (Banks, Blough, & Negus, 2013).

4.3. Safety

Studies cited earlier provide evidence to suggest that medications functioning as DAT inhibitors or substrates may have efficacy to decrease abuse-related effects of cocaine in animals and to decrease stimulant use by addicted humans. However, the clinical utility of these medications will depend not only on their efficacy but also on their safety. This issue has been addressed in detail by others (Grabowski et al., 2004; Mariani et al., 2012), but three points will be highlighted here. First, many DAT inhibitors and substrates are already available for treatment of other disorders including obesity,

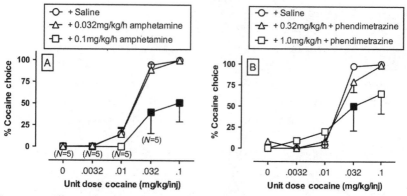

Figure 4.5 Effects of 14-day treatment with either amphetamine or phendimetrazine on choice between cocaine and food by rhesus monkeys. Cocaine injections and food pellets were available simultaneously during daily experimental sessions consisting of five sequential components, with the available cocaine dose increasing from 0 (no injection) to 0.1 mg/kg/injection across components. Continuous infusion with amphetamine ($N=6$) or phendimetrazine ($N=4$) produced rightward shifts in the cocaine-choice dose–effect curve and promoted reallocation of behavior away from cocaine choice and toward food choice. Filled points indicate a significant effect of amphetamine or phendimetrazine versus saline as determined by two-way analysis of variance followed by the LSD multiple comparisons post hoc test. Notations of "$N=5$" in the left panel indicate that five of six monkeys contributed to the point during treatment with 0.1 mg/kg/h amphetamine, and one monkey failed to respond for either food or cocaine. *Adapted from Banks et al. (2013).*

narcolepsy, and ADHD, and particularly for the last of these indications, treatment involves chronic administration to a wide range of subjects including children. Consequently, there is already substantial clinical experience in the use of these medications that could guide strategies for their use to treat addiction. Second, the constellation of undesirable effects associated with these medications is well established and, in particular, includes cardiovascular effects and abuse liability. Although these effects would remain a clear concern given the risk of diversion and in patients being treated for addiction, existing data suggest that histories of stimulant abuse sufficient to warrant pharmacotherapy are likely to render patients tolerant to the cardiovascular effects and abuse liability of these compounds. For example, one recent study found that subjects with a history of "crack" cocaine use were tolerant to abuse-related subjective effects of amphetamine (Comer et al., 2013). More generally, it will be important to weigh risks associated with treatment against risks associated with continued use of the abused stimulant. Lastly, data from both preclinical and clinical studies cited earlier

suggest that subjects can be safely maintained on DAT inhibitors or substrates despite continued access to cocaine or other abuse stimulants. In particular, preclinical studies that show selective and sustained decreases in
cocaine self-administration with lesser or no effect on food-maintained
responding provide compelling evidence to suggest that reductions in
cocaine self-administration can be achieved without general disruption of
other adaptive behaviors (Mello & Negus, 1996). Moreover, data from
choice studies suggest that these medications may not only reduce cocaine
use but also promote reallocation of behavior toward responding maintained
by nondrug alternative reinforcers (Banks & Negus, 2012; Haney and
Spealman, 2008; Vocci & Appel, 2007).

5. CONCLUSION

Monoamine transporters, in general, and DATs, in particular, are critical molecular targets that mediate abuse-related effects of psychostimulants
such as cocaine and amphetamine. Moreover, chronic administration of
psychostimulants can cause enduring changes in neurobiology reflected in
dysregulation of monoamine neurochemistry and behavior. Findings
observed in stimulant abusers document significant dysregulation of dopamine systems that are associated with brain metabolic changes in areas
involved in reward circuitry and cognition. The current review has evaluated abundant evidence for the efficacy of monoamine transporter inhibitors
and releasers to reduce abuse-related effects of stimulants in preclinical assays
of stimulant self-administration, drug discrimination, and reinstatement,
providing a strong rationale for developing monoamine transporter inhibitors and releasers as medications for the treatment of stimulant addiction.
Amphetamine maintenance has shown strong translational evidence of efficacy and safety to reduce cocaine self-administration and warrants further
consideration as a candidate agonist medication for treatment of cocaine
addiction. In general, inhibitors produce less selective decreases than substrates in cocaine- versus food-maintained responding, and inhibitors
have been less effective than releasers in human laboratory studies and clinical trials of cocaine dependence. However, it remains to be determined
whether transporter inhibitors are more effective in the treatment of dependence to substrate-type stimulants such as amphetamine and methamphetamine. A possible limitation to the use of DAT inhibitors and substrates as
medications for treatment of cocaine addiction is their potential for abuse,
given their documented reinforcing effects. Previous approaches to mitigate

this concern have included pharmacokinetic considerations of medications with slow onset and extended duration of action and mixed-action compounds that target DAT and SERT. Future directions in drug discovery should identify novel medications that retain efficacy to decrease cocaine use but possess lower abuse liability and evaluate the degree to which efficacious medications can attenuate or reverse neurobiological effects of chronic cocaine use.

CONFLICT OF INTEREST

The authors have no conflicts of interest to declare.

ACKNOWLEDGMENTS

The authors would like to thank Susan Marshall for technical assistance in preparation of the chapter. This work is supported by Office of Research Infrastructure Programs/OD P51OD11132 (L. L. H.), DA 031246 (L. L. H.), and DA026946 (S. S. N.).

REFERENCES

Amara, S. G., & Kuhar, M. J. (1993). Neurotransmitter transporters: Recent progress. *Annual Review of Neuroscience, 16*, 73–93.

American_Psychiatric_Association, (2013). *Diagnostic and statistical manual of mental disorders* (5th ed.). Arlington, VA: American Psychiatric Publishing.

Andersen, M. L., Kessler, E., Murnane, K. S., McClung, J. C., Tufik, S., & Howell, L. L. (2010). Dopamine transporter-related effects of modafinil in rhesus monkeys. *Psychopharmacology, 210*, 439–448.

Anderson, A. L., Reid, M. S., Li, S. H., Holmes, T., Shemanski, L., Slee, A., et al. (2009). Modafinil for the treatment of cocaine dependence. *Drug and Alcohol Dependence, 104*, 133–139.

Arndt, I. O., Dorozynsky, L., Woody, G. E., McLellan, A. T., & O'Brien, C. P. (1992). Desipramine treatment of cocaine dependence in methadone-maintained patients. *Archives of General Psychiatry, 49*, 888–893.

Astier, B., Van Bockstaele, E. J., Aston-Jones, G., & Pieribone, V. A. (1990). Anatomical evidence for multiple pathways leading from the rostral ventrolateral medulla (nucleus paragigantocellularis) to the locus coeruleus in rat. *Neuroscience Letters, 118*, 141–146.

Ator, N. A., & Griffiths, R. R. (2003). Principles of drug abuse liability assessment in laboratory animals. *Drug and Alcohol Dependence, 70*, S55–S72.

Baker, D. A., Tran-Nguyen, T. L., Fuchs, R. A., & Neisewander, J. L. (2001). Influence of individual differences and chronic fluoxetine treatment on cocaine-seeking behavior in rats. *Psychopharmacology, 155*, 18–26.

Banks, M. L., Blough, B. E., Fennel, T. R., Snyder, R. W., & Negus, S. S. (2013). Effects of phendimetrazine treatment on cocaine vs food choice and extended-access cocaine consumption in rhesus monkeys. *Neuropsychopharmacology, 38*, 2698–2707.

Banks, M. L., Blough, B. E., & Negus, S. S. (2011). Effects of monoamine releasers with varying selectivity for releasing dopamine/norepinephrine versus serotonin on choice between cocaine and food in rhesus monkeys. *Behavioural Pharmacology, 22*, 824–836.

Banks, M. L., Blough, B. E., & Negus, S. S. (2013). Effects of 14-day treatment with the schedule III anorectic phendimetrazine on choice between cocaine and food in rhesus monkeys. *Drug and Alcohol Dependence, 131*, 204–213.

Banks, M. L., Czoty, P. W., Gage, H. D., Bounds, M. C., Garg, P. K., Garg, S., et al. (2008). Effects of cocaine and MDMA self-administration on serotonin transporter availability in monkeys. *Neuropsychopharmacology, 33*, 219–225.

Banks, M. L., & Negus, S. S. (2012). Preclinical determinants of drug choice under concurrent schedules of drug self-administration. *Advances in Pharmacological Sciences, 2012*, 281768.

Barnes, N. M., & Sharp, T. (1999). A review of central 5-HT receptors and their function. *Neuropharmacology, 38*, 1083–1152.

Barrett, R. J., Caul, W. F., & Smith, R. (2005). Withdrawal, tolerance, and sensitization to dopamine mediated interoceptive cues in rats trained on a three-lever drug-discrimination task. *Pharmacology, Biochemistry and Behavior, 81*, 1–8.

Bauer, C. T., Banks, M. L., Blough, B. E., & Negus, S. S. (2013). Use of intracranial self-stimulation to evaluate abuse-related and abuse-limiting effects of monoamine releasers in rats. *British Journal of Pharmacology, 168*, 850–862.

Baumann, M. H., Ayestas, M. A., Dersch, C. M., Brockington, A., Rice, K. C., & Rothman, R. B. (2000). Effects of phentermine and fenfluramine on extracellular dopamine and serotonin in rat nucleus accumbens: Therapeutic implications. *Synapse, 36*, 102–113.

Baumann, M. H., Ayestas, M. A., Jr., Partilla, J. S., Sink, J. R., Shulgin, A. T., Daley, P. F., et al. (2012). The designer methcathinone analogs, mephedrone and methylone, are substrates for monoamine transporters in brain tissue. *Neuropsychopharmacology, 37*, 1192–1203.

Baumann, M. H., & Rothman, R. B. (1998). Alterations in serotonergic responsiveness during cocaine withdrawal in rats: Similarities to major depression in humans. *Biological Psychiatry, 44*, 578–591.

Bergman, J., Kamien, J. B., & Spealman, R. D. (1990). Antagonism of cocaine self-administration by selective dopamine D(1) and D(2) antagonists. *Behavioural Pharmacology, 1*, 355–363.

Bergman, J., Madras, B. K., Johnson, S. E., & Spealman, R. D. (1989). Effects of cocaine and related drugs in nonhuman primates. III. Self-administration by squirrel monkeys. *The Journal of Pharmacology and Experimental Therapeutics, 251*, 150–155.

Biebuyck, J. (1990). Pharmacology and therapeutic applications of cocaine. *Anesthesiology, 73*, 518–531.

Boulay, D., Duterte-Boucher, D., Leroux-Nicollet, I., Naudon, L., & Costentin, J. (1996). Locomotor sensitization and decrease in [3H]mazindol binding to the dopamine transporter in the nucleus accumbens are delayed after chronic treatments by GBR12783 or cocaine. *The Journal of Pharmacology and Experimental Therapeutics, 278*, 330–337.

Bradberry, C. W. (2000). Acute and chronic dopamine dynamics in a nonhuman primate model of recreational cocaine use. *The Journal of Neuroscience, 20*, 7109–7115.

Burmeister, J. J., Lungren, E. M., & Neisewander, J. L. (2003). Effects of fluoxetine and d-fenfluramine on cocaine-seeking behavior in rats. *Psychopharmacology, 168*, 146–154.

Caine, S. B., & Koob, G. F. (1994). Effects of dopamine D-1 and D-2 antagonists on cocaine self-administration under different schedules of reinforcement in the rat. *The Journal of Pharmacology and Experimental Therapeutics, 270*, 209–218.

Caine, S. B., Negus, S. S., Mello, N. K., & Bergman, J. (2000). Effects of dopamine D1-like and D2-like agonists in rats trained to discriminate cocaine from saline: Influence of experimental history. *Experimental and Clinical Psychopharmacology, 8*, 404–414.

Campbell, J. L., Thomas, H. M., Gabrielli, W., Liskow, B. I., & Powell, B. J. (1994). Impact of desipramine or carbamazepine on patient retention in outpatient cocaine treatment: Preliminary findings. *Journal of Addictive Diseases, 13*, 191–199.

Carlezon, W. A., Jr., & Nestler, E. J. (2002). Elevated levels of GluR1 in the midbrain: A trigger for sensitization to drugs of abuse? *Trends in Neurosciences, 25,* 610–615.

Carpenter, M. B., & Sutin, J. (1983). *Human neuroanatomy.* Baltimore: Williams & Wilkins.

Carrasco, G. A., & Battaglia, G. (2007). Withdrawal from a single exposure to cocaine increases 5-HT2A receptor and G protein function. *Neuroreport, 18,* 51–55.

Carrasco, G. A., Van de Kar, L. D., Sullivan, N. R., Landry, M., Garcia, F., Muma, N. A., et al. (2006). Cocaine-mediated supersensitivity of 5-HT2A receptors in hypothalamic paraventricular nucleus is a withdrawal-induced phenomenon. *Neuroscience, 143,* 7–13.

Carroll, F. I., Howell, L. L., & Kuhar, M. J. (1999). Pharmacotherapies for treatment of cocaine abuse: Preclinical aspects. *Journal of Medicinal Chemistry, 42,* 2721–2736.

Carroll, M. E., Lac, S. T., Asencio, M., & Kragh, R. (1990). Fluoxetine reduces intravenous cocaine self-administration in rats. *Pharmacology, Biochemistry and Behavior, 35,* 237–244.

Carter, L. P., & Griffiths, R. R. (2009). Principles of laboratory assessment of drug abuse liability and implications for clinical development. *Drug and Alcohol Dependence, 105*(Suppl. 1), S14–S25.

Catterall, W. A., & Mackie, K. (2005). Local anesthetics. In J. G. Hardman & L. E. Limbird (Eds.), *The pharmacological basis of therapeutics* (pp. 369–388). New York: McGraw-Hill.

Chi, L., & Reith, M. E. (2003). Substrate-induced trafficking of the dopamine transporter in heterologously expressing cells and in rat striatal synaptosomal preparations. *The Journal of Pharmacology and Experimental Therapeutics, 307,* 729–736.

Chiodo, K. A., Lack, C. M., & Roberts, D. C. (2008). Cocaine self-administration reinforced on a progressive ratio schedule decreases with continuous D-amphetamine treatment in rats. *Psychopharmacology, 200,* 465–473.

Claye, L. H., Akunne, H. C., Davis, M. D., DeMattos, S., & Soliman, K. F. (1995). Behavioral and neurochemical changes in the dopaminergic system after repeated cocaine administration. *Molecular Neurobiology, 11,* 55–66.

Colpaert, F. C. (1999). Drug discrimination in neurobiology. *Pharmacology, Biochemistry and Behavior, 64,* 337–345.

Comer, S. D., Ashworth, J. B., Foltin, R. W., Johanson, C. E., Zacny, J. P., & Walsh, S. L. (2008). The role of human drug self-administration procedures in the development of medications. *Drug and Alcohol Dependence, 96,* 1–15.

Comer, S. D., Mogali, S., Saccone, P. A., Askalsky, P., Martinez, D., Walker, E. A., et al. (2013). Effects of acute oral naltrexone on the subjective and physiological effects of oral d-amphetamine and smoked cocaine in cocaine abusers. *Neuropsychopharmacology, 38,* 2427–2438.

Corwin, R. L., Woolverton, W. L., Schuster, C. R., & Johanson, C. E. (1987). Anorectics: Effects on food intake and self-administration in rhesus monkeys. *Alcohol and Drug Research, 7,* 351–361.

Cunningham, K. A., Paris, J. M., & Goeders, N. E. (1992). Chronic cocaine enhances serotonin autoregulation and serotonin uptake binding. *Synapse, 11,* 112–123.

Czoty, P. W., Gage, H. D., & Nader, M. A. (2005). PET imaging of striatal dopamine D2 receptors in nonhuman primates: Increases in availability produced by chronic raclopride treatment. *Synapse, 58,* 215–219.

Czoty, P. W., Ginsburg, B. C., & Howell, L. L. (2002). Serotonergic attenuation of the reinforcing and neurochemical effects of cocaine in squirrel monkeys. *The Journal of Pharmacology and Experimental Therapeutics, 300,* 831–837.

Czoty, P. W., Martelle, J. L., Garrett, B. E., & Nader, M. A. (2008). Chronic d-amphetamine alters food-reinforced responding and cocaine self-administration under a progressive-ratio schedule in rhesus monkeys. *FASEB Journal, 22,* 713–714.

Czoty, P. W., Martelle, S. E., Gould, R. W., & Nader, M. A. (2013). Effects of chronic methylphenidate on cocaine self-administration under a progressive-ratio schedule of reinforcement in rhesus monkeys. *The Journal of Pharmacology and Experimental Therapeutics, 345*, 374–382.

Czoty, P. W., Morgan, D., Shannon, E. E., Gage, H. D., & Nader, M. A. (2004). Characterization of dopamine D1 and D2 receptor function in socially housed cynomolgus monkeys self-administering cocaine. *Psychopharmacology, 174*, 381–388.

Czoty, P. W., Reboussin, B. A., Calhoun, T. L., Nader, S. H., & Nader, M. A. (2007). Long-term cocaine self-administration under fixed-ratio and second-order schedules in monkeys. *Psychopharmacology, 191*, 287–295.

Dackis, C. A., Kampman, K. M., Lynch, K. G., Pettinati, H. M., & O'Brien, C. P. (2005). A double-blind, placebo-controlled trial of modafinil for cocaine dependence. *Neuropsychopharmacology, 30*, 205–211.

Dackis, C. A., Kampman, K. M., Lynch, K. G., Plebani, J. G., Pettinati, H. M., Sparkman, T., et al. (2012). A double-blind, placebo-controlled trial of modafinil for cocaine dependence. *Journal of Substance Abuse Treatment, 43*, 303–312.

Dackis, C. A., Lynch, K. G., Yu, E., Samaha, F. F., Kampman, K. M., Cornish, J. W., et al. (2003). Modafinil and cocaine: A double-blind, placebo-controlled drug interaction study. *Drug and Alcohol Dependence, 70*, 29–37.

Daws, L. C., Callaghan, P. D., Moron, J. A., Kahlig, K. M., Shippenberg, T. S., Javitch, J. A., et al. (2002). Cocaine increases dopamine uptake and cell surface expression of dopamine transporters. *Biochemical and Biophysical Research Communications, 290*, 1545–1550.

Ding, Y. S., Singhal, T., Planeta-Wilson, B., Gallezot, J. D., Nabulsi, N., Labaree, D., et al. (2010). PET imaging of the effects of age and cocaine on the norepinephrine transporter in the human brain using (S, S)-[(11)C]O-methylreboxetine and HRRT. *Synapse, 64*, 30–38.

D'Mello, G. D., & Stolerman, I. P. (1977). Comparison of the discriminative stimulus properties of cocaine and amphetamine in rats. *British Journal of Pharmacology, 61*, 415–422.

Do Carmo, G. P., Mello, N. K., Rice, K. C., Folk, J. E., & Negus, S. S. (2006). Effects of the selective delta opioid agonist SNC80 on cocaine- and food-maintained responding in rhesus monkeys. *European Journal of Pharmacology, 547*, 92–100.

Dwoskin, L. P., Peris, J., Yasuda, R. P., Philpott, K., & Zahniser, N. R. (1988). Repeated cocaine administration results in supersensitivity of striatal D-2 dopamine autoreceptors to pergolide. *Life Sciences, 42*, 255–262.

Epstein, D. H., Preston, K. L., Stewart, J., & Shaham, Y. (2006). Toward a model of drug relapse: An assessment of the validity of the reinstatement procedure. *Psychopharmacology, 189*, 1–16.

Erickson, J. D., Eiden, L. E., & Hoffman, B. J. (1992). Expression cloning of a reserpine-sensitive vesicular monoamine transporter. *Proceedings of the National Academy of Sciences of the United States of America, 89*, 10993–10997.

Ferster, C. B., & Skinner, B. F. (1957). *Schedules of reinforcement.* New York: Appleton-Century-Crofts.

Fischman, M. W., Schuster, C. R., Resnekov, L., Shick, J. F., Krasnegor, N. A., Fennell, W., et al. (1976). Cardiovascular and subjective effects of intravenous cocaine administration in humans. *Archives of General Psychiatry, 33*, 983–989.

Fleckenstein, A. E., Gibb, J. W., & Hanson, G. R. (2000). Differential effects of stimulants on monoaminergic transporters: Pharmacological consequences and implications for neurotoxicity. *European Journal of Pharmacology, 406*, 1–13.

Furman, C. A., Chen, R., Guptaroy, B., Zhang, M., Holz, R. W., & Gnegy, M. (2009). Dopamine and amphetamine rapidly increase dopamine transporter trafficking to the surface: Live-cell imaging using total internal reflection fluorescence microscopy. *The Journal of Neuroscience, 29*, 3328–3336.

Gerber, G. J., & Stretch, R. (1975). Drug-induced reinstatement of extinguished self-administration behavior in monkeys. *Pharmacology, Biochemistry and Behavior, 3*, 1055–1061.

Ginsburg, B. C., Kimmel, H. L., Carroll, F. I., Goodman, M. M., & Howell, L. L. (2005). Interaction of cocaine and dopamine transporter inhibitors on behavior and neurochemistry in monkeys. *Pharmacology, Biochemistry and Behavior, 80*, 481–491.

Glatz, A. C., Ehrlich, M., Bae, R. S., Clarke, M. J., Quinlan, P. A., Brown, E. C., et al. (2002). Inhibition of cocaine self-administration by fluoxetine or D-fenfluramine combined with phentermine. *Pharmacology, Biochemistry and Behavior, 71*, 197–204.

Glennon, R. A., & Young, R. (2011). *Drug discrimination: Applications to medicinal chemistry and drug studies*. Hoboken, NJ: John Wiley and Sons.

Glowa, J. R., Fantegrossi, W. E., Lewis, D. B., Matecka, D., Rice, K. C., & Rothman, R. B. (1996). Sustained decrease in cocaine-maintained responding in rhesus monkeys with 1-[2-[bis(4-fluorophenyl)methoxy]ethyl]-4-(3-hydroxy-3-phenylpropyl) piperazinyl decanoate, a long-acting ester derivative of GBR 12909. *Journal of Medicinal Chemistry, 39*, 4689–4691.

Glowa, J. R., Wojnicki, F. H., Matecka, D., & Bacher, J. D. (1995). Effects of dopamine reuptake inhibitors on food- and cocaine-maintained responding: I. Dependence on unit dose of cocaine. *Experimental and Clinical Psychopharmacology, 3*, 219–231.

Goeders, N. E., & Kuhar, M. J. (1987). Chronic cocaine administration induces opposite changes in dopamine receptors in the striatum and nucleus accumbens. *Alcohol and Drug Research, 7*, 207–216.

Gold, L. H., & Balster, R. L. (1996). Evaluation of the cocaine-like discriminative stimulus effects and reinforcing effects of modafinil. *Psychopharmacology, 126*, 286–292.

Gould, R. W., Duke, A. N., & Nader, M. A. (2013). PET studies in nonhuman primate models of cocaine abuse: Translational research related to vulnerability and neuroadaptations. *Neuropharmacology*.

Gould, R. W., Gage, H. D., Banks, M. L., Blaylock, B. L., Czoty, P. W., & Nader, M. A. (2011). Differential effects of cocaine and MDMA self-administration on cortical serotonin transporter availability in monkeys. *Neuropharmacology, 61*, 245–251.

Gould, R. W., Gage, H. D., & Nader, M. A. (2012). Effects of chronic cocaine self-administration on cognition and cerebral glucose utilization in Rhesus monkeys. *Biological Psychiatry, 72*, 856–863.

Grabowski, J., Rhoades, H., Elk, R., Schmitz, J., Davis, C., Creson, D., et al. (1995). Fluoxetine is ineffective for treatment of cocaine dependence or concurrent opiate and cocaine dependence: Two placebo-controlled double-blind trials. *Journal of Clinical Psychopharmacology, 15*, 163–174.

Grabowski, J., Rhoades, H., Schmitz, J., Stotts, A., Daruzska, L. A., Creson, D., et al. (2001). Dextroamphetamine for cocaine-dependence treatment: A double-blind randomized clinical trial. *Journal of Clinical Psychopharmacology, 21*, 522–526.

Grabowski, J., Shearer, J., Merrill, J., & Negus, S. S. (2004). Agonist-like, replacement pharmacotherapy for stimulant abuse and dependence. *Addictive Behaviors, 29*, 1439–1464.

Grant, S. J., Aston-Jones, G., & Redmond, D. E., Jr. (1988). Responses of primate locus coeruleus neurons to simple and complex sensory stimuli. *Brain Research Bulletin, 21*, 401–410.

Greengard, P. (2001). The neurobiology of dopamine signaling. *Bioscience Reports, 21*, 247–269.

Greenwald, M. K., Lundahl, L. H., & Steinmiller, C. L. (2010). Sustained release d-amphetamine reduces cocaine but not 'speedball'-seeking in buprenorphine-maintained volunteers: A test of dual-agonist pharmacotherapy for cocaine/heroin polydrug abusers. *Neuropsychopharmacology, 35*, 2624–2637.

Haney, M., & Spealman, R. (2008). Controversies in translational research: Drug self-administration. *Psychopharmacology, 199*, 403–419.

Hart, C. L., Haney, M., Vosburg, S. K., Rubin, E., & Foltin, R. W. (2008). Smoked cocaine self-administration is decreased by modafinil. *Neuropsychopharmacology*, *33*, 761–768.

Heal, D. J., Buckley, N. W., Gosden, J., Slater, N., France, C. P., & Hackett, D. (2013). A preclinical evaluation of the discriminative and reinforcing properties of lisdexamfetamine in comparison to d-amfetamine, methylphenidate and modafinil. *Neuropharmacology*, *73C*, 348–358.

Henry, P. K., Murnane, K. S., Votaw, J. R., & Howell, L. L. (2010). Acute brain metabolic effects of cocaine in rhesus monkeys with a history of cocaine use. *Brain Imaging and Behavior*, *4*, 212–219.

Hiranita, T., Soto, P. L., Newman, A. H., & Katz, J. L. (2009). Assessment of reinforcing effects of benztropine analogs and their effects on cocaine self-administration in rats: Comparisons with monoamine uptake inhibitors. *The Journal of Pharmacology and Experimental Therapeutics*, *329*, 677–686.

Hoffman, B. J., Hansson, S. R., Mezey, E., & Palkovits, M. (1998). Localization and dynamic regulation of biogenic amine transporters in the mammalian central nervous system. *Frontiers in Neuroendocrinology*, *19*, 187–231.

Howell, L. L., & Byrd, L. D. (1991). Characterization of the effects of cocaine and GBR 12909, a dopamine uptake inhibitor, on behavior in the squirrel monkey. *The Journal of Pharmacology and Experimental Therapeutics*, *258*, 178–185.

Howell, L. L., & Byrd, L. D. (1995). Serotonergic modulation of the behavioral effects of cocaine in the squirrel monkey. *The Journal of Pharmacology and Experimental Therapeutics*, *275*, 1551–1559.

Howell, L. L., Carroll, F. I., Votaw, J. R., Goodman, M. M., & Kimmel, H. L. (2007). Effects of combined dopamine and serotonin transporter inhibitors on cocaine self-administration in rhesus monkeys. *The Journal of Pharmacology and Experimental Therapeutics*, *320*, 757–765.

Howell, L. L., Czoty, P. W., & Byrd, L. D. (1997). Pharmacological interactions between serotonin and dopamine on behavior in the squirrel monkey. *Psychopharmacology*, *131*, 40–48.

Howell, L. L., Czoty, P. W., Kuhar, M. J., & Carrol, F. I. (2000). Comparative behavioral pharmacology of cocaine and the selective dopamine uptake inhibitor RTI-113 in the squirrel monkey. *The Journal of Pharmacology and Experimental Therapeutics*, *292*, 521–529.

Howell, L. L., Hoffman, J. M., Votaw, J. R., Landrum, A. M., Wilcox, K. M., & Lindsey, K. P. (2002). Cocaine-induced brain activation determined by positron emission tomography neuroimaging in conscious rhesus monkeys. *Psychopharmacology*, *159*, 154–160.

Howell, L. L., & Kimmel, H. L. (2008). Monoamine transporters and psychostimulant addiction. *Biochemical Pharmacology*, *75*, 196–217.

Howell, L. L., Votaw, J. R., Goodman, M. M., & Lindsey, K. P. (2010). Cortical activation during cocaine use and extinction in rhesus monkeys. *Psychopharmacology*, *208*, 191–199.

Howell, L. L., & Wilcox, K. M. (2001). The dopamine transporter and cocaine medication development: Drug self-administration in nonhuman primates. *The Journal of Pharmacology and Experimental Therapeutics*, *298*, 1–6.

Hoyer, D., Hannon, J. P., & Martin, G. R. (2002). Molecular, pharmacological and functional diversity of 5-HT receptors. *Pharmacology, Biochemistry and Behavior*, *71*, 533–554.

Huang, C. C., Liang, Y. C., Lee, C. C., Wu, M. Y., & Hsu, K. S. (2009). Repeated cocaine administration decreases 5-HT(2A) receptor-mediated serotonergic enhancement of synaptic activity in rat medial prefrontal cortex. *Neuropsychopharmacology*, *34*, 1979–1992.

Jacobs, B. L., & Azmitia, E. C. (1992). Structure and function of the brain serotonin system. *Physiological Reviews*, *72*, 165–229.

Jacobsen, L. K., Staley, J. K., Malison, R. T., Zoghbi, S. S., Seibyl, J. P., Kosten, T. R., et al. (2000). Elevated central serotonin transporter binding availability in acutely abstinent cocaine-dependent patients. *The American Journal of Psychiatry*, *157*, 1134–1140.

Jasinski, D. R. (2000). An evaluation of the abuse potential of modafinil using methylphenidate as a reference. *Journal of Psychopharmacology, 14*, 53–60.

Johanson, C. E., & Fischman, M. W. (1989). The pharmacology of cocaine related to its abuse. *Pharmacological Reviews, 41*, 3–52.

Johanson, C. E., Frey, K. A., Lundahl, L. H., Keenan, P., Lockhart, N., Roll, J., et al. (2006). Cognitive function and nigrostriatal markers in abstinent methamphetamine abusers. *Psychopharmacology, 185*, 327–338.

Katz, J. L. (1989). Drugs as reinforcers: Pharmacological and behavioural factors. In J. M. Liebman & S. J. Cooper (Eds.), *The neuropharmacological basis of reward* (pp. 164–213). Oxford: Clarendon Press.

Katz, J. L., & Higgins, S. T. (2003). The validity of the reinstatement model of craving and relapse to drug use. *Psychopharmacology, 168*, 21–30.

Katz, J. L., Izenwasser, S., & Terry, P. (2000). Relationships among dopamine transporter affinities and cocaine-like discriminative-stimulus effects. *Psychopharmacology, 148*, 90–98.

Kimmel, H. L., Joyce, A. R., Carroll, F. I., & Kuhar, M. J. (2001). Dopamine D1 and D2 receptors influence dopamine transporter synthesis and degradation in the rat. *The Journal of Pharmacology and Experimental Therapeutics, 298*, 129–140.

Kimmel, H. L., Negus, S. S., Wilcox, K. M., Ewing, S. B., Stehouwer, J., Goodman, M. M., et al. (2008). Relationship between rate of drug uptake in brain and behavioral pharmacology of monoamine transporter inhibitors in rhesus monkeys. *Pharmacology, Biochemistry and Behavior, 90*, 453–462.

Kimmel, H. L., O'Connor, J. A., Carroll, F. I., & Howell, L. L. (2007). Faster onset and dopamine transporter selectivity predict stimulant and reinforcing effects of cocaine analogs in squirrel monkeys. *Pharmacology, Biochemistry and Behavior, 86*, 45–54.

Kirkland Henry, P., Davis, M., & Howell, L. L. (2009). Effects of cocaine self-administration history under limited and extended access conditions on in vivo striatal dopamine neurochemistry and acoustic startle in rhesus monkeys. *Psychopharmacology, 205*, 237–247.

Kittler, K., Lau, T., & Schloss, P. (2010). Antagonists and substrates differentially regulate serotonin transporter cell surface expression in serotonergic neurons. *European Journal of Pharmacology, 629*, 63–67.

Kleven, M. S., Anthony, E. W., & Woolverton, W. L. (1990). Pharmacological characterization of the discriminative stimulus effects of cocaine in rhesus monkeys. *The Journal of Pharmacology and Experimental Therapeutics, 254*, 312–317.

Kleven, M. S., Perry, B. D., Woolverton, W. L., & Seiden, L. S. (1990). Effects of repeated injections of cocaine on D1 and D2 dopamine receptors in rat brain. *Brain Research, 532*, 265–270.

Kleven, M. S., & Woolverton, W. L. (1990). Effects of bromocriptine and desipramine on behavior maintained by cocaine or food presentation in rhesus monkeys. *Psychopharmacology, 101*, 208–213.

Kleven, M. S., & Woolverton, W. L. (1993). Effects of three monoamine uptake inhibitors on behavior maintained by cocaine or food presentation in rhesus monkeys. *Drug and Alcohol Dependence, 31*, 149–158.

Kohut, S. J., Fivel, P. A., Blough, B. E., Rothman, R. B., & Mello, N. K. (2013). Effects of methcathinone and 3-Cl-methcathinone (PAL-434) in cocaine discrimination or self-administration in rhesus monkeys. *The International Journal of Neuropsychopharmacology, 16*, 1985–1998.

Koob, G. F. (1992). Neural mechanisms of drug reinforcement. *Annals of the New York Academy of Sciences, 654*, 171–191.

Kuhar, M. J., & Pilotte, N. S. (1996). Neurochemical changes in cocaine withdrawal. *Trends in Pharmacological Sciences, 17*, 260–264.

Langer, S. Z., & Galzin, A. M. (1988). Studies on the serotonin transporter in platelets. *Experientia, 44*, 127–130.

Letchworth, S. R., Daunais, J. B., Hedgecock, A. A., & Porrino, L. J. (1997). Effects of chronic cocaine administration on dopamine transporter mRNA and protein in the rat. *Brain Research, 750*, 214–222.

Letchworth, S. R., Nader, M. A., Smith, H. R., Friedman, D. P., & Porrino, L. J. (2001). Progression of changes in dopamine transporter binding site density as a result of cocaine self-administration in rhesus monkeys. *The Journal of Neuroscience, 21*, 2799–2807.

Letchworth, S. R., Sexton, T., Childers, S. R., Vrana, K. E., Vaughan, R. A., Davies, H. M., et al. (1999). Regulation of rat dopamine transporter mRNA and protein by chronic cocaine administration. *Journal of Neurochemistry, 73*, 1982–1989.

Levin, F. R., & Lehman, A. F. (1991). Meta-analysis of desipramine as an adjunct in the treatment of cocaine addiction. *Journal of Clinical Psychopharmacology, 11*, 374–378.

Lile, J., & Nader, M. (2003). The abuse liability and therapeutic potential of drugs evaluated for cocaine addiction as predicted by animal models. *Current Neuropharmacology, 1*, 21–46.

Lima, M. S., Reisser, A. A., Soares, B. G., & Farrell, M. (2003). Antidepressants for cocaine dependence. *Cochrane Database of Systematic Reviews*, CD002950.

Lin, Z., Canales, J. J., Bjorgvinsson, T., Thomsen, M., Qu, H., Liu, Q. R., et al. (2011). Monoamine transporters: Vulnerable and vital doorkeepers. *Progress in Molecular Biology and Translational Science, 98*, 1–46.

Lindsey, K. P., Wilcox, K. M., Votaw, J. R., Goodman, M. M., Plisson, C., Carroll, F. I., et al. (2004). Effects of dopamine transporter inhibitors on cocaine self-administration in rhesus monkeys: Relationship to transporter occupancy determined by positron emission tomography neuroimaging. *The Journal of Pharmacology and Experimental Therapeutics, 309*, 959–969.

Little, K. Y., Elmer, L. W., Zhong, H., Scheys, J. O., & Zhang, L. (2002). Cocaine induction of dopamine transporter trafficking to the plasma membrane. *Molecular Pharmacology, 61*, 436–445.

Little, K. Y., Kirkman, J. A., Carroll, F. I., Clark, T. B., & Duncan, G. E. (1993). Cocaine use increases [3H]WIN 35428 binding sites in human striatum. *Brain Research, 628*, 17–25.

Loder, M. K., & Melikian, H. E. (2003). The dopamine transporter constitutively internalizes and recycles in a protein kinase C-regulated manner in stably transfected PC12 cell lines. *The Journal of Biological Chemistry, 278*, 22168–22174.

Malison, R. T., Best, S. E., van Dyck, C. H., McCance, E. F., Wallace, E. A., Laruelle, M., et al. (1998). Elevated striatal dopamine transporters during acute cocaine abstinence as measured by [123I] beta-CIT SPECT. *The American Journal of Psychiatry, 155*, 832–834.

Mariani, J. J., Pavlicova, M., Bisaga, A., Nunes, E. V., Brooks, D. J., & Levin, F. R. (2012). Extended-release mixed amphetamine salts and topiramate for cocaine dependence: A randomized controlled trial. *Biological Psychiatry, 72*, 950–956.

Martinez, D., Narendran, R., Foltin, R. W., Slifstein, M., Hwang, D. R., Broft, A., et al. (2007). Amphetamine-induced dopamine release: Markedly blunted in cocaine dependence and predictive of the choice to self-administer cocaine. *The American Journal of Psychiatry, 164*, 622–629.

Martinez, D., Slifstein, M., Narendran, R., Foltin, R. W., Broft, A., Hwang, D. R., et al. (2009). Dopamine D1 receptors in cocaine dependence measured with PET and the choice to self-administer cocaine. *Neuropsychopharmacology, 34*, 1774–1782.

Martin-Fardon, R., & Weiss, F. (2013). Modeling relapse in animals. *Current Topics in Behavioral Neurosciences, 13*, 403–432.

Mash, D. C., Staley, J. K., Izenwasser, S., Basile, M., & Ruttenber, A. J. (2000). Serotonin transporters upregulate with chronic cocaine use. *Journal of Chemical Neuroanatomy, 20*, 271–280.

Mateo, Y., Lack, C. M., Morgan, D., Roberts, D. C., & Jones, S. R. (2005). Reduced dopamine terminal function and insensitivity to cocaine following cocaine binge self-administration and deprivation. *Neuropsychopharmacology, 30,* 1455–1463.

McCann, U. D., Kuwabara, H., Kumar, A., Palermo, M., Abbey, R., Brasic, J., et al. (2008). Persistent cognitive and dopamine transporter deficits in abstinent methamphetamine users. *Synapse, 62,* 91–100.

McCann, U. D., Szabo, Z., Scheffel, U., Dannals, R. F., & Ricaurte, G. A. (1998). Positron emission tomographic evidence of toxic effect of MDMA ("Ecstasy") on brain serotonin neurons in human beings. *Lancet, 352,* 1433–1437.

McClung, J., Fantegrossi, W., & Howell, L. L. (2010). Reinstatement of extinguished amphetamine self-administration by 3,4-methylenedioxymethamphetamine (MDMA) and its enantiomers in rhesus monkeys. *Psychopharmacology, 210,* 75–83.

Mello, N. K., Lukas, S. E., Bree, M. P., & Mendelson, J. H. (1990). Desipramine effects on cocaine self-administration by rhesus monkeys. *Drug and Alcohol Dependence, 26,* 103–116.

Mello, N. K., & Negus, S. S. (1996). Preclinical evaluation of pharmacotherapies for treatment of cocaine and opioid abuse using drug self-administration procedures. *Neuropsychopharmacology, 14,* 375–424.

Meltzer, P. C., Liu, S., Blanchette, H., Blundell, P., & Madras, B. K. (2002). Design and synthesis of an irreversible dopamine-sparing cocaine antagonist. *Bioorganic & Medicinal Chemistry, 10,* 3583–3591.

Moeller, F. G., Schmitz, J. M., Steinberg, J. L., Green, C. M., Reist, C., Lai, L. Y., et al. (2007). Citalopram combined with behavioral therapy reduces cocaine use: A double-blind, placebo-controlled trial. *The American Journal of Drug and Alcohol Abuse, 33,* 367–378.

Moeller, F. G., Steinberg, J. L., Schmitz, J. M., Ma, L., Liu, S., Kjome, K. L., et al. (2010). Working memory fMRI activation in cocaine-dependent subjects: Association with treatment response. *Psychiatry Research, 181,* 174–182.

Mooney, M. E., Herin, D. V., Schmitz, J. M., Moukaddam, N., Green, C. E., & Grabowski, J. (2009). Effects of oral methamphetamine on cocaine use: A randomized, double-blind, placebo-controlled trial. *Drug and Alcohol Dependence, 101,* 34–41.

Moore, R. J., Vinsant, S. L., Nader, M. A., Porrino, L. J., & Friedman, D. P. (1998a). Effect of cocaine self-administration on dopamine D2 receptors in rhesus monkeys. *Synapse, 30,* 88–96.

Moore, R. J., Vinsant, S. L., Nader, M. A., Porrino, L. J., & Friedman, D. P. (1998b). Effect of cocaine self-administration on striatal dopamine D1 receptors in rhesus monkeys. *Synapse, 28,* 1–9.

Morgan, D., Grant, K. A., Gage, H. D., Mach, R. H., Kaplan, J. R., Prioleau, O., et al. (2002). Social dominance in monkeys: Dopamine D2 receptors and cocaine self-administration. *Nature Neuroscience, 5,* 169–174.

Murnane, K. S., & Howell, L. L. (2010). Development of an apparatus and methodology for conducting functional magnetic resonance imaging (fMRI) with pharmacological stimuli in conscious rhesus monkeys. *Journal of Neuroscience Methods, 191,* 11–20.

Nader, M. A., Daunais, J. B., Moore, T., Nader, S. H., Moore, R. J., Smith, H. R., et al. (2002). Effects of cocaine self-administration on striatal dopamine systems in rhesus monkeys: Initial and chronic exposure. *Neuropsychopharmacology, 27,* 35–46.

Nader, M. A., Grant, K. A., Davies, H. M., Mach, R. H., & Childers, S. R. (1997). The reinforcing and discriminative stimulus effects of the novel cocaine analog 2beta-propanoyl-3beta-(4-tolyl)-tropane in rhesus monkeys. *The Journal of Pharmacology and Experimental Therapeutics, 280,* 541–550.

Nader, M. A., Morgan, D., Gage, H. D., Nader, S. H., Calhoun, T. L., Buchheimer, N., et al. (2006). PET imaging of dopamine D2 receptors during chronic cocaine self-administration in monkeys. *Nature Neuroscience, 9,* 1050–1056.

Nader, M. A., Nader, S. H., Czoty, P. W., Riddick, N. V., Gage, H. D., Gould, R. W., et al. (2012). Social dominance in female monkeys: Dopamine receptor function and cocaine reinforcement. *Biological Psychiatry, 72,* 414–421.

Natarajan, R., & Yamamoto, B. K. (2011). The basal ganglia as a substrate for the multiple actions of amphetamines. *Basal Ganglia, 1,* 49–57.

Negus, S. S. (2003). Rapid assessment of choice between cocaine and food in rhesus monkeys: Effects of environmental manipulations and treatment with d-amphetamine and flupenthixol. *Neuropsychopharmacology, 28,* 919–931.

Negus, S. S., & Banks, M. L. (2011). Making the right choice: Lessons from drug discrimination for research on drug reinforcement and drug self-administration. In R. Glennon & R. Young (Eds.), *Drug discrimination: Applications to medicinal chemistry and drug studies* (pp. 361–388). Hoboken, NJ: John Wiley and Sons.

Negus, S. S., Baumann, M. H., Rothman, R. B., Mello, N. K., & Blough, B. E. (2009). Selective suppression of cocaine- versus food-maintained responding by monoamine releasers in rhesus monkeys: Benzylpiperazine, (+)phenmetrazine, and 4-benzylpiperidine. *The Journal of Pharmacology and Experimental Therapeutics, 329,* 272–281.

Negus, S. S., Brandt, M. R., & Mello, N. K. (1999). Effects of the long-acting monoamine reuptake inhibitor indatraline on cocaine self-administration in rhesus monkeys. *The Journal of Pharmacology and Experimental Therapeutics, 291,* 60–69.

Negus, S. S., & Mello, N. K. (2002). Effects of mu-opioid agonists on cocaine- and food-maintained responding and cocaine discrimination in rhesus monkeys: Role of mu-agonist efficacy. *The Journal of Pharmacology and Experimental Therapeutics, 300,* 1111–1121.

Negus, S. S., & Mello, N. K. (2003a). Effects of chronic d-amphetamine treatment on cocaine- and food-maintained responding under a progressive-ratio schedule in rhesus monkeys. *Psychopharmacology, 167,* 324–332.

Negus, S. S., & Mello, N. K. (2003b). Effects of chronic d-amphetamine treatment on cocaine- and food-maintained responding under a second-order schedule in rhesus monkeys. *Drug and Alcohol Dependence, 70,* 39–52.

Negus, S. S., & Mello, N. K. (2004). Effects of chronic methadone treatment on cocaine- and food-maintained responding under second-order, progressive-ratio and concurrent-choice schedules in rhesus monkeys. *Drug and Alcohol Dependence, 74,* 297–309.

Negus, S. S., Mello, N. K., Blough, B. E., Baumann, M. H., & Rothman, R. B. (2007). Monoamine releasers with varying selectivity for dopamine/norepinephrine versus serotonin release as candidate "agonist" medications for cocaine dependence: Studies in assays of cocaine discrimination and cocaine self-administration in rhesus monkeys. *The Journal of Pharmacology and Experimental Therapeutics, 320,* 627–636.

Negus, S. S., Mello, N. K., Kimmel, H. L., Howell, L. L., & Carroll, F. I. (2009). Effects of the monoamine uptake inhibitors RTI-112 and RTI-113 on cocaine- and food-maintained responding in rhesus monkeys. *Pharmacology, Biochemistry and Behavior, 91,* 333–338.

Negus, S. S., Mello, N. K., Lamas, X., & Mendelson, J. H. (1996). Acute and chronic effects of flupenthixol on the discriminative stimulus and reinforcing effects of cocaine in rhesus monkeys. *The Journal of Pharmacology and Experimental Therapeutics, 278,* 879–890.

Negus, S. S., Mello, N. K., Portoghese, P. S., & Lin, C. E. (1997). Effects of kappa opioids on cocaine self-administration by rhesus monkeys. *The Journal of Pharmacology and Experimental Therapeutics, 282,* 44–55.

Newman, J. L., Negus, S. S., Lozama, A., Prisinzano, T. E., & Mello, N. K. (2010). Behavioral evaluation of modafinil and the abuse-related effects of cocaine in rhesus monkeys. *Experimental and Clinical Psychopharmacology, 18*, 395–408.

Norman, A. B., Norman, M. K., Hall, J. F., & Tsibulsky, V. L. (1999). Priming threshold: A novel quantitative measure of the reinstatement of cocaine self-administration. *Brain Research, 831*, 165–174.

O'Brien, C. P. (2006). Drug addiction and drug abuse. In L. Brunton, J. Lazo, & K. Parker (Eds.), *Goodman and Gilman's The pharmacological basis of therapeutics* (pp. 607–628). New York: McGraw-Hill.

Oliveto, A., Poling, J., Mancino, M. J., Williams, D. K., Thostenson, J., Pruzinsky, R., et al. (2012). Sertraline delays relapse in recently abstinent cocaine-dependent patients with depressive symptoms. *Addiction, 107*, 131–141.

Overton, D. A. (1987). Applications and limitations of the drug discrimination method for the study of drug abuse. In M. J. Bozarth (Ed.), *Methods of assessing the reinforcing properties of abused drugs* (pp. 291–340). New York: Springer Verlag.

Peltier, R. L., Li, D. H., Lytle, D., Taylor, C. M., & Emmett-Oglesby, M. W. (1996). Chronic d-amphetamine or methamphetamine produces cross-tolerance to the discriminative and reinforcing stimulus effects of cocaine. *The Journal of Pharmacology and Experimental Therapeutics, 277*, 212–218.

Pilotte, N. S., Sharpe, L. G., & Kuhar, M. J. (1994). Withdrawal of repeated intravenous infusions of cocaine persistently reduces binding to dopamine transporters in the nucleus accumbens of Lewis rats. *The Journal of Pharmacology and Experimental Therapeutics, 269*, 963–969.

Platt, D. M., Rowlett, J. K., & Spealman, R. D. (2007). Noradrenergic mechanisms in cocaine-induced reinstatement of drug seeking in squirrel monkeys. *The Journal of Pharmacology and Experimental Therapeutics, 322*, 894–902.

Preston, K. L., Sullivan, J. T., Berger, P., & Bigelow, G. E. (1993). Effects of cocaine alone and in combination with mazindol in human cocaine abusers. *The Journal of Pharmacology and Experimental Therapeutics, 267*, 296–307.

Reivich, M., Alavi, A., Wolf, A., Fowler, J., Russell, J., Arnett, C., et al. (1985). Glucose metabolic rate kinetic model parameter determination in humans: The lumped constants and rate constants for [18F]fluorodeoxyglucose and [11C]deoxyglucose. *Journal of Cerebral Blood Flow and Metabolism, 5*, 179–192.

Ricci, L. A., Stellar, J. R., & Todtenkopf, M. S. (2004). Subregion-specific down-regulation of 5-HT3 immunoreactivity in the nucleus accumbens shell during the induction of cocaine sensitization. *Pharmacology, Biochemistry and Behavior, 77*, 415–422.

Ritz, M. C., & Kuhar, M. J. (1989). Relationship between self-administration of amphetamine and monoamine receptors in brain: Comparison with cocaine. *The Journal of Pharmacology and Experimental Therapeutics, 248*, 1010–1017.

Ritz, M. C., Lamb, R. J., Goldberg, S. R., & Kuhar, M. J. (1987). Cocaine receptors on dopamine transporters are related to self-administration of cocaine. *Science, 237*, 1219–1223.

Robinson, T. E., & Berridge, K. C. (2000). The psychology and neurobiology of addiction: An incentive-sensitization view. *Addiction, 95*(Suppl. 2), S91–S117.

Rothman, R. B., Baumann, M. H., Dersch, C. M., Romero, D. V., Rice, K. C., Carroll, F. I., et al. (2001). Amphetamine-type central nervous system stimulants release norepinephrine more potently than they release dopamine and serotonin. *Synapse, 39*, 32–41.

Rothman, R. B., Becketts, K. M., Radesca, L. R., de Costa, B. R., Rice, K. C., Carroll, F. I., et al. (1993). Studies of the biogenic amine transporters. II. A brief study on the use of [3H]DA-uptake-inhibition to transporter-binding-inhibition ratios for the in vitro evaluation of putative cocaine antagonists. *Life Sciences, 53*, L267–L272.

Rothman, R. B., Blough, B. E., & Baumann, M. H. (2002). Appetite suppressants as agonist substitution therapies for stimulant dependence. *Annals of the New York Academy of Sciences*, *965*, 109–126.

Rothman, R. B., Blough, B. E., & Baumann, M. H. (2007). Dual dopamine/serotonin releasers as potential medications for stimulant and alcohol addictions. *The AAPS Journal*, *9*, E1–E10.

Rothman, R. B., Blough, B. E., & Baumann, M. H. (2008). Dual dopamine/serotonin releasers: Potential treatment agents for stimulant addiction. *Experimental and Clinical Psychopharmacology*, *16*, 458–474.

Rothman, R. B., Blough, B. E., Woolverton, W. L., Anderson, K. G., Negus, S. S., Mello, N. K., et al. (2005). Development of a rationally designed, low abuse potential, biogenic amine releaser that suppresses cocaine self-administration. *The Journal of Pharmacology and Experimental Therapeutics*, *313*, 1361–1369.

Rothman, R. B., Clark, R. D., Partilla, J. S., & Baumann, M. H. (2003). (+)-Fenfluramine and its major metabolite, (+)-norfenfluramine, are potent substrates for norepinephrine transporters. *The Journal of Pharmacology and Experimental Therapeutics*, *305*, 1191–1199.

Rothman, R. B., Dersch, C. M., Ananthan, S., & Partilla, J. S. (2009). Studies of the biogenic amine transporters. 13. Identification of "agonist" and "antagonist" allosteric modulators of amphetamine-induced dopamine release. *The Journal of Pharmacology and Experimental Therapeutics*, *329*, 718–728.

Rothman, R. B., & Glowa, J. R. (1995). A review of the effects of dopaminergic agents on humans, animals, and drug-seeking behavior, and its implications for medication development. Focus on GBR 12909. *Molecular Neurobiology*, *11*, 1–19.

Rothman, R. B., Katsnelson, M., Vu, N., Partilla, J. S., Dersch, C. M., Blough, B. E., et al. (2002). Interaction of the anorectic medication, phendimetrazine, and its metabolites with monoamine transporters in rat brain. *European Journal of Pharmacology*, *447*, 51–57.

Rudnick, G. (1997). Mechanisms of biogenic amine transporters. In M. Reith (Ed.), *Neurotransmitter transporters: Structure, function, and regulation* (pp. 73–100). Totowa, NY: Humana Press.

Rudnick, G., & Clark, J. (1993). From synapse to vesicle: The reuptake and storage of biogenic amine neurotransmitters. *Biochimica et Biophysica Acta*, *1144*, 249–263.

Rush, C. R., Stoops, W. W., Sevak, R. J., & Hays, L. R. (2010). Cocaine choice in humans during D-amphetamine maintenance. *Journal of Clinical Psychopharmacology*, *30*, 152–159.

Sawyer, E. K., Mun, J., Nye, J. A., Kimmel, H. L., Voll, R. J., Stehouwer, J. S., et al. (2012). Neurobiological changes mediating the effects of chronic fluoxetine on cocaine use. *Neuropsychopharmacology*, *37*, 1816–1824.

Schama, K. F., Howell, L. L., & Byrd, L. D. (1997). Serotonergic modulation of the discriminative-stimulus effects of cocaine in squirrel monkeys. *Psychopharmacology*, *132*, 27–34.

Schechter, M. D. (1990). Rats become acutely tolerant to cathine after amphetamine or cathinone administration. *Psychopharmacology*, *101*, 126–131.

Schenk, S., Hely, L., Gittings, D., Lake, B., & Daniela, E. (2008). Effects of priming injections of MDMA and cocaine on reinstatement of MDMA- and cocaine-seeking in rats. *Drug and Alcohol Dependence*, *96*, 249–255.

Schenk, S., & Partridge, B. (1999). Cocaine-seeking produced by experimenter-administered drug injections: Dose-effect relationships in rats. *Psychopharmacology*, *147*, 285–290.

Schindler, C. W., Panlilio, L. V., & Thorndike, E. B. (2009). Effect of rate of delivery of intravenous cocaine on self-administration in rats. *Pharmacology, Biochemistry and Behavior*, *93*, 375–381.

Schmitz, J. M., Averill, P., Stotts, A. L., Moeller, F. G., Rhoades, H. M., & Grabowski, J. (2001). Fluoxetine treatment of cocaine-dependent patients with major depressive disorder. *Drug and Alcohol Dependence*, *63*, 207–214.

Schuldiner, S., Shirvan, A., & Linial, M. (1995). Vesicular neurotransmitter transporters: From bacteria to humans. *Physiological Reviews, 75*, 369–392.

Schuster, C. R., & Johanson, C. E. (1988). Relationship between the discriminative stimulus properties and subjective effects of drugs. *Psychopharmacology Series, 4*, 161–175.

Sekine, Y., Iyo, M., Ouchi, Y., Matsunaga, T., Tsukada, H., Okada, H., et al. (2001). Methamphetamine-related psychiatric symptoms and reduced brain dopamine transporters studied with PET. *The American Journal of Psychiatry, 158*, 1206–1214.

Shaham, Y., Shalev, U., Lu, L., De Wit, H., & Stewart, J. (2003). The reinstatement model of drug relapse: History, methodology and major findings. *Psychopharmacology, 168*, 3–20.

Skinner, B. F. (1938). *The behavior of organisms.* New York: Appleton-Century-Crofts.

Spealman, R. D. (1993). Modification of behavioral effects of cocaine by selective serotonin and dopamine uptake inhibitors in squirrel monkeys. *Psychopharmacology, 112*, 93–99.

Spealman, R. D. (1995). Noradrenergic involvement in the discriminative stimulus effects of cocaine in squirrel monkeys. *The Journal of Pharmacology and Experimental Therapeutics, 275*, 53–62.

Spealman, R. D., Barrett-Larimore, R. L., Rowlett, J. K., Platt, D. M., & Khroyan, T. V. (1999). Pharmacological and environmental determinants of relapse to cocaine-seeking behavior. *Pharmacology, Biochemistry and Behavior, 64*, 327–336.

Staley, J. K., Hearn, W. L., Ruttenber, A. J., Wetli, C. V., & Mash, D. C. (1994). High affinity cocaine recognition sites on the dopamine transporter are elevated in fatal cocaine overdose victims. *The Journal of Pharmacology and Experimental Therapeutics, 271*, 1678–1685.

Stine, S. M., Krystal, J. H., Kosten, T. R., & Charney, D. S. (1995). Mazindol treatment for cocaine dependence. *Drug and Alcohol Dependence, 39*, 245–252.

Stoops, W. W., & Rush, C. R. (2013). Agonist replacement for stimulant dependence: A review of clinical research. *Current Pharmaceutical Design.*

Tella, S. R. (1995). Effects of monoamine reuptake inhibitors on cocaine self-administration in rats. *Pharmacology, Biochemistry and Behavior, 51*, 687–692.

Tella, S. R., Ladenheim, B., Andrews, A. M., Goldberg, S. R., & Cadet, J. L. (1996). Differential reinforcing effects of cocaine and GBR-12909: Biochemical evidence for divergent neuroadaptive changes in the mesolimbic dopaminergic system. *The Journal of Neuroscience, 16*, 7416–7427.

Thomsen, M., Barrett, A. C., Negus, S. S., & Caine, S. B. (2013). Cocaine versus food choice procedure in rats: Environmental manipulations and effects of amphetamine. *Journal of the Experimental Analysis of Behavior, 99*, 211–233.

Thomsen, M., Hall, F. S., Uhl, G. R., & Caine, S. B. (2009). Dramatically decreased cocaine self-administration in dopamine but not serotonin transporter knock-out mice. *The Journal of Neuroscience, 29*, 1087–1092.

Thomsen, M., Han, D. D., Gu, H. H., & Caine, S. B. (2009). Lack of cocaine self-administration in mice expressing a cocaine-insensitive dopamine transporter. *The Journal of Pharmacology and Experimental Therapeutics, 331*, 204–211.

Vanover, K. E., Nader, M. A., & Woolverton, W. L. (1992). Evaluation of the discriminative stimulus and reinforcing effects of sertraline in rhesus monkeys. *Pharmacology, Biochemistry and Behavior, 41*, 789–793.

Vocci, F. J., & Appel, N. M. (2007). Approaches to the development of medications for the treatment of methamphetamine dependence. *Addiction, 102*(Suppl. 1), 96–106.

Volkow, N. D., Chang, L., Wang, G. J., Fowler, J. S., Ding, Y. S., Sedler, M., et al. (2001). Low level of brain dopamine D2 receptors in methamphetamine abusers: Association with metabolism in the orbitofrontal cortex. *The American Journal of Psychiatry, 158*, 2015–2021.

Volkow, N. D., Chang, L., Wang, G. J., Fowler, J. S., Franceschi, D., Sedler, M., et al. (2001a). Loss of dopamine transporters in methamphetamine abusers recovers with protracted abstinence. *The Journal of Neuroscience, 21,* 9414–9418.

Volkow, N. D., Chang, L., Wang, G. J., Fowler, J. S., Franceschi, D., Sedler, M. J., et al. (2001b). Higher cortical and lower subcortical metabolism in detoxified methamphetamine abusers. *The American Journal of Psychiatry, 158,* 383–389.

Volkow, N. D., Chang, L., Wang, G. J., Fowler, J. S., Leonido-Yee, M., Franceschi, D., et al. (2001). Association of dopamine transporter reduction with psychomotor impairment in methamphetamine abusers. *The American Journal of Psychiatry, 158,* 377–382.

Volkow, N. D., & Fowler, J. S. (2000). Addiction, a disease of compulsion and drive: Involvement of the orbitofrontal cortex. *Cerebral Cortex, 10,* 318–325.

Volkow, N. D., Fowler, J. S., Logan, J., Alexoff, D., Zhu, W., Telang, F., et al. (2009). Effects of modafinil on dopamine and dopamine transporters in the male human brain: Clinical implications. *JAMA, 301,* 1148–1154.

Volkow, N. D., Fowler, J. S., Wang, G. J., & Swanson, J. M. (2004). Dopamine in drug abuse and addiction: Results from imaging studies and treatment implications. *Molecular Psychiatry, 9,* 557–569.

Volkow, N. D., Fowler, J. S., Wolf, A. P., Hitzemann, R., Dewey, S., Bendriem, B., et al. (1991). Changes in brain glucose metabolism in cocaine dependence and withdrawal. *The American Journal of Psychiatry, 148,* 621–626.

Volkow, N. D., Mullani, N., Gould, K. L., Adler, S., & Krajewski, K. (1988). Cerebral blood flow in chronic cocaine users: A study with positron emission tomography. *The British Journal of Psychiatry, 152,* 641–648.

Volkow, N. D., Wang, G. J., Fischman, M. W., Foltin, R. W., Fowler, J. S., Abumrad, N. N., et al. (1997). Relationship between subjective effects of cocaine and dopamine transporter occupancy. *Nature, 386,* 827–830.

Volkow, N. D., Wang, G. J., Fowler, J. S., Logan, J., Angrist, B., Hitzemann, R., et al. (1997). Effects of methylphenidate on regional brain glucose metabolism in humans: Relationship to dopamine D2 receptors. *The American Journal of Psychiatry, 154,* 50–55.

Vosburg, S. K., Hart, C. L., Haney, M., Rubin, E., & Foltin, R. W. (2010). Modafinil does not serve as a reinforcer in cocaine abusers. *Drug and Alcohol Dependence, 106,* 233–236.

Votaw, J. R., Howell, L. L., Martarello, L., Hoffman, J. M., Kilts, C. D., Lindsey, K. P., et al. (2002). Measurement of dopamine transporter occupancy for multiple injections of cocaine using a single injection of [F-18]FECNT. *Synapse, 44,* 203–210.

Walsh, S. L., Middleton, L. S., Wong, C. J., Nuzzo, P. A., Campbell, C. L., Rush, C. R., et al. (2013). Atomoxetine does not alter cocaine use in cocaine dependent individuals: Double blind randomized trial. *Drug and Alcohol Dependence, 130,* 150–157.

Walsh, S. L., Preston, K. L., Sullivan, J. T., Fromme, R., & Bigelow, G. E. (1994). Fluoxetine alters the effects of intravenous cocaine in humans. *Journal of Clinical Psychopharmacology, 14,* 396–407.

Wee, S., Anderson, K. G., Baumann, M. H., Rothman, R. B., Blough, B. E., & Woolverton, W. L. (2005). Relationship between the serotonergic activity and reinforcing effects of a series of amphetamine analogs. *The Journal of Pharmacology and Experimental Therapeutics, 313,* 848–854.

Westerink, R. H. (2006). Targeting exocytosis: Ins and outs of the modulation of quantal dopamine release. *CNS & Neurological Disorders Drug Targets, 5,* 57–77.

Wilcox, K. M., Kimmel, H. L., Lindsey, K. P., Votaw, J. R., Goodman, M. M., & Howell, L. L. (2005). In vivo comparison of the reinforcing and dopamine transporter effects of local anesthetics in rhesus monkeys. *Synapse, 58,* 220–228.

Wilcox, K. M., Lindsey, K. P., Votaw, J. R., Goodman, M. M., Martarello, L., Carroll, F. I., et al. (2002). Self-administration of cocaine and the cocaine analog RTI-113:

Relationship to dopamine transporter occupancy determined by PET neuroimaging in rhesus monkeys. *Synapse, 43*, 78–85.

Wilson, J. M., Nobrega, J. N., Corrigall, W. A., Coen, K. M., Shannak, K., & Kish, S. J. (1994). Amygdala dopamine levels are markedly elevated after self- but not passive-administration of cocaine. *Brain Research, 668*, 39–45.

Wimalasena, K. (2011). Vesicular monoamine transporters: Structure-function, pharmacology, and medicinal chemistry. *Medicinal Research Reviews, 31*, 483–519.

Winstanley, E. L., Bigelow, G. E., Silverman, K., Johnson, R. E., & Strain, E. C. (2011). A randomized controlled trial of fluoxetine in the treatment of cocaine dependence among methadone-maintained patients. *Journal of Substance Abuse Treatment, 40*, 255–264.

Wojnicki, F. H., Rothman, R. B., Rice, K. C., & Glowa, J. R. (1999). Effects of phentermine on responding maintained under multiple fixed-ratio schedules of food and cocaine presentation in the rhesus monkey. *The Journal of Pharmacology and Experimental Therapeutics, 288*, 550–560.

Wolf, M. E., Sun, X., Mangiavacchi, S., & Chao, S. Z. (2004). Psychomotor stimulants and neuronal plasticity. *Neuropharmacology, 47*(Suppl. 1), 61–79.

Woolverton, W. L. (1987). Evaluation of the role of norepinephrine in the reinforcing effects of psychomotor stimulants in rhesus monkeys. *Pharmacology, Biochemistry and Behavior, 26*, 835–839.

Woolverton, W. L., Cervo, L., & Johanson, C. E. (1984). Effects of repeated methamphetamine administration on methamphetamine self-administration in rhesus monkeys. *Pharmacology, Biochemistry and Behavior, 21*, 737–741.

Woolverton, W. L., & Johnson, K. M. (1992). Neurobiology of cocaine abuse. *Trends in Pharmacological Sciences, 13*, 193–200.

Woolverton, W. L., & Weiss, S. R. B. (1998). Tolerance and sensitization to cocaine: An integrated view. In S. Higgens & J. Katz (Eds.), *Cocaine abuse: Behavior, pharmacology, and clinical applications* (pp. 107–134). San Diego: Academic Press.

Young, A. M., & Herling, S. (1986). Drugs as reinforcers: Studies in laboratory animals. In S. R. Goldberg & I. P. Stolerman (Eds.), *Behavioral analysis of drug dependence* (pp. 9–67). Orlando, FL: Academic Press.

Zolkowska, D., Jain, R., Rothman, R. B., Partilla, J. S., Roth, B. L., Setola, V., et al. (2009). Evidence for the involvement of dopamine transporters in behavioral stimulant effects of modafinil. *The Journal of Pharmacology and Experimental Therapeutics, 329*, 738–746.

CHAPTER FIVE

Bupropion and Bupropion Analogs as Treatments for CNS Disorders

F. Ivy Carroll[*,1], Bruce E. Blough[*], S. Wayne Mascarella[*], Hernán A. Navarro[†], Ronald J. Lukas[‡], M. Imad Damaj[§]

[*]Center for Organic and Medicinal Chemistry, Research Triangle Institute, Research Triangle Park, North Carolina, USA
[†]Discovery Sciences, Research Triangle Institute, Research Triangle Park, North Carolina, USA
[‡]Division of Neurobiology, St. Joseph's Hospital and Medical Center, Barrow Neurological Institute, Phoenix, Arizona, USA
[§]Pharmacology and Toxicology, Virginia Commonwealth University, Richmond, Virginia, USA
[1]Corresponding author: e-mail address: fic@rti.org

Contents

Abstract

Bupropion, introduced as an antidepressant in the 1980s, is also effective as a smoking cessation aid and is beneficial in the treatment of methamphetamine addiction, cocaine dependence, addictive behaviors such as pathological gambling, and attention deficit hyperactivity disorder. (2S,3S)-hydroxybupropion is an active metabolite of bupropion produced in humans that contributes to antidepressant and smoking cessation efficacy and perhaps benefits in other CNS disorders. Mechanisms underlying its antidepressant and smoking abstinence remain elusive. However, it seems likely that efficacy is due to a combination of the effects of bupropion and/or its active metabolite (2S,3S)-hydroxybupropion involving the inhibition of reuptake of dopamine (DA) and NE in reward centers of the brain and the noncompetitive antagonism of $\alpha4\beta2$- and $\alpha3\beta4^*$-nAChRs. These combined effects of bupropion and its active metabolite may be responsible for its ability to decrease nicotine reward and withdrawal.

Advances in Pharmacology, Volume 69
ISSN 1054-3589
http://dx.doi.org/10.1016/B978-0-12-420118-7.00005-6

Studies directed toward development of a bupropion analog for treatment of cocaine addiction led to compounds, typified by 2-(N-cyclopropylamino)-3′-chloropropiophenone (RTI-6037-39), thought to act as indirect DA agonists. In addition, (2S,3S)-hydroxybupropion analogs were developed, which had varying degrees of DA and NE uptake inhibition and antagonism of nAChRs. These compounds will be valuable tools for animal behavioral studies and as clinical candidates.

Here, we review the (1) early studies leading to the development of bupropion, (2) bupropion metabolism and the identification of (2S,3R)-hydroxybupropion as an active metabolite, (3) mechanisms of bupropion and metabolite action, (4) effects in animal behavioral studies, (5) results of clinical studies, and (6) development of bupropion analogs as potential pharmacotherapies for treating nicotine and cocaine addiction.

ABBREVIATIONS

[^{125}I]SADU-3-72 (±)-2-(N-tert-butylamino)-3′-[^{125}I]iodo-4′-azidopropiophenone
ADHD attention deficit hyperactivity disorder
AUC area under the curve
CYP2B6 cytochrome P450 2B6
DA dopamine
DAT dopamine transporter
FR fixed ratio
Meth methamphetamine
nAChR nicotinic acetylcholine receptor(s)
NE norepinephrine
NET norepinephrine transporter
PET positron emission tomography
PR progressive ratio
SAR structure activity relationship
SSRI serotonin selective reuptake inhibitor

1. INTRODUCTION

(±)-2-(tert-Butylamino)-3′-chloropropiophenone (**1**, Fig. 5.1) (bupropion, Wellbutrin®) was developed as a new structural-type antidepressant with pharmacological properties different from those of tricyclic antidepressants. Unlike tricyclic antidepressants, bupropion does not possess sympathomimetic or anticholinergic activity and does not inhibit monoamine oxidase (Fabre, Louis, & McLendon, 1978; Ferris et al., 1981; Maxwell, 1985; Maxwell, Mehta, Tucker, Schroeder, & Stern, 1981; Soroko, Mehta, Maxwell, Ferris, & Schroeder, 1977). Unlike other stimulants, bupropion shows little or no undesirable psychostimulant activity in humans (Fann, Schroeder, Metha, Soroko, & Maxwell, 1978).

The potential antidepressant activity of bupropion was initially determined by its activity in mouse tests of depression where it reversed sedation and ptosis induced by tetrabenazine and hypothermia induced by reserpine (Ascher et al., 1995). In addition, several studies reported that bupropion decreased immobility in the Porsolt forced-swim test (Cooper, Hester, & Maxwell, 1980; Cooper et al., 1994; Foley & Cozzi, 2003). Activity in these tests is thought to be predictive of a compound's antidepressant effects in humans. Because bupropion is a racemic mixture, the (+)- and (−)-enantiomers, (+)- and (−)-**1** (Fig. 5.2), respectively, were synthesized and their biological properties compared to those of bupropion (Musso et al., 1993). The (+)- and (−)-isomers of bupropion had ED_{50} values of 23 and 17 mg/kg (i.p.), respectively, compared to 18 mg/kg for bupropion in the tetrabenazine test (Table 5.1). Bupropion and its two enantiomers are weak (μM) dopamine (DA) and norepinephrine (NE) uptake inhibitors *in vitro* (Table 5.1). Biological tests showed (-)-bupropion racemizes *in vivo*,

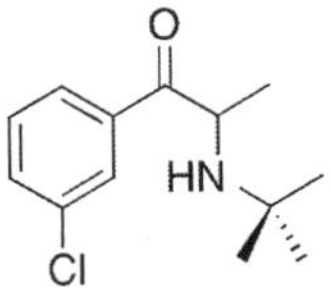

1

Figure 5.1 Structure of bupropion.

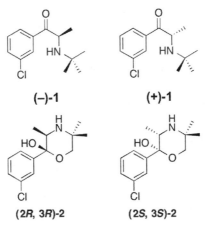

(−)-**1**   (+)-**1**

(2*R*, 3*R*)-**2**   (2*S*, 3*S*)-**2**

Figure 5.2 Structures of (+)- and (−)-bupropion and (2*R*,3*R*)- and (2*S*,3*S*)-hydroxybupropion.

Table 5.1 Biological data for (±)-, (+)-, and (−)-bupropion

Compound	Antitetrabenazine activity ED_{50} mg/kg i.p. + SE	Biogenic amine uptake inhibition IC_{50} (μM or %) at 10^{-5} M	
		NE	DA
Bupropion	18±3	6.7±1.9	2.1±0.8
(+)-1 Bupropion	23±4	4.0±1.1	2.3±0.9
(−)-1 Bupropion	17±4	10.5±3.2	4.2±1.9

Data from Musso et al. (1993).

so the lack of greater enantiomeric specificity in the previous studies may be due to racemization (Musso et al., 1993).

A more convenient synthesis of (+)- and (-)-bupropion was developed, which made the enantiomers readily available (Fang et al., 2000). The synthesis also established that (+)- and (-)-isomers had (S)- and (R)-configurations, respectively. However, due to the rapid racemization, there has been very little interest in studies directed toward the individual isomers.

2. METABOLISM OF BUPROPION

An understanding of bupropion's therapeutic utility requires knowledge about its kinetics and metabolism in animals and in humans. In a 1987 study, bupropion was reported to be extensively metabolized in mice, rats, dogs, and humans with approximately 85% of the administered dose excreted in urine of rats and humans (Welch, Lai, & Schroeder, 1987). The predominant metabolites in rat urine are m-chlorobenzoic acid and the corresponding glycine conjugate, m-chlorohippuric acid (Fig. 5.3). These data suggest that the rat metabolizes bupropion primarily by side-chain cleavage. In contrast, mice, dogs, and humans hydroxylate one of the tert-butyl methyl groups to give a hydroxy intermediate (BW306U, not isolated), which spontaneously cyclizes to give hydroxybupropion (Fig. 5.3). Pharmacokinetic studies following a single oral administration of 100 mg of bupropion in humans showed that the plasma concentration area under the curve (AUC) for hydroxybupropion exceeded that of bupropion by a factor of 16 (Fig. 5.4), whereas in rat, the AUC for bupropion (single oral administration of 200 mg/kg) exceeded that for hydroxybupropion by a factor of 3.4 (Fig. 5.5). Pharmacokinetic studies in mice showed that the AUC for hydroxybupropion was about

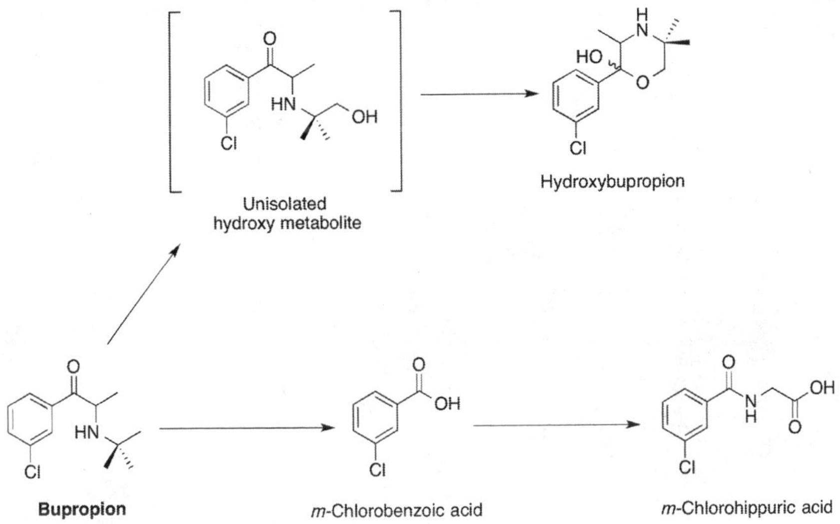

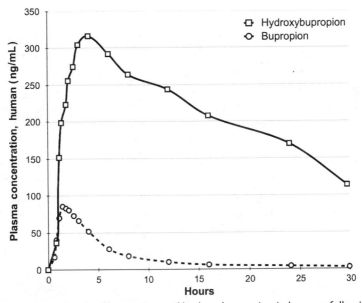

Figure 5.3 Identified metabolites of bupropion in mice, rats, dogs, and humans.

Figure 5.4 Plasma levels of bupropion and hydroxybupropion in humans following the oral administration.

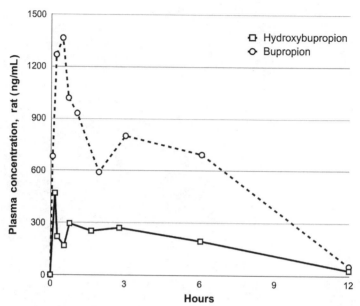

Figure 5.5 Comparative plasma levels of bupropion and hydroxybupropion in rats after a single oral dose of bupropion.

$2.9 \times$ greater than that for bupropion (single oral administration of 150 mg/kg; Fig. 5.6). Thus, acute effects seen on a single administration could be strongly influenced by substantial differences in bupropion metabolism and levels of it and its metabolites across species, with the mouse being a better model than the rat for pharmacokinetics in humans.

Administration (200 mg/kg daily for 14 days) of bupropion to rat or mouse also resulted in major differences in the relative amount of bupropion and hydroxybupropion (Welch et al., 1987) (Table 5.2). In rats, the AUC for bupropion at day 14 was reduced to only 5.8% of that observed on day 1, and the $t_{1/2}$ was reduced from 1.6 to 0.8 h (Table 5.2). In mice treated with 150 mg/kg bupropion daily for 14 days, plasma levels of bupropion declined ninefold by the last day of treatment, and the $t_{1/2}$ was reduced from 1.8 to 0.28 h. In contrast to the rat, little change was observed in the AUC for the metabolite hydroxybupropion (Table 5.2). The ratio of hydroxybupropion to bupropion on day 14 increased to 20.5, whereas the ratio in rats for treatment with bupropion was 1.7. These findings suggest that longer-term dosing in mice or rats also produces a different spectrum of bupropion and metabolite concentrations.

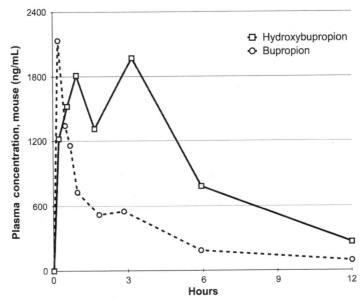

Figure 5.6 Comparative plasma levels of bupropion and hydroxybupropion in mice after a single oral dose of bupropion.

Table 5.2 Effect of pretreatment with high daily doses of bupropion on the plasma concentration and half-life of bupropion and its major metabolite hydroxybupropion in rat and mouse

	First day		14 Daily doses	
	AUC[a]	$t_{1/2}$[a]	AUC[a]	$t_{1/2}$[a]
Rat (200 mg/kg)				
Bupropion	7614 ± 2642	1.6 ± 0.70	442 ± 157	0.8 ± 0.20
Hydroxybupropion	2211 ± 296	1.1 ± 0.16	760 ± 215	1.0 ± 0.03
Mouse (150 mg/kg)				
Bupropion	4815 ± 885	1.8 ± 0.20	489 ± 97	0.28 ± 0.1
Hydroxybupropion	$13,081 \pm 1563$	1.5 ± 0.10	$10,055 \pm 2413$	1.49 ± 8.1

[a]AUC given in ng h mL^{-1} and $t_{1/2}$ in h.
Male rats and mice were dosed orally with bupropion daily for 14 days. The area under the plasma curves (AUC$_0^\infty$, ng h mL^{-1}) and the plasma half-lives (h) of bupropion and its major metabolite hydroxybupropion were determined on day 1 and day 14. Results are expressed as the mean (±SD) values from 12 to 24 mice and rats.
Data from Welch et al. (1987).

Hydroxybupropion is an active metabolite that contributes to the biological efficacy of bupropion in rat (Bondarev, Bondareva, Young, & Glennon, 2003; Damaj et al., 2004). Peak plasma and cerebrospinal fluid hydroxybupropion concentrations exceed those of bupropion by four- to sevenfold, hydroxybupropion has a longer elimination half-life than bupropion, and the hydroxybupropion/bupropion AUC versus time ratio after a single dose is 10 or greater.

The hydroxylation of bupropion to form hydroxybupropion occurs by cytochrome P450 2B6 (*CYP2B6*) oxidation (Faucette et al., 2000; Faucette, Hawke, Shord, Lecluyse, & Lindley, 2001; Hesse et al., 2000), and the subsequent cyclization results in the creation of a second chiral center with the potential for the generation of two diastereomers (Suckow, Zhang, & Cooper, 1997). Interestingly, only the *trans*-diastereomers, (2S,3S)- and (2R,3R)-hydroxybupropion (**2a** and **2b**, respectively), have been found in plasma in humans and when synthesized *de novo* (Fang et al., 2000), indicating that they are the thermodynamically more stable isomers. Steric hindrance greatly reduces cyclization to the *cis*-diastereomers, (2R,3S)- and (2S,3R)-hydroxybupropion (Suckow et al., 1997). The chirality of the second stereocenters is determined by the configuration of the existing stereocenter alpha to the ketone derived from either (S)- or (R)- bupropion.

The plasma concentration in humans of (2R,3R)-hydroxybupropion is approximately 20-fold greater than that of (2S,3S)-hydroxybupropion (Coles & Kharasch, 2007; Suckow et al., 1997; Xu, Loboz, Gross, & McLachlan, 2007). In both cases, the (R)-isomers predominate in plasma. The plasma hydroxybupropion/bupropion AUC ratio was 15-fold lower for (S)- versus (R)-enantiomers in humans (Kharasch, Mitchell, & Coles, 2008), indicating that a small amount of (2S,3S)-hydroxybupropion is present compared to the other compounds.

3. MECHANISM OF BUPROPION THERAPEUTIC PROPERTIES

Ascher et al. (1995) published an early review on the mechanism of antidepressant activity of bupropion. The review summarized studies on bupropion and hydroxybupropion in inhibition of NE uptake, reduction of noradrenergic firing rates, reversal of tetrabenazine-induced sedation in mice, antidepressant effects on the behavioral despair test in rats, inhibition of DA uptake, stimulation of locomotor activity, and reduction of A9 and

A10 dopaminergic neuronal firing rates. The review concluded that bupropion was an atypical antidepressant that demonstrates a significant and unusual pattern of noradrenergic activity and produces a unique spectrum of biochemical effects that differ significantly from those produced by all other antidepressants used at that time and that the mild dopaminergic effects may be especially beneficial in some patients. The authors concluded, "The exact mechanism by which bupropion produces its antidepressant effects is still not completely understood." The authors also pointed out, "It is believed that bupropion metabolites, hydroxybupropion in particular, will be found to play an important role in the antidepressant activity of bupropion."

Four different studies have been conducted to determine dopamine transporter (DAT) occupancy after dosing patients with bupropion or bupropion SR. These studies were conducted to gain information concerning the contribution of inhibition of the DAT to the pharmacological mechanism of action of bupropion.

In the first study, positron emission tomography (PET) with [^{11}C]RTI-32 was used to determine the striatal DAT binding potential of eight depressed patients before and during treatment with bupropion (Meyer et al., 2002). DAT occupancy after bupropion treatment was 14% (confidence interval 6–22%). This low DAT occupancy raised questions as to the importance of DAT inhibition contribution to bupropion's mechanism of action and suggested that CNS targets other than the DAT may contribute to bupropion's mechanism of action.

In another PET imaging study, Learned-Coughlin et al. (2003) reported that dosing with bupropion SR-inhibited striatal uptake of [^{11}C]-N-ω-fluoroalkyl-2β-carboxy-3β-(4-iodophenyl)nortropane ester was consistent with 26% DAT occupancy, a level that was maintained through the last PET assessment at 24 h after dosing. These authors concluded that their data were consistent with the hypothesis that DA reuptake inhibition may in part be responsible for the therapeutic effects of bupropion SR.

In a 2005 SPECT study using ^{99}Tc-TRODAT-1, 20.8% DAT occupancy during bupropion treatment was observed (Argyelan et al., 2005). In contrast with the PET study using [^{11}C]RTI-32 (Meyer et al., 2002), this study did not find a significant difference between baseline DAT occupancies in depressed patients relative to that in healthy volunteers. Thus, several studies are consistent with an ∼20% DAT occupancy of bupropion or its metabolites during bupropion exposure.

[^{11}C]raclopride was used to determine whether bupropion administration increases extracellular DA levels in the rat and human striatum (Egerton et al., 2010). In rats, bupropion administration decreased striatal [^{11}C]raclopride-specific binding, consistent with increases in extracellular DA concentrations resulting from inhibition of DA reuptake. However, when this approach was translated to humans, bupropion administration did not decrease striatal [^{11}C]raclopride BP$_{ND}$, indicating that extracellular DA levels were not increased to levels detectable using this approach. These results suggest that in humans, bupropion's therapeutic efficacy is unlikely to principally derive from marked increases in striatal dopaminergic transmission.

Imaging studies with (2S,3S)-hydroxybupropion (2) (radafaxine) showed that peak DAT blockade of 22% occurred at about 4 h (Volkow et al., 2005). The study showed that there was slow onset of DAT blockade by (2S,3S)-hydroxybupropion and block was long-lasting. Similar to bupropion, the relatively low potency of DAT blockade by (2S,3S)-hydroxybupropion combined with its slow onset suggests that it would not have reinforcing effects. The lack of reinforcing effects is supported by PET imaging studies showing that other DAT-blocking drugs are not reinforcing if they block less than 50% of DAT within a relatively short period and clear the brain rapidly (Volkow et al., 1995, 1997, 1998).

A 2004 review of preclinical and clinical data covering the period 1965 to May 2002 concluded that bupropion acts via dual inhibition of NE and DA reuptake, which constituted a then-novel mechanism of antidepressant action (Stahl et al., 2004).

With regard to treatment of nicotine dependence, Fryer and Lukas (1999) reported the first study that bupropion blocks function of human nicotinic acetylcholine receptor (nAChR). Bupropion inhibited carbamylcholine (1 mM)-induced ^{86}Rb$^+$ efflux from human neuroblastoma cells expressing the ganglionic α3β4*-nAChR subtype (* indicates that subunits other than those specified are known or possible assembly partners in the complex) (Lukas et al., 1999) at an IC$_{50}$ = 10.5 μM and or from human clonal cells expressing the α1*-, muscle-type nAChR at an IC$_{50}$ = 1.5 μM (Fryer & Lukas, 1999). nAChR inhibition at both subtypes was shown to be noncompetitive. Studies in humans have shown that peak plasma levels of bupropion (Hsyu et al., 1997) and its active metabolite hydroxybupropion (Golden et al., 1988) reach levels of 0.52 and 4 μM, respectively, and their long half-life (see Ascher et al., 1995) suggested that the pharmacological properties in humans of bupropion could in part be due to the inhibition of nAChR function.

In 1999, Damaj et al. reported that bupropion antagonized nicotine-induced antinociception in the tail-flick test in the mouse after systemic administration with an $AD_{50} = 8$ μmol/kg, suggesting that the activity was due to nAChR antagonism (Damaj, Slemmer, Carroll, & Martin, 1999). In a follow-up study, bupropion was found to block nicotine's antinociceptive (in two tests), motor, hypothermic, and convulsive effects with different potencies, suggesting that bupropion possesses some selectivity for neuronal nicotinic receptors underlying these various nicotinic effects (Slemmer, Martin, & Damaj, 2000). In addition, bupropion inhibited acetylcholine (ACh, 1 μM) activation at rat α3β2- and α4β2-nAChRs with IC_{50} values of 1.3 and 8 μM, respectively, expressed in Xenopus oocytes. The inhibition of α3β2- and α4β2-nAChRs was shown to be noncompetitive (Slemmer et al., 2000).

In another study, bupropion was shown to inhibit nicotine-induced tritium overflow from superfused rat striatal slices preloaded with [^{3}H]dopamine ([^{3}H]DA) and nicotine-induced tritium overflow from hippocampal slices preloaded with [^{3}H]norepinephrine ([^{3}H]NE) with IC_{50} values of 1.27 and 0.323 μM, respectively, at bupropion concentrations well below those eliciting intrinsic activity (Miller, Sumithran, & Dwoskin, 2002). Thus, IC_{50} values are similar to the IC_{50} values of 2 and 5 μM at which bupropion inhibits [^{3}H]DA and [^{3}H]NE uptake into rat striatal and hypothalamus synaptosomes, respectively (Ascher et al., 1995; Ferris & Cooper, 1993).

4. ANIMAL BEHAVIORAL STUDIES OF BUPROPION

A detailed review of the pharmacology of bupropion was published in 2006 (Dwoskin, Rauhut, King-Pospisil, & Bardo, 2006). A summary of these studies along with more recent studies is presented. Bupropion administration in rats was found to generalize to CNS stimulants and catecholamine uptake inhibitors including (+)-amphetamine, caffeine, cocaine, methylphenidate, mazindol, nomifensine, and GBR 12909 (Blitzer & Becker, 1985; Jones, Howard, & McBennett, 1980; Terry & Katz, 1997). In addition, nicotine and bupropion were shown to share a similar discriminative stimulus effect in rats (Young & Glennon, 2002).

Studies have shown that bupropion alleviates nicotine withdrawal symptoms in rodents and humans (Cryan, Bruijnzeel, Skjei, & Markou, 2003;

Damaj et al., 2010; Malin, 2001; Shiffman et al., 2000). However, studies examining the effects of bupropion on the rewarding properties of nicotine are inconclusive. Both increases (Shoaib et al., 2002) and decreases (Glick, Maisonneuve, & Kitchen, 2002) in responding for nicotine under fixed ratio (FR) schedules of reinforcement have been reported. Interestingly, while bupropion pretreatment decreased nicotine self-administration, it enhanced cue-reinstated nicotine seeking in rats (Liu, Caggiula, Palmatier, Donny, & Sved, 2008).

A study designed to investigate the effects of bupropion on the reinforcing properties of nicotine and food in rats showed that high doses of bupropion decrease reinforcing properties of nicotine, relative to those of food, in rats, as measured under a FR schedule of self-administration, while having no apparent effects on breaking points for nicotine under a progressive ratio (PR) schedule that reflects both reinforcing properties and the motivation to obtain nicotine (Bruijnzeel & Markou, 2003). Based on these results, the authors suggested that bupropion might help in smoking cessation not only by reducing the negative affective and somatic signs of nicotine withdrawal but also, at high doses, by decreasing the reinforcing properties of nicotine, possibly by serving as a substitute for nicotine (Cryan et al., 2003; Malin, 2001). In another self-administration study in rats, high doses of bupropion were found to decrease responding nonspecifically, whereas low doses selectively increased responding for nicotine (Rauhut, Neugebauer, Dwoskin, & Bardo, 2003). The authors suggested that the increase in nicotine self-administration was likely due to inhibition of DAT and norepinephrine transporter (NET), combined with inhibition of nAChR. However, it should be cautioned that these studies were in rats where little of the active hydroxybupropion metabolite is formed, demonstrating that bupropion's effect on intravenous nicotine self-administration in some (Bruijnzeel & Markou, 2003; Glick et al., 2002) but not all studies (Rauhut et al., 2003; Shoaib, Sidhpura, & Shafait, 2003) could be related to its actions at nAChR. In an interesting study designed to "dissect" the involvement of various pharmacological targets related to the mechanism of action of bupropion in a nicotine rat i.v. self-administration model (FR and PR schedules of reinforcement), Coen, Adamson, and Corrigall (2009) suggested that noradrenergic–nicotinic cholinergic interactions may be involved in the effects of bupropion on nicotine reinforcement. In addition, they showed that an enhanced effect on reinforced responding following inhibition of DAT may be important aspects of the effects of bupropion-like compounds in rats.

Several studies suggest that the effectiveness of bupropion on smoking cessation could be attributed to reversal of the depressive symptoms of nicotine withdrawal, thus facilitating abstinence. In support of this, bupropion reversed both the affective and somatic aspects of nicotine withdrawal in rats (Kotlyar, Golding, Hatsukami, & Jamerson, 2001) and mice (Damaj et al., 2010). However, antidepressants acting by different mechanisms of action are not effective in the treatment of smoking cessation, suggesting that bupropion possesses a unique constellation of pharmacological effects, such as its actions at nAChR, that make it useful to treat nicotine addiction.

Using intracranial self-stimulation studies in rats, Cryan et al. (2003) found that bupropion reduces the expression of somatic signs of withdrawal and increases brain reward function under baseline conditions in non-withdrawing rats (Cryan et al., 2003). At low doses, bupropion blocks rewarding effects of nicotine. In addition, bupropion reverses negative affective aspects of nicotine withdrawal. The results from this study demonstrate that the utility of bupropion as an aid to smoking cessation may be due to its ability to alter the rewarding aspects of acute nicotine and to reverse the negative affective and somatic aspects of the nicotine withdrawal syndrome.

Malin et al. (2006) reported that bupropion attenuated nicotine abstinence syndrome in rats. In one experiment, they found that infusion of nicotine and bupropion had significantly fewer mecamylamine-precipitated abstinence signs than rats infused with nicotine alone. In a second experiment, they found that bupropion pretreatment significantly reduced the aversiveness of mecamylamine-precipitated nicotine abstinence, and in a third experiment, they found that a single bupropion injection dose-dependently alleviated spontaneous nicotine abstinence syndrome. Damaj et al. recently showed that (2S,3S)-hydroxybupropion is more effective than bupropion in blocking several measures of nicotine reward, withdrawal, tolerance, and discrimination in mice (Damaj et al., 2010; Grabus, Carroll, & Damaj, 2012). This amelioration observed with (2S,3S)-hydroxybupropion is correlated with an increase in its selectivity toward nAChRs compared to DAT/NET (Damaj et al., 2004).

In summary, the precise mechanism of action of bupropion as a smoking cessation agent remains unclear. The studies summarized earlier suggest that reduction of nicotine withdrawal may be an important component in bupropion efficacy in nicotine dependence. This effect could be mediated by the bupropion's action on DA and NE. Its ability to antagonize nAChR may prevent relapse by attenuating the reinforcing properties of nicotine. However, most behavioral studies on nicotine dependence were conducted on rats. A further exploration of bupropion metabolites and their role in withdrawal, reinforcement, and relapse is warranted in species other than rats given the difference in metabolism pathways. Greater elucidation of the effects of bupropion metabolites could lead to the development of new drugs even more beneficial in promoting smoking abstinence. Some studies suggest that the antidepressant effects of bupropion could be due to its effects on the noradrenergic system (Ascher et al., 1995; Cryan et al., 2001) similar to clinically used antidepressants such as Effexor® and Cymbalta®. However, unlike many other antidepressants, bupropion also acts as a DAT inhibitor (Ascher et al., 1995). Other studies suggest that bupropion acts as a functional antagonist at nAChR (Fryer & Lukas, 1999; Slemmer et al., 2000). Thus, bupropion could act to attenuate the rewarding effects of nicotine, thus increasing the likelihood of smoking cessation.

5. CLINICAL STUDIES WITH BUPROPION

A number of excellent reviews have been published on clinical studies with bupropion, bupropion SR, and bupropion XL (Davidson & Connor, 1998; Dhillon, Yang, & Curran, 2008; Dwoskin et al., 2006; Goldstein, 1998; Hays & Ebbert, 2003; Kotlyar et al., 2001; Tonstad, 2002; Tonstad & Johnston, 2004; Warner & Shoaib, 2005; Wilkes, 2008). The reader is referred to these reviews and references cited for details concerning clinical studies with bupropion. A brief summary of some of the studies along with a little more details concerning more recent clinical studies is presented. A very thorough review of bupropion's use in the management of major depressive disorders was published in 2008 (Dhillon et al., 2008). Generally, some advantages of the use of bupropion as an antidepressant relative to selective serotonin reuptake inhibitors (SSRIs) are that bupropion causes less sexual dysfunction than SSRIs and does not result in weight gain typically seen with SSRIs. The bulk of the review here of bupropion's clinical utility concerns other indications for its use, focusing on it as a smoking cessation aid.

A number of clinical studies have shown that bupropion SR is an effective treatment for smoking cessation in a wide range of patients and treatment settings (reviewed in Tonstad & Johnston, 2004). These include community volunteers, patients with chronic obstructive pulmonary disease and cardiovascular disease, relapsed smokers, individuals with a history of depression, women, and the elderly. Beyond randomized clinical trials, the effectiveness of bupropion has been shown in clinical practice and managed care settings.

Hurt et al. (1997) reported that bupropion was an effective smoking cessation aid; at 12 months, the abstinence rates were 23% among subjects assigned to receive 300 mg of bupropion per day for 7 weeks and 12% among subjects assigned to receive placebo. Jorenby et al. (1999) found that treatment with sustained-release bupropion alone or in combination with a nicotine patch resulted in significantly higher long-term rates of smoking cessation than the use of either the nicotine patch alone or the placebo. Treatment with both bupropion and the nicotine patch was not significantly better than treatment with bupropion alone. Treatment with the nicotine patch, the nicotine patch and bupropion, and bupropion alone all resulted in less severe withdrawal symptoms and less weight gain after smoking cessation.

Five randomized, controlled clinical studies have been published that evaluate the efficacy of bupropion SR in the treatment of tobacco dependence (reviewed in Hays & Ebbert, 2003). It was concluded from the studies that bupropion SR is an effective and safe treatment for tobacco use dependence.

In a study designed to examine the effects of bupropion on nicotine craving and withdrawal, the results indicated that bupropion may alleviate some symptoms of nicotine withdrawal and may improve some measures of performance during smoking cessation (Shiffman et al., 2000). However, the study suggested that bupropion's effects on craving and withdrawal are more modest than its effects on abstinence (refraining from smoking), suggesting that other mechanisms are also involved.

Clinical trial studies with bupropion SR indicate that the drug is an effective treatment of tobacco dependence in various populations of smokers who may experience difficulty in quitting smoking. Bupropion is a useful first-line treatment of tobacco dependence in smokers with pulmonary or cardiovascular disease as well as those with a history of depression or alcoholism (reviewed by Tonstad, 2002).

In the first smoking cessation clinical trial for cancer patients, the conclusions were that cancer patients with depression symptoms who smoke may benefit from bupropion, while cancer patients without depression symptoms who smoke may be effectively treated with counseling and nicotine replacement therapy (Schnoll et al., 2010).

The *CYP2B6* enzyme, which hydroxylates bupropion, is the primary enzyme involved in its metabolism (Faucette et al., 2000), and the

$CYP2B6^{*}5$ and $^{*}6$ allele variants are associated with slower bupropion metabolism (Hesse et al., 2004; Loboz et al., 2006). In a recent double-blind placebo, randomized smoking cessation clinical study, plasma levels of bupropion and hydroxybupropion were determined (Zhu et al., 2012). The study demonstrated that increasing hydroxybupropion levels, but not bupropion levels, increased smoking cessation rates. Genetic variation in $CYP2B6$, the enzyme that mediates bupropion hydroxylation, was identified as a significant source of variation in hydroxybupropion levels. The results from this study indicate that personalized stratified bupropion therapy based on hydroxybupropion levels or $CYP2B6$ genotype may substantially improve bupropion's therapeutic efficacy (Zhu et al., 2012).

Bupropion SR was evaluated for the treatment of hypoactive sexual desire disorder (HSDD) in premenopausal women. The study showed that bupropion has a positive effect on various aspects of sexual function in women diagnosed with HSDD (Segraves, Clayton, Croft, Wolf, & Warnock, 2004).

The results from a 2005 multisite controlled clinical trial showed that bupropion XL significantly improved attention deficit hyperactivity disorder (ADHD) symptoms in adults, as measured by multiple end points (Wilens et al., 2005). Earlier studies demonstrated efficacy of bupropion in open (Hudziak, Brigidi, Bergersen, Stanger, & Marte, 2000; Simeon, Ferguson, & Van Wyck Fleet, 1986) and controlled (Barrickman et al., 1995; Conners et al., 1996) ADHD trials in children and adolescents as well as open (Wender & Reimherr, 1990) and controlled studies (Kuperman et al., 2001; Reimherr et al., 2000; Wilens, 2003) in adults.

In a clinical trial using bupropion for cocaine abuse, an exploratory analysis suggested that a subgroup of patients with depression at the beginning of the trial may have benefited from bupropion treatment (Margolin et al., 1995). In a follow-up clinical study, bupropion augmented contingency management for cocaine dependence in methadone-maintained patients, but there was no evidence that bupropion, alone, was effective at treating cocaine dependence (Poling et al., 2006).

Bupropion showed promising results on methamphetamine (Meth) craving in a clinical study reported by Newton et al. (2006). In a 2008 study using a larger number of subjects, bupropion failed to support the earlier beneficial effects seen on Meth use (Shoptaw et al., 2008). However, a second 2008 study (Elkashef et al., 2008) suggested that bupropion may be effective selectively in male subjects with low to moderate Meth dependence.

In a follow-up study to an open-label trial of 22 patients, which suggested that bupropion SR may be an effective and well-tolerated treatment of neuropathic pain (Semenchuk & Davis, 2000), placebo-controlled crossover trials showed that bupropion SR (150–300 mg daily) was effective and well-tolerated for the treatment of neuropathic pain (Semenchuk, Sherman, & Davis, 2001).

Restless legs syndrome (RLS), a movement disorder that interferes with sleep, is reported to affect 2–15% of the population (Lee, Erdos, Wilkosz, LaPlante, & Wagoner, 2009). Patients with this disorder are usually treated with DA agonists. Clinical studies suggested that bupropion XL may be a treatment option for RLS patients who are unable to tolerate DA agonists (Lee et al., 2009).

(2S,3S)-hydroxybupropion [(2S,3S)-2, radafaxine] has been studied clinically for RLS, bipolar disorder, depression, obesity, fibromyalgia, and neuropathic pain (Australasian Drug Information Service (2008)), and results can be found at ClinicalTrials.Gov.

6. BUPROPION nAChR BINDING SITE

Bupropion presumably acts at the site of substrate translocation similar to other DAT and NET inhibitors, but the site of action of bupropion at nAChRs is less certain. Although direct observation of the bupropion/nAChR binding interaction via X-ray crystallography is not available at this time, significant progress toward understanding the location and geometry of bupropion binding pocket has been made. These insights into the details of the site and possible mechanism of bupropion binding have been provided by a variety of methods including those involving electrophysiology, affinity chromatography, photoaffinity ligand labeling, and molecular modeling (docking and molecular dynamics).

Electrophysiological studies confirmed that bupropion directly inhibits agonist-activated Ca^{2+} influx. Furthermore, these studies indicated that bupropion acts not by merely blocking the ion channel but by preferentially binding to the muscle-type nAChR resting state and then both inhibiting ion-channel opening and subsequently accelerating the receptor desensitization rate (Arias et al., 2009).

Affinity chromatography using immobilized nAChR columns confirmed that the bupropion (and other noncompetitive inhibitors) binding site is distinct from the agonist (ACh) binding site. In this system, mecamylamine, a known noncompetitive inhibitor that binds within the ion channel, displaces other noncompetitive inhibitors such as bupropion and ketamine. In addition, agonists, such as nicotine, did not displace bupropion from immobilized nAChRs (Jozwiak, Haginaka, Moaddel, & Wainer, 2002; Jozwiak, Ravichandran, Collins, Moaddel, & Wainer, 2007).

Specific amino acid residues adjacent to the bupropion binding pocket within the nAChR were revealed by the use of a radiolabeled, photoreactive analog of bupropion, $[^{125}I]$-SADU-3-72. These photoaffinity labeling studies identified two pharmacologically relevant bupropion/nAChR binding sites: one near the middle of the ion channel occupied in the resting and desensitized state and a second at the extracellular end of the α-subunit M1 helix occupied in the desensitized state. The photoaffinity labeling of the ion-channel site by the bupropion analog $[^{125}I]$-SADU-3-72 was inhibited by the parent compound (bupropion), other noncompetitive inhibitors such as TCP, and known ion-channel blockers such as tetracaine (Arias et al., 2012; Pandhare et al., 2012).

Computational docking and molecular dynamics studies have provided a detailed view of the bupropion/nAChR ligand/receptor complex that is in good agreement with experimental results (Arias, 2010; Arias et al., 2009; Jozwiak et al., 2007; Jozwiak, Ravichandran, Collins, & Wainer, 2004). The pharmacological, electrophysiological, affinity chromatographic, and photoaffinity ligand studies combined with computational studies provide a coherent picture of the location and mechanism of bupropion binding to nAChRs. Bupropion apparently binds preferentially to either the resting or desensitized state of the receptor at a specific site within the lumen of the ion channel shared with other noncompetitive inhibitors such as PCP. In addition, the binding of bupropion with the receptor promotes the conformational transition to the desensitized receptor state.

To determine whether the active metabolite of bupropion, radafaxine ((2S,3S)-hydroxybupropion), could share the same binding pocket, molecular docking studies were done (unpublished results) using a model of the human $\alpha3\beta4$-nAChR transmembrane region (Jozwiak et al., 2004). As illustrated by Fig. 5.7, the modeling suggests that radafaxine and bupropion associate with the same binding pocket.

A direct observation of the conformational transition from the resting to the activated receptor state of the nAChR was recently published by Unwin and Fujiyoshi (2012). This new picture of the mechanics of nAChR ion-channel gating provides important implications regarding the possible mechanism by which bupropion stabilizes the resting (closed) receptor state. In the resting state, the transmembrane M2 helices are closely associated in a

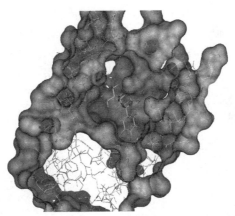

Figure 5.7 The *S,S*-isomer of the bupropion metabolite (radafaxine) docked with a model of the α3β4-nAChR. (For color version of this figure, the reader is referred to the online version of this chapter.)

symmetrical arrangement. These helix-to-helix interactions cause each M2 helix to be slightly bent toward the center of the ion channel thus obstructing the passage of ions at the critical hydrophobic gating region. This metastable conformation is disrupted by agonist binding, which causes key helix-to-helix interactions to weaken and thus allows the strained, bent M2 helix geometry to relax to a lower-energy linear geometry. These relatively large-scale conformational changes result in opening of the ion channel. This observed gating mechanism suggests that bupropion (and bupropion analogs), by binding within the nAChR lumen near the critical ion-channel gating region, functions to consolidate the helix-to-helix interactions that hold the five M2 helices in the bent, closed orientation. This picture of the bupropion binding event provides further support for the concept that bupropion and its analogs operate not as simple channel blockers but as conformational "wedges" that lock the receptor in a closed state.

7. BUPROPION AND HYDROXYBUPROPION ANALOG CLINICAL DEVELOPMENT

Starting in the early 1990s, considerable effort was directed toward the development of compounds that were DAT inhibitors and, thus, acted as indirect DA agonists and as potential pharmacotherapies for cocaine dependence. Because bupropion was a DAT uptake inhibitor *in vitro* and in animal behavioral pharmacology studies, it induced locomotor activity (Nielsen, Shannon, Bero, & Moore, 1986; Nomikos, Damsma, Wenkstern, & Fibiger, 1992), generalized to cocaine and amphetamine in drug discrimination studies (Jones et al., 1980; Lamb & Griffiths, 1990); produced conditioned place preference (Ortmann, 1985); was self-administered in both rats (Tella, Ladenheim, & Cadet, 1997) and nonhuman primates (Lamb & Griffiths, 1990); and increased responding on a fixed-interval (FI) schedule stimulus-shock termination study in squirrel monkeys (Spealman, Madras, & Bergman, 1989), and a structure activity relationship (SAR) study to identify analogs with better overall pharmacological properties than bupropion was conducted (Carroll et al., 2009). The goal was to develop a bupropion analog with increased potency in blockade of DAT and reduced NE uptake potency and having a slow onset and long duration effects on dopaminergic systems so as to reduce abuse potential (Gorelick, 1998; Quinn, Wodak, & Day, 1997; Volkow, 2006; Volkow et al., 1995). The study involved the characterization of monoamine transporter binding properties, functional monoamine uptake inhibition efficacy, locomotor activity, and drug discrimination properties of 30 bupropion analogs and comparison to those effects to those of bupropion and cocaine.

Results showed that 2-(N-*tert*-butylamino)-3'-chlorobutyrophenone (RTI-6037-12), 2-(N-*tert*-butylamino-3'-chloropentanophenone (RTI-6037-13), 2-(N-*tert*-(butylamino)-3'-chlorohexanophenone (RTI-6037-17), and 2-(N-cyclopropylamino)-3'-chloropropiophenone (RTI-6037-39) overall had the most promise as for cocaine addiction pharmacotherapy. Analogs RTI-6037-12, RTI-6037-13, or RTI-6037-17 obtained by replacing the α-methyl group in bupropion with an ethyl, propyl, or butyl group, respectively, had DAT IC_{50} values of 31, 33, and 69 nM compared to 945 nM for bupropion (Table 5.3). Analog RTI-6037-39, which has the N-*tert*-butyl group of bupropion replaced with an N-cyclopropyl group, had an $IC_{50} = 265$ nM for DA uptake inhibition. Overall, 11 bupropion analogs from the study had lower IC_{50} values for DA uptake inhibition ($IC_{50} = 31$–650 nM) than bupropion ($IC_{50} = 945$). The study also showed that RTI-6037-12 and RTI-6037-39 had the desired lower efficacy for NE uptake inhibition relative to bupropion and that RTI-6037-17 and RTI-6037-13 had IC_{50} values similar to that for bupropion.

A study of the locomotor stimulant effects of RTI-6037-12, RTI-6037-13, RTI-6037-17, and RTI-6037-39 showed that these ligands had 62%, 108%, 136%, and 82% maximal effects as a percent of cocaine's maximum effect, respectively (Table 5.4). All four compounds had very long duration of locomotor activity (350–480 min). In a drug discrimination test for generalization to cocaine after i.p. administration in rats using a standard 2-lever

Table 5.3 Comparison of dopamine, serotonin, and norepinephrine transporter binding and uptake studies in C6hDAT, HEK-hSERT, and HEK-hNET cells for bupropion analogs[a]

RTI-6037-12, R_1 = C_2H_5, R_2 = $(CH_3)_3C$
RTI-6037-13, R_1 = C_3H_7, R_2 = $(CH_3)_3C$
RTI-6037-17, R_1 = C_4H_9, R_2 = $(CH_3)_3C$
RTI-6037-39, R_1 = CH_3, R_2 = Cyclopropyl

Compound	R_1	R_2	Binding, K_i (nM)			Uptake, IC_{50} (nM)		
			DAT	SERT	NET	[³H]DA	[³H]5-HT	[³H]NE
Cocaine			272 ± 60	601 ± 130	830 ± 147	267 ± 47	318 ± 57	385 ± 40
Bupropion (**1**)	CH_3	$C(CH_3)_3$	871 ± 126	$>10\ \mu M$	6970 ± 2620	945 ± 213	–[b]	443 ± 245
RTI-6037-12	C_2H_5	$C(CH_3)_3$	459 ± 50	$>10\ \mu M$	3195 ± 145	31 ± 9	–[b]	969 ± 410
RTI-6037-13	C_3H_7	$C(CH_3)_3$	96 ± 20	$>10\ \mu M$	1171 ± 260	33 ± 7	–[b]	472 ± 93
RTI-6037-17	C_4H_9	$C(CH_3)_3$	350 ± 100	$>10\ \mu M$	3190 ± 850	69 ± 23	–[b]	400 ± 190
RTI-6037-39	CH_3	$CH(CH_2CH_2)$	1150 ± 370	3420 ± 260	4000 ± 1200	265 ± 94	3180 ± 170	2150 ± 850

[a]Values for the mean ± standard error of three independent experiments, each conducted with triplicate determination.
[b]Not determined.
Data from Carroll et al. (2009) supplied through the NIDA Cocaine Treatment Discovery Program (CTDP).

Table 5.4 Comparison of locomotor stimulant effects for bupropion analogs

Compound	ED_{50}^{a} (mg/kg)	95% CI^{b}	% Peak[c] cocaine	Time of max effect[d] (min)	Duration[e] (min)
Cocaine	7.8 ± 0.45^{f}		100	0–30	40–100
Bupropion (1)	5.5	(3.4, 8.9)	87	0–30	130–270
RTI-6037-12	18.6	(10.7, 31.6)	62	0–30	360
RTI-6037-13	15.5	(10.5, 22.9)	108	90–120	210–480
RTI-6037-17	10.2	(5.5, 19.0)	136	0–30	40–460
RTI-6037-39	16.6	(11.9, 22.9)	82	0–30	350

[a]Dose producing 50% of the compound's maximal effect.
[b]95% confidence interval based on logistic fit to ascending portion of dose response.
[c]Compound's maximal effect as a percent of cocaine's maximal effect.
[d]The 30 min period in which the maximal effect occurred.
[e]Duration of stimulant effect for one or more doses on ascending portion of dose response.
[f]Mean ± SD for 28 evaluations of cocaine's stimulant effect.
Data from Carroll et al. (2009) supplied through the NIDA CTDP.

operant chamber with pretreatment intervals adjusted based on studies of locomotor activity, analogs RTI-6037-12, RTI-6037-13, and RTI-6037-17 all showed full generalization at a dose of 25 mg/kg (Table 5.5). Similar to bupropion, RTI-6037-39 showed partial generalization from 5 to 25 mg/kg. Several other analogs also showed full or partial generalization (Carroll et al., 2009). All four analogs tested in the drug discrimination time-course study showed full generalization in at least one time point after oral administration (Table 5.6). Analog RTI-6037-39 showed partial generalization at 45 min following a 10 mg/kg and 25 mg/kg dose and full generalization at 90 and 180 min at a 25 mg/kg dose. Similar to bupropion, analog RTI-6037-17 showed full generalization at one time point at a dose of 50 mg/kg. Analog RTI-6037-13 showed full generalization at a dose of 100 mg/kg.

The clinical efficacy of bupropion for smoking cessation/nicotine addiction was discovered serendipitously while being used as an antidepressant, which suggests that it may not be the best compound for smoking cessation in the drug class. Since only about one-fifth of smokers are able to maintain long-term (12 months) abstinence with any of the present pharmacotherapies (Hesse et al., 2000; Johnston et al., 2002), new and improved drugs are needed for treating smoking cessation, including a better bupropion-based pharmacotherapy. Both bupropion and hydroxybupropion were found to be noncompetitive antagonists at the $\alpha 4\beta 2$- and $\alpha 3\beta 4^{*}$-nAChRs

Table 5.5 Effect of bupropion analogs in rats trained to discriminate cocaine after i.p. administration

Compound	Pretreatment time (min)	Dose (mg/kg), % cocaine-lever responding									ED$_{50}$ (mg/kg)	Comments[a]
		Vehicle	Cocaine	1	2.5	5	10	25	50	100		
Bupropion (1)	15	0	83	24.1	0.7	0	67.1	66.3	66.7			A
RTI-6037-12	15	19	83		0.6	33.4	50	100			7.8 (4.9–12.5)	B
RTI-6037-13	15	0	100		0.2	17.2	33.3	83.3			12.2 (7.4–20.1)	C
RTI-6037-17	30	11	100		0	17.2	66.6	100			7.8 (5.7–10.7)	D
RTI-6037-39	15	1	100	21.5	39.5	67.2	66.7	66.3				E
Cocaine ($n=66$)		4.5	89.1	14.7	39.2	60.6	84.9				3.2 (2.7–3.8)	

[a]Response rate comments: A = The average response rate was increased relative to vehicle control following 5–25 mg/kg with a maximum effect at 5 mg/kg (127% of vehicle control). The average response rate decreased to 30% of vehicle control following 50 mg/kg bupropion. B = Response rate was decreased following 100 mg/kg. C = Response rate increased following 25 mg/kg. D = Response rate was increased following 5 mg/kg. E = Response rate was reduced following 50–100 mg/kg. Data from Carroll et al. (2009) supplied through the NIDA CTDP.

Table 5.6 Drug discrimination effects of bupropion analogs in rats (p.o.) in a time-course study

Compound	Pretreatment time	Dose (mg/kg), % cocaine-lever responding								ED_{50} (mg/kg)	Comments[a]
		Vehicle	2.5	5	10	25	50	100	200		
Bupropion (1)	45	0	0	33	17	50	83			22.8	A
	90		0	0	1	0	50			(12.0–43.2)	
	180			2.5	0	22	17				
	360		0	0	0	1	0				
RTI-6037-13	45	0	0	17	33	33[b]	50[c]	100[d]		23.2	B
	90		0	0	0	33[b]	17[c]	100[d]		(11.9–45.4)	
	180		0	22	33	0[b]	17[c]	50[d]			
	360		0	0	0	0[b]	16[c]	1[d]			
RTI-6037-17	45	0		17	0	0	83			46.9[e]	C
	90			0	0	0	17				
	180			26	29	0	17				
	360			0	0	0	0				

RTI-6037-39[f]			34	34	74	67	12.8	D
90	0		0	0	33	83	(8.2–19.9)	
180			34	0	33	99		
360			0	0	0	0		

[a]Response rate comments: A = No significant change in response rate. B = Response rate was decreased following 2.5 and 5 mg/kg at 45 min. C = Response rate was increased relative to vehicle control 45 min following 10 mg/kg. D = Response rate failed to show significant change at the 90 min pretreatment interval. I = Decreased food consumption was observed following 25 mg/kg (1/24 rats) and 50 mg/kg (1/24 rats).

[b]Dose = 20 mg/kg.

[c]Dose = 40 mg/kg.

[d]Dose = 80 mg/kg.

[e]Confidence intervals could not be calculated.

[f]RTI-6037-39 was also studied at other doses. At 0.25 mg/kg, the % cocaine lever responding was 0 for all time points except 360 min, when it was 34%. At 0.5 mg/kg, the % cocaine lever responding was 1, 16, 0, and 2 at 45, 90, 180, and 360 min, respectively. At 1 mg/kg, the % cocaine lever responding was 0 at all time points.

Data from Carroll et al. (2009) supplied through the NIDA CTDP.

as discussed earlier and are believed to at least partially explain the clinical efficacy for smoking cessation. DAT and NET inhibition properties of bupropion and hydroxybupropion may also play a role in the clinical efficacy of bupropion, but it is difficult to tease apart their respective roles. Since bupropion was originally developed as a DAT and/or NET inhibitor for depression, and since several studies have shown that uptake inhibitors alone are not effective smoking cessation drugs, the goal for developing improved compounds for smoking cessation concentrated on the antagonist activity of both chemotypes at α3β4- and α4β2-nAChRs as well as DA and NE uptake inhibition, a multitarget approach (Carroll et al., 2010; Lukas et al., 2010).

Table 5.7 Inhibition of monoamine uptake and nicotinic acetylcholine receptor (nAChR) function for bupropion and analogs—ordered by α3β4*-nAChR inhibition

Compound	R	X	Y	Monoamine uptake inhibition[a] IC_{50} (μM)			nAChR inhibition[b] IC_{50} (μM)	
				[³H]DA	[³H]NE	[³H]SERT[c]	α3β4*-	α4β2-
Bupropion	CH_3	Cl	H	0.658	1.850	IA	1.8	12
RTI-9736-6	C_2H_5	Cl	Cl	0.118	0.389	1.090	0.51	10
RTI-6037-12	C_2H_5	Cl	H	0.209	0.607	16.000	0.58	8.6
RTI-9736-14	C_3H_7	Cl	Cl	0.031	0.180	2.300	0.62	9.8
RTI-9736-20	CH_3	Cl	CH_3	0.410	2.040	IA	0.65	9.2
RTI-6037-13	C_3H_7	Cl	H	0.056	0.370	IA	0.70	7.7
RTI-9736-1	CH_3	Br	H	0.511	5.600	IA	1.3	15
RTI-9736-2	CH_3	H	Br	0.689	2.540	4.508	1.4	23
RTI-9736-15	CH_3	CH_3	H	1.470	6.200	IA	1.5	19

[a]Values for three independent experiments, each conducted with triplicate determination.
[b]Mean micromolar IC_{50} values (to two significant digits) for bupropion and the indicated analogs from three independent experiments for inhibition of functional responses to an EC_{80}–EC_{90} concentration of carbamylcholine mediated by nAChR subtypes composed of the indicated subunits (where * indicates that additional subunits are or may be additional assembly partners with the subunits specified).
[c]IA = inactive.
Data from Carroll et al. (2010).

Table 5.7 (ordered by potency for inhibition at a3β4*-nAChR) lists the results obtained for eight bupropion analogs of a total of 33 analogs studied (Carroll et al., 2010), which had the best overall balance of potency for DA and NE uptake inhibition combined with antagonism at α3β4*- and α4β2-nAChRs. Bupropion is more potent as an antagonist of α3β4*- than α4β2-nAChR. Five of the eight bupropion analogs (RTI-6037-12, RTI-6037-13, RTI-9736-6, RTI-9736-14, and RTI-9736-20) shown in Table 5.7 had potency for inhibiting activity at α3β4*-nAChR 2–3 × better than bupropion. The ability to improve DA and NE uptake inhibition potency was even better. With the exception of RTI-9736-20, all five analogs were more potent than bupropion at DA and NE uptake inhibition. 2-(*tert*-Butylamino)-3′,4′-dichloropentanophenone (RTI-9736-14) with IC_{50} values of 0.031 and 0.180 μM for DA and NE uptake inhibition, respectively, and $IC_{50} = 0.62$ and 9.8 μM for antagonism of α3β4*- and α4β2-nAChRs, respectively, had the best overall *in vitro* profile relative to bupropion. From a structure activity relationship (SAR) perspective, a longer side chain (R_1) (see Table 5.7 for structures) and the addition of a *para* chloro group seemed to improve potency as DA and NE uptake inhibitors, as well as α3β4*- and α4β2-nAChR antagonist activity. These results show that novel ligands based on the bupropion template can be developed that have greater affinity and selectivity for DA and NE uptake inhibition and/or α3β4*-nAChR antagonism than bupropion (Carroll et al., 2010).

Table 5.8 (ordered by potency for inhibition at α3β4*-nAChR) lists the results obtained for nine hydroxybupropion analogs that had the best overall balance of potency for DA and NE uptake inhibition combined with antagonism at α3β4*- and α4β2-nAChRs of a total of 23 analogs studied (Lukas et al., 2010). In contrast to bupropion, (2S,3S)-hydroxybupropion (the more potent of the two enantiomers) is more potent as an antagonist at α4β2-nAChRs than at α3β4*-nAChRs (Lukas et al., 2010). Likewise, most analogs of hydroxybupropion were also more selective for α4β2-nAChRs over α3β4*-nAChRs. Most of the nine hydroxybupropion analogs shown in Table 5.8 were more potent than bupropion at α4β2-nAChR, some by more than an order of magnitude. Only analogs RTI-9736-54, RTI-9736-53, RTI-9736-70, and RTI-9736-89 were more potent antagonists of α4β2-nAChRs than the metabolite (2S,3S)-hydroxybupropion. The bromophenyl analog RTI-9736-53 with an IC_{50} value of 0.55 μM was the most potent α4β2-nAChR antagonist. The most selective analog as far as nAChR to DA/NE function is concerned was RTI-9736-89, which was relatively potent at both α3β4*- and α4β2-nAChRs

Table 5.8 Inhibition of monoamine uptake and nAChR function for hydroxybupropion analogs—ordered by $\alpha3\beta4^*$-nAChR inhibition

Compound[a]	R	X	Y	Monoamine uptake inhibition[b] IC_{50} (μM)			nAChR inhibition[c] IC_{50} (μM)	
				[³H]DA	[³H]NE	[³H]5HT[a]	$\alpha3\beta4^*$	$\alpha4\beta2$
Bupropion	–			0.660	1.850	IA	1.8	12
(2R,3R)-2	CH₃	Cl	H	IA	9.900	IA	6.5	31
(2S,3S)-2	CH₃	Cl	H	0.630	0.241	IA	11	3.3
RTI-6037-89	CH₃	H	C₆H₅	IA	10.300	IA	1.3	1.8
RTI-6037-16	CH₃	Cl	Cl	0.070	0.114	0.360	2.6	20
RTI-6037-53	CH₃	Br	H	3.340	0.920	IA	3.2	0.55
RTI-6037-70	C₂H₅	Cl	H	0.204	0.043	2.500	4.3	2.9
RTI-6037-71	C₃H₇	Cl	H	0.030	0.031	4.130	4.8	7.5
RTI-6037-88	CH₃	H	Cl	0.285	0.830	4.600	5.1	9.2
RTI-6037-91	CH₃	H	CH₃	0.832	1.680	IA	8.6	12
RTI-6037-57	CH₃	CH₃	H	2.600	1.130	IA	8.6	6.0
RTI-6037-54	CH₃	F	H	1.380	0.740	IA	15	1.3

[a]IA, inactive.
[b]Values for three independent experiments, each conducted with triplicate determination.
[c]Mean micromolar IC_{50} values (to two significant digits) for bupropion and the indicated analogs from three independent experiments for inhibition of functional responses to an EC_{80}–EC_{90} concentration of carbamylcholine mediated by nAChR subtypes composed of the indicated subunits (where * indicates that additional subunits are or may be additional assembly partners with the subunits specified). Data from Lukas et al. (2010).

with respective IC_{50} values of 1.3 and 1.8 μM while completely lacking transporter activity. RTI-9736-89 is therefore a good pharmacological behavioral tool for dissecting the contributions of $\alpha3\beta4^*$- and $\alpha4\beta2$-nAChRs relative to transporter inhibition and a good lead structure for further development. From an SAR perspective, as with the bupropion analogs, a longer side chain (R_1) (see Table 5.8 for structures) and the addition

Table 5.9 Pharmacological evaluation of bupropion and hydroxybupropion analogs as noncompetitive nicotinic antagonists

Compd	AD$_{50}$ (mg/kg)[a,b]			
	Tail-flick	Hot-plate	Locomotion	Hypothermia
Bupropion	1.2 (1–1.8)	15 (6–19)	4.9 (0.9–46)	9.2 (4–23)
RTI-9736-1	0.12 (0.03–0.5)	14.9 (6.5–34)	27.1 (2.9–46)	11.5 (8.2–16.1)
RTI-9736-6	0.05 (0.03–0.2)	6.8 (4.2–11.1)	4.3 (0.7–28)	7.8 (7.4–8.2)
RTI-9736-2	0.15 (0.04–0.6)	23.5 (12.3–44.6)	IA	29 (11.8–69.1)
RTI-9736-20	0.2 (0.13–1.3)	7.2 (0.13–13)	11 (1.5–83)	10 (5.1–18.2)
RTI-6037-12	0.5 (0.1–2.1)	IA	11.7	IA
RTI-6037-13	10 (3.7–26)	IA	IA	IA
RTI-9736-15	0.05 (0.03–0.8)	IA	IA	IA
RTI-9736-14	0.13 (0.06–0.3)	15 (0.9–25)	IA	17.5 (13–24)
(2S,3S)-hydroxybupropion	0.2 (0.1–1.1)	1.0 (0.5–4.5)	0.9 (0.38–1.1)	1.5 (0.95–2.6)
(2R,3R)-hydroxybupropion	2.5 (1.7–3.5)	10.3 (8.9–15)	IA	IA
RTI-9736-54	0.012 (0.002–0.16)	8.6 (0.7–10.5)	IA	4.4 (1.3–14.5)
RTI-9736-53	0.16 (0.05–0.6)	4.3 (1.8–9.8)	2.6 (0.7–10.1)	1.7 (0.5–6.8)
RTI-9736-57	0.054 (0.04–0.066)	7.6 (2–29)	IA	2.3 (0.4–1.)
RTI-9736-88	0.019 (0.063–0.1)	IA	IA	IA
RTI-9736-91	0.004 (0.002–0.012)	IA	IA	IA
RTI-9736-16	8.8 (4.3–18)	IA	IA	IA
RTI-9736-70	0.004 (0.001–0.03)	3.7 (0.8–17)	10.3 (1.4–75)	7 (4.5–10.8)

Continued

Table 5.9 Pharmacological evaluation of bupropion and hydroxybupropion analogs as noncompetitive nicotinic antagonists—cont'd

| Compd | AD_{50} (mg/kg)[a,b] | | | |
	Tail-flick	Hot-plate	Locomotion	Hypothermia
RTI-9736-71	0.004 (0.001–0.03)	IA	4.7	IA
RTI-9736-89	0.021 (0.005–0.1)	IA	IA	IA

[a]Results were expressed as AD_{50} (mg/kg) ± confidence limits (CL) or % effect at the highest dose tested. Dose–response curves were determined using a minimum of four different doses of test compound, and at least eight mice were used per dose group.
[b]IA = inactive.
Data from Carroll et al. (2010) and Lukas et al. (2010).

of a *para* chloro group improved transporter inhibition potencies as seen with RTI-9736-16 and RTI-9736-71, while a biphenyl group-eliminated transporter activity as seen with RTI-9736-89 improved nAChR potencies, especially for α3β4*-nAChR relative to (2S,3S)-hydroxybupropion.

The bupropion and hydroxybupropion analogs in Tables 5.7 and 5.8 were all tested for their ability to block nicotine-induced effects in tail-flick, hot-plate, locomotor activity, and hypothermia assays (Table 5.9). All of the bupropion analogs were either equipotent to or less active than bupropion at blocking the hot-plate, locomotor stimulation, and hypothermia assay effects (bupropion AD_{50} values were 15, 4.9, and 9.2 mg/kg, respectively). By contrast, all of the compounds except RTI-6037-13 were more potent than bupropion at blocking the effects of nicotine-induced antinociception in the tail-flick assay. The most potent compounds were RTI-9736-6 and RTI-9736-15 (AD_{50} values of 0.05 mg/kg or 24-fold more potent than bupropion). However, the underlying mechanistic rationale is unclear. There was no correlation between these results and *in vitro* nAChR or DA and NE uptake inhibition data.

Similar findings were observed with the hydroxybupropion compounds. The lead structure, (2S,3S)-hydroxybupropion, was the most potent compound at blocking nicotine-induced effects in the hot-plate, locomotor stimulation, and hypothermia assays with AD_{50} values of 1.0, 0.9, and 1.5, respectively, including in comparison of its effects to those of its (2R,3R)-isomer. As was the case for bupropion analogs, all of the hydroxybupropion analogs except RTI-9736-16 were more active at blocking the effects of nicotine in the tail-flick assay than (2S,3S)-hydroxybupropion. The most potent compounds were RTI-9736-70, RTI-9736-71, and

RTI-9736-91, all with AD_{50} values of 0.004. These compounds were $50 \times$ more potent than (2S,3S)-hydroxybupropion and $300 \times$ more potent than bupropion at blocking the effects of nicotine in the tail-flick assay. As was the case with bupropion analogs, no correlation was found between the behavioral data and the *in vitro* data.

Although measuring antinociceptive and hypothermic responses after acute administration of nicotine may not directly relate to nicotine and smoking dependence, it provided a quantitative measure of the *in vivo* potency of bupropion analogs to block nAChRs. In addition, the importance of measured acute effects of nicotine lies in the fact that pathways and mechanisms leading to more relevant complex behavioral effects of nicotine are initiated by binding to relevant nAChR subtypes in the brain. Moreover, both responses of nicotine (antinociception and hypothermia) are mediated to a large extent by neuronal $\alpha 4 \beta 2^*$ nicotine receptors (Marubio et al., 1999; Tritto et al., 2004), which play an important role in nicotine dependence. It can be challenging to relate *in vitro* to *in vivo* activities of ligands in the absence of data about ligand pharmacokinetics and actual free concentrations at their behaviorally relevant sites of action. However, the higher potencies of analogs of both chemotypes in blockade of nicotine's effects in the tail-flick assay suggest that it is possible to find new ligands that are better clinical candidates than bupropion for antagonism of effects of nicotine, possibly including those relevant to smoking cessation. As noted, since bupropion was designed as a DAT-based antidepressant, the likelihood is very low that bupropion is the best possible drug candidate for smoking cessation, especially given the probable involvement of nAChR in such effects. Perhaps more importantly, the finding that increased hydroxybupropion plasma levels and increased bupropion metabolism through *CYP2B6* are associated with increased rates of smoking cessation (Zhu et al., 2012) suggests that the smoking cessation efficacy of bupropion is really attributed to actions of (2S,3S)-hydroxybupropion. Combined, the data point to (2S,3S)-hydroxybupropion as the best scaffold for smoking cessation drug development.

As noted earlier, (2S,3S)-hydroxybupropion [(2S,3S)-**2**, radafaxine] has been recently studied clinically for RLS, bipolar disorder, depression, obesity, fibromyalgia, and neuropathic pain (Australasian Drug Information Service (2008)), supporting the notion that the hydroxybupropion analogs may have clinical utility. No smoking cessation clinical studies using (2S,3S)-hydroxybupropion have been conducted to our knowledge. A series of hydroxybupropion analogs were explored leading to the development of 1555U88, a

3,5-difluoro hydroxybupropion analog selective for inhibiting NE reuptake ($IC_{50} = 70$ nM) (Kelley, Musso, Boswell, Soroko, & Cooper, 1996). Compound 1555U88 was found to be more potent than bupropion in the tetrabenazine assay for depression in both rats and mice. The nAChR activity of 1555U88 was not determined at that time since these compounds were not known to interact with nAChR, but a related 3,5-difluorohydroxybupropion analog was found to be a slightly more potent antagonist of $\alpha 4\beta 2$-nAChRs than the metabolite (2S,3S)-hydroxybupropion with an IC_{50} value of 6.3 µM (Lukas et al., 2010). Additional hydroxybupropion metabolite analogs have also been described in which the hydroxyl group has been removed in order to lock the molecule into the cyclic form (Boswell, Musso, Kelley, Soroko, & Cooper, 1996). These compounds also have antidepressant activity as measured by the tetrabenazine assay in mice, but not any better than 1555U88.

8. CONCLUSION

Bupropion is an atypical antidepressant with smoking cessation activity that seems to be related in humans to concentrations of its (2S,3S)-hydroxymetabolite and not due to antidepressant effects. Clinical efficacy of bupropion in several other indications, including Meth and cocaine addiction and in several neuropsychiatric disorders, is evident, but more work is needed to determine whether these effects also are more closely related to metabolite levels. Some improvements have been achieved in in vitro activity of bupropion or (2S,3S)-hydroxybupropion as inhibitors of DAT, NET, and/or $\alpha 3\beta 4$- or $\alpha 4\beta 2$-nAChR, and insights have been gained as to mechanisms and atomic-level sites of ligand action at DAT, NET, and nAChR targets. Even more substantial improvements have been made in potency of such analogs in behavioral pharmacological animal studies thought to be relevant to addictions and neuropsychiatric maladies such as ADHD and depression. However, relationships between in vitro activity and effects in blockade of some fundamental effects of nicotine on locomotor behavior, temperature, and antinociception are not yet obvious. One possibility is that its efficacy as a smoking cessation agent results from both inhibition in some combination of DAT, NET, and nAChR. Since clinical activity of "bupropion" may be due to its effects on a combination of targets, much more work is needed to lay a rational and scientifically sound basis for understanding its rich pharmacodynamic and pharmacokinetic properties, its potential therapeutic utility, toward development of agents that have superior clinical efficacy and safety. Whether for treatment of dependence on cocaine, Meth, or nicotine, the balance of the evidence suggests that (2S,3S)-hydroxybupropion appears to be the most viable and promising scaffold for clinical development.

Even though a number of studies have been directed toward determining the mechanism by which bupropion increases abstinence rates in smokers, questions remain to be answered. One possibility is that its efficacy as a smoking cessation agent results from both inhibition of the reuptake of both DA and NE and the noncompetitive antagonism of nAChR. It is likely that the bupropion metabolite (2S,3S)-hydroxybupropion, which also inhibits DA and NE reuptake and antagonizes nAChR, also plays an important role in the mechanism of action. Recent clinical studies show that (2S,3S)-hydroxybupropion is likely a major contributor to bupropion's smoking cessation effects.

The studies directed toward the development of a bupropion analog as a better pharmacotherapy for cocaine additions showed that analogs RTI-6037-12, RTI-6037-13, RTI-6037-17, and RTI-6037-39 had the best overall profiles, with RTI-6037-39 being the most interesting. Importantly, RTI-6037-39 was more potent than bupropion in the time-course discrimination study and had a slower onset and longer duration of action. The *in vitro* efficacy and animal behavioral properties thought to be necessary for an indirect DA agonist pharmacotherapy for treating abuse of cocaine, Meth, and nicotine are both better for RTI-6037-39 than for bupropion.

The study directed toward the development of bupropion analogs for nicotine addiction showed that eight analogs that are better antagonists at $\alpha3\beta4^*$-nAChR than bupropion were developed. Seven of the eight analogs were more potent in blocking nicotine-induced antinociception. Six hydroxybupropion analogs had potency for inhibition of $\alpha3\beta4^*$-nAChR that were $2–8.5 \times$ greater than hydroxybupropion. Three analogs were equal to or more potent $\alpha4\beta2$-nAChR antagonists. Four and three analogs were more potent DA and NE uptake inhibitors, respectively. Similar to bupropion, all compounds except one were more potent as antagonists of nicotine-induced antinociception in the tail-flick test.

Hydroxybupropion appears to be the most viable and promising scaffold for clinical development. In addition, RTI-9736-89, which was selective for nAChRs relative to the DAT, NET, and SERT, will be a useful pharmacological tool for future studies.

CONFLICT OF INTEREST

The authors have no conflicts of interest to declare.

ACKNOWLEDGMENTS

This work was supported by National Institutes of Health National Cooperative Drug Discovery Group Grant U19 DA019377.

REFERENCES

Argyelan, M., Szabo, Z., Kanyo, B., Tanacs, A., Kovacs, Z., Janka, Z., et al. (2005). Dopamine transporter availability in medication free and in bupropion treated depression: A 99mTc-TRODAT-1 SPECT study. *Journal of Affective Disorders, 89*(1–3), 115–123.

Arias, H. R. (2010). Molecular interaction of bupropion with nicotinic acetylcholine receptors. *Journal of Pediatric Biochemistry, 1,* 185–197.

Arias, H. R., Feuerbach, D., Targowska-Duda, K. M., Aggarwal, S., Lapinsky, D. J., & Jozwiak, K. (2012). Structural and functional interaction of (+/-)-2-(N-tert-butylamino)-3'-iodo-4'-azidopropiophenone, a photoreactive bupropion derivative, with nicotinic acetylcholine receptors. *Neurochemistry International, 61*(8), 1433–1441.

Arias, H. R., Gumilar, F., Rosenberg, A., Targowska-Duda, K. M., Feuerbach, D., Jozwiak, K., et al. (2009). Interaction of bupropion with muscle-type nicotinic acetylcholine receptors in different conformational states. *Biochemistry, 48*(21), 4506–4518.

Ascher, J. A., Cole, J. O., Colin, J. N., Feighner, J. P., Ferris, R. M., Fibiger, H. C., et al. (1995). Bupropion: A review of its mechanism of antidepressant activity. *Journal of Clinical Psychiatry, 56*(9), 395–401.

Australasian Drug Information Service. (2008). *Radafaxine.* Retrieved from the ADIS R&D Insight database 6/26/2013.

Barrickman, L. L., Perry, P. J., Allen, A. J., Kuperman, S., Arndt, S. V., Herrmann, K. J., et al. (1995). Bupropion versus methylphenidate in the treatment of attention-deficit hyperactivity disorder. *Journal of the American Academy of Child & Adolescent Psychiatry, 34*(5), 649–657.

Blitzer, R. D., & Becker, R. E. (1985). Characterization of the bupropion cue in the rat: Lack of evidence for a dopaminergic mechanism. *Psychopharmacology (Berlin), 85*(2), 173–177.

Bondarev, M. L., Bondareva, T. S., Young, R., & Glennon, R. A. (2003). Behavioral and biochemical investigations of bupropion metabolites. *European Journal of Pharmacology, 474*(1), 85–93.

Boswell, G. E., Musso, D. L., Kelley, J. L., Soroko, F. E., & Cooper, B. R. (1996). Synthesis and anti-tetrabenazine activity of c-3 analogues of dimethyl-2-phenylmorpholines. *Journal of Heterocyclic Chemistry, 33*(1), 33–39.

Bruijnzeel, A. W., & Markou, A. (2003). Characterization of the effects of bupropion on the reinforcing properties of nicotine and food in rats. *Synapse, 50*(1), 20–28.

Carroll, F. I., Blough, B., Abraham, P., Mills, A. C., Holleman, J. A., Wolckenhauer, S. A., et al. (2009). Synthesis and biological evaluation of bupropion analogues as potential pharmacotherapies for cocaine addiction. *Journal of Medicinal Chemistry, 52*(21), 6768–6781.

Carroll, F. I., Blough, B. E., Mascarella, S. W., Navarro, H. A., Eaton, J. B., Lukas, R. J., et al. (2010). Synthesis and biological evaluation of bupropion analogues as potential pharmacotherapies for smoking cessation. *Journal of Medicinal Chemistry, 53*(5), 2204–2214.

Coen, K. M., Adamson, K. L., & Corrigall, W. A. (2009). Medication-related pharmacological manipulations of nicotine self-administration in the rat maintained on fixed- and progressive-ratio schedules of reinforcement. *Psychopharmacology, 201*(4), 557–568.

Coles, R., & Kharasch, E. D. (2007). Stereoselective analysis of bupropion and hydroxybupropion in human plasma and urine by LC/MS/MS. *Journal of Chromatography, B: Analytical Technologies in the Biomedical and Life Sciences, 857*(1), 67–75.

Conners, C. K., Casat, C. D., Gualtieri, C. T., Weller, E., Reader, M., Reiss, A., et al. (1996). Bupropion hydrochloride in attention deficit disorder with hyperactivity. *Journal of the American Academy of Child & Adolescent Psychiatry, 35*(10), 1314–1321.

Cooper, B. R., Hester, T. J., & Maxwell, R. A. (1980). Behavioral and biochemical effects of the antidepressant bupropion (Wellbutrin): Evidence for selective blockade of dopamine uptake in vivo. *Journal of Pharmacology and Experimental Therapeutics, 215*(1), 127–134.

Cooper, B. R., Wang, C. M., Cox, R. F., Norton, R., Shea, V., & Ferris, R. M. (1994). Evidence that the acute behavioral and electrophysiological effects of bupropion (Wellbutrin) are mediated by a noradrenergic mechanism. *Neuropsychopharmacology, 11*(2), 133–141.

Cryan, J. F., Bruijnzeel, A. W., Skjei, K. L., & Markou, A. (2003). Bupropion enhances brain reward function and reverses the affective and somatic aspects of nicotine withdrawal in the rat. *Psychopharmacology (Berlin), 168*(3), 347–358.

Cryan, J. F., Dalvi, A., Jin, S. H., Hirsch, B. R., Lucki, I., & Thomas, S. A. (2001). Use of dopamine-beta-hydroxylase-deficient mice to determine the role of norepinephrine in the mechanism of action of antidepressant drugs. *Journal of Pharmacology and Experimental Therapeutics, 298*(2), 651–657.

Damaj, M. I., Carroll, F. I., Eaton, J. B., Navarro, H. A., Blough, B. E., Mirza, S., et al. (2004). Enantioselective effects of hydroxy metabolites of bupropion on behavior and on function of monoamine transporters and nicotinic receptors. *Molecular Pharmacology, 66*(3), 675–682.

Damaj, M. I., Grabus, S. D., Navarro, H. A., Vann, R. E., Warner, J. A., King, L. S., et al. (2010). Effects of hydroxymetabolites of bupropion on nicotine dependence behavior in mice. *Journal of Pharmacology and Experimental Therapeutics, 334*, 1087–1095.

Damaj, M. I., Slemmer, J. E., Carroll, F. I., & Martin, B. R. (1999). Pharmacological characterization of nicotine's interaction with cocaine and cocaine analogs. *Journal of Pharmacology and Experimental Therapeutics, 289*(3), 1229–1236.

Davidson, J. R. T., & Connor, K. M. (1998). Bupropion sustained release: A therapeutic overview. *Journal of Clinical Psychiatry, 59*(Suppl. 4), 25–31.

Dhillon, S., Yang, L. P., & Curran, M. P. (2008). Bupropion: A review of its use in the management of major depressive disorder. *Drugs, 68*(5), 653–689.

Dwoskin, L. P., Rauhut, A. S., King-Pospisil, K. A., & Bardo, M. T. (2006). Review of the pharmacology and clinical profile of bupropion, an antidepressant and tobacco use cessation agent. *CNS Drug Reviews, 12*(3–4), 178–207.

Egerton, A., Shotbolt, J. P., Stokes, P. R., Hirani, E., Ahmad, R., Lappin, J. M., et al. (2010). Acute effect of the anti-addiction drug bupropion on extracellular dopamine concentrations in the human striatum: An [11C]raclopride PET study. *NeuroImage, 50*(1), 260–266.

Elkashef, A. M., Rawson, R. A., Anderson, A. L., Li, S. H., Holmes, T., Smith, E. V., et al. (2008). Bupropion for the treatment of methamphetamine dependence. *Neuropsychopharmacology, 33*(5), 1162–1170.

Fabre, J., Louis, F., & McLendon, D. M. (1978). Double-blind placebo-controlled study of bupropion hydrochloride (Wellbutrin®) in the treatment of depressed in-patients. *Current Therapeutic Research, 23*(3), 393 (section 2).

Fang, Q. K., Han, Z., Grover, P., Kessler, D., Senanayake, C. H., & Wald, S. A. (2000). Rapid access to enantiopure bupropion and its major metabolite by stereospecific nucleophilic substitution on an a-ketotriflate. *Tetrahedron: Asymmetry*, *11*, 3659–3663.

Fann, W. E., Schroeder, D. H., Metha, N. B. S., Soroko, F. E., & Maxwell, R. A. (1978). Clinical trial of bupropion HCl in treatment of depression. *Current Therapeutic Research*, *23*(2), 222 (section 2).

Faucette, S. R., Hawke, R. L., Lecluyse, E. L., Shord, S. S., Yan, B., Laethem, R. M., et al. (2000). Validation of bupropion hydroxylation as a selective marker of human cytochrome P450 2B6 catalytic activity. *Drug Metabolism and Disposition: The Biological Fate of Chemicals*, *28*(10), 1222–1230.

Faucette, S. R., Hawke, R. L., Shord, S. S., Lecluyse, E. L., & Lindley, C. M. (2001). Evaluation of the contribution of cytochrome P450 3A4 to human liver microsomal bupropion hydroxylation. *Drug Metabolism and Disposition: The Biological Fate of Chemicals*, *29*(8), 1123–1129.

Ferris, R. M., & Cooper, B. R. (1993). Mechanism of antidepressant activity of bupropion. *Journal of Clinical Psychiatry Monograph*, *11*, 2–14.

Ferris, R. M., White, H. L., Cooper, B. R., Maxwell, R. A., Tang, F. L. M., Beaman, O. J., et al. (1981). Some neurochemical properties of a new antidepressant, bupropion hydrochloride (Wellbutrin®). *Drug Development Research*, *1*, 21–35.

Foley, K. F., & Cozzi, N. V. (2003). Novel aminopropiophenones as potential antidepressants. *Drug Development Research*, *60*(4), 252–260.

Fryer, J. D., & Lukas, R. J. (1999). Noncompetitive functional inhibition at diverse, human nicotinic acetylcholine receptor subtypes by bupropion, phencyclidine, and ibogaine. *Journal of Pharmacology and Experimental Therapeutics*, *288*(1), 88–92.

Glick, S. D., Maisonneuve, I. M., & Kitchen, B. A. (2002). Modulation of nicotine self-administration in rats by combination therapy with agents blocking alpha 3 beta 4 nicotinic receptors. *European Journal of Pharmacology*, *448*(2–3), 185–191.

Golden, R. N., De Vane, C. L., Laizure, S. C., Rudorfer, M. V., Sherer, M. A., & Potter, W. Z. (1988). Bupropion in depression. II. The role of metabolites in clinical outcome. *Archives of General Psychiatry*, *45*(2), 145–149.

Goldstein, M. G. (1998). Bupropion sustained release and smoking cessation. *Journal of Clinical Psychiatry*, *59*(Suppl. 4), 66–72.

Gorelick, D. A. (1998). The rate hypothesis and agonist substitution approaches to cocaine abuse treatment. *Advances in Pharmacology*, *42*, 995–997.

Grabus, S. D., Carroll, F. I., & Damaj, M. I. (2012). Bupropion and its main metabolite reverse nicotine chronic tolerance in the mouse. *Nicotine and Tobacco Research*, *14*(11), 1356–1361.

Hays, J. T., & Ebbert, J. O. (2003). Bupropion sustained release for treatment of tobacco dependence. *Mayo Clinic Proceedings*, *78*(8), 1020–1024, quiz 1024.

Hesse, L. M., He, P., Krishnaswamy, S., Hao, Q., Hogan, K., von Moltke, L. L., et al. (2004). Pharmacogenetic determinants of interindividual variability in bupropion hydroxylation by cytochrome P450 2B6 in human liver microsomes. *Pharmacogenetics*, *14*(4), 225–238.

Hesse, L. M., Venkatakrishnan, K., Court, M. H., von Moltke, L. L., Duan, S. X., Shader, R. I., et al. (2000). CYP2B6 mediates the in vitro hydroxylation of bupropion: Potential drug interactions with other antidepressants. *Drug Metabolism and Disposition: The Biological Fate of Chemicals*, *28*(10), 1176–1183.

Hsyu, P. H., Singh, A., Giargiari, T. D., Dunn, J. A., Ascher, J. A., & Johnston, J. A. (1997). Pharmacokinetics of bupropion and its metabolites in cigarette smokers versus nonsmokers. *Journal of Clinical Pharmacology*, *37*(8), 737–743.

Hudziak, J. J., Brigidi, B. D., Bergersen, T., Stanger, C., & Marte, B. (2000). *The use of bupropion SR in ritalin responsive adolescents with ADHD.* Chicago, IL: American Psychiatric Association.

Hurt, R. D., Sachs, D. P., Glover, E. D., Offord, K. P., Johnston, J. A., Dale, L. C., et al. (1997). A comparison of sustained-release bupropion and placebo for smoking cessation. *New England Journal of Medicine, 337*(17), 1195–1202.

Johnston, A. J., Ascher, J., Leadbetter, R., Schmith, V. D., Patel, D. K., Durcan, M., et al. (2002). Pharmacokinetic optimisation of sustained-release bupropion for smoking cessation. *Drugs, 62*(Suppl. 2), 11–24.

Jones, C. N., Howard, J. L., & McBennett, S. T. (1980). Stimulus properties of antidepressants in the rat. *Psychopharmacology (Berlin), 67*(2), 111–118.

Jorenby, D. E., Leischow, S. J., Nides, M. A., Rennard, S. I., Johnston, J. A., Hughes, A. R., et al. (1999). A controlled trial of sustained-release bupropion, a nicotine patch, or both for smoking cessation. *New England Journal of Medicine, 340*(9), 685–691.

Jozwiak, K., Haginaka, J., Moaddel, R., & Wainer, I. W. (2002). Displacement and nonlinear chromatographic techniques in the investigation of interaction of noncompetitive inhibitors with an immobilized alpha3beta4 nicotinic acetylcholine receptor liquid chromatographic stationary phase. *Analytical Chemistry, 74*(18), 4618–4624.

Jozwiak, K., Ravichandran, S., Collins, J. R., Moaddel, R., & Wainer, I. W. (2007). Interaction of noncompetitive inhibitors with the alpha3beta2 nicotinic acetylcholine receptor investigated by affinity chromatography and molecular docking. *Journal of Medicinal Chemistry, 50*(24), 6279–6283.

Jozwiak, K., Ravichandran, S., Collins, J. R., & Wainer, I. W. (2004). Interaction of noncompetitive inhibitors with an immobilized alpha3beta4 nicotinic acetylcholine receptor investigated by affinity chromatography, quantitative-structure activity relationship analysis, and molecular docking. *Journal of Medicinal Chemistry, 47*(16), 4008–4021.

Kelley, J. L., Musso, D. L., Boswell, G. E., Soroko, F. E., & Cooper, B. R. (1996). (2S,3S,5R)-2-(3,5-difluorophenyl)-3,5-dimethyl-2-morpholinol: A novel antidepressant agent and selective inhibitor of norepinephrine uptake. *Journal of Medicinal Chemistry, 39*(2), 347–349.

Kharasch, E. D., Mitchell, D., & Coles, R. (2008). Stereoselective bupropion hydroxylation as an in vivo phenotypic probe for cytochrome P4502B6 (CYP2B6) activity. *Journal of Clinical Pharmacology, 48*(4), 464–474.

Kotlyar, M., Golding, M., Hatsukami, D. K., & Jamerson, B. D. (2001). Effect of non-nicotine pharmacotherapy on smoking behavior. *Pharmacotherapy, 21*(12), 1530–1548.

Kuperman, S., Perry, P. J., Gaffney, G. R., Lund, B. C., Bever-Stille, K. A., Arndt, S., et al. (2001). Bupropion SR vs. methylphenidate vs. placebo for attention deficit hyperactivity disorder in adults. *Annals of Clinical Psychiatry, 13*(3), 129–134.

Lamb, R. J., & Griffiths, R. R. (1990). Self-administration in baboons and the discriminative stimulus effects in rats of bupropion, nomifensine, diclofensine and imipramine. *Psychopharmacology (Berlin), 102*(2), 183–190.

Learned-Coughlin, S. M., Bergstrom, M., Savitcheva, I., Ascher, J., Schmith, V. D., & Langstrom, B. (2003). In vivo activity of bupropion at the human dopamine transporter as measured by positron emission tomography. *Biological Psychiatry, 54*(8), 800–805.

Lee, J. J., Erdos, J., Wilkosz, M. F., LaPlante, R., & Wagoner, B. (2009). Bupropion as a possible treatment option for restless legs syndrome. *Annals of Pharmacotherapy, 43*(2), 370–374.

Liu, X., Caggiula, A. R., Palmatier, M. I., Donny, E. C., & Sved, A. F. (2008). Cue-induced reinstatement of nicotine-seeking behavior in rats: Effect of bupropion, persistence over repeated tests, and its dependence on training dose. *Psychopharmacology (Berlin), 196*(3), 365–375.

Loboz, K. K., Gross, A. S., Williams, K. M., Liauw, W. S., Day, R. O., Blievernicht, J. K., et al. (2006). Cytochrome P450 2B6 activity as measured by bupropion hydroxylation: Effect of induction by rifampin and ethnicity. *Clinical Pharmacology and Therapeutics*, *80*(1), 75–84.

Lukas, R. J., Changeux, J. P., Le Novere, N., Albuquerque, E. X., Balfour, D. J., Berg, D. K., et al. (1999). International Union of Pharmacology. XX. Current status of the nomenclature for nicotinic acetylcholine receptors and their subunits. *Pharmacological Reviews*, *51*(2), 397–401.

Lukas, R. J., Muresan, A. Z., Damaj, M. I., Blough, B. E., Huang, X., Navarro, H. A., et al. (2010). Synthesis and characterization of in vitro and in vivo profiles of hydroxybupropion analogues: Aids to smoking cessation. *Journal of Medicinal Chemistry*, *53*(12), 4731–4748.

Malin, D. H. (2001). Nicotine dependence: Studies with a laboratory model. *Pharmacology, Biochemistry, and Behavior*, *70*(4), 551–559.

Malin, D. H., Lake, J. R., Smith, T. D., Khambati, H. N., Meyers-Paal, R. L., Montellano, A. L., et al. (2006). Bupropion attenuates nicotine abstinence syndrome in the rat. *Psychopharmacology (Berlin)*, *184*(3–4), 494–503.

Margolin, A., Kosten, T. R., Avants, S. K., Wilkins, J., Ling, W., Beckson, M., et al. (1995). A multicenter trial of bupropion for cocaine dependence in methadone-maintained patients. *Drug and Alcohol Dependence*, *40*(2), 125–131.

Marubio, L. M., del Mar Arroyo-Jimenez, M., Cordero-Erausquin, M., Lena, C., Le Novere, N., de Kerchove d'Exaerde, A., et al. (1999). Reduced antinociception in mice lacking neuronal nicotinic receptor subunits. *Nature*, *398*(6730), 805–810.

Maxwell, R. A. (1985). The pharmacological rationale for bupropion. In P. Pichot, P. Berner, R. Wolf, & K. Thau (Eds.), *Psychiatry: The state of the art*, (Vol. 3, pp. 135–140). New York: Plenum Press.

Maxwell, R. A., Mehta, N. B., Tucker, W. E., Jr., Schroeder, D. H., & Stern, W. C. (1981). Bupropion. In M. E. Goldberg (Ed.), *Pharmacological and biochemical properties of substances: Vol. 3*, (pp. 1–55). Washington, DC: American Pharmaceutical Association.

Meyer, J. H., Goulding, V. S., Wilson, A. A., Hussey, D., Christensen, B. K., & Houle, S. (2002). Bupropion occupancy of the dopamine transporter is low during clinical treatment. *Psychopharmacology (Berlin)*, *163*(1), 102–105.

Miller, D. K., Sumithran, S. P., & Dwoskin, L. P. (2002). Bupropion inhibits nicotine-evoked [(3)H]overflow from rat striatal slices preloaded with [(3)H]dopamine and from rat hippocampal slices preloaded with [(3)H]norepinephrine. *Journal of Pharmacology and Experimental Therapeutics*, *302*(3), 1113–1122.

Musso, D. L., Mehta, N. B., Soroko, F. E., Ferris, R. M., Hollingsworth, E. B., & Kenney, B. T. (1993). Synthesis and evaluation of the antidepressant activity of the enantiomers of bupropion. *Chirality*, *5*(7), 495–500.

Newton, T. F., Roache, J. D., De La Garza, R., 2nd., Fong, T., Wallace, C. L., Wallace, C., et al. (2006). Bupropion reduces methamphetamine-induced subjective effects and cue-induced craving. *Neuropsychopharmacology*, *31*(7), 1537–1544.

Nielsen, J. A., Shannon, N. J., Bero, L., & Moore, K. E. (1986). Effects of acute and chronic bupropion on locomotor activity and dopaminergic neurons. *Pharmacology, Biochemistry, and Behavior*, *24*(4), 795–799.

Nomikos, G. G., Damsma, G., Wenkstern, D., & Fibiger, H. C. (1992). Effects of chronic bupropion on interstitial concentrations of dopamine in rat nucleus accumbens and striatum. *Neuropsychopharmacology*, *7*(1), 7–14.

Ortmann, R. (1985). The conditioned place preference paradigm in rats: Effect of bupropion. *Life Sciences*, *37*(21), 2021–2027.

Pandhare, A., Hamouda, A. K., Staggs, B., Aggarwal, S., Duddempudi, P. K., Lever, J. R., et al. (2012). Bupropion binds to two sites in the Torpedo nicotinic acetylcholine receptor transmembrane domain: A photoaffinity labeling study with the bupropion analogue [(125)I]-SADU-3-72. *Biochemistry*, *51*(12), 2425–2435.

Poling, J., Oliveto, A., Petry, N., Sofuoglu, M., Gonsai, K., Gonzalez, G., et al. (2006). Six-month trial of bupropion with contingency management for cocaine dependence in a methadone-maintained population. *Archives of General Psychiatry, 63*(2), 219–228.

Quinn, D. I., Wodak, A., & Day, R. O. (1997). Pharmacokinetic and pharmacodynamic principles of illicit drug use and treatment of illicit drug users. *Clinical Pharmacokinetics, 33*(5), 344–400.

Rauhut, A. S., Neugebauer, N., Dwoskin, L. P., & Bardo, M. T. (2003). Effect of bupropion on nicotine self-administration in rats. *Psychopharmacology (Berlin), 169*(1), 1–9.

Reimherr, F. W., Hedges, D. W., Strong, R. E., Marchant, B., Williams, E. D., & Wender, P. H. (2000). *Six-week, double-blind, placebo-controlled trial of bupropion SR for the treatment of adults with attention deficit hyperactivity disorder (ADHD)*. Chicago, IL: American Psychiatric Association.

Schnoll, R. A., Martinez, E., Tatum, K. L., Weber, D. M., Kuzla, N., Glass, M., et al. (2010). A bupropion smoking cessation clinical trial for cancer patients. *Cancer Causes and Control, 21*(6), 811–820.

Segraves, R. T., Clayton, A., Croft, H., Wolf, A., & Warnock, J. (2004). Bupropion sustained release for the treatment of hypoactive sexual desire disorder in premenopausal women. *Journal of Clinical Psychopharmacology, 24*(3), 339–342.

Semenchuk, M. R., & Davis, B. (2000). Efficacy of sustained-release bupropion in neuropathic pain: An open-label study. *Clinical Journal of Pain, 16*(1), 6–11.

Semenchuk, M. R., Sherman, S., & Davis, B. (2001). Double-blind, randomized trial of bupropion SR for the treatment of neuropathic pain. *Neurology, 57*(9), 1583–1588.

Shiffman, S., Johnston, J. A., Khayrallah, M., Elash, C. A., Gwaltney, C. J., Paty, J. A., et al. (2000). The effect of bupropion on nicotine craving and withdrawal. *Psychopharmacology (Berlin), 148*(1), 33–40.

Shoaib, M., Gommans, J., Morley, A., Stolerman, I. P., Grailhe, R., & Changeux, J. P. (2002). The role of nicotinic receptor beta-2 subunits in nicotine discrimination and conditioned taste aversion. *Neuropharmacology, 42*(4), 530–539.

Shoaib, M., Sidhpura, N., & Shafait, S. (2003). Investigating the actions of bupropion on dependence-related effects of nicotine in rats. *Psychopharmacology (Berlin), 165*(4), 405–412.

Shoptaw, S., Heinzerling, K. G., Rotheram-Fuller, E., Steward, T., Wang, J., Swanson, A. N., et al. (2008). Randomized, placebo-controlled trial of bupropion for the treatment of methamphetamine dependence. *Drug and Alcohol Dependence, 96*(3), 222–232.

Simeon, J. G., Ferguson, H. B., & Van Wyck Fleet, J. (1986). Bupropion effects in attention deficit and conduct disorders. *Canadian Journal of Psychiatry, 31*(6), 581–585.

Slemmer, J. E., Martin, B. R., & Damaj, M. I. (2000). Bupropion is a nicotinic antagonist. *Journal of Pharmacology and Experimental Therapeutics, 295*(1), 321–327.

Soroko, F. E., Mehta, N. B., Maxwell, R. A., Ferris, R. M., & Schroeder, D. H. (1977). Bupropion hydrochloride ((+/-) alpha-t-butylamino-3-chloropropiophenone HCl): A novel antidepressant agent. *Journal of Pharmacy and Pharmacology, 29*(12), 767–770.

Spealman, R. D., Madras, B. K., & Bergman, J. (1989). Effects of cocaine and related drugs in nonhuman primates. II. Stimulant effects on schedule-controlled behavior. *Journal of Pharmacology and Experimental Therapeutics, 251*(1), 142–149.

Stahl, S. M., Pradko, J. F., Haight, B. R., Modell, J. G., Rockett, C. B., & Learned-Coughlin, S. (2004). A review of the neuropharmacology of bupropion, a dual norepinephrine and dopamine reuptake inhibitor. *Primary Care Companion to the Journal of Clinical Psychiatry, 6*(4), 159–166.

Suckow, R. F., Zhang, M. F., & Cooper, T. B. (1997). Enantiomeric determination of the phenylmorpholinol metabolite of bupropion in human plasma using coupled achiral-chiral liquid chromatography. *Biomedical Chromatography, 11*(3), 174–179.

Tella, S. R., Ladenheim, B., & Cadet, J. L. (1997). Differential regulation of dopamine transporter after chronic self-administration of bupropion and nomifensine. *Journal of Pharmacology and Experimental Therapeutics, 281*(1), 508–513.

Terry, P., & Katz, J. L. (1997). Dopaminergic mediation of the discriminative stimulus effects of bupropion in rats. *Psychopharmacology (Berlin), 134*(2), 201–212.

Tonstad, S. (2002). Use of sustained-release bupropion in specific patient populations for smoking cessation. *Drugs, 62*(Suppl. 2), 37–43.

Tonstad, S., & Johnston, J. A. (2004). Does bupropion have advantages over other medical therapies in the cessation of smoking? *Expert Opinion on Pharmacotherapy, 5*(4), 727–734.

Tritto, T., McCallum, S. E., Waddle, S. A., Hutton, S. R., Paylor, R., Collins, A. C., et al. (2004). Null mutant analysis of responses to nicotine: Deletion of beta2 nicotinic acetylcholine receptor subunit but not alpha7 subunit reduces sensitivity to nicotine-induced locomotor depression and hypothermia. *Nicotine & Tobacco Research, 6*(1), 145–158.

Unwin, N., & Fujiyoshi, Y. (2012). Gating movement of acetylcholine receptor caught by plunge-freezing. *Journal of Molecular Biology, 422*(5), 617–634.

Volkow, N. D. (2006). Stimulant medications: How to minimize their reinforcing effects? *American Journal of Psychiatry, 163*(3), 359–361.

Volkow, N. D., Ding, Y. S., Fowler, J. S., Wang, G. J., Logan, J., Gatley, J. S., et al. (1995). Is methylphenidate like cocaine? Studies on their pharmacokinetics and distribution in the human brain. *Archives of General Psychiatry, 52*(6), 456–463.

Volkow, N. D., Wang, G. J., Fischman, M. W., Foltin, R. W., Fowler, J. S., Abumrad, N. N., et al. (1997). Relationship between subjective effects of cocaine and dopamine transporter occupancy. *Nature, 386*(6627), 827–830.

Volkow, N. D., Wang, G. J., Fowler, J. S., Gatley, S. J., Logan, J., Ding, Y. S., et al. (1998). Dopamine transporter occupancies in the human brain induced by therapeutic doses of oral methylphenidate. *American Journal of Psychiatry, 155*(10), 1325–1331.

Volkow, N. D., Wang, G. J., Fowler, J. S., Learned-Coughlin, S., Yang, J., Logan, J., et al. (2005). The slow and long-lasting blockade of dopamine transporters in human brain induced by the new antidepressant drug radafaxine predict poor reinforcing effects. *Biological Psychiatry, 57*(6), 640–646.

Warner, C., & Shoaib, M. (2005). How does bupropion work as a smoking cessation aid? *Addiction Biology, 10*(3), 219–231.

Welch, R. M., Lai, A. A., & Schroeder, D. H. (1987). Pharmacological significance of the species differences in bupropion metabolism. *Xenobiotica, 17*(3), 287–298.

Wender, P. H., & Reimherr, F. W. (1990). Bupropion treatment of attention-deficit hyperactivity disorder in adults. *American Journal of Psychiatry, 147*(8), 1018–1020.

Wilens, T. E. (2003). Drug therapy for adults with attention-deficit hyperactivity disorder. *Drugs, 63*(22), 2395–2411.

Wilens, T. E., Haight, B. R., Horrigan, J. P., Hudziak, J. J., Rosenthal, N. E., Connor, D. F., et al. (2005). Bupropion XL in adults with attention-deficit/hyperactivity disorder: A randomized, placebo-controlled study. *Biological Psychiatry, 57*(7), 793–801.

Wilkes, S. (2008). The use of bupropion SR in cigarette smoking cessation. *International Journal of Chronic Obstructive Pulmonary Disease, 3*(1), 45–53.

Xu, H., Loboz, K. K., Gross, A. S., & McLachlan, A. J. (2007). Stereoselective analysis of hydroxybupropion and application to drug interaction studies. *Chirality, 19*(3), 163–170.

Young, R., & Glennon, R. A. (2002). Nicotine and bupropion share a similar discriminative stimulus effect. *European Journal of Pharmacology, 443*(1–3), 113–118.

Zhu, A. Z., Cox, L. S., Nollen, N., Faseru, B., Okuyemi, K. S., Ahluwalia, J. S., et al. (2012). CYP2B6 and bupropion's smoking-cessation pharmacology: The role of hydroxybupropion. *Clinical Pharmacology and Therapeutics, 92*(6), 771–777.

CHAPTER SIX

The Role of Guanfacine as a Therapeutic Agent to Address Stress-Related Pathophysiology in Cocaine-Dependent Individuals

Helen Fox[1], Rajita Sinha
Yale Stress Center, Yale University School of Medicine, New Haven Connecticut USA
[1]Corresponding author: e-mail address: helen.fox@yale.edu

Contents

Abstract

The pathophysiology of cocaine addiction is linked to changes within neural systems and brain regions that are critical mediators of stress system sensitivity and behavioral processes associated with the regulation of adaptive goal-directed behavior. This is characterized by the upregulation of core adrenergic and corticotropin-releasing factor mechanisms that subserve negative affect and anxiety and impinge upon intracellular pathways in the prefrontal cortex underlying cognitive regulation of stress and negative emotional state. Not only are these mechanisms essential to the severity of cocaine withdrawal symptoms, and hence the trajectory of clinical outcome, but also they may be particularly pertinent to the demography of cocaine dependence. The ability

Advances in Pharmacology, Volume 69
ISSN 1054-3589
http://dx.doi.org/10.1016/B978-0-12-420118-7.00006-8

217

of guanfacine to target overlapping stress, reward, and anxiety pathophysiology suggests that it may be a useful agent for attenuating the stress- and cue-induced craving state not only in women but also in men. This is supported by recent research findings from our own laboratory. Additionally, the ability of guanfacine to improve regulatory mechanisms that are key to exerting cognitive and emotional control over drug-seeking behavior also suggests that guanfacine may be an effective medication for reducing craving and relapse vulnerability in many drugs of abuse. As cocaine-dependent individuals are typically polydrug abusers and women may be at a greater disadvantage for compulsive drug use than men, it is plausible that medications that target catecholaminergic frontostriatal inhibitory circuits and simultaneously reduce stress system arousal may provide added benefits for attenuating cocaine dependence.

1. INTRODUCTION

While cocaine dependence is one of the most preventable health-care problems in the United States, no effective FDA-approved medication currently exists that addresses the high rates of craving and cocaine relapse (Kang et al., 1991; O'Brien & Anthony, 2005; Sinha, 2001). This may be due in part to many tested medications showing high abuse potential and focusing predominantly on targeting reward attenuation (Amato et al., 2011; Sofuoglu, 2010; Vocci & Ling, 2005). On the basis of prior findings, we propose that affect and behavioral regulation in the face of both internal and external stressors may also represent a process integral to the acquisition, maintenance, and outcome of dependence for multiple drugs of abuse in both men and women (Albein-Urios et al., 2012; Carelli & West, 2013; Fox, Hong, et al., 2009; Koob & Volkow, 2010). As such, these processes may provide effective targets for medications development. This is important in terms of the demography of cocaine use. First, cocaine-dependent individuals typically abuse multiple drugs, including nicotine and alcohol (Patkar et al., 2006; Wiseman & McMillan, 1998). Moreover, cigarette smoking is more prevalent in cocaine abusers than alcohol and marijuana (Budney, Higgins, Hughes, & Bickel, 1993; Sees & Clark, 1991) and may serve to increase craving (Epstein, Marrone, Heishman, Schmittner, & Preston, 2010; Reid, Mickalian, Delucchi, Hall, & Berger, 1998) and relapse vulnerability (Dackis & O'Brien, 2001; McKay, Alterman, Mulvaney, & Koppenhaver, 1999). Second, recent changes in gender socialization and gender roles and recent gains within the labor force (Bullers, 2012) mean that the traditional gender gap in both licit and street drug consumption has become much smaller (Degenhardt et al., 2008). For example, increases in the prevalence of single, divorced women either living alone or cohabiting and a greater number of women in nontraditional occupations have been associated with gender convergence in substance use (McPherson, Casswell, & Pledger, 2004). Moreover, a number of sex-specific risk factors (e.g., stress and sex steroid hormones) set women at a disadvantage for compulsive drug use (Becker & Hu, 2008; Fattore, Altea, & Fratta, 2008) and the negative consequences of drug use in females often appear accelerated or "telescoped" (Back, Brady, Jackson, Salstrom, & Zinzow, 2005). As such, the development of an FDA-approved medication that targets this vulnerability in women and men who abuse multiple drugs alongside cocaine is imperative.

On this basis, we present data on the nonstimulant alpha-2 adrenergic agonist guanfacine HCL, with regard to its role as a viable agent for (a) attenuating many of the sex-specific and anxiety- and stress-related factors underpinning craving and relapse for cocaine and other substances (Fox, Hong, et al., 2009; Fox, Hong, Siedlarz, & Sinha, 2008) and (b) strengthening cognitive, behavioral, and emotional regulatory processes associated with improved prefrontal network connectivity (Arnsten, 2011b; Arnsten & Jin, 2012; Arnsten & Pliszka, 2011) and substance abuse outcome (Blume & Marlatt, 2009; Williams, Simpson, Simpson, & Nahas, 2009; Witkiewitz & Marlatt, 2005). Initially, therefore, it may be necessary to discuss the relationship between stress system sensitization, anxiety, prefrontal control mechanisms, and compulsive cocaine use in order to subsequently determine the efficacy of guanfacine in targeting stress and negative emotion sensitization and regulation through the mediation of peripheral and central sympathetic arousal (Scahill et al., 2009; Wang, Ji, & Li, 2004). Research data from our laboratory will be presented in order to assess the effects of guanfacine on stress system dysregulation and regulatory function in comorbid cocaine-dependent men and women.

1.1. Stress system dysregulation underlying compulsive cocaine seeking, cocaine craving, and relapse

Cocaine dependence has been described as a chronic stress state (Fox, Hong, et al., 2009; Goeders, 2002; Sinha, 2001) characterized socially by a high prevalence of cumulative lifetime stress (Sinha, 2008), early childhood abuse, and traumatic stress (Hyman et al., 2008; Hyman, Paliwal, & Sinha, 2007; Viola, Tractenberg, Pezzi, Kristensen, & Grassi-Oliveira, 2013) and biophysiologically as comprising decreased dopamine (DA) activity in the mesolimbic pathways (Everitt & Wolf, 2002; Kalivas & Stewart, 1991; Piazza & Le Moal, 1997) and a recruitment of the brain stress systems that include mutual anxiogenic pathophysiology (Dunn & Swiergiel, 2008b; Dunn, Swiergiel, & Palamarchouk, 2004; Koob, 2009a). Due to the overlap in brain stress and reward pathways, these neuroadaptations have been associated with the motivational effects of cocaine (Koob, Caine, Markou, Pulvirenti, & Weiss, 1994; Kuhar, Ritz, & Boja, 1991), including behavioral sensitization (de Jong, Steenbergen, & de Kloet, 2009; Shalev, Grimm, & Shaham, 2002), persistent cocaine craving (Fox, Hong, Siedlarz, & Sinha, 2008; Sinha et al., 2003), and cocaine seeking (Anderson & Pierce, 2005; Bossert, Ghitza, Lu, Epstein, & Shaham, 2005; Sinha, Garcia, Paliwal, Kreek, & Rounsaville, 2006).

The activation of the dopaminergic pathway from the ventral tegmental area (VTA) to the nucleus accumbens (NAc) is thought to be critical for cocaine reward (Bardo, 1998; Johanson & Fischman, 1989; Koob, 1992; Tzschentke, 2001). Specifically, both repeated stress and the maintenance of psychostimulant dependence have been associated with alterations to these mesocorticolimbic DA systems (Everitt & Wolf, 2002; Kalivas & Stewart, 1991; Piazza & Le Moal, 1997) particularly in the NAc and the medial prefrontal cortex (mPFC) (Di Chiara & Imperato, 1988; Kalivas & Duffy, 1990; Koob & Le Moal, 2001) via glutamatergic corticolimbic circuitry (Everitt & Robbins, 2005; Saal, Dong, Bonci, & Malenka, 2003) and the effects of CRF stress systems on glutamate and DA release in the VTA (Ungless, Whistler, Malenka, & Bonci, 2001; Wang et al., 2005). According to the allostatic model of addiction, a sustained increase in the secretion over time of DA may culminate in increased allostatic load and result in a decrease in the function of normal reward-related neurocircuitry and persistence or sensitivity of the stress-related systems (Koob & Le Moal, 2005). Furthermore, chronic cocaine-related adaptations in the noradrenergic system have been implicated in the withdrawal/abstinence and compulsive drug-seeking aspects of cocaine dependence (Aston-Jones & Kalivas, 2008). Both animal and human studies have shown that neuroadaptations to these core stress systems and the persistent nature of an enhanced stress state may modulate the propensity for individuals to misuse many drugs of abuse including cocaine, alcohol, opioids, and nicotine (De Jong & De Kloet, 2004; Fox, Hong, et al., 2009).

Growing preclinical research has shown that the responsiveness of central noradrenergic systems to stress and central activation of noradrenergic transmission, via alpha-2 antagonism, reinstate extinguished cocaine seeking (Feltenstein & See, 2006; Lee, Tiefenbacher, Platt, & Spealman, 2004; Mantsch et al., 2010; Vranjkovic, Hang, Baker, & Mantsch, 2012). Research from our own laboratory has also indicated that in cocaine-dependent individuals, exposure to stressors results in 15% increases in plasma norepinephrine and 20–25% increases in plasma epinephrine, with little indication of normalization/return to baseline even 1 h poststress induction (Sinha et al., 2003). Moreover, these increases in catecholamines were accompanied by augmented craving and anxiety and associated with a greater chance of relapse. Findings from subsequent studies have also indicated that elevations in sympathetic and HPA axis tone are associated with a dysregulated emotional, interoceptive, and biophysiological response to stress provocation, shown to characterize the craving state and predict increased subsequent relapse risk in both cocaine- and alcohol-dependent individuals (Bergquist, Fox, & Sinha, 2010; Chaplin et al., 2010; Fox, Bergquist, Hong, & Sinha, 2007; Fox, Bergquist, Peihua, & Rajita, 2010; Fox, Hong, Paliwal, Morgan, & Sinha, 2008; Sinha, Fox, et al., 2011; Sinha et al., 2006). As increased stress-related adrenergic sensitivity may be involved in the transition from controlled to compulsive drug seeking in cocaine-dependent individuals, medications such as guanfacine, which block central norepinephrine activity, may also serve to attenuate stress-related cocaine craving and relapse rates.

1.2. The role of anxiety symptomatology in compulsive cocaine seeking, cocaine craving, and relapse

During early recovery from cocaine, clinical studies also highlight persistent and dysfunctional aspects of anxiety processing in dependent individuals (Chaplin et al., 2010; Fox, Hong, Paliwal, Morgan, & Sinha, 2008; Harris & Aston-Jones, 1993; Kampman et al., 2001; Lejuez et al., 2008). Although there is a paucity of data regarding the prevalence of comorbid anxiety disorders, possibly due to the fact that cocaine is less commonly thought to be consumed in individuals with a predisposition for anxiety, a NESARC survey documented that 31% of individuals with cocaine dependence reported lifetime anxiety disorders (Conway, Compton, Stinson, & Grant, 2006) and paranoia has also been documented as occurring in 68–84% of patients using cocaine (Morton, 1999). The clinical relevance of this is highlighted by the fact that the severity of withdrawal-related anxiety has been found to impact the course, treatment outcome, and prognosis of both syndromes (Naifeh, Tull, & Gratz, 2012; O'Leary et al., 2000) (Sanchez-Hervas & Llorente del Pozo, 2012), particularly in women (Ambrose-Lanci, Sterling, & Van Bockstaele, 2010; Back et al., 2005; Chaplin, Hong, Bergquist, & Sinha, 2008; Fox & Sinha, 2009). In both genders, higher resting anxiety in alcoholics has been shown to be associated with greater stress and cue-induced alcohol craving and anxiety and higher ACTH and cortisol levels (Sinha, Hong, Seo, Fox, & Bergquist, 2010). Higher stress-induced anxiety also predicts less treatment engagement in after care following inpatient treatment (Sinha, Fox, et al., 2011). Notably, in substance-abusing women, enhanced emotional- and anxiety-related sensitivity to stress has been a dissociable and defining factor of the craving state compared with men and may reflect a vulnerability pathway to relapse in women. For example, significantly elevated stress-induced anxiety ratings documented in women compared with men have been observed in social drinkers (Chaplin, Hong, Bergquist, & Sinha, 2008), alcoholics (Fox et al., 2007), and comorbid cocaine- and alcohol-dependent individuals (Fox, Hong, et al., 2009). In all cases, this sensitized anxiety response was accompanied by significantly higher ratings of both stress-induced and drug cue-induced craving.

With regard to treatment development, it is notable that despite chronic cocaine-related adaptations to core stress and anxiety pathophysiology, few studies have focused directly on treating withdrawal and stress-related anxiety sensitivity. Chronic cocaine use and abuse of other substances, including alcohol and nicotine, all reflect upregulation of CRF and NE feedforward circuitry (Marcinkiewcz et al., 2009; Smith & Aston-Jones, 2008) and elevated noradrenergic transporter binding in the hypothalamus, brain stem, hippocampus, midbrain, and limbic forebrain regions and a desensitization of the alpha-2 adrenoceptors in the prefrontal cortex (PFC) (Baumann, Milchanowski, & Rothman, 2004; Beveridge, Smith, Nader, & Porrino, 2005; Goldstein & Volkow, 2002; Porrino, Lyons, Smith, Daunais, & Nader, 2004). In addition, anxiety involves upregulated extrahypothalamic CRF and NE circuits involving the amygdala and bed nucleus of the stria terminalis (BNST) and downregulated medial prefrontal circuits, which, in turn, result in changes in stress-related pathways involving the hypothalamic paraventricular nucleus and locus coeruleus (LC) to construct a powerful "feedforward" loop that contributes to increased anxiety and stress responses (Dunn & Berridge, 1990; Dunn & Swiergiel, 2008a; Dunn et al., 2004; Koob, 2009a; Kushner, Abrams, & Borchardt, 2000).

Therefore, in addition to playing an integral role in underlying stress-induced craving, these central noradrenergic systems are also key in terms of inducing anxiety, dysphoria, and autonomous panic attacks during early withdrawal from cocaine (McDougle et al., 1994). For example, placebo-corrected adrenergic challenge using alpha-2 antagonist, yohimbine, has been shown to elicit elevated levels of norepinephrine metabolite, 3-methoxy-4-hydroxyphenylglycol, and augmented fear and panic attacks during early recovery in cocaine-addicted individuals (McDougle et al., 1994). As such, adrenergic medications that focus on attenuating the upregulation of central norepinephrine feedforward circuitry, known to underlie chronic cocaine use, withdrawal symptoms, craving, relapse vulnerability, and mutual anxiety pathophysiology, may reduce stress-related compulsive cocaine seeking by targeting the negative anxiogenic reinforcing aspects of cocaine.

1.3. The role of guanfacine and alpha-2 receptor agonists in reducing stress-related anxiety, negative mood, and compulsive drug seeking

Guanfacine is an alpha-2 adrenergic agonist, known to inhibit NE centrally (Shaham, Shalev, Lu, De Wit, & Stewart, 2003) by stimulating presynaptic alpha-2 adrenergic receptors (Arnsten, 2007) and significantly by reducing peripheral sympathetic stress system arousal response and drug seeking (Erb, Shaham, & Stewart, 1998; Erb et al., 2000; Highfield, Yap, Grimm, Shalev, & Shaham, 2001). The enhancement of cognitive performance by guanfacine may be associated with the drug's ability to mimic the enhancing effects of norepinephrine at postsynaptic $\alpha(2A)$ receptors in the PFC (Arnsten, 2011a; Ramos & Arnsten, 2007) and decreasing excitatory post-synaptic transmission in the mPFC and BNST (Ji, Ji, Zhang, & Li, 2008; Le et al., 2011; Shields, Wang, & Winder, 2009). Although the specific mechanisms of action are not fully known with regard to the anxiolytic effects of guanfacine, the indirect downregulation of DA turnover has been documented (Jetmalani, 2010), as well as feedback inhibition of noradrenaline release via presynaptic $\alpha 2$ receptors in humans (Mosqueda-Garcia, 1990; Sorkin & Heel, 1986). It may therefore be of benefit to cocaine-dependent individuals with a susceptibility to upregulated stress dysregulation secondary to chronic cocaine abuse and in women whose stress-related cocaine-craving state may typically be characterized by elevated levels of anxiety symptomatology. In support of this, there is a burgeoning body of research that, taken together, indicates that chronic relapse-related adaptations in the noradrenergic system can be reversed by decreasing norepinephrine centrally, thereby reducing sympathetic arousal and anxiety and, ultimately, attenuating compulsive drug seeking in cocaine dependence.

By downregulating sympathomimetic outflow from the vasomotor center of the brain to the heart and stimulating peripheral alpha (2) receptors (Scahill, 2009; Sica, 2007), guanfacine may decrease the anxiogenic and negative reinforcing components of the craving state for several drugs of abuse, including cocaine. Several animal studies have modeled this noradrenergic mediation of anxiety-like behavior, which emerges after withdrawal of cocaine, predicts relapse (Ambrose-Lanci et al., 2010; Kampman, Volpicelli, et al., 2001; O'Leary et al., 2000), and is attenuated by alpha-2 adrenergic receptor agonists. For example, several recent studies from the animal and human literature have examined the ability of alpha-2 adrenergic agonists including guanfacine, clonidine, and lofexidine to attenuate stress-induced craving, cocaine seeking, and relapse and other negative reinforcing components of the craving state including negative affect and anxiety (Sinha, Shaham, & Heilig, 2011). Shaham and colleagues have shown that α2-adrenergic receptor agonists (clonidine, lofexidine, and guanfacine) modulate the sympathetic stress response, decrease norepinephrine cell firing, and release centrally (Shaham et al., 2003; Sinha, Fox, et al., 2011) and block footshock stress-induced reinstatement of cocaine seeking (Erb et al., 2000, 1998; Highfield et al., 2001). Clonidine at low doses has also been shown to block forced swim-induced reinstatement of cocaine in mice (Mantsch et al., 2010). In addition, clonidine has been shown to block stress-induced reinstatement of speedball seeking (Highfield et al., 2001) and yohimbine-induced cocaine reinstatement after extinction (Lee et al., 2004). Guanfacine has also successfully attenuated cue-induced self-administration of cocaine in laboratory rats (Smith & Aston-Jones, 2011).

A recent preclinical study by Buffalari and colleagues (Buffalari, Baldwin, & See, 2012) also examined the relationship between cocaine withdrawal anxiety symptoms with reinstatement in laboratory rats by using alpha-2 agonist guanfacine and alpha-2 antagonist yohimbine to modulate anxiety and impact cocaine seeking. Findings indicated that anxiety-type behaviors, measured using the elevated plus maze and shock-probe burying behavior, were significantly correlated with cocaine-primed reinstatement. In addition, yohimbine treatment increased reinstatement to cues while guanfacine reduced yohimbine-related reinstatement, emphasizing both the potential utility of withdrawal-related anxiety and related reinstatement of cocaine seeking as a target for medications development and guanfacine as a possible treatment.

While the effects of guanfacine on drinking behaviors in humans have been less well studied, several studies have examined its effects on alcohol seeking in laboratory animals. Furthermore, as alcohol dependence is highly comorbid with anxiety-related disorders (Kessler et al., 1997; Schneider et al., 2001) and acute alcohol withdrawal and protracted abstinence involves noradrenergic dysregulation (Patkar et al., 2003, 2004; Rasmussen, Wilkinson, & Raskind, 2006), it is likely that guanfacine may also provide a viable pharmacotherapeutic treatment for attenuating anxiety-related drinking, or comorbid drinking, in addicted humans. In support of this, early preclinical studies indicated that both clonidine and guanfacine were able to reduce ethanol intake in ethanol-preferring rats having free choice between 10% ethanol and water (Opitz, 1990) and attenuate the appearance and incidence of ethanol withdrawal symptoms (Parale & Kulkarni, 1986; Washton & Resnick, 1981). More recently, preclinical studies' have also shown that activation of alpha-2 adrenoceptors mediates stress- and anxiety-induced reinstatement of alcohol seeking. In one study, guanfacine was shown to attenuate yohimbine-induced reinstatement of alcohol in laboratory rats (Le et al., 2011), and in another, pretreatment with lofexidine was observed to reduce stress-related reinstatement of alcohol seeking and decrease alcohol self-administration.

In terms of smoking, while several clinical and preclinical studies have assessed the effects of alpha-2 adrenergic stimulation on stress-induced reinstatement and withdrawal-related symptoms using clonidine and dexmedetomidine, the effects of guanfacine, per se, have not been well assessed. Despite this, early studies investigating the effects of alpha-2 agonists on nicotine withdrawal-related symptoms served to highlight the salience of noradrenergic transmission in terms of underpinning the anxiolytic, negative reinforcing and possibly control-related aspects of craving. They also demonstrated the sex specificity of noradrenergic mediation of the stress-related craving state. For example, Glassman and colleagues first showed that while clonidine demonstrated similar efficacy to alprazolam in reducing anxiety, tension, irritability, and restlessness during nicotine withdrawal in 15 heavy smokers, only clonidine successfully reduced cigarette craving (Glassman, Jackson, Walsh, Roose, & Rosenfeld, 1984). In a slightly later study, Glassman and colleagues also showed that clonidine was significantly efficacious in reducing nicotine withdrawal and promoting smoking cessation in women compared to men (Covey & Glassman, 1991; Glassman et al., 1988) and particularly in vulnerable women (Glassman et al., 1993). Recent preclinical research holds support for these studies showing that intracentral nucleus of the amygdala (CeA) infusion of clonidine and dexmedetomidine in rats attenuates stress-induced reinstatement of nicotine seeking, possibly via synaptic connections between noradrenergic terminals and CRF neurons (Yamada & Bruijnzeel, 2011).

A recent meta-analysis reviewing 24 studies comprising a total of 1631 participants also investigated the efficacy of alpha-2 agonists for the management of opioid withdrawal (Gowing, Farrell, Ali, & White, 2009). Overall findings indicated that the alpha-2 adrenergic agonists, clonidine and lofexidine, were both more effective than placebo in managing withdrawal from heroin, although the chances of completing withdrawal were no different to those associated with reducing doses of methadone (Gowing et al., 2009). Importantly, however, many clinical trials have indicated that cocaine use is also prevalent in approximately 50% of individuals receiving opioid maintenance treatment (Castells et al., 2009; Grella, Anglin, & Wugalter, 1995; Kosten, Rounsaville, & Kleber, 1987; Peles, Kreek, Kellogg, & Adelson, 2006). Furthermore, the coabuse of cocaine is known to be associated with poorer outcomes in heroin users, suggesting that addressing both cocaine and opioid dependence may be an optimal strategy. In view of this, findings from our own laboratory indicated that lofexidine successfully attenuated stress- and drug cue-related opiate and cocaine craving in opiate-dependent individuals also treated with naltrexone (Sinha, Kimmerling, Doebrick, & Kosten, 2007).

2. GUANFACINE AS A MEDICATION FOR SUBSTANCE ABUSE COMPARED WITH OTHER ALPHA-2 ADRENERGIC AGONISTS

In view of these previous clinical and preclinical findings, we subsequently proposed to examine the effects of guanfacine on stress system adaptations underlying the craving state in cocaine-dependent individuals who also abuse alcohol and nicotine. Compared with other alpha-2 adrenergic agonists, such as clonidine and lofexidine, guanfacine was deemed to have a more preferable pharmacodynamic profile (Balldin, Berggren, Eriksson, Lindstedt, & Sundkler, 1993; Bearn, Gossop, & Strang, 1996; Chappell et al., 1995; Kahn, Mumford, Rogers, & Beckford, 1997). First, early preclinical studies have indicated that guanfacine is 8–10 times more selective than clonidine for alpha-2 adrenoceptors (Jarrott, Louis, & Summers, 1982; Seedat, 1985; Summers, Jarrott, & Louis, 1981). Second, clonidine has consistently shown greater side effects compared with both guanfacine and lofexidine in terms of orthostatic hypotension, sexual dysfunction, and withdrawal syndrome following cessation (Gish, Miller, Honey, & Johnson,

2010; Sorkin & Heel, 1986). In addition, guanfacine has been shown to enhance selective executive and inhibitory control processes underlying impulsivity and other behavioral factors associated with outcome in substance abuse (Brady, Gray, & Tolliver, 2011; Sofuoglu, DeVito, Waters, & Carroll, 2013) in nonhuman primates (Franowicz & Arnsten, 2002), healthy volunteers (Jakala, Riekkinen, Sirvio, Koivisto, Kejonen, et al., 1999; Jakala, Riekkinen, Sirvio, Koivisto, & Riekkinen, 1999), and other clinical populations (Swartz, McDonald, Patel, & Torgersen, 2008). Conversely, although few studies assessing the cognitive profile of lofexidine have been conducted, one study documented decreased cognitive efficiency after lofexidine administration compared with placebo, in 14 opioid-dependent individuals stabilized on methadone (Schroeder et al., 2007). As our studies comprised experimental paradigms conducted across only a few days, we also proposed to use the generic preparation of guanfacine, rather than extended-release formula.

Consistent with our previous studies (Fox et al., 2006; Fox, Hong, Siedlarz, & Sinha, 2008; Fox et al., 2005; Sinha et al., 2009), we used a personalized guided imagery paradigm in order to induce a distress state in 29 early abstinent treatment-seeking substance-abusing men and women. Of the 29 cocaine-dependent individuals, 17 were randomized to guanfacine (2 or 3 mg) and 12 to placebo after a 12-day dosing titration period. Two doses were incorporated into the paradigm as there was little previous research regarding the optimal guanfacine dosing levels for drug craving-related outcomes. The laboratory challenge studies were conducted following approximately 21 days of abstinence during which patients resided on an inpatient treatment research unit. All participants were exposed to three 10 min guided imagery conditions (stress, cocaine cue, and combined stress and cocaine cue), once per day, consecutively in a random, counterbalanced order. Subjective craving, anxiety, and arousal and cardiovascular output were assessed at baseline, immediately following imagery exposure and at repeated recovery time points until 1 h post imagery (Fox, Seo, et al., 2012).

As anticipated, guanfacine attenuated sympathetic tone in cocaine-dependent individuals, characterized by significantly lower heart rate levels ($p = 0.001$) and blood pressure (SBP: $p = 0.002$; DBP: $p = 0.01$) compared with the placebo group. In terms of phasic response, the guanfacine group also demonstrated reduced cue-related cocaine craving and nicotine craving following exposure to all three imagery conditions. In addition, negative reinforcing effects of cocaine, such as anxiety and arousal, were also decreased in the guanfacine group compared with the placebos following exposure to the cocaine cue imagery condition (see Fig. 6.1A–D) (Fox, Seo, et al., 2012). Although guanfacine did not impact phasic heart rate and blood pressure response, its efficacy in lowering autonomic tone may itself represent a key sympathetic mechanism underlying the changes in subjective response to stress and cue. For example, upregulated heart rate and blood pressure are often characteristic of the nonspecific physiological adaptations observed in chronic cocaine dependence, especially during early abstinence (Fox, Hong, et al., 2009). In addition, high tonic autonomic arousal per se may act as a cue or trigger for cocaine craving and increased anxiety during early abstinence (Kampman et al., 2006). As such, the guanfacine-related decrease in peripheral physiological arousal observed in this study may contribute to decreasing subjective anxiety, arousal, and craving response to provocation.

While the combined doses of 2 and 3 mg of guanfacine seemed to produce more robust effects in terms of attenuating cue-related cocaine craving and accompanying negative reinforcing aspects, a preliminary dose analysis showed that the higher 3 mg dose of guanfacine was also beneficial in decreasing stress-induced cocaine craving, stress-induced alcohol craving, and stress-induced nicotine craving (see Fig. 6.2).

As an extension of the same project, additional data were subsequently collected in 27 cocaine-dependent males and 13 cocaine-dependent females in order to better ascertain sex differences in these cocaine-related stress system neuroadaptations (Fox, Morgan, & Sinha, 2013). As mentioned earlier, many prior studies show robust sex variation in the stress- and cue-induced craving state (Brady et al., 2006; Colamussi, Bovbjerg, & Erblich, 2007; Fox, Hong, et al., 2009; Kajantie & Phillips, 2006; Saladin et al., 2012; Waldrop, Back, Verduin, & Brady, 2007; Waldrop et al., 2010) with women generally reporting significantly higher ratings of anxiety, stress, and negative affect (Back et al., 2005; Chaplin et al., 2008; Fox, Hong, Siedlarz, & Sinha, 2008; Fox & Sinha, 2009) alongside unique sympathetic dysregulation patterns compared with those of men (Fox et al., 2006; Fox, Hong, et al., 2009). Preclinical studies have also shown sex diversity, with female rats displaying longer HPA axis activation and greater norepinephrine response to stressors compared to male rats (Heinsbroek et al., 1990; Heinsbroek, Van Haaren, Van de Poll, & Steenbergen, 1991). We therefore hypothesized that guanfacine's effects would be sex-specific with women potentially showing enhanced benefit from adrenergic medication compared with males.

In response to the three provocation conditions described in the preceding text, multiple medications by sex interactions revealed a significantly

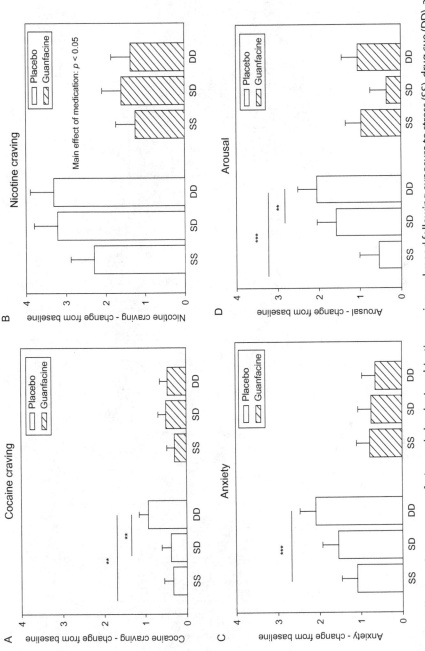

Figure 6.1 Differences between guanfacine and placebo in subjective craving and mood following exposure to stress (SS), drug cue (DD), and combined stress and drug cue (SD). Note: SS, stress/stress condition; SD, stress/drug cue condition; DD, drug cue/drug cue condition. Group differences: **, $p \leq 0.01$; ***, $p < 0.0001$.

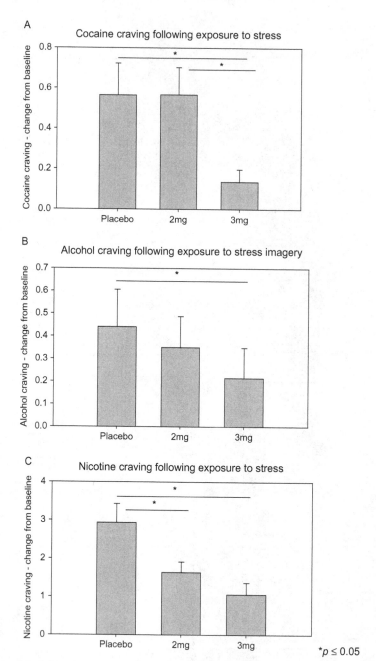

Figure 6.2 Subjective craving responses following exposure to stress imagery, by guanfacine dose.

greater benefit of guanfacine in cocaine-dependent women compared to men (Fig. 6.3). Guanfacine significantly attenuated cocaine craving, alcohol craving, anxiety, and negative emotion in women administered guanfacine compared with women given placebo. This discrepancy was not observed between the male guanfacine and placebo groups. Guanfacine also significantly reduced sympathetic tone and stress-induced and cue-induced blood pressure and nicotine craving in both males and females.

The significant reduction observed in craving, anxiety, and negative emotion in the guanfacine female group stemmed predominantly from the significantly higher ratings reported in all measures by the placebo females compared with both the guanfacine females and the placebo males. This is again consistent with extensive research showing that both cocaine-dependent and cocaine-nondependent females report significantly higher, anxiety, stress, and negative mood during distress compared with males (Back et al., 2005; Chaplin et al., 2008; Eisenberg et al., 1991; Fox, Hong,

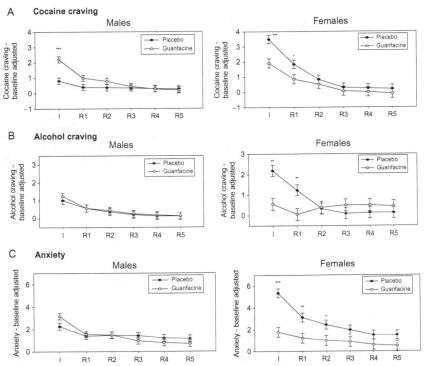

Figure 6.3 Medication (guanfacine vs. placebo) differences by gender following exposure to all three imagery conditions combined. I, imagery exposure; R, recovery time points.

Paliwal, Morgan, & Sinha, 2008; Kelly, Tyrka, Anderson, Price, & Carpenter, 2008) and experience negative emotions at a greater frequency and intensity than men (Craske, 2003; Nolen-Hoeksema, Larson, & Grayson, 1999). Findings also support clinical data indicating that US women are markedly overrepresented with regard to stress-related psychopathology, including anxiety and mood disorders (Blanchard, 1998; Brady, Grice, Dustan, & Randall, 1993; McCance-Katz, Carroll, & Rounsaville, 1999; Rounsaville et al., 1991). In view of this, potentiated stress and cue-related negative mood and anxiety might represent a salient motivational component of the provoked craving state in dependent women (Chaplin et al., 2008; Fox, Hong, et al., 2009; Fox & Sinha, 2009). As an adrenergic agonist, guanfacine targets core anxiety-related CRH and NE sympathetic pathways (Arnsten, 2011a; Sica, 2007; van Zwieten, 1999), and this mechanism may therefore underlie its efficacy in reducing anxiety, negative emotion, and, thus, craving for multiple drugs of abuse in dependent females.

In summary, research from both our own laboratory and those of others demonstrates that alpha-2 adrenergic agonists such as guanfacine may represent a viable medication for reducing peripheral autonomic and emotional arousal mechanisms pertinent to stress-related compulsive cocaine seeking, especially in cocaine-dependent women. It is likely that such attenuation of stress system arousal may be related to central noradrenergic mediation of anxiety-like behavior, which emerges after the withdrawal of cocaine (Buffalari et al., 2012; El Hage et al., 2012; Kampman et al., 2001, 1998), is associated with craving and relapse factors (Ahmadi, Kampman, & Dackis, 2006; Ahmadi et al., 2009; Erb, 2010; Fox, Hong, Siedlarz, & Sinha, 2008), and is sensitive to gender (Ambrose-Lanci et al., 2010; Back et al., 2005; Chaplin et al., 2008; Fox, Hong, Siedlarz, & Sinha, 2008). This is clinically important as anxiety sensitivity may be enhanced in females (Chaplin et al., 2008; Fox, Hong, et al., 2008; Frye, Petralia, & Rhodes, 2000) and be directly related to their increased relapse severity compared with men (Ambrose-Lanci et al., 2010). Furthermore, findings from this initial body of research are particularly salient as polydrug use is a common feature of cocaine dependence (McCance-Katz et al., 1999; Patkar et al., 2006), and women are especially vulnerable to the acquisition, maintenance, and outcome of addiction (Quinones-Jenab, 2006).

2.1. Prefrontal regulatory function and cocaine dependence

In addition to reducing peripheral and central arousal mechanisms underlying the affective and anxiolytic aspects of cocaine addiction, guanfacine is also a powerful modulator of catecholaminergic frontostriatal regulatory circuits (Arnsten & Li, 2005; Ma, Arnsten, & Li, 2005). Dysregulation of emotion and desires/cravings is related to a general diminished ability to recruit frontal systems including the anterior cingulate and PFC (Goldstein & Volkow, 2002; Kalivas & Volkow, 2005; Paulus, Tapert, & Schuckit, 2005; Sinha, 2001) and often underpins the eventual loss of control over drug seeking and consumption. For example, the ability to regulate affect and desires may underlie thoughtful, more adaptive goal-directed behaviors (Gallagher, McMahan, & Schoenbaum, 1999; Kuhl & Koole, 2004; Tice, Bratslavsky, & Baumeister, 2001), including planning, organizational skills, self-control, self-monitoring, and decision-making, which, in turn, are necessary to change substance abuse behaviors and promote better treatment outcome (Blume & Marlatt, 2009; Verdejo-Garcia & Perez-Garcia, 2007). Specifically, poor inhibitory control processes may be a central mechanism of distractibility and impulsive behaviors (Fishbein et al., 2005; Marlatt & Gordon, 1985; Witkiewitz & Marlatt, 2005) and impulsive behavior may cause one to use cocaine despite the negative consequences (Garavan & Hester, 2007). In addition, poor cognitive control may also be related to an inability to resist environmental cues that might trigger drug use (de Wit & Richards, 2004).

Not only is cognitive, emotional, and behavioral self-regulation key to characterizing and determining the trajectory of many substance use disorders (Blume & Marlatt, 2009), but also regulatory strategies are psychologically effortful, and under demanding or stressful situations, volitional behavior may be jeopardized due to a reduction in either mental or motivational capacity (Kuhl & Koole, 2004). According to theorists, this may be the result of conflict in different regulatory goals. While the self-monitoring of impulses and urges may be beneficial for an individual to focus on longer-term priorities, uncontrollable, cumulative, and persistent stressors shift attention toward more immediate often pleasure-seeking goals (Baumeister, Stillwell, & Heatherton, 1994). Notably then, managing such conflicts in regulatory goals has vital implications for treatment attrition, particularly in a population of dependent individuals defined by a high prevalence of lifetime cumulative stress (Ansell, Rando, Tuit, Guarnaccia, & Sinha, 2012) and chronic stress system upregulation (Fox et al., 2010; Fox, Hong, et al., 2009), where stress may literally deplete the psychological resources required for effective emotional and behavioral control.

In view of this, substance-dependent individuals may be extremely vulnerable to stress-induced prefrontal impairment. For example, cocaine use impinges functionally (Goldstein et al., 2009), structurally (Franklin et al., 2002; Lim, Choi, Pomara, Wolkin, & Rotrosen, 2002), and metabolically (Thanos, Michaelides, Benveniste, Wang, & Volkow, 2008; Volkow, Fowler, Wang, & Swanson, 2004) upon regulatory prefrontal executive control systems of the brain and memory-related corticostriatal and hippo-campal regions (Rabbitt, 1997; Roberts, Robbins, & Weiskrantz, 1998). Furthermore, with regard to the efficacy of guanfacine, these brain areas are also rich in DA and norepinephrine innervations (Aston-Jones, Aston-Jones, & Koob, 1984; Foote, Bloom, & Aston-Jones, 1983) and crit-ical to the arousal state (Sara, 2009). This is important as optimal levels of norepinephrine acting at presynaptic $\alpha(2A)$-adrenoceptors serve to enhance neuronal "signals" in the PFC and optimal levels of DA at D1 receptors serve to reduce "noise" in the PFC by suppressing neuronal processing of irrele-vant information (Brennan & Arnsten, 2008; Gamo & Arnsten, 2011; Levy, 2008) and hence strengthen regulatory function and reduce distractibility. In effect, moderate levels of norepinephrine and DA under optimal arousal conditions may serve to facilitate the suppression of irrelevant noise while enhancing relevant signals (Gamo & Arnsten, 2011). Cocaine-related changes to these powerful attentional catecholaminergic systems may there-fore impact related regulatory behaviors including executive (Sawaguchi & Goldman-Rakic, 1994; Zahrt, Taylor, Mathew, & Arnsten, 1997) and inhibitory control processes (Woodward, Mansbach, Carroll, & Balster, 1991). In addition, cocaine-related changes to DA-dependent corticostriatal interconnectivity with the PFC may also alter stimulus–response-associative learning processes that are associated with habit formation (Everitt, Dickinson, & Robbins, 2001; Everitt & Robbins, 2005; Haber, Fudge, & McFarland, 2000) and may also impinge on one's ability to regulate both emotion and behavior under challenging circumstances.

2.2. Prefrontal regulatory dysfunction as targets for alpha-2 adrenergic agonists

As guanfacine is an alpha-2 adrenergic agonist, known to stimulate presyn-aptic receptors in the PFC, it may serve to enhance regulatory cognitive–affective function by means of several putative processes and mechanisms. First, as already discussed, the attenuation of central and peripheral sympa-thetic mechanisms (Erb et al., 2000, 1998; Shaham et al., 2003) may serve to assist with the reduction of anxiety and negative affective state (Ambrose-Lanci et al., 2010; Fox, Seo, et al., 2012) and, hence, attenuate potential con-flict in regulatory goals (Koole & Jostmann, 2004). This may subsequently facilitate cognitive reappraisal during negative emotional experiences (Albein-Urios et al., 2012) known to impact drug-seeking behavior. In addition, guanfacine's ability to optimize catecholamine levels in the PFC and strengthen prefrontal connectivity via the stimulation of alpha-2 receptors and inhibition of cAMP–potassium channel signaling in postsynaptic spines (Arnsten & Li, 2005; Arnsten & Pliszka, 2011; Ramos, Stark, Verduzco, van Dyck, & Arnsten, 2006; Wang et al., 2007) may also improve executive and inhibitory function (Arnsten, 2009, 2011b; Mao, Arnsten, & Li, 1999) and hence goal-directed behaviors integral to outcome factors (Blume & Marlatt, 2009).

In support of this, animal studies using monkeys have indicated that guanfacine-related improvements to delayed response and spatial working memory are accompanied by enhanced regional blood flow to discreet regions of the PFC including the dorsolateral PFC (Avery, Franowicz, Studholme, van Dyck, & Arnsten, 2000), which is associated with inhibitory control, planning (Lazeron et al., 2000), and associative memory deficits (Petrides & Milner, 1982; Sahakian et al., 1988). Other preclinical studies have also demonstrated guanfacine-improved delayed response performance in adult and elderly monkeys (Arnsten, Cai, & Goldman-Rakic, 1988; Mao et al., 1999; Rama, Linnankoski, Tanila, Pertovaara, & Carlson, 1996; Ramos et al., 2006) and rats (Ramos et al., 2006). Furthermore, while yohimbine (an alpha-2 adrenergic antagonist) has been shown to increase distractibility and impulsiveness in rodents, guanfacine improves attention, working memory, inhibitory control, and orbitofrontal reversal learning in nonhuman primates (Arnsten & Li, 2005; Ma, Arnsten, & Li, 2005; Steere & Arnsten, 1997).

In humans, guanfacine treatment has also been efficacious in decreasing impulsivity in children and adults with ADHD and tic disorders (Chappell et al., 1995; Hunt, Arnsten, & Asbell, 1995; Scahill et al., 2001; Taylor & Russo, 2001). With regard to healthy volunteers, however, findings demonstrating working memory enhancement have been ambiguous, with several studies showing guanfacine-related improvements in selective function, including planning and associative learning (Jakala, Riekkinen, Sirvio, Koivisto, Kejonen, et al., 1999; Jakala, Sirvio, et al., 1999), and other studies failing to document any improvements (Birnbaum, Podell, & Arnsten, 2000; Muller et al., 2005). It has therefore been suggested that the effects of guanfacine on executive and regulatory mechanisms may be more likely observed in conditions characterized by catecholaminergic dysfunction (Arnsten, Steere, Jentsch, & Li, 1998; Franowicz & Arnsten, 1998;

Milstein, Lehmann, Theobald, Dalley, & Robbins, 2007). As cocaine withdrawal and ADHD both share a common pathophysiology associated with prefrontal dysregulation and interactions with the caudate and catecholamine system (Arnsten, Steere, & Hunt, 1996; El Hage et al., 2012; Ernst, Zametkin, Matochik, Jons, & Cohen, 1998), guanfacine treatment may be particularly effective at enhancing inhibitory control processes in cocaine-dependent individuals.

Notably, enhancing these prefrontal cognitive processes that are integral to exerting control over drug-seeking behaviors may highlight one of the major benefits of guanfacine compared with several other adrenergic agents. For example, while a number of clinical studies have evaluated the effects of anxiolytic noradrenergic agents in decreasing cocaine withdrawal-related stress on cocaine outcomes, they have not found positive effects on either craving or relapse. While, Kampman and colleagues showed positive effects of propranolol on cocaine severity and withdrawal (Kampman, Alterman, et al., 2001; Kampman et al., 1998), a larger study found no effects of propranolol on cocaine abstinence (Kampman et al., 2006; Kampman, Volpicelli, et al., 2001).

It is also important to emphasize that stress-signaling pathways are responsible for taking the PFC "off-line" by increasing excess catecholamine release into the PFC and modulating ionic regulation of microcircuits (Gamo & Arnsten, 2011). For example, during periods of heightened and uncontrollable stress, potassium channels are opened by elevated cAMP signaling, which reduces persistent firing and weakens prefrontal network activity (Arnsten & Jin, 2012). This is extremely pertinent in chronic stress-related disorders such as cocaine dependence due to the fact that stimulation of α(2A) receptors on prefrontal spines, by agents such as guanfacine, is known to inhibit cAMP signals and increases delay-related firing (Wang et al., 2007). This, in turn, may serve to improve control-related and purpose-driven regulatory behaviors under challenging and stressful situations, common to dependent populations (Sinha, 2008).

Previous research findings from our own laboratory have provided some initial support for this by demonstrating that the ability to optimize dorsolateral and ventromedial function in the face of stress and/or environmental challenge may highlight an important pharmacotherapeutic mechanism associated with guanfacine. In addition to the laboratory component of our double-blind placebo-controlled study (Fox, Seo, et al., 2012), a subsample of 15 cocaine-dependent individuals (nine placebo/six guanfacine) also completed an fMRI component. In the fMRI session, six 2 min imagery scripts (stress, two; cue, two; and neutral, two) were presented in a quasi-randomized manner across one testing session. It was ensured that trials of the same imagery conditions were not presented consecutively. Functional MRI scans during six 5 min trials were acquired, with each trial comprising a 1.5 min quiet baseline period followed by a 2.5 min imagery period (2 min of read imagery) and a 1 min quiet recovery period as in our previous studies (Jastreboff et al., 2011; Li, Kosten, & Sinha, 2005; Seo et al., 2011; Sinha et al., 2005). During the baseline, participants were instructed to stay still without engaging in any mental activity. During the recovery period, participants were asked to stop imagining and lie still in the scanner. Each script was presented only once and scripts from the same condition were not presented consecutively. Between fMRI blocks, all subjects participated in progressive relaxation for 2 min in order to normalize any residual anxiety or craving from previous trials.

Following voxel-based analysis using AFNI, findings showed that guanfacine treatment increased activation in specific regions of the medial and lateral PFC in response to stress and drug cue exposure and increasing insula activation during stress imagery exposure compared with placebo. Most importantly, these increases in regional blood flow occurred in the prefrontal regions typically implicated with distractibility and alertness (Sara, 2009) and the cognitive and emotional regulatory mechanisms underpinning craving, interoceptive function, and treatment outcome (Aron, 2007; Kober, Kross, Mischel, Hart, & Ochsner, 2010; Li, Luo, Yan, Bergquist, & Sinha, 2009; Sinha et al., 2005).

3. OTHER POTENTIAL ANXIOLYTICS AND COGNITIVE ENHANCERS

Much converging evidence suggests that reducing central stress system function and enhancing regulatory processes by stimulating adrenergic transmission within frontostriatal systems may be an important mechanism for reducing craving and relapse in cocaine-dependent individuals who also abuse alcohol and nicotine. However, in order to fully ascertain the efficacy of guanfacine in terms of outcome and abuse potential, it may be necessary to briefly evaluate these factors against additional agents including other anxiolytics and cognitive enhancers.

As many of the subjective and reinforcing effects of cocaine have traditionally been attributed to dopaminergic deficiencies within the mesocorticolimbic pathways (Koob, 2003; Volkow, Fowler, Wang, &

Goldstein, 2002), potentiating DA transmission via "agonist therapy" has provided an important therapeutic target for reducing withdrawal symptoms and preventing relapse (Verrico, Haile, Newton, Kosten, & De La Garza, 2013). However, many of these candidate medications have been limited due to their high abuse liability and high prevalence of side effects (Diana, 2011; Thanos et al., 2004). While the development of both partial agonists and dual DA/5-HT (serotonin) releasers has provided some feasible means of preventing deleterious effects caused by the activation of mesolimbic DA neurons (Grabowski, Shearer, Merrill, & Negus, 2004; Rothman & Baumann, 2003; Rothman et al., 2005), there are still problems regarding long-term use.

For example, while the "antistimulant" effects of increasing levels of 5-HT with DA agonists have been shown to decrease cocaine self-administration behavior in rats and rhesus monkeys (Carroll, Lac, Asencio, & Kragh, 1990; Peltier & Schenk, 1993; Rothman, Blough, & Baumann, 2008), findings in humans have been mixed (Batki, Washburn, Delucchi, & Jones, 1996; Covi, Hess, Kreiter, & Haertzen, 1995; Shorter & Kosten, 2011). Furthermore, 5-HT releasing agents, including SSRIs such as fenfluramine, have also been associated with unpleasant side effects and rare but serious conditions such as cardiac valve disease (Fitzgerald et al., 2000; Rothman et al., 2000), serotonergic depletion and neurotoxicity, and primary pulmonary hypertension (Rothman & Baumann, 2002). Although important steps have been made to develop monoamine releasers that isolate the desirable qualities of DA stimulation on cocaine self-administration while eliminating the reinforcing stimulant effects, such as PAL-287 (Rothman & Baumann, 2009; Rush & Stoops, 2012), future studies still need to assess the potential of these medications with regard to increasing risk for cardiac valve and pulmonary heart disease.

In contrast, while initial reactions to guanfacine are common, most symptoms are mild and include fatigue, sedation, light-headedness, dizziness, and vertigo and tend to disappear either on continued dosing or following dose adjustment (Strang, Bearn, & Gossop, 1999). In fact, one major advantage of guanfacine over other alpha-2 adrenergic agonists such as clonidine is that it is less sedating with less hypotensive potential in both children and adults (Balldin et al., 1993; Bearn et al., 1996; Chappell et al., 1995; Kahn et al., 1997; Scahill et al., 2001). No serious side effects have been noted in adult populations, between the ages 18 and 65 and there are no reported differences in responses between elderly and younger populations. The most serious side effects in pediatric patients are reports of mania and aggressive behavior in pediatric subjects with ADHD (Horrigan & Barnhill, 1998). This side effect has not been documented within adult populations and there is no evidence that guanfacine poses a greater risk than those seen in children and adults with ADHD. In our own laboratory studies using guanfacine for cocaine dependence, the most common side effects of tiredness and fatigue were reported as being mild to moderate and dissipated within the initial 2 weeks of inpatient stay. There were also no significant differences in reported side effects between the experimental group and the placebos (Fox et al., 2013; Fox, Seo, et al., 2012).

Other anxiolytic medications have frequently been used as relapse prevention medications, typically administered in order to reduce cocaine reinforcement following the attainment of a short abstinence period (Kampman, 2008). However, while these agents show promise in terms of preventing relapse to cocaine, they are often associated with high levels of sedation and subsequent problems pertaining to attention, memory, and language. For example, in two clinical trials, the GABA uptake inhibitor tiagabine demonstrated promise with regard to decreasing cocaine use (Gonzales et al., 2003), potentially via anxiolytic mechanisms (Schwartz & Nihalani, 2006). However, several studies also documented clear evidence for tiagabine-induced cognitive impairment in adults and children (Ijff & Aldenkamp, 2013). Similarly, while GABAB receptor agonist, baclofen, has been observed to reduce cocaine administration (Roberts, 2005; Roberts & Brebner, 2000) and cocaine seeking in rats (Di Ciano & Everitt, 2003) and craving for cocaine, tobacco, and marijuana in humans (Brebner, Childress, & Roberts, 2002; Ling, Shoptaw, & Majewska, 1998), it has also worsened cognitive performance during marijuana withdrawal in humans (Haney et al., 2010) and induced sedation in mice (Li et al., 2013). In addition, while controlled pilot trials for topiramate have shown it to be efficacious in terms of maintaining abstinence (Kampman et al., 2004), it is also known to induce sedation and memory problems, particularly with regard to verbal fluency and reaction time (Sommer, Mitchell, & Wroolie, 2013).

In view of this, noradrenergic medications that attenuate sympathetic function are also worth reporting as several have shown some ability to decrease anxiety and cocaine use and limit the effects of psychostimulants without being mediated by severe side effects (Blanc et al., 1994). For example, several studies have shown that alpha-1 antagonist prazosin versus placebo decreases anxiety and arousal symptoms, particularly nightmares and sleep disturbances in PTSD and other anxiety disorders (Boynton, Bentley, Strachan, Barbato, & Raskind, 2009; Fraleigh, Hendratta, Ford, & Connor, 2009; Raskind et al., 2007; Taylor, Freeman, & Cates, 2008). Both prazosin and doxazosin have also been shown to attenuate stress-induced alcohol craving (Fox, Anderson, et al., 2012), fewer drinking days compared with placebo during a 6-week pilot study (Simpson et al., 2009), and a greater number of cocaine-negative urines in a 13-week placebo-controlled pilot study (Shorter, Lindsay, & Kosten, 2013) with minimal side effects. Similarly, in alcohol-related preclinical work, prazosin is effective in decreasing alcohol consumption in dependent animals (Rasmussen, Alexander, Raskind, & Froehlich, 2009).

In addition to alpha receptors, other studies have indicated that nonselective beta-adrenergic blockers such as propranolol may additionally represent a promising pharmacotherapeutic strategy for abstinence initiation in individuals with severe cocaine withdrawal symptoms and heightened anxiety. Clinical trials in humans have documented increases in cocaine treatment retention and attenuation of severity of withdrawal symptoms (Kampman, Alterman, et al., 2001; Kampman et al., 2006, 1999). Again, however, while findings for adrenergic medications show initial promise, beta-adrenergic blockers have been shown to induce sedation and impaired memory consolidation as a possible function of their therapeutic effects (Kampman, 2008; McGaugh, 1989) and alpha-1 adrenergic receptor blockers have also been associated with sedation and behavioral inactivity (Lapiz & Morilak, 2006), perhaps indicating less promise in terms of cognitive enhancement, although this has yet to be determined.

As executive functions such as inhibitory/regulatory control may be an essential component of behaviors underlying treatment outcome (Blume & Marlatt, 2009; Fox, Jackson, & Sinha, 2009), it may become necessary to start assessing the benefits of cognitive enhancers as potential therapies for substance abuse. Several agents including guanfacine, such as glutamatergic mediators (memantine and minocycline), monoamine transporter inhibitors (methylphenidate and atomoxetine), and cholinergic agents (galantamine and varenicline), may show some promise (see Sofuoglu et al., 2013, for full review). Moreover, cognitive-enhancing agents that also target depressive and anxiety symptomatology may be particularly efficacious. For example, selective NET inhibitors such as atomoxetine have been used successfully to improve attention and visual memory performance in children with ADHD (Shang & Gau, 2012) and outcome in children with ADHD, with (Gabriel & Violato, 2011) or without (Durell et al., 2013) comorbid partially responsive anxiety symptoms. However, although atomoxetine may show initial potential in terms of attenuating some of the negative reinforcing effects of cocaine and enhancing regulatory function, the drug has yet to be tested in clinical trials for substance abuse. Similarly, preclinical studies using modafinil have shown both dose- and delay-dependent cognitive improvements and cognitive-enhancing properties in substance abusers (Heinzerling et al., 2010; Mereu, Bonci, Newman, & Tanda, 2013) alongside low abuse potential. This is thought to be due to the fact that modafinil has a markedly lower affinity for DAT binding compared with other stimulants (Minzenberg & Carter, 2008). However, the literature remains ambiguous with regard to modafinil's anxiolytic properties, and several studies have indicated that modafinil may *increase* the levels of anxiety in a range of human populations (Randall, Shneerson, Plaha, & File, 2003; Taneja, Haman, Shelton, & Robertson, 2007; Wong et al., 1999), making it a potentially less viable medication than guanfacine for substance-abusing females.

4. LONG-TERM MAINTENANCE OF GUANFACINE

One of the major benefits of guanfacine in terms of the long-tem potential may be based around the fact that guanfacine represents a medication targeting core regulatory stress systems underlying combined anxiety and addiction pathology. Substance abuse and anxiety disorders are highly comorbid and treatment and health-care burdens are higher for comorbid groups. Using an integrated medication with the potential to uniquely target common stress systems through which substance abuse and anxiety disorders co-occur at highly prevalent rates may therefore help individuals address both disorders simultaneously. Most importantly, several studies comparing integrated with nonintegrated treatment programs have reported significantly greater improvement in substance abuse outcomes for individuals receiving long-term integrated treatments (Barrowclough et al., 2001; Drake, Yovetich, Bebout, Harris, & McHugo, 1997; Godley, Godley, Pratt, & Wallace, 1994) compared with short-term intensive treatment (Brunette, Drake, Woods, & Hartnett, 2001). The requirement for longer-term treatments in comorbid substance abusers is also highlighted by the fact that short periods of abstinence are typically followed by a more challenging and qualitatively different phase of sustained abstinence (Kampman et al., 2006; Marlatt & George, 1984). Moreover, the potential utility of extended-release guanfacine in this context may be highlighted by the fact that optimal cognitive skills may be considered a lynch pin of successful relapse prevention (Blume, Schmaling, & Marlatt, 2005; Marlatt & Gordon, 1985).

In light of these studies, as guanfacine is a nonstimulant agent with minimal treatment-limiting side effects, the extended-release formula may additionally offer long-term therapeutic potential in substance abusers comorbid for anxiety and dysregulatory behaviors. In support of this, to date, studies examining the long-term tolerability of extended-release guanfacine in children with ADHD have been successful in maintaining the attenuation of symptoms safely, over 2 years, with minimal and transient side effects (Biederman et al., 2008; Sallee et al., 2009). Extended-release guanfacine administered across 8 weeks has also been shown to safely improve traumatic stress, anxiety, and ADHD symptoms in children and adolescents (Connor, Grasso, Slivinsky, Pearson, & Banga, 2013).

5. CONCLUSION

Cocaine dependence is a chronic stress state characterized by compulsive and often uncontrollable, drug seeking and drug use despite debilitating negative consequences (Goldstein & Volkow, 2002). Moreover, compared with many other drugs of abuse, there are few efficacious medications that address the high rates of craving and cocaine relapse (Kang et al., 1991; O'Brien, 2005; Sinha, 2001). Notably, the chronic use of cocaine is associated with robust adaptations to core neural stress systems that mediate stress sensitivity, anxiety pathophysiology, and prefrontal regulatory function (Fox & Sinha, 2009). Specifically, these include upregulated extrahypothalamic CRF and norepinephrine circuits involving the amygdala and BNST and downregulated medial prefrontal circuits, which, in turn, result in changes to hypothalamic paraventricular nucleus and LC connections. Over time, these changes may reflect a powerful feedforward loop that contributes to sex-specific changes in anxiety and stress sensitivity (Dunn & Berridge, 1990; Dunn & Swiergiel, 2008b; Dunn et al., 2004; Koob, 2009b; Kushner et al., 2000). These catecholaminergic frontostriatal circuits are also important components of executive and regulatory processes known to underpin goal-directed behaviors, critical to treatment outcome (Blume & Marlatt, 2009).

As an alpha-2 adrenergic agonist, guanfacine's ability to target such overlapping stress, reward, and anxiety pathophysiology suggests that it may be a useful long-term agent for attenuating the stress and cue-induced craving state not only in women but also in men. This is supported by recent research findings from our own laboratory (Fox et al., 2013). The ability of guanfacine to improve regulatory mechanisms that are key to exerting cognitive and emotional control over drug-seeking behavior (Verdejo-Garcia & Perez-Garcia, 2007) also suggests that guanfacine may be an effective medication for reducing craving and relapse vulnerability in many drugs of abuse. As cocaine-dependent individuals are typically polydrug abusers and women may be at a greater disadvantage for compulsive drug use than men (Becker & Hu, 2008), it is plausible that medications that target catecholaminergic frontostriatal regulatory circuits and simultaneously reduce stress system arousal may provide added benefits for attenuating cocaine dependence.

CONFLICT OF INTEREST

The authors have no conflicts of interest to declare.

REFERENCES

Ahmadi, J., Kampman, K., & Dackis, C. (2006). Outcome predictors in cocaine dependence treatment trials. *The American Journal on Addictions*, *15*(6), 434–439. http://dx.doi.org/10.1080/10550490600998476, [Research Support, N.I.H., Extramural].

Ahmadi, J., Kampman, K. M., Oslin, D. M., Pettinati, H. M., Dackis, C., & Sparkman, T. (2009). Predictors of treatment outcome in outpatient cocaine and alcohol dependence treatment. *The American Journal on Addictions*, *18*(1), 81–86. http://dx.doi.org/10.1080/10550490802545174, [Randomized Controlled Trial Research Support, N.I.H., Extramural].

Albein-Urios, N., Verdejo-Roman, J., Asensio, S., Soriano-Mas, C., Martinez-Gonzalez, J. M., & Verdejo-Garcia, A. (2012). Re-appraisal of negative emotions in cocaine dependence: Dysfunctional corticolimbic activation and connectivity. *Addiction Biology* http://dx.doi.org/10.1111/j.1369-1600.2012.00497.x.

Amato, L., Minozzi, S., Pani, P. P., Solimini, R., Vecchi, S., Zuccaro, P., et al. (2011). Dopamine agonists for the treatment of cocaine dependence. *Cochrane Database of Systematic Reviews*, (12), CD003352. http://dx.doi.org/10.1002/14651858.CD003352.pub3, [Meta-Analysis Review].

Ambrose-Lanci, L. M., Sterling, R. C., & Van Bockstaele, E. J. (2010). Cocaine withdrawal-induced anxiety in females: Impact of circulating estrogen and potential use of delta-opioid receptor agonists for treatment. *Journal of Neuroscience Research*, *88*(4), 816–824. http://dx.doi.org/10.1002/jnr.22259, [Research Support, N.I.H., Extramural].

Anderson, S. M., & Pierce, R. C. (2005). Cocaine-induced alterations in dopamine receptor signaling: Implications for reinforcement and reinstatement. *Pharmacology & Therapeutics*, *106*(3), 389–403. http://dx.doi.org/10.1016/j.pharmthera.2004.12.004, [Research Support, N.I.H., Extramural Research Support, U.S. Gov't, P.H.S. Review].

Ansell, E. B., Rando, K., Tuit, K., Guarnaccia, J., & Sinha, R. (2012). Cumulative adversity and smaller gray matter volume in medial prefrontal, anterior cingulate, and insula regions. *Biological Psychiatry*, *72*(1), 57–64. http://dx.doi.org/10.1016/j.biopsych.2011.11.022, [Research Support, N.I.H., Extramural].

Arnsten, A. F. (2007). Catecholamine and second messenger influences on prefrontal cortical networks of "representational knowledge": A rational bridge between genetics and the symptoms of mental illness. *Cerebral Cortex*, *17*(Suppl. 1), i6–i15. http://dx.doi.org/10.1093/cercor/bhm033, [Research Support, N.I.H., Extramural Research Support, Non-U.S. Gov't Review].

Arnsten, A. F. (2009). Ameliorating prefrontal cortical dysfunction in mental illness: Inhibition of phosphotidyl inositol-protein kinase C signaling. *Psychopharmacology, 202*(1–3), 445–455. http://dx.doi.org/10.1007/s00213-008-1274-9, [Research Support, N.I.H., Extramural Review].

Arnsten, A. F. (2011a). Catecholamine influences on dorsolateral prefrontal cortical networks. *Biological Psychiatry, 69*(12), e89–e99. http://dx.doi.org/10.1016/j.biopsych.2011.01.027, [Research Support, N.I.H., Extramural Research Support, Non-U.S. Gov't Review].

Arnsten, A. F. (2011b). Prefrontal cortical network connections: Key site of vulnerability in stress and schizophrenia. *International Journal of Developmental Neuroscience, 29*(3), 215–223. http://dx.doi.org/10.1016/j.ijdevneu.2011.02.006, [Research Support, N.I.H., Extramural Research Support, Non-U.S. Gov't Review].

Arnsten, A. F., Cai, J. X., & Goldman-Rakic, P. S. (1988). The alpha-2 adrenergic agonist guanfacine improves memory in aged monkeys without sedative or hypotensive side effects: Evidence for alpha-2 receptor subtypes. *The Journal of Neuroscience, 8*(11), 4287–4298, [Research Support, Non-U.S. Gov't Research Support, U.S. Gov't, P.H.S.].

Arnsten, A. F., & Jin, L. E. (2012). Guanfacine for the treatment of cognitive disorders: A century of discoveries at Yale. *Yale Journal of Biology and Medicine, 85*(1), 45–58, [Historical Article Review].

Arnsten, A. F., & Li, B. M. (2005). Neurobiology of executive functions: Catecholamine influences on prefrontal cortical functions. *Biological Psychiatry, 57*(11), 1377–1384. http://dx.doi.org/10.1016/j.biopsych.2004.08.019, [Research Support, N.I.H., Extramural Research Support, Non-U.S. Gov't Research Support, U.S. Gov't, P.H.S. Review].

Arnsten, A. F., & Pliszka, S. R. (2011). Catecholamine influences on prefrontal cortical function: Relevance to treatment of attention deficit/hyperactivity disorder and related disorders. *Pharmacology, Biochemistry and Behavior, 99*(2), 211–216. http://dx.doi.org/10.1016/j.pbb.2011.01.020, [Research Support, N.I.H., Extramural Research Support, Non-U.S. Gov't Review].

Arnsten, A. F., Steere, J. C., & Hunt, R. D. (1996). The contribution of alpha 2-noradrenergic mechanisms of prefrontal cortical cognitive function. Potential significance for attention-deficit hyperactivity disorder. *Archives of General Psychiatry, 53*(5), 448–455, [Research Support, U.S. Gov't, P.H.S. Review].

Arnsten, A. F., Steere, J. C., Jentsch, D. J., & Li, B. M. (1998). Noradrenergic influences on prefrontal cortical cognitive function: Opposing actions at postjunctional alpha 1 versus alpha 2-adrenergic receptors. *Advances in Pharmacology, 42*, 764–767, [Research Support, U.S. Gov't, P.H.S.].

Aron, A. R. (2007). The neural basis of inhibition in cognitive control. *The Neuroscientist, 13*(3), 214–228. http://dx.doi.org/10.1177/1073858407299288, [Review].

Aston-Jones, S., Aston-Jones, G., & Koob, G. F. (1984). Cocaine antagonizes anxiolytic effects of ethanol. *Psychopharmacology, 84*(1), 28–31, [Research Support, U.S. Gov't, P.H.S.].

Aston-Jones, G., & Kalivas, P. W. (2008). Brain norepinephrine rediscovered in addiction research. *Biological Psychiatry, 63*(11), 1005–1006. http://dx.doi.org/10.1016/j.biopsych.2008.03.016, [Comment].

Avery, R. A., Franowicz, J. S., Studholme, C., van Dyck, C. H., & Arnsten, A. F. (2000). The alpha-2A-adrenoceptor agonist, guanfacine, increases regional cerebral blood flow in dorsolateral prefrontal cortex of monkeys performing a spatial working memory task. *Neuropsychopharmacology, 23*(3), 240–249. http://dx.doi.org/10.1016/S0893-133X(00)00111-1.

Back, S. E., Brady, K. T., Jackson, J. L., Salstrom, S., & Zinzow, H. (2005). Gender differences in stress reactivity among cocaine-dependent individuals. *Psychopharmacology*, *180*(1), 169–176. http://dx.doi.org/10.1007/s00213-004-2129-7.

Balldin, J., Berggren, U., Eriksson, E., Lindstedt, G., & Sundkler, A. (1993). Guanfacine as an alpha-2-agonist inducer of growth hormone secretion–a comparison with clonidine. *Psychoneuroendocrinology*, *18*(1), 45–55, [Clinical Trial Comparative Study Randomized Controlled Trial Research Support, Non-U.S. Gov't].

Bardo, M. T. (1998). Neuropharmacological mechanisms of drug reward: Beyond dopamine in the nucleus accumbens. *Critical Reviews in Neurobiology*, *12*(1–2), 37–67.

Barrowclough, C., Haddock, G., Tarrier, N., Lewis, S. W., Moring, J., O'Brien, R., et al. (2001). Randomized controlled trial of motivational interviewing, cognitive behavior therapy, and family intervention for patients with comorbid schizophrenia and substance use disorders. *The American Journal of Psychiatry*, *158*(10), 1706–1713, [Clinical Trial Randomized Controlled Trial Research Support, Non-U.S. Gov't].

Batki, S. L., Washburn, A. M., Delucchi, K., & Jones, R. T. (1996). A controlled trial of fluoxetine in crack cocaine dependence. *Drug and Alcohol Dependence*, *41*(2), 137–142, [Clinical Trial Randomized Controlled Trial Research Support, U.S. Gov't, P.H.S.].

Baumann, M. H., Milchanowski, A. B., & Rothman, R. B. (2004). Evidence for alterations in alpha2-adrenergic receptor sensitivity in rats exposed to repeated cocaine administration. *Neuroscience*, *125*(3), 683–690. http://dx.doi.org/10.1016/j.neuroscience.2004.02.013.

Baumeister, R. F., Stillwell, A. M., & Heatherton, T. F. (1994). Guilt: An interpersonal approach. *Psychological Bulletin*, *115*(2), 243–267, [Research Support, Non-U.S. Gov't Review].

Bearn, J., Gossop, M., & Strang, J. (1996). Randomised double-blind comparison of lofexidine and methadone in the in-patient treatment of opiate withdrawal. *Drug and Alcohol Dependence*, *43*(1–2), 87–91, [Clinical Trial Comparative Study Randomized Controlled Trial Research Support, Non-U.S. Gov't].

Becker, J. B., & Hu, M. (2008). Sex differences in drug abuse. *Frontiers in Neuroendocrinology*, *29*(1), 36–47. http://dx.doi.org/10.1016/j.yfrne.2007.07.003, [Research Support, N.I.H., Extramural Review].

Bergquist, K. L., Fox, H. C., & Sinha, R. (2010). Self-reports of interoceptive responses during stress and drug cue-related experiences in cocaine- and alcohol-dependent individuals. *Experimental and Clinical Psychopharmacology*, *18*(3), 229–237. http://dx.doi.org/10.1037/a0019451, [Research Support, N.I.H., Extramural].

Beveridge, T. J., Smith, H. R., Nader, M. A., & Porrino, L. J. (2005). Effects of chronic cocaine self-administration on norepinephrine transporters in the nonhuman primate brain. *Psychopharmacology*, *180*(4), 781–788. http://dx.doi.org/10.1007/s00213-005-2162-1, [Comparative Study Research Support, N.I.H., Extramural Research Support, U.S. Gov't, P.H.S.].

Biederman, J., Melmed, R. D., Patel, A., McBurnett, K., Donahue, J., & Lyne, A. (2008). Long-term, open-label extension study of guanfacine extended release in children and adolescents with ADHD. *CNS Spectrums*, *13*(12), 1047–1055, [Clinical Trial Research Support, Non-U.S. Gov't].

Birnbaum, S. G., Podell, D. M., & Arnsten, A. F. (2000). Noradrenergic alpha-2 receptor agonists reverse working memory deficits induced by the anxiogenic drug, FG7142, in rats. *Pharmacology, Biochemistry and Behavior*, *67*(3), 397–403, [Research Support, U.S. Gov't, P.H.S.].

Blanc, G., Trovero, F., Vezina, P., Herve, D., Godeheu, A. M., Glowinski, J., et al. (1994). Blockade of prefronto-cortical alpha 1-adrenergic receptors prevents locomotor hyperactivity induced by subcortical D-amphetamine injection. *The European Journal of Neuroscience*, *6*(3), 293–298, [Research Support, Non-U.S. Gov't].

Blanchard, D. C. (1998). Stress-related psychopathology as a vulnerability factor in drug taking: The role of sex. In C. L. Weatherington & A. B. Roman (Eds.), *Drug addiction research and the health of women* (pp. 151–164). Bethesda: National Institute on Drug Abuse, NIH.

Blume, A. W., & Marlatt, G. A. (2009). The role of executive cognitive functions in changing substance use: What we know and what we need to know. *Annals of Behavioral Medicine*, *37*(2), 117–125. http://dx.doi.org/10.1007/s12160-009-9093-8, [Review].

Blume, A. W., Schmaling, K. B., & Marlatt, G. A. (2005). Memory, executive cognitive function, and readiness to change drinking behavior. *Addictive Behaviors*, *30*(2), 301–314. http://dx.doi.org/10.1016/j.addbeh.2004.05.019, [Research Support, Non-U.S. Gov't Research Support, U.S. Gov't, P.H.S.].

Bossert, J. M., Ghitza, U. E., Lu, L., Epstein, D. H., & Shaham, Y. (2005). Neurobiology of relapse to heroin and cocaine seeking: An update and clinical implications. *European Journal of Pharmacology*, *526*(1–3), 36–50. http://dx.doi.org/10.1016/j.ejphar.2005.09.030, [Review].

Boynton, L., Bentley, J., Strachan, E., Barbato, A., & Raskind, M. (2009). Preliminary findings concerning the use of prazosin for the treatment of posttraumatic nightmares in a refugee population. *Journal of Psychiatric Practice*, *15*(6), 454–459. http://dx.doi.org/10.1097/01.pra.0000364287.63210.92, [Case Reports Clinical Trial].

Brady, K. T., Back, S. E., Waldrop, A. E., McRae, A. L., Anton, R. F., Upadhyaya, H. P., et al. (2006). Cold pressor task reactivity: Predictors of alcohol use among alcohol-dependent individuals with and without comorbid posttraumatic stress disorder. *Alcoholism, Clinical and Experimental Research*, *30*(6), 938–946. http://dx.doi.org/10.1111/j.1530-0277.2006.00097.x, [Research Support, N.I.H., Extramural].

Brady, K. T., Gray, K. M., & Tolliver, B. K. (2011). Cognitive enhancers in the treatment of substance use disorders: Clinical evidence. *Pharmacology, Biochemistry and Behavior*, *99*(2), 285–294. http://dx.doi.org/10.1016/j.pbb.2011.04.017, [Review].

Brady, K. T., Grice, D. E., Dustan, L., & Randall, C. (1993). Gender differences in substance use disorders. *The American Journal of Psychiatry*, *150*(11), 1707–1711.

Brebner, K., Childress, A. R., & Roberts, D. C. (2002). A potential role for GABA(B) agonists in the treatment of psychostimulant addiction. *Alcohol and Alcoholism*, *37*(5), 478–484, [Review].

Brennan, A. R., & Arnsten, A. F. (2008). Neuronal mechanisms underlying attention deficit hyperactivity disorder: The influence of arousal on prefrontal cortical function. *Annals of the New York Academy of Sciences*, *1129*, 236–245. http://dx.doi.org/10.1196/annals.1417.007, [Research Support, N.I.H., Extramural Review].

Brunette, M. F., Drake, R. E., Woods, M., & Hartnett, T. (2001). A comparison of long-term and short-term residential treatment programs for dual diagnosis patients. *Psychiatric Services*, *52*(4), 526–528, [Comparative Study Evaluation Studies Research Support, U.S. Gov't, P.H.S.].

Budney, A. J., Higgins, S. T., Hughes, J. R., & Bickel, W. K. (1993). Nicotine and caffeine use in cocaine-dependent individuals. *Journal of Substance Abuse*, *5*(2), 117–130, [Research Support, U.S. Gov't, P.H.S.].

Buffalari, D. M., Baldwin, C. K., & See, R. E. (2012). Treatment of cocaine withdrawal anxiety with guanfacine: Relationships to cocaine intake and reinstatement of cocaine seeking in rats. *Psychopharmacology*, *223*(2), 179–190. http://dx.doi.org/10.1007/s00213-012-2705-1, [Research Support, N.I.H., Extramural].

Bullers, S. (2012). An exploratory study of gender and changes in alcohol consumption: A qualitative approach. *Sociation Today*, *10*(1).

Carelli, R. M., & West, E. A. (2013). When a good taste turns bad: Neural mechanisms underlying the emergence of negative affect and associated natural reward devaluation by cocaine. *Neuropharmacology* http://dx.doi.org/10.1016/j.neuropharm.2013.04.025.

Carroll, M. E., Lac, S. T., Asencio, M., & Kragh, R. (1990). Intravenous cocaine self-administration in rats is reduced by dietary L-tryptophan. *Psychopharmacology, 100*(3), 293–300, [Research Support, U.S. Gov't, P.H.S.].

Castells, X., Kosten, T. R., Capella, D., Vidal, X., Colom, J., & Casas, M. (2009). Efficacy of opiate maintenance therapy and adjunctive interventions for opioid dependence with comorbid cocaine use disorders: A systematic review and meta-analysis of controlled clinical trials. *The American Journal of Drug and Alcohol Abuse, 35*(5), 339–349. http://dx.doi.org/10.1080/00952990903108215, [Meta-Analysis Research Support, Non-U.S. Gov't].

Chaplin, T. M., Hong, K., Bergquist, K., & Sinha, R. (2008). Gender differences in response to emotional stress: An assessment across subjective, behavioral, and physiological domains and relations to alcohol craving. *Alcoholism, Clinical and Experimental Research, 32*(7), 1242–1250. http://dx.doi.org/10.1111/j.1530-0277.2008.00679.x, ACER679 [pii].

Chaplin, T. M., Hong, K., Fox, H. C., Siedlarz, K. M., Bergquist, K., & Sinha, R. (2010). Behavioral arousal in response to stress and drug cue in alcohol and cocaine addicted individuals versus healthy controls. *Human Psychopharmacology, 25*(5), 368–376. http://dx.doi.org/10.1002/hup.1127, [Research Support, N.I.H., Extramural].

Chappell, P. B., Riddle, M. A., Scahill, L., Lynch, K. A., Schultz, R., Arnsten, A., et al. (1995). Guanfacine treatment of comorbid attention-deficit hyperactivity disorder and Tourette's syndrome: Preliminary clinical experience. *Journal of the American Academy of Child and Adolescent Psychiatry, 34*(9), 1140–1146. http://dx.doi.org/10.1097/00004583-199509000-00010, [Research Support, U.S. Gov't, P.H.S.].

Colamussi, L., Bovbjerg, D. H., & Erblich, J. (2007). Stress- and cue-induced cigarette craving: Effects of a family history of smoking. *Drug and Alcohol Dependence, 88*(2–3), 251–258. http://dx.doi.org/10.1016/j.drugalcdep.2006.11.006, [Research Support, N.I.H., Extramural Research Support, Non-U.S. Gov't].

Connor, D. F., Grasso, D. J., Slivinsky, M. D., Pearson, G. S., & Banga, A. (2013). An open-label study of guanfacine extended release for traumatic stress related symptoms in children and adolescents. *Journal of Child and Adolescent Psychopharmacology, 23*(4), 244–251. http://dx.doi.org/10.1089/cap.2012.0119, [Research Support, Non-U.S. Gov't].

Conway, K. P., Compton, W., Stinson, F. S., & Grant, B. F. (2006). Lifetime comorbidity of DSM-IV mood and anxiety disorders and specific drug use disorders: results from the national epidemiologic survey on alcohol and related conditions. *The Journal of Clinical Psychiatry, 67*(2), 247–257, [Comparative Study Research Support, N.I.H., Extramural].

Covey, L. S., & Glassman, A. H. (1991). A meta-analysis of double-blind placebo-controlled trials of clonidine for smoking cessation. *British Journal of Addiction, 86*(8), 991–998, [Clinical Trial Meta-Analysis].

Covi, L., Hess, J. M., Kreiter, N. A., & Haertzen, C. A. (1995). Effects of combined fluoxetine and counseling in the outpatient treatment of cocaine abusers. *The American Journal of Drug and Alcohol Abuse, 21*(3), 327–344. http://dx.doi.org/10.3109/00952999509002701, [Clinical Trial Comparative Study Randomized Controlled Trial].

Craske, M. G. (2003). *Origins of phobias and anxiety disorders: Why women more than men?* Oxford: Elsevier.

Dackis, C. A., & O'Brien, C. P. (2001). Cocaine dependence: A disease of the brain's reward centers. *Journal of Substance Abuse Treatment, 21*(3), 111–117, [Review].

De Jong, I. E. M., & De Kloet, E. R. (2004). Glucocorticoids and vulnerability to psychostimulant drugs: Toward substrate and mechanism. *Annals of the New York Academy of Sciences, 1018,* 192–198.

de Jong, I. E., Steenbergen, P. J., & de Kloet, E. R. (2009). Behavioral sensitization to cocaine: Cooperation between glucocorticoids and epinephrine. *Psychopharmacology, 204*(4), 693–703. http://dx.doi.org/10.1007/s00213-009-1498-3, [Research Support, Non-U.S. Gov't].

de Wit, H., & Richards, J. B. (2004). Dual determinants of drug use in humans: Reward and impulsivity. *Nebraska Symposium on Motivation, 50,* 19–55, [Research Support, U.S. Gov't, P.H.S. Review].

Degenhardt, L., Chiu, W. T., Sampson, N., Kessler, R. C., Anthony, J. C., Angermeyer, M., et al. (2008). Toward a global view of alcohol, tobacco, cannabis, and cocaine use: Findings from the WHO World Mental Health Surveys. *PLoS Medicine, 5*(7), e141. http://dx. doi.org/10.1371/journal.pmed.0050141, [Comparative Study Research Support, N.I.H., Extramural Research Support, Non-U.S. Gov't].

Di Chiara, G., & Imperato, A. (1988). Drugs abused by humans preferentially increase synaptic dopamine concentrations in the mesolimbic system of freely moving rats. *Proceedings of the National Academy of Sciences, 85*(14), 5274–5278.

Di Ciano, P., & Everitt, B. J. (2003). The GABA(B) receptor agonist baclofen attenuates cocaine- and heroin-seeking behavior by rats. *Neuropsychopharmacology, 28*(3), 510–518. http://dx.doi.org/10.1038/sj.npp.1300088, [Research Support, Non-U.S. Gov't].

Diana, M. (2011). The dopamine hypothesis of drug addiction and its potential therapeutic value. *Front Psychiatry, 2,* 64. http://dx.doi.org/10.3389/fpsyt.2011.00064.

Drake, R. E., Yovetich, N. A., Bebout, R. R., Harris, M., & McHugo, G. J. (1997). Integrated treatment for dually diagnosed homeless adults. *The Journal of Nervous and Mental Disease, 185*(5), 298–305, [Clinical Trial Comparative Study Controlled Clinical Trial Research Support, U.S. Gov't, P.H.S.].

Dunn, A. J., & Berridge, C. W. (1990). Physiological and behavioral responses to corticotropin-releasing factor administration: Is CRF a mediator of anxiety or stress responses? *Brain Research Brain Research Reviews, 15*(2), 71–100, [Research Support, U.S. Gov't, P.H.S. Review].

Dunn, A. J., & Swiergiel, A. H. (2008a). Effects of acute and chronic stressors and CRF in rat and mouse tests for depression. *Annals of the New York Academy of Sciences, 1148,* 118–126. http://dx.doi.org/10.1196/annals.1410.022, [Research Support, N.I.H., Extramural Research Support, Non-U.S. Gov't].

Dunn, A. J., & Swiergiel, A. H. (2008b). The role of corticotropin-releasing factor and noradrenaline in stress-related responses, and the inter-relationships between the two systems. *European Journal of Pharmacology, 583*(2–3), 186–193. http://dx.doi.org/10.1016/ j.ejphar.2007.11.069, [Research Support, N.I.H., Extramural Review].

Dunn, A. J., Swiergiel, A. H., & Palamarchouk, V. (2004). Brain circuits involved in corticotropin-releasing factor-norepinephrine interactions during stress. *Annals of the New York Academy of Sciences, 1018,* 25–34. http://dx.doi.org/10.1196/annals.1296.003, [Review].

Durell, T. M., Adler, L. A., Williams, D. W., Deldar, A., McGough, J. J., Glaser, P. E., et al. (2013). Atomoxetine treatment of attention-deficit/hyperactivity disorder in young adults with assessment of functional outcomes: A randomized, double-blind, placebo-controlled clinical trial. *Journal of Clinical Psychopharmacology, 33*(1), 45–54. http://dx. doi.org/10.1097/JCP.0b013e31827d8a23, [Multicenter Study Randomized Controlled Trial Research Support, Non-U.S. Gov't].

Eisenberg, N., Fabes, R. A., Schaller, M., Miller, P., Carlo, G., Poulin, R., et al. (1991). Personality and socialization correlates of vicarious emotional responding. *Journal of Personality and Social Psychology, 61*(3), 459–470, [Research Support, U.S. Gov't, Non-P.H.S. Research Support, U.S. Gov't, P.H.S.].

El Hage, C., Rappeneau, V., Etievant, A., Morel, A. L., Scarna, H., Zimmer, L., et al. (2012). Enhanced anxiety observed in cocaine withdrawn rats is associated with altered reactivity of the dorsomedial prefrontal cortex. *PLoS One, 7*(8), e43535. http://dx.doi.org/ 10.1371/journal.pone.0043535, [Research Support, Non-U.S. Gov't].

Epstein, D. H., Marrone, G. F., Heishman, S. J., Schmittner, J., & Preston, K. L. (2010). Tobacco, cocaine, and heroin: Craving and use during daily life. *Addictive Behaviors*, *35*(4), 318–324. http://dx.doi.org/10.1016/j.addbeh.2009.11.003, [Research Support, N.I.H., Intramural].

Erb, S. (2010). Evaluation of the relationship between anxiety during withdrawal and stress-induced reinstatement of cocaine seeking. *Progress in Neuro-Psychopharmacology & Biological Psychiatry*, *34*(5), 798–807. http://dx.doi.org/10.1016/j.pnpbp.2009.11.025, [Review].

Erb, S., Hitchcott, P. K., Rajabi, H., Mueller, D., Shaham, Y., & Stewart, J. (2000). Alpha-2 adrenergic receptor agonists block stress-induced reinstatement of cocaine seeking. *Neuropsychopharmacology*, *23*(2), 138–150. http://dx.doi.org/10.1016/S0893-133X(99) 00158-X, [Research Support, Non-U.S. Gov't].

Erb, S., Shaham, Y., & Stewart, J. (1998). The role of corticotropin-releasing factor and corticosterone in stress- and cocaine-induced relapse to cocaine seeking in rats. *The Journal of Neuroscience*, *18*(14), 5529–5536, [Research Support, Non-U.S. Gov't Research Support, U.S. Gov't, P.H.S.].

Ernst, M., Zametkin, A. J., Matochik, J. A., Jons, P. H., & Cohen, R. M. (1998). DOPA decarboxylase activity in attention deficit hyperactivity disorder adults. A [fluorine-18]fluorodopa positron emission tomographic study. *The Journal of Neuroscience*, *18*(15), 5901–5907.

Everitt, B. J., Dickinson, A., & Robbins, T. W. (2001). The neuropsychological basis of addictive behaviour. *Brain Research Brain Research Reviews*, *36*(2–3), 129–138, [Research Support, Non-U.S. Gov't Review].

Everitt, B. J., & Robbins, T. W. (2005). Neural systems of reinforcement for drug addiction: From actions to habits to compulsion. *Nature Neuroscience*, *8*(11), 1481–1489. http://dx. doi.org/10.1038/nn1579, [Research Support, Non-U.S. Gov't Review].

Everitt, B. J., & Wolf, M. E. (2002). Psychomotor stimulant addiction: A neural systems perspective. *The Journal of Neuroscience*, *22*(9), 3312–3320, [Research Support, Non-U.S. Gov't Research Support, U.S. Gov't, P.H.S. Review], 20026356.

Fattore, L., Altea, S., & Fratta, W. (2008). Sex differences in drug addiction: A review of animal and human studies. *Women's Health (London, England)*, *4*, 51–65. http://dx.doi. org/10.2217/17455057.4.1.51, [Review].

Feltenstein, M. W., & See, R. E. (2006). Potentiation of cue-induced reinstatement of cocaine-seeking in rats by the anxiogenic drug yohimbine. *Behavioural Brain Research*, *174*(1), 1–8. http://dx.doi.org/10.1016/j.bbr.2006.06.039, [Comparative Study Research Support, N.I.H., Extramural].

Fishbein, D. H., Eldreth, D. L., Hyde, C., Matochik, J. A., London, E. D., Contoreggi, C., et al. (2005). Risky decision making and the anterior cingulate cortex in abstinent drug abusers and nonusers. *Brain Research Cognitive Brain Research*, *23*(1), 119–136. http://dx. doi.org/10.1016/j.cogbrainres.2004.12.010, [Clinical Trial Research Support, U.S. Gov't, Non-P.H.S.].

Fitzgerald, L. W., Burn, T. C., Brown, B. S., Patterson, J. P., Corjay, M. H., Valentine, P. A., et al. (2000). Possible role of valvular serotonin 5-HT(2B) receptors in the cardiopathy associated with fenfluramine. *Molecular Pharmacology*, *57*(1), 75–81.

Foote, S. L., Bloom, F. E., & Aston-Jones, G. (1983). Nucleus locus ceruleus: New evidence of anatomical and physiological specificity. *Physiological Reviews*, *63*(3), 844–914, [Research Support, U.S. Gov't, P.H.S. Review].

Fox, H. C., Anderson, G. M., Tuit, K., Hansen, J., Kimmerling, A., Siedlarz, K. M., et al. (2012). Prazosin effects on stress- and cue-induced craving and stress response in alcohol-dependent individuals: Preliminary findings. *Alcoholism, Clinical and Experimental Research*, *36*(2), 351–360. http://dx.doi.org/10.1111/j.1530-0277.2011.01628.x, [Randomized Controlled Trial Research Support, N.I.H., Extramural Research Support, Non-U.S. Gov't].

Fox, H. C., Bergquist, K. L., Hong, K. I., & Sinha, R. (2007). Stress-induced and alcohol cue-induced craving in recently abstinent alcohol-dependent individuals. *Alcoholism, Clinical and Experimental Research, 31*(3), 395–403. http://dx.doi.org/10.1111/j.1530-0277.2006.00320.x, [Research Support, N.I.H., Extramural].

Fox, H. C., Bergquist, K. L., Peihua, G., & Rajita, S. (2010). Interactive effects of cumulative stress and impulsivity on alcohol consumption. *Alcoholism, Clinical and Experimental Research, 34*(8), 1376–1385. http://dx.doi.org/10.1111/j.1530-0277.2010.01221.x, [Comparative Study Research Support, N.I.H., Extramural].

Fox, H. C., Garcia, M., Jr., Kemp, K., Milivojevic, V., Kreek, M. J., & Sinha, R. (2006). Gender differences in cardiovascular and corticoadrenal response to stress and drug cues in cocaine dependent individuals. *Psychopharmacology, 185*(3), 348–357. http://dx.doi.org/10.1007/s00213-005-0303-1, [Research Support, N.I.H., Extramural].

Fox, H. C., Hong, K. A., Paliwal, P., Morgan, P. T., & Sinha, R. (2008). Altered levels of sex and stress steroid hormones assessed daily over a 28-day cycle in early abstinent cocaine-dependent females. *Psychopharmacology, 195*(4), 527–536. http://dx.doi.org/10.1007/s00213-007-0936-3, [Research Support, N.I.H., Extramural].

Fox, H. C., Hong, K. I., Siedlarz, K. M., Bergquist, K., Anderson, G., Kreek, M. J., et al. (2009). Sex-specific dissociations in autonomic and HPA responses to stress and cues in alcohol-dependent patients with cocaine abuse. *Alcohol and Alcoholism, 44*(6), 575–585. http://dx.doi.org/10.1093/alcalc/agp060, [Comparative Study Research Support, N.I.H., Extramural].

Fox, H. C., Hong, K. I., Siedlarz, K., & Sinha, R. (2008). Enhanced sensitivity to stress and drug/alcohol craving in abstinent cocaine-dependent individuals compared to social drinkers. *Neuropsychopharmacology, 33*(4), 796–805. http://dx.doi.org/10.1038/sj.npp.1301470, [Comparative Study Research Support, N.I.H., Extramural].

Fox, H. C., Jackson, E. D., & Sinha, R. (2009). Elevated cortisol and learning and memory deficits in cocaine dependent individuals: Relationship to relapse outcomes. *Psychoneuroendocrinology, 34*(8), 1198–1207. http://dx.doi.org/10.1016/j.psyneuen.2009.03.007, [Research Support, N.I.H., Extramural].

Fox, H. C., Morgan, P. T., & Sinha, R. (2013). Sex differences in guanfacine effects on drug craving and stress arousal in cocaine dependent individuals. *Neuropsychopharmacology.*

Fox, H. C., Seo, D., Tuit, K., Hansen, J., Kimmerling, A., Morgan, P. T., et al. (2012). Guanfacine effects on stress, drug craving and prefrontal activation in cocaine dependent individuals: Preliminary findings. *Journal of Psychopharmacology, 26*(7), 958–972. http://dx.doi.org/10.1177/0269881111430746, [Randomized Controlled Trial Research Support, N.I.H., Extramural Research Support, Non-U.S. Gov't].

Fox, H. C., & Sinha, R. (2009). Sex differences in drug-related stress-system changes: Implications for treatment in substance-abusing women. *Harvard Review of Psychiatry, 17*(2), 103–119. http://dx.doi.org/10.1080/10673220902899680.

Fox, H. C., Talih, M., Malison, R., Anderson, G. M., Kreek, M. J., & Sinha, R. (2005). Frequency of recent cocaine and alcohol use affects drug craving and associated responses to stress and drug-related cues. *Psychoneuroendocrinology, 30*(9), 880–891. http://dx.doi.org/10.1016/j.psyneuen.2005.05.002, [Clinical Trial Comparative Study Randomized Controlled Trial Research Support, N.I.H., Extramural Research Support, U.S. Gov't, P.H.S.].

Fraleigh, L. A., Hendratta, V. D., Ford, J. D., & Connor, D. F. (2009). Prazosin for the treatment of posttraumatic stress disorder-related nightmares in an adolescent male. *Journal of Child and Adolescent Psychopharmacology, 19*(4), 475–476. http://dx.doi.org/10.1089/cap.2009.0002, [Case Reports Letter].

Franklin, T. R., Acton, P. D., Maldjian, J. A., Gray, J. D., Croft, J. R., Dackis, C. A., et al. (2002). Decreased gray matter concentration in the insular, orbitofrontal, cingulate, and temporal cortices of cocaine patients. *Biological Psychiatry, 51*(2), 134–142, [Research Support, U.S. Gov't, P.H.S.].

Franowicz, J. S., & Arnsten, A. F. (1998). The alpha-2a noradrenergic agonist, guanfacine, improves delayed response performance in young adult rhesus monkeys. *Psychopharmacology*, *136*(1), 8–14.

Franowicz, J. S., & Arnsten, A. F. (2002). Actions of alpha-2 noradrenergic agonists on spatial working memory and blood pressure in rhesus monkeys appear to be mediated by the same receptor subtype. *Psychopharmacology*, *162*(3), 304–312. http://dx.doi.org/10.1007/s00213-002-1110-6, [Research Support, U.S. Gov't, P.H.S.].

Frye, C. A., Petralia, S. M., & Rhodes, M. E. (2000). Estrous cycle and sex differences in performance on anxiety tasks coincide with increases in hippocampal progesterone and 3alpha,5alpha-THP. *Pharmacology, Biochemistry and Behavior*, *67*(3), 587–596, [Research Support, Non-U.S. Gov't Research Support, U.S. Gov't, Non-P.H.S.].

Gabriel, A., & Violato, C. (2011). Adjunctive atomoxetine to SSRIs or SNRIs in the treatment of adult ADHD patients with comorbid partially responsive generalized anxiety (GA): An open-label study. *Attention Deficit and Hyperactivity Disorders*, *3*(4), 319–326. http://dx.doi.org/10.1007/s12402-011-0063-1, [Clinical Trial].

Gallagher, M., McMahan, R. W., & Schoenbaum, G. (1999). Orbitofrontal cortex and representation of incentive value in associative learning. *The Journal of Neuroscience*, *19*(15), 6610–6614, [Research Support, U.S. Gov't, P.H.S.].

Gamo, N. J., & Arnsten, A. F. (2011). Molecular modulation of prefrontal cortex: Rational development of treatments for psychiatric disorders. *Behavioral Neuroscience*, *125*(3), 282–296. http://dx.doi.org/10.1037/a0023165, [Review].

Garavan, H., & Hester, R. (2007). The role of cognitive control in cocaine dependence. *Neuropsychology Review*, *17*(3), 337–345. http://dx.doi.org/10.1007/s11065-007-9034-x, [Review].

Gish, E. C., Miller, J. L., Honey, B. L., & Johnson, P. N. (2010). Lofexidine, an {alpha}2-receptor agonist for opioid detoxification. *Annals of Pharmacotherapy*, *44*(2), 343–351. http://dx.doi.org/10.1345/aph.1M347, [Review].

Glassman, A. H., Covey, L. S., Dalack, G. W., Stetner, F., Rivelli, S. K., Fleiss, J., et al. (1993). Smoking cessation, clonidine, and vulnerability to nicotine among dependent smokers. *Clinical Pharmacology and Therapeutics*, *54*(6), 670–679, [Clinical Trial Randomized Controlled Trial Research Support, Non-U.S. Gov't Research Support, U.S. Gov't, P.H.S.].

Glassman, A. H., Jackson, W. K., Walsh, B. T., Roose, S. P., & Rosenfeld, B. (1984). Cigarette craving, smoking withdrawal, and clonidine. *Science*, *226*(4676), 864–866, [Clinical Trial].

Glassman, A. H., Stetner, F., Walsh, B. T., Raizman, P. S., Fleiss, J. L., Cooper, T. B., et al. (1988). Heavy smokers, smoking cessation, and clonidine. Results of a double-blind, randomized trial. *JAMA*, *259*(19), 2863–2866, [Clinical Trial Randomized Controlled Trial Research Support, Non-U.S. Gov't].

Godley, S. H., Godley, M. D., Pratt, A., & Wallace, J. L. (1994). Case management services for adolescent substance abusers: A program description. *Journal of Substance Abuse Treatment*, *11*(4), 309–317, [Research Support, Non-U.S. Gov't Review].

Goeders, N. E. (2002). Stress and cocaine addiction. *The Journal of Pharmacology and Experimental Therapeutics*, *301*(3), 785–789, [Research Support, U.S. Gov't, P.H.S. Review].

Goldstein, R. Z., Alia-Klein, N., Tomasi, D., Carrillo, J. H., Maloney, T., Woicik, P. A., et al. (2009). Anterior cingulate cortex hypoactivations to an emotionally salient task in cocaine addiction. *Proceedings of the National Academy of Sciences of the United States of America*, *106*(23), 9453–9458. http://dx.doi.org/10.1073/pnas.0900491106, [Research Support, N.I.H., Extramural].

Goldstein, R. Z., & Volkow, N. D. (2002). Drug addiction and its underlying neurobiological basis: Neuroimaging evidence for the involvement of the frontal cortex. *The American Journal of Psychiatry*, *159*(10), 1642–1652, [Research Support, U.S. Gov't, Non-P.H.S. Research Support, U.S. Gov't, P.H.S. Review].

Gonzales, G., Sevarino, K., Sofuoglu, M., Poling, J., Oliveto, A., Gonsai, K., et al. (2003). Tiagabine increases cocaine-free urines in cocaine-dependent methadone-treated patients: Results of a randomized pilot study. *Addiction*, *98*, 1625–1632.

Gowing, L., Farrell, M., Ali, R., & White, J. M. (2009). Alpha2-adrenergic agonists for the management of opioid withdrawal. *Cochrane Database of Systematic Reviews*, (2), CD002024. http://dx.doi.org/10.1002/14651858.CD002024.pub3, [Meta-Analysis Review].

Grabowski, J., Shearer, J., Merrill, J., & Negus, S. S. (2004). Agonist-like, replacement pharmacotherapy for stimulant abuse and dependence. *Addictive Behaviors*, *29*(7), 1439–1464. http://dx.doi.org/10.1016/j.addbeh.2004.06.018, [Research Support, U.S. Gov't, P.H.S. Review].

Grella, C. E., Anglin, M. D., & Wugalter, S. E. (1995). Cocaine and crack use and HIV risk behaviors among high-risk methadone maintenance clients. *Drug and Alcohol Dependence*, *37*(1), 15–21, [Research Support, U.S. Gov't, P.H.S.].

Haber, S. N., Fudge, J. L., & McFarland, N. R. (2000). Striatonigrostriatal pathways in primates form an ascending spiral from the shell to the dorsolateral striatum. *The Journal of Neuroscience*, *20*(6), 2369–2382, [Research Support, U.S. Gov't, P.H.S.].

Haney, M., Hart, C. L., Vosburg, S. K., Comer, S. D., Reed, S. C., Cooper, Z. D., et al. (2010). Effects of baclofen and mirtazapine on a laboratory model of marijuana withdrawal and relapse. *Psychopharmacology*, *211*(2), 233–244. http://dx.doi.org/10.1007/s00213-010-1888-6, [Controlled Clinical Trial Research Support, N.I.H., Extramural].

Harris, G. C., & Aston-Jones, G. (1993). Beta-adrenergic antagonists attenuate withdrawal anxiety in cocaine- and morphine-dependent rats. *Psychopharmacology*, *113*(1), 131–136, [Research Support, U.S. Gov't, P.H.S.].

Heinsbroek, R. P., van Haaren, F., Feenstra, M. G., van Galen, H., Boer, G., & van de Poll, N. E. (1990). Sex differences in the effects of inescapable footshock on central catecholaminergic and serotonergic activity. *Pharmacology, Biochemistry and Behavior*, *37*(3), 539–550.

Heinsbroek, R. P., Van Haaren, F., Van de Poll, N. E., & Steenbergen, H. L. (1991). Sex differences in the behavioral consequences of inescapable footshocks depend on time since shock. *Physiology and Behavior*, *49*(6), 1257–1263.

Heinzerling, K. G., Swanson, A. N., Kim, S., Cederblom, L., Moe, A., Ling, W., et al. (2010). Randomized, double-blind, placebo-controlled trial of modafinil for the treatment of methamphetamine dependence. *Drug and Alcohol Dependence*, *109*(1–3), 20–29. http://dx.doi.org/10.1016/j.drugalcdep.2009.11.023, [Randomized Controlled Trial Research Support, N.I.H., Extramural].

Highfield, D., Yap, J., Grimm, J. W., Shalev, U., & Shaham, Y. (2001). Repeated lofexidine treatment attenuates stress-induced, but not drug cues-induced reinstatement of a heroin-cocaine mixture (speedball) seeking in rats. *Neuropsychopharmacology*, *25*(3), 320–331. http://dx.doi.org/10.1016/S0893-133X(01)00227-5, [Research Support, Non-U.S. Gov't Research Support, U.S. Gov't, P.H.S.].

Horrigan, J. P., & Barnhill, L. J. (1998). Does guanfacine trigger mania in children? *Journal of Child and Adolescent Psychopharmacology*, *8*(2), 149–150, [Case Reports Letter].

Hunt, R. D., Arnsten, A. F., & Asbell, M. D. (1995). An open trial of guanfacine in the treatment of attention-deficit hyperactivity disorder. *Journal of the American Academy of Child and Adolescent Psychiatry*, *34*(1), 50–54. http://dx.doi.org/10.1097/00004583-199501000-00013.

Hyman, S. M., Paliwal, P., Chaplin, T. M., Mazure, C. M., Rounsaville, B. J., & Sinha, R. (2008). Severity of childhood trauma is predictive of cocaine relapse outcomes in women but not men. *Drug and Alcohol Dependence*, *92*(1–3), 208–216. http://dx.doi.org/10.1016/j.drugalcdep.2007.08.006, [Research Support, N.I.H., Extramural].

Hyman, S. M., Paliwal, P., & Sinha, R. (2007). Childhood maltreatment, perceived stress, and stress-related coping in recently abstinent cocaine dependent adults. *Psychology of*

Addictive Behaviors, 21(2), 233–238. http://dx.doi.org/10.1037/0893-164X.21.2.233, [Research Support, N.I.H., Extramural].

Ijff, D. M., & Aldenkamp, A. P. (2013). Cognitive side-effects of antiepileptic drugs in children. *Handbook of Clinical Neurology, 111*, 707–718. http://dx.doi.org/10.1016/B978-0-444-52891-9.00073-7.

Jakala, P., Riekkinen, M., Sirvio, J., Koivisto, E., Kejonen, K., Vanhanen, M., et al. (1999). Guanfacine, but not clonidine, improves planning and working memory performance in humans. *Neuropsychopharmacology, 20*(5), 460–470. http://dx.doi.org/10.1016/S0893-133X(98)00127-4, [Clinical Trial Comparative Study Randomized Controlled Trial].

Jakala, P., Riekkinen, M., Sirvio, J., Koivisto, E., & Riekkinen, P., Jr. (1999). Clonidine, but not guanfacine, impairs choice reaction time performance in young healthy volunteers. *Neuropsychopharmacology, 21*(4), 495–502. http://dx.doi.org/10.1016/S0893-133X(99) 00048-2, [Clinical Trial Comparative Study Randomized Controlled Trial Research Support, Non-U.S. Gov't].

Jakala, P., Sirvio, J., Riekkinen, M., Koivisto, E., Kejonen, K., Vanhanen, M., et al. (1999). Guanfacine and clonidine, alpha 2-agonists, improve paired associates learning, but not delayed matching to sample, in humans. *Neuropsychopharmacology, 20*(2), 119–130. http://dx.doi.org/10.1016/S0893-133X(98)00055-4, [Clinical Trial Randomized Controlled Trial Research Support, Non-U.S. Gov't].

Jarrott, B., Louis, W. J., & Summers, R. J. (1982). [3H]-guanfacine: A radioligand that selectively labels high affinity alpha2-adrenoceptor sites in homogenates of rat brain. *British Journal of Pharmacology, 75*(2), 401–408, [In Vitro Research Support, Non-U.S. Gov't].

Jastreboff, A. M., Potenza, M. N., Lacadie, C., Hong, K. A., Sherwin, R. S., & Sinha, R. (2011). Body mass index, metabolic factors, and striatal activation during stressful and neutral-relaxing states: An FMRI study. *Neuropsychopharmacology, 36*(3), 627–637. http://dx.doi.org/10.1038/npp.2010.194, [Research Support, N.I.H., Extramural].

Jetmalani, A. N. (2010). Tourette Syndrome. In K. Cheng & K. M. Myers (Eds.), *Child and adolescent psychiatry: The essentials* (2nd ed., pp. 160–175). New York, Philadelphia, London: Wolters and Kluwer health Lippincott Williams and Wilkins.

Ji, X. H., Ji, J. Z., Zhang, H., & Li, B. M. (2008). Stimulation of alpha2-adrenoceptors suppresses excitatory synaptic transmission in the medial prefrontal cortex of rat. *Neuropsychopharmacology, 33*(9), 2263–2271. http://dx.doi.org/10.1038/sj.npp.1301603, [In Vitro Research Support, Non-U.S. Gov't].

Johanson, C. E., & Fischman, M. W. (1989). The pharmacology of cocaine related to its abuse. *Pharmacological Reviews, 41*(1), 3–52.

Kahn, A., Mumford, J. P., Rogers, G. A., & Beckford, H. (1997). Double-blind study of lofexidine and clonidine in the detoxification of opiate addicts in hospital. *Drug and Alcohol Dependence, 44*(1), 57–61, [Clinical Trial Comparative Study Randomized Controlled Trial].

Kajantie, E., & Phillips, D. I. (2006). The effects of sex and hormonal status on the physiological response to acute psychosocial stress. *Psychoneuroendocrinology, 31*(2), 151–178. http://dx.doi.org/10.1016/j.psyneuen.2005.07.002, [Research Support, Non-U.S. Gov't Review].

Kalivas, P. W., & Duffy, P. (1990). Effect of acute and daily cocaine treatment on extracellular dopamine in the nucleus accumbens. *Synapse (New York, N.Y.), 5*(1), 48–58.

Kalivas, P. W., & Stewart, J. (1991). Dopamine transmission in the initiation and expression of drug- and stress-induced sensitization of motor activity. *Brain Research Brain Research Reviews, 16*(3), 223–244, [Research Support, Non-U.S. Gov't Research Support, U.S. Gov't, P.H.S. Review].

Kalivas, P. W., & Volkow, N. D. (2005). The neural basis of addiction: A pathology of motivation and choice. *The American Journal of Psychiatry, 162*(8), 1403–1413. http://dx.doi.org/10.1176/appi.ajp.162.8.1403, [Research Support, N.I.H., Extramural Research Support, U.S. Gov't, P.H.S. Review].

Kampman, K. M. (2008). The search for medications to treat stimulant dependence. *Addiction Science & Clinical Practice*, 4(2), 28–35.

Kampman, K. M., Alterman, A. I., Volpicelli, J. R., Maany, I., Muller, E. S., Luce, D. D., et al. (2001). Cocaine withdrawal symptoms and initial urine toxicology results predict treatment attrition in outpatient cocaine dependence treatment. *Psychology of Addictive Behaviors*, 15(1), 52–59, [Research Support, U.S. Gov't, Non-P.H.S. Research Support, U.S. Gov't, P.H.S.].

Kampman, K. M., Dackis, C., Lynch, K. G., Pettinati, H., Tirado, C., Gariti, P., et al. (2006). A double-blind, placebo-controlled trial of amantadine, propranolol, and their combination for the treatment of cocaine dependence in patients with severe cocaine withdrawal symptoms. *Drug and Alcohol Dependence*, 85(2), 129–137. http://dx.doi.org/10.1016/j.drugalcdep.2006.04.002, [Randomized Controlled Trial Research Support, N.I.H., Extramural].

Kampman, K. M., Pettinati, H., Lynch, K. G., Dackis, C., Sparkman, T., Weigley, C., et al. (2004). A pilot trial of topiramate for the treatment of cocaine dependence. *Drug and Alcohol Dependence*, 75(3), 233–240. http://dx.doi.org/10.1016/j.drugalcdep.2004.03.008, [Comparative Study Research Support, U.S. Gov't, P.H.S.].

Kampman, K. M., Rukstalis, M., Ehrman, R., McGinnis, D. E., Gariti, P., Volpicelli, J. R., et al. (1999). Open trials as a method of prioritizing medications for inclusion in controlled trials for cocaine dependence. *Addictive Behaviors*, 24(2), 287–291, [Clinical Trial Controlled Clinical Trial Research Support, U.S. Gov't, P.H.S.].

Kampman, K. M., Volpicelli, J. R., McGinnis, D. E., Alterman, A. I., Weinrieb, R. M., D'Angelo, L., et al. (1998). Reliability and validity of the Cocaine Selective Severity Assessment. *Addictive Behaviors*, 23(4), 449–461, [Research Support, U.S. Gov't, Non-P.H.S. Research Support, U.S. Gov't, P.H.S.].

Kampman, K. M., Volpicelli, J. R., Mulvaney, F., Alterman, A. I., Cornish, J., Gariti, P., et al. (2001). Effectiveness of propranolol for cocaine dependence treatment may depend on cocaine withdrawal symptom severity. *Drug and Alcohol Dependence*, 63(1), 69–78, [Clinical Trial Randomized Controlled Trial Research Support, U.S. Gov't, Non-P. H.S. Research Support, U.S. Gov't, P.H.S.].

Kang, S. Y., Kleinman, P. H., Woody, G. E., Millman, R. B., Todd, T. C., Kemp, J., et al. (1991). Outcomes for cocaine abusers after once-a-week psychosocial therapy. *The American Journal of Psychiatry*, 148(5), 630–635, [Clinical Trial Comparative Study Randomized Controlled Trial Research Support, U.S. Gov't, P.H.S.].

Kelly, M. M., Tyrka, A. R., Anderson, G. M., Price, L. H., & Carpenter, L. L. (2008). Sex differences in emotional and physiological responses to the Trier Social Stress Test. *Journal of Behavior Therapy and Experimental Psychiatry*, 39(1), 87–98. http://dx.doi.org/10.1016/j.jbtep.2007.02.003, [Comparative Study Research Support, Non-U.S. Gov't].

Kessler, R. C., Crum, R. M., Warner, L. A., Nelson, C. B., Schulenberg, J., & Anthony, J. C. (1997). Lifetime co-occurrence of DSM-III-R alcohol abuse and dependence with other psychiatric disorders in the National Comorbidity Survey. *Archives of General Psychiatry*, 54(4), 313–321, [Research Support, Non-U.S. Gov't Research Support, P.H.S.].

Kober, H., Kross, E. F., Mischel, W., Hart, C. L., & Ochsner, K. N. (2010). Regulation of craving by cognitive strategies in cigarette smokers. *Drug and Alcohol Dependence*, 106(1), 52–55. http://dx.doi.org/10.1016/j.drugalcdep.2009.07.017, [Research Support, N.I.H., Extramural].

Koob, G. F. (1992). Neural mechanisms of drug reinforcement. *Annals of the New York Academy of Sciences*, 654, 171–191, [Research Support, U.S. Gov't, P.H.S. Review].

Koob, G. F., & Le Moal, M. (2001). Drug addiction, dysregulation of reward, and allostasis. *Neuropsychopharmacology*, 24(2), 97–129.

Koob, G. F. (2003). Neuroadaptive mechanisms of addiction: Studies on the extended amygdala. *European Neuropsychopharmacology, 13*(6), 442–452, [Research Support, U.S. Gov't, P.H.S. Review].

Koob, G. F. (2009a). Brain stress systems in the amygdala and addiction. *Brain Research, 1293*, 61–75. http://dx.doi.org/10.1016/j.brainres.2009.03.038, [Research Support, N.I.H., Extramural Research Support, Non-U.S. Gov't Review].

Koob, G. F. (2009b). New dimensions in human laboratory models of addiction. *Addiction Biology, 14*(1), 1–8. http://dx.doi.org/10.1111/j.1369-1600.2008.00127.x, [Editorial Introductory Research Support, N.I.H., Extramural].

Koob, G. F., Caine, B., Markou, A., Pulvirenti, L., & Weiss, F. (1994). Role for the mesocortical dopamine system in the motivating effects of cocaine. *NIDA Research Monograph, 145*, 1–18, [Research Support, Non-U.S. Gov't Research Support, U.S. Gov't, P.H.S. Review].

Koob, G. F., & Le Moal, M. (2005). Plasticity of reward neurocircuitry and the 'dark side' of drug addiction. *Nature Neuroscience, 8*(11), 1442–1444. http://dx.doi.org/10.1038/nn1105-1442.

Koob, G. F., & Volkow, N. D. (2010). Neurocircuitry of addiction. *Neuropsychopharmacology, 35*(1), 217–238. http://dx.doi.org/10.1038/npp.2009.110, [Research Support, N.I.H., Extramural Review].

Koole, S. L., & Jostmann, N. B. (2004). Getting a grip on your feelings: Effects of action orientation and external demands on intuitive affect regulation. *Journal of Personality and Social Psychology, 87*(6), 974–990. http://dx.doi.org/10.1037/0022-3514.87.6.974, [Research Support, Non-U.S. Gov't].

Kosten, T. R., Rounsaville, B. J., & Kleber, H. D. (1987). A 2.5-year follow-up of cocaine use among treated opioid addicts. Have our treatments helped? *Archives of General Psychiatry, 44*(3), 281–284, [Research Support, U.S. Gov't, P.H.S.].

Kuhar, M. J., Ritz, M. C., & Boja, J. W. (1991). The dopamine hypothesis of the reinforcing properties of cocaine. *Trends in Neurosciences, 14*(7), 299–302, [Review].

Kuhl, J., & Koole, S. L. (2004). Workings of the will. In J. Greenberg, S. L. Koole, & T. Pyszczynski (Eds.), *Handbook of experimental existential psychology* (pp. 411–430). New York: Guildford Press.

Kushner, M. G., Abrams, K., & Borchardt, C. (2000). The relationship between anxiety disorders and alcohol use disorders: A review of major perspectives and findings. *Clinical Psychology Review, 20*(2), 149–171, [Research Support, U.S. Gov't, P.H.S. Review].

Lapiz, M. D., & Morilak, D. A. (2006). Noradrenergic modulation of cognitive function in rat medial prefrontal cortex as measured by attentional set shifting capability. *Neuroscience, 137*(3), 1039–1049. http://dx.doi.org/10.1016/j.neuroscience.2005.09.031, [Research Support, N.I.H., Extramural].

Lazeron, R. H., Rombouts, S. A., Machielsen, W. C., Scheltens, P., Witter, M. P., Uylings, H. B., et al. (2000). Visualizing brain activation during planning: The tower of London test adapted for functional MR imaging. *American Journal of Neuroradiology, 21*(8), 1407–1414, [Research Support, Non-U.S. Gov't].

Le, A. D., Funk, D., Juzytsch, W., Coen, K., Navarre, B. M., Cifani, C., et al. (2011). Effect of prazosin and guanfacine on stress-induced reinstatement of alcohol and food seeking in rats. *Psychopharmacology, 218*(1), 89–99. http://dx.doi.org/10.1007/s00213-011-2178-7, [Research Support, N.I.H., Extramural Research Support, N.I.H., Intramural].

Lee, B., Tiefenbacher, S., Platt, D. M., & Spealman, R. D. (2004). Pharmacological blockade of alpha2-adrenoceptors induces reinstatement of cocaine-seeking behavior in squirrel monkeys. *Neuropsychopharmacology, 29*(4), 686–693. http://dx.doi.org/10.1038/sj.npp.1300391, [Comparative Study Research Support, U.S. Gov't, P.H.S.].

Lejuez, C. W., Zvolensky, M. J., Daughters, S. B., Bornovalova, M. A., Paulson, A., Tull, M. T., et al. (2008). Anxiety sensitivity: A unique predictor of dropout among inner-city heroin and crack/cocaine users in residential substance use treatment. *Behaviour Research and Therapy, 46*(7), 811–818. http://dx.doi.org/10.1016/j.brat.2008.03.010.

Levy, F. (2008). Pharmacological and therapeutic directions in ADHD: Specificity in the PFC. *Behavioral and Brain Functions, 4,* 12. http://dx.doi.org/10.1186/1744-9081-4-12.

Li, C. S., Kosten, T. R., & Sinha, R. (2005). Sex differences in brain activation during stress imagery in abstinent cocaine users: A functional magnetic resonance imaging study. *Biological Psychiatry, 57*(5), 487–494. http://dx.doi.org/10.1016/j.biopsych.2004.11.048, [Comparative Study Research Support, Non-U.S. Gov't Research Support, U.S. Gov't, P.H.S.].

Li, C. S., Luo, X., Yan, P., Bergquist, K., & Sinha, R. (2009). Altered impulse control in alcohol dependence: Neural measures of stop signal performance. *Alcoholism, Clinical and Experimental Research, 33*(4), 740–750. http://dx.doi.org/10.1111/j.1530-0277.2008.00891.x, [Research Support, N.I.H., Extramural Research Support, Non-U.S. Gov't].

Li, X., Risbrough, V. B., Cates-Gatto, C., Kaczanowska, K., Finn, M. G., Roberts, A. J., et al. (2013). Comparison of the effects of the GABAB receptor positive modulator BHF177 and the GABAB receptor agonist baclofen on anxiety-like behavior, learning, and memory in mice. *Neuropharmacology, 70,* 156–167. http://dx.doi.org/10.1016/j.neuropharm.2013.01.018, [Research Support, N.I.H., Extramural].

Lim, K. O., Choi, S. J., Pomara, N., Wolkin, A., & Rotrosen, J. P. (2002). Reduced frontal white matter integrity in cocaine dependence: A controlled diffusion tensor imaging study. *Biological Psychiatry, 51*(11), 890–895, [Research Support, U.S. Gov't, Non-P.H.S.].

Ling, W., Shoptaw, S., & Majewska, D. (1998). Baclofen as a cocaine anti-craving medication: A preliminary clinical study. *Neuropsychopharmacology, 18*(5), 403–404. http://dx.doi.org/10.1016/S0893-133X(97)00128-0, [Clinical Trial Letter Research Support, U.S. Gov't, P.H.S.].

Ma, C. L., Arnsten, A. F., & Li, B. M. (2005). Locomotor hyperactivity induced by blockade of prefrontal cortical alpha2-adrenoceptors in monkeys. *Biological Psychiatry, 57*(2), 192–195. http://dx.doi.org/10.1016/j.biopsych.2004.11.004, [Research Support, Non-U.S. Gov't].

Mantsch, J. R., Weyer, A., Vranjkovic, O., Beyer, C. E., Baker, D. A., & Caretta, H. (2010). Involvement of noradrenergic neurotransmission in the stress- but not cocaine-induced reinstatement of extinguished cocaine-induced conditioned place preference in mice: Role for beta-2 adrenergic receptors. *Neuropsychopharmacology, 35*(11), 2165–2178. http://dx.doi.org/10.1038/npp.2010.86, [Comparative Study Research Support, N.I.H., Extramural].

Mao, Z. M., Arnsten, A. F., & Li, B. M. (1999). Local infusion of an alpha-1 adrenergic agonist into the prefrontal cortex impairs spatial working memory performance in monkeys. *Biological Psychiatry, 46*(9), 1259–1265, [Research Support, Non-U.S. Gov't].

Marcinkiewcz, C. A., Prado, M. M., Isaac, S. K., Marshall, A., Rylkova, D., & Bruijnzeel, A. W. (2009). Corticotropin-releasing factor within the central nucleus of the amygdala and the nucleus accumbens shell mediates the negative affective state of nicotine withdrawal in rats. *Neuropsychopharmacology, 34*(7), 1743–1752. http://dx.doi.org/10.1038/npp.2008.231, [Research Support, N.I.H., Extramural].

Marlatt, G. A., & George, W. H. (1984). Relapse prevention: Introduction and overview of the model. *British Journal of Addiction, 79*(3), 261–273.

Marlatt, G. A., & Gordon, J. R. (1985). *Relapse prevention: Maintenance strategies in the treatment of addictive behaviors.* New York: Guildford Press.

McCance-Katz, E. F., Carroll, K. M., & Rounsaville, B. J. (1999). Gender differences in treatment-seeking cocaine abusers–implications for treatment and prognosis. *The American Journal on Addictions, 8*(4), 300–311, [Research Support, Non-U.S. Gov't Research Support, U.S. Gov't, P.H.S.].

McDougle, C. J., Black, J. E., Malison, R. T., Zimmermann, R. C., Kosten, T. R., Heninger, G. R., et al. (1994). Noradrenergic dysregulation during discontinuation of cocaine use in addicts. *Archives of General Psychiatry, 51*(9), 713–719, [Clinical Trial Randomized Controlled Trial Research Support, Non-U.S. Gov't Research Support, U.S. Gov't, P.H.S.].

McGaugh, J. L. (1989). Dissociating learning and performance: Drug and hormone enhancement of memory storage. *Brain Research Bulletin, 23*(4–5), 339–345, [Research Support, U.S. Gov't, Non-P.H.S. Research Support, U.S. Gov't, P.H.S. Review].

McKay, J. R., Alterman, A. I., Mulvaney, F. D., & Koppenhaver, J. M. (1999). Predicting proximal factors in cocaine relapse and near miss episodes: Clinical and theoretical implications. *Drug and Alcohol Dependence, 56*(1), 67–78, [Research Support, U.S. Gov't, Non-P.H.S. Research Support, U.S. Gov't, P.H.S.].

McPherson, M., Casswell, S., & Pledger, M. (2004). Gender convergence in alcohol consumption and related problems: Issues and outcomes from comparisons of New Zealand survey data. *Addiction, 99*(6), 738–748. http://dx.doi.org/10.1111/j.1360-0443.2004.00758.x.

Mereu, M., Bonci, A., Newman, A. H., & Tanda, G. (2013). The neurobiology of modafinil as an enhancer of cognitive performance and a potential treatment for substance use disorders. *Psychopharmacology, 229*(3), 415–434. http://dx.doi.org/10.1007/s00213-013-3232-4, [Comparative Study Research Support, Non-U.S. Gov't].

Milstein, J. A., Lehmann, O., Theobald, D. E., Dalley, J. W., & Robbins, T. W. (2007). Selective depletion of cortical noradrenaline by anti-dopamine beta-hydroxylase-saporin impairs attentional function and enhances the effects of guanfacine in the rat. *Psychopharmacology, 190*(1), 51–63. http://dx.doi.org/10.1007/s00213-006-0594-x, [Research Support, Non-U.S. Gov't].

Minzenberg, M. J., & Carter, C. S. (2008). Modafinil: A review of neurochemical actions and effects on cognition. *Neuropsychopharmacology, 33*(7), 1477–1502. http://dx.doi.org/10.1038/sj.npp.1301534, [Research Support, N.I.H., Extramural Research Support, Non-U.S. Gov't Review].

Morton, W. A. (1999). Cocaine and psychiatric symptoms. *Primary Care Companion to the Journal of Clinical Psychiatry, 1*(4), 109–113.

Mosqueda-Garcia, R. (1990). Guanfacine: A second generation alpha 2-adrenergic blocker. *The American Journal of the Medical Sciences, 299*(1), 73–76, [Comparative Study Review].

Muller, U., Clark, L., Lam, M. L., Moore, R. M., Murphy, C. L., Richmond, N. K., et al. (2005). Lack of effects of guanfacine on executive and memory functions in healthy male volunteers. *Psychopharmacology, 182*(2), 205–213. http://dx.doi.org/10.1007/s00213-005-0078-4, [Randomized Controlled Trial Research Support, Non-U.S. Gov't].

Naifeh, J. A., Tull, M. T., & Gratz, K. L. (2012). Anxiety sensitivity, emotional avoidance, and PTSD symptom severity among crack/cocaine dependent patients in residential treatment. *Cognitive Therapy and Research, 36*(3), 247–257. http://dx.doi.org/10.1007/s10608-010-9337-8.

Nolen-Hoeksema, S., Larson, J., & Grayson, C. (1999). Explaining the gender difference in depressive symptoms. *Journal of Personality and Social Psychology, 77*(5), 1061–1072, [Research Support, U.S. Gov't, P.H.S.].

O'Brien, C. P. (2005). Anticraving medications for relapse prevention: A possible new class of psychoactive medications. *The American Journal of Psychiatry, 162*(8), 1423–1431. http://dx.doi.org/10.1176/appi.ajp.162.8.1423, [Research Support, N.I.H., Extramural Research Support, U.S. Gov't, P.H.S. Review].

O'Brien, M. S., & Anthony, J. C. (2005). Risk of becoming cocaine dependent: Epidemiological estimates for the United States, 2000-2001. *Neuropsychopharmacology, 30*(5), 1006–1018. http://dx.doi.org/10.1038/sj.npp.1300681, [Research Support, U.S. Gov't, P.H.S.].

O'Leary, T. A., Rohsenow, D. J., Martin, R., Colby, S. M., Eaton, C. A., & Monti, P. M. (2000). The relationship between anxiety levels and outcome of cocaine abuse treatment. *The American Journal of Drug and Alcohol Abuse, 26*(2), 179–194.

Opitz, K. (1990). The effect of clonidine and related substances on voluntary ethanol consumption in rats. *Drug and Alcohol Dependence, 25*(1), 43–48, [Comparative Study].

Parale, M. P., & Kulkarni, S. K. (1986). Studies with alpha 2-adrenoceptor agonists and alcohol abstinence syndrome in rats. *Psychopharmacology, 88*(2), 237–239, [Comparative Study Research Support, Non-U.S. Gov't].

Patkar, A. A., Gopalakrishnan, R., Naik, P. C., Murray, H. W., Vergare, M. J., & Marsden, C. A. (2003). Changes in plasma noradrenaline and serotonin levels and craving during alcohol withdrawal. *Alcohol and Alcoholism, 38*(3), 224–231, [Research Support, Non-U.S. Gov't].

Patkar, A. A., Mannelli, P., Peindl, K., Murray, H. W., Meier, B., & Leone, F. T. (2006). Changes in tobacco smoking following treatment for cocaine dependence. *The American Journal of Drug and Alcohol Abuse, 32*(2), 135–148. http://dx.doi.org/10.1080/00952990500479209, [Research Support, N.I.H., Extramural].

Patkar, A. A., Marsden, C. A., Naik, P. C., Kendall, D. A., Gopalakrishnan, R., Vergare, M. J., et al. (2004). Differences in peripheral noradrenergic function among actively drinking and abstinent alcohol-dependent individuals. *The American Journal on Addictions, 13*(3), 225–235. http://dx.doi.org/10.1080/10550490490459898, [Research Support, Non-U.S. Gov't].

Paulus, M. P., Tapert, S. F., & Schuckit, M. A. (2005). Neural activation patterns of methamphetamine-dependent subjects during decision making predict relapse. *Archives of General Psychiatry, 62*(7), 761–768. http://dx.doi.org/10.1001/archpsyc.62.7.761, [Research Support, N.I.H., Extramural Research Support, U.S. Gov't, P.H.S.].

Peles, E., Kreek, M. J., Kellogg, S., & Adelson, M. (2006). High methadone dose significantly reduces cocaine use in methadone maintenance treatment (MMT) patients. *Journal of Addictive Diseases, 25*(1), 43–50. http://dx.doi.org/10.1300/J069v25n01_07, [Research Support, N.I.H., Extramural Research Support, Non-U.S. Gov't].

Peltier, R., & Schenk, S. (1993). Effects of serotonergic manipulations on cocaine self-administration in rats. *Psychopharmacology, 110*(4), 390–394, [Comparative Study Research Support, U.S. Gov't, P.H.S.].

Petrides, M., & Milner, B. (1982). Deficits on subject-ordered tasks after frontal- and temporal-lobe lesions in man. *Neuropsychologia, 20*(3), 249–262, [Research Support, Non-U.S. Gov't].

Piazza, P. V., & Le Moal, M. (1997). Glucocorticoids as a biological substrate of reward: Physiological and pathophysiological implications. *Brain Research Brain Research Reviews, 25*(3), 359–372, [Research Support, Non-U.S. Gov't Review].

Porrino, L. J., Lyons, D., Smith, H. R., Daunais, J. B., & Nader, M. A. (2004). Cocaine self-administration produces a progressive involvement of limbic, association, and sensori-motor striatal domains. *The Journal of Neuroscience, 24*(14), 3554–3562. http://dx.doi.org/10.1523/JNEUROSCI.5578-03.2004, [Research Support, U.S. Gov't, P.H.S.].

Quinones-Jenab, V. (2006). Why are women from Venus and men from Mars when they abuse cocaine? *Brain Research, 1126*(1), 200–203. http://dx.doi.org/10.1016/j.brainres.2006.08.109, [Research Support, N.I.H., Extramural Review].

Rabbitt, P. (1997). Methodologies and models in the study of executive function. In P. Rabbitt (Ed.), *Methodology of frontal and executive function*. East Sussex: Psychology Press Ltd.

Rama, P., Linnankoski, I., Tanila, H., Pertovaara, A., & Carlson, S. (1996). Medetomidine, atipamezole, and guanfacine in delayed response performance of aged monkeys. *Pharmacology, Biochemistry and Behavior, 55*(3), 415–422, [Comparative Study Research Support, Non-U.S. Gov't].

Ramos, B. P., & Arnsten, A. F. (2007). Adrenergic pharmacology and cognition: Focus on the prefrontal cortex. *Pharmacology & Therapeutics, 113*(3), 523–536. http://dx.doi.org/10.1016/j.pharmthera.2006.11.006, [Research Support, N.I.H., Extramural Review].

Ramos, B. P., Stark, D., Verduzco, L., van Dyck, C. H., & Arnsten, A. F. (2006). Alpha2A-adrenoceptor stimulation improves prefrontal cortical regulation of behavior through inhibition of cAMP signaling in aging animals. *Learning and Memory, 13*(6), 770–776. http://dx.doi.org/10.1101/lm.298006, [Comparative Study Research Support, N.I.H., Extramural Research Support, Non-U.S. Gov't].

Randall, D. C., Shneerson, J. M., Plaha, K. K., & File, S. E. (2003). Modafinil affects mood, but not cognitive function, in healthy young volunteers. *Human Psychopharmacology, 18*(3), 163–173. http://dx.doi.org/10.1002/hup.456, [Clinical Trial Randomized Controlled Trial].

Raskind, M. A., Peskind, E. R., Hoff, D. J., Hart, K. L., Holmes, H. A., Warren, D., et al. (2007). A parallel group placebo controlled study of prazosin for trauma nightmares and sleep disturbance in combat veterans with post-traumatic stress disorder. *Biological Psychiatry, 61*(8), 928–934. http://dx.doi.org/10.1016/j.biopsych.2006.06.032, [Evaluation Studies Randomized Controlled Trial Research Support, N.I.H., Extramural Research Support, U.S. Gov't, Non-P.H.S.].

Rasmussen, D. D., Alexander, L. L., Raskind, M. A., & Froehlich, J. C. (2009). The alpha1-adrenergic receptor antagonist, prazosin, reduces alcohol drinking in alcohol-preferring (P) rats. *Alcoholism, Clinical and Experimental Research, 33*(2), 264–272. http://dx.doi.org/10.1111/j.1530-0277.2008.00829.x, [Research Support, N.I.H., Extramural].

Rasmussen, D. D., Wilkinson, C. W., & Raskind, M. A. (2006). Chronic daily ethanol and withdrawal: 6. Effects on rat sympathoadrenal activity during "abstinence" *Alcohol, 38*(3), 173–177. http://dx.doi.org/10.1016/j.alcohol.2006.06.007, [Research Support, N.I.H., Extramural Research Support, U.S. Gov't, Non-P.H.S.].

Reid, M. S., Mickalian, J. D., Delucchi, K. L., Hall, S. M., & Berger, S. P. (1998). An acute dose of nicotine enhances cue-induced cocaine craving. *Drug and Alcohol Dependence, 49*(2), 95–104, [Clinical Trial Randomized Controlled Trial Research Support, U.S. Gov't, P.H.S.].

Roberts, D. C. (2005). Preclinical evidence for GABAB agonists as a pharmacotherapy for cocaine addiction. *Physiology and Behavior, 86*(1–2), 18–20. http://dx.doi.org/10.1016/j.physbeh.2005.06.017, [Comparative Study Review].

Roberts, D. C., & Brebner, K. (2000). GABA modulation of cocaine self-administration. *Annals of the New York Academy of Sciences, 909*, 145–158, [Research Support, Non-U.S. Gov't Research Support, U.S. Gov't, P.H.S. Review].

Roberts, A. C., Robbins, T. W., & Weiskrantz, L. (1998). *The prefrontal cortex executive and cognitive functions.* Oxford: Oxford University Press.

Rothman, R. B., & Baumann, M. H. (2002). Serotonin releasing agents. Neurochemical, therapeutic and adverse effects. *Pharmacology, Biochemistry and Behavior, 71*(4), 825–836, [Review].

Rothman, R. B., & Baumann, M. H. (2003). Monoamine transporters and psychostimulant drugs. *European Journal of Pharmacology, 479*(1–3), 23–40, [Review].

Rothman, R. B., & Baumann, M. H. (2009). Serotonergic drugs and valvular heart disease. *Expert Opinion on Drug Safety, 8*(3), 317–329. http://dx.doi.org/10.1517/14740330902931524, [Research Support, N.I.H., Intramural Review].

Rothman, R. B., Blough, B. E., & Baumann, M. H. (2008). Dual dopamine/serotonin releasers: Potential treatment agents for stimulant addiction. *Experimental and Clinical Psychopharmacology, 16*(6), 458–474. http://dx.doi.org/10.1037/a0014103, [Research Support, N.I.H., Extramural Research Support, N.I.H., Intramural Review].

Rothman, R. B., Blough, B. E., Woolverton, W. L., Anderson, K. G., Negus, S. S., Mello, N. K., et al. (2005). Development of a rationally designed, low abuse potential, biogenic amine releaser that suppresses cocaine self-administration. *The Journal of Pharmacology and Experimental Therapeutics, 313*(3), 1361–1369. http://dx.doi.org/10.1124/jpet.104.082503, [Research Support, N.I.H., Extramural Research Support, U.S. Gov't, P.H.S.].

Rothman, R. B., Partilla, J. S., Dersch, C. M., Carroll, F. I., Rice, K. C., & Baumann, M. H. (2000). Methamphetamine dependence: Medication development efforts based on the dual deficit model of stimulant addiction. *Annals of the New York Academy of Sciences, 914*, 71–81, [Comparative Study Review].

Rounsaville, B. J., Anton, S. F., Carroll, K., Budde, D., Prusoff, B. A., & Gawin, F. (1991). Psychiatric diagnoses of treatment-seeking cocaine abusers. *Archives of General Psychiatry, 48*(1), 43–51, [Research Support, U.S. Gov't, P.H.S.].

Rush, C. R., & Stoops, W. W. (2012). Agonist replacement therapy for cocaine dependence: A translational review. *Future Medicinal Chemistry, 4*(2), 245–265. http://dx.doi.org/10.4155/fmc.11.184, [Research Support, N.I.H., Extramural Review].

Saal, D., Dong, Y., Bonci, A., & Malenka, R. C. (2003). Drugs of abuse and stress trigger a common synaptic adaptation in dopamine neurons. *Neuron, 37*(4), 577–582, doi: S0896627303000217 [pii].

Sahakian, B. J., Morris, R. G., Evenden, J. L., Heald, A., Levy, R., Philpot, M., et al. (1988). A comparative study of visuospatial memory and learning in Alzheimer-type dementia and Parkinson's disease. *Brain, 111*(Pt. 3), 695–718, [Comparative Study Research Support, Non-U.S. Gov't].

Saladin, M. E., Gray, K. M., Carpenter, M. J., LaRowe, S. D., DeSantis, S. M., & Upadhyaya, H. P. (2012). Gender differences in craving and cue reactivity to smoking and negative affect/stress cues. *The American Journal on Addictions, 21*(3), 210–220. http://dx.doi.org/10.1111/j.1521-0391.2012.00232.x, [Research Support, N.I.H., Extramural].

Sallee, F. R., McGough, J., Wigal, T., Donahue, J., Lyne, A., & Biederman, J. (2009). Guanfacine extended release in children and adolescents with attention-deficit/hyperactivity disorder: A placebo-controlled trial. *Journal of the American Academy of Child and Adolescent Psychiatry, 48*(2), 155–165. http://dx.doi.org/10.1097/CHI.0b013e318191769e, [Multicenter Study Randomized Controlled Trial Research Support, Non-U.S. Gov't].

Sanchez-Hervas, E., & Llorente del Pozo, J. M. (2012). Relapse in cocaine addiction: A review. *Adicciones, 24*(3), 269–279, Review.

Sara, S. J. (2009). The locus coeruleus and noradrenergic modulation of cognition. *Nature Reviews Neuroscience, 10*(3), 211–223. http://dx.doi.org/10.1038/nrn2573, [Research Support, Non-U.S. Gov't Review].

Sawaguchi, T., & Goldman-Rakic, P. S. (1994). The role of D1-dopamine receptor in working memory: Local injections of dopamine antagonists into the prefrontal cortex of rhesus monkeys performing an oculomotor delayed-response task. *Journal of Neurophysiology, 71*(2), 515–528.

Scahill, L. (2009). Alpha-2 adrenergic agonists in children with inattention, hyperactivity and impulsiveness. *CNS Drugs, 23*(Suppl. 1), 43–49. http://dx.doi.org/10.2165/00023210-200923000-00006, [Review].

Scahill, L., Aman, M. G., McDougle, C. J., Arnold, L. E., McCracken, J. T., Handen, B., et al. (2009). Trial design challenges when combining medication and parent training in children with pervasive developmental disorders. *Journal of Autism and Developmental Disorders, 39*(5), 720–729. http://dx.doi.org/10.1007/s10803-008-0675-2, [Randomized Controlled Trial Research Support, N.I.H., Extramural].

Scahill, L., Chappell, P. B., Kim, Y. S., Schultz, R. T., Katsovich, L., Shepherd, E., et al. (2001). A placebo-controlled study of guanfacine in the treatment of children with tic disorders and attention deficit hyperactivity disorder. *The American Journal of Psychiatry,*

158(7), 1067–1074, [Clinical Trial Randomized Controlled Trial Research Support, Non-U.S. Gov't Research Support, U.S. Gov't, P.H.S.].

Schneider, U., Altmann, A., Baumann, M., Bernzen, J., Bertz, B., Bimber, U., et al. (2001). Comorbid anxiety and affective disorder in alcohol-dependent patients seeking treatment: The first Multicentre Study in Germany. *Alcohol and Alcoholism, 36*(3), 219–223, [Multicenter Study].

Schroeder, J. R., Schmittner, J., Bleiberg, J., Epstein, D. H., Krantz, M. J., & Preston, K. L. (2007). Hemodynamic and cognitive effects of lofexidine and methadone coadministration: A pilot study. *Pharmacotherapy, 27*(8), 1111–1119. http://dx.doi.org/10.1592/phco.27.8.1111, [Clinical Trial, Phase I Research Support, N.I.H., Intramural].

Schwartz, T. L., & Nihalani, N. (2006). Tiagabine in anxiety disorders. *Expert Opinion on Pharmacotherapy, 7*(14), 1977–1987. http://dx.doi.org/10.1517/14656566.7.14.1977, [Review].

Seedat, Y. K. (1985). Clonidine and guanfacine—Comparison of their effects on haemodynamics in hypertension. *South African Medical Journal, 67*(14), 557–559, [Comparative Study Review].

Sees, K. L., & Clark, H. W. (1991). Substance abusers want to stop smoking!. *Alcoholism, Clinical and Experimental Research, 15,* 152.

Seo, D., Jia, Z., Lacadie, C. M., Tsou, K. A., Bergquist, K., & Sinha, R. (2011). Sex differences in neural responses to stress and alcohol context cues. *Human Brain Mapping, 32*(11), 1998–2013. http://dx.doi.org/10.1002/hbm.21165, [Research Support, N.I.H., Extramural].

Shaham, Y., Shalev, U., Lu, L., De Wit, H., & Stewart, J. (2003). The reinstatement model of drug relapse: History, methodology and major findings. *Psychopharmacology, 168*(1–2), 3–20. http://dx.doi.org/10.1007/s00213-002-1224-x, [Review].

Shalev, U., Grimm, J. W., & Shaham, Y. (2002). Neurobiology of relapse to heroin and cocaine seeking: A review. *Pharmacological Reviews, 54*(1), 1–42, [Research Support, U.S. Gov't, P.H.S. Review].

Shang, C. Y., & Gau, S. S. (2012). Improving visual memory, attention, and school function with atomoxetine in boys with attention-deficit/hyperactivity disorder. *Journal of Child and Adolescent Psychopharmacology, 22*(5), 353–363. http://dx.doi.org/10.1089/cap.2011.0149, [Research Support, Non-U.S. Gov't].

Shields, A. D., Wang, Q., & Winder, D. G. (2009). Alpha2a-adrenergic receptors heterosynaptically regulate glutamatergic transmission in the bed nucleus of the stria terminalis. *Neuroscience, 163*(1), 339–351. http://dx.doi.org/10.1016/j.neuroscience.2009.06.022, [Research Support, N.I.H., Extramural].

Shorter, D., & Kosten, T. R. (2011). Novel pharmacotherapeutic treatments for cocaine addiction. *BMC Medicine, 9*(119). http://dx.doi.org/10.1186/1741-7015-9-119, [Research Support, N.I.H., Extramural Research Support, U.S. Gov't, Non-P.H.S. Review].

Shorter, D., Lindsay, J. A., & Kosten, T. R. (2013). The alpha-1 adrenergic antagonist doxazosin for treatment of cocaine dependence: A pilot study. *Drug and Alcohol Dependence, 131*(1–2), 66–70. http://dx.doi.org/10.1016/j.drugalcdep.2012.11.021, [Research Support, N.I.H., Extramural].

Sica, D. A. (2007). Centrally acting antihypertensive agents: An update. *Journal of Clinical Hypertension (Greenwich, Conn), 9*(5), 399–405, [Review].

Simpson, T. L., Saxon, A. J., Meredith, C. W., Malte, C. A., McBride, B., Ferguson, L. C., et al. (2009). A pilot trial of the alpha-1 adrenergic antagonist, prazosin, for alcohol dependence. *Alcoholism, Clinical and Experimental Research, 33*(2), 255–263. http://dx.doi.org/10.1111/j.1530-0277.2008.00807.x, [Randomized Controlled Trial Research Support, Non-U.S. Gov't].

Sinha, R. (2001). How does stress increase risk of drug abuse and relapse? *Psychopharmacology*, *158*(4), 343–359. http://dx.doi.org/10.1007/s002130100917, [Research Support, U.S. Gov't, P.H.S. Review].

Sinha, R. (2008). Chronic stress, drug use, and vulnerability to addiction. *Annals of the New York Academy of Sciences*, *1141*, 105–130.

Sinha, R., Fox, H. C., Hong, K. A., Bergquist, K., Bhagwagar, Z., & Siedlarz, K. M. (2009). Enhanced negative emotion and alcohol craving, and altered physiological responses following stress and cue exposure in alcohol dependent individuals. *Neuropsychopharmacology*, *34*(5), 1198–1208. http://dx.doi.org/10.1038/npp.2008.78, [Research Support, N.I.H., Extramural].

Sinha, R., Fox, H. C., Hong, K. I., Hansen, J., Tuit, K., & Kreek, M. J. (2011). Effects of adrenal sensitivity, stress- and cue-induced craving, and anxiety on subsequent alcohol relapse and treatment outcomes. *Archives of General Psychiatry*, *68*(9), 942–952. http://dx. doi.org/10.1001/archgenpsychiatry.2011.49, [Research Support, N.I.H., Extramural].

Sinha, R., Garcia, M., Paliwal, P., Kreek, M. J., & Rounsaville, B. J. (2006). Stress-induced cocaine craving and hypothalamic-pituitary-adrenal responses are predictive of cocaine relapse outcomes. *Archives of General Psychiatry*, *63*(3), 324–331. http://dx.doi.org/ 10.1001/archpsyc.63.3.324, [Comparative Study Research Support, N.I.H., Extramural].

Sinha, R., Hong, A. K., Seo, D., Fox, H. C., & Bergquist, K. L. (2010). Neural and endocrine predictions of alcohol relapse risk. *Alcoholism, Clinical and Experimental Research*, *34*(6), 290A, Supplement.

Sinha, R., Kimmerling, A., Doebrick, C., & Kosten, T. R. (2007). Effects of lofexidine on stress-induced and cue-induced opioid craving and opioid abstinence rates: Preliminary findings. *Psychopharmacology*, *190*(4), 569–574. http://dx.doi.org/10.1007/s00213-006-0640-8, [Randomized Controlled Trial Research Support, N.I.H., Extramural].

Sinha, R., Lacadie, C., Skudlarski, P., Fulbright, R. K., Rounsaville, B. J., Kosten, T. R., et al. (2005). Neural activity associated with stress-induced cocaine craving: A functional magnetic resonance imaging study. *Psychopharmacology*, *183*(2), 171–180. http://dx.doi. org/10.1007/s00213-005-0147-8, [Comparative Study Research Support, N.I.H., Extramural].

Sinha, R., Shaham, Y., & Heilig, M. (2011). Translational and reverse translational research on the role of stress in drug craving and relapse. *Psychopharmacology*, *218*(1), 69–82. http://dx.doi.org/10.1007/s00213-011-2263-y, [Research Support, N.I.H., Extramural Research Support, N.I.H., Intramural Review].

Sinha, R., Talih, M., Malison, R., Cooney, N., Anderson, G. M., & Kreek, M. J. (2003). Hypothalamic-pituitary-adrenal axis and sympatho-adreno-medullary responses during stress-induced and drug cue-induced cocaine craving states. *Psychopharmacology*, *170*(1), 62–72. http://dx.doi.org/10.1007/s00213-003-1525-8, [Research Support, Non-U.S. Gov't Research Support, U.S. Gov't, P.H.S.].

Smith, R. J., & Aston-Jones, G. (2008). Noradrenergic transmission in the extended amygdala: Role in increased drug-seeking and relapse during protracted drug abstinence. *Brain Structure and Function*, *213*(1–2), 43–61. http://dx.doi.org/10.1007/s00429-008-0191-3, [Review].

Smith, R. J., & Aston-Jones, G. (2011). Alpha(2) adrenergic and imidazoline receptor agonists prevent cue-induced cocaine seeking. *Biological Psychiatry*, *70*(8), 712–719. http:// dx.doi.org/10.1016/j.biopsych.2011.06.010, [Research Support, N.I.H., Extramural].

Sofuoglu, M. (2010). Cognitive enhancement as a pharmacotherapy target for stimulant addiction. *Addiction*, *105*(1), 38–48. http://dx.doi.org/10.1111/j.1360-0443.2009.02791.x, [Research Support, N.I.H., Extramural Research Support, U.S. Gov't, Non-P.H.S. Review].

Sofuoglu, M., DeVito, E. E., Waters, A. J., & Carroll, K. M. (2013). Cognitive enhancement as a treatment for drug addictions. *Neuropharmacology*, *64*, 452–463. http://dx.doi.org/

10.1016/j.neuropharm.2012.06.021, [Research Support, N.I.H., Extramural Research Support, U.S. Gov't, Non-P.H.S. Review].

Sommer, B. R., Mitchell, E. L., & Wroolie, T. E. (2013). Topiramate: Effects on cognition in patients with epilepsy, migraine headache and obesity. *Therapeutic Advances in Neurological Disorders, 6*(4), 211–227. http://dx.doi.org/10.1177/1756285613481257.

Sorkin, E. M., & Heel, R. C. (1986). Guanfacine. A review of its pharmacodynamic and pharmacokinetic properties, and therapeutic efficacy in the treatment of hypertension. *Drugs, 31*(4), 301–336, [Review].

Steere, J. C., & Arnsten, A. F. (1997). The alpha-2A noradrenergic receptor agonist guanfacine improves visual object discrimination reversal performance in aged rhesus monkeys. *Behavioral Neuroscience, 111*(5), 883–891.

Strang, J. J., Bearn, J., & Gossop, M. (1999). Lofexidine for opiate detoxification: Review of recent randomised and open controlled trials. *The American Journal on Addictions, 8*(4), 337–348.

Summers, R. J., Jarrott, B., & Louis, W. J. (1981). Comparison of [3H]clonidine and [3H] guanfacine binding to alpha 2 adrenoceptors in membranes from rat cerebral cortex. *Neuroscience Letters, 25*(1), 31–36, [Research Support, Non-U.S. Gov't].

Swartz, B. E., McDonald, C. R., Patel, A., & Torgersen, D. (2008). The effects of guanfacine on working memory performance in patients with localization-related epilepsy and healthy controls. *Clinical Neuropharmacology, 31*(5), 251–260. http://dx.doi.org/10.1097/WNF.0b013e3181633461, [Comparative Study].

Taneja, I., Haman, K., Shelton, R. C., & Robertson, D. (2007). A randomized, double-blind, crossover trial of modafinil on mood. *Journal of Clinical Psychopharmacology, 27*(1), 76–79. http://dx.doi.org/10.1097/jcp.0b013e31802eb7ea, [Randomized Controlled Trial Research Support, N.I.H., Extramural].

Taylor, H. R., Freeman, M. K., & Cates, M. E. (2008). Prazosin for treatment of nightmares related to posttraumatic stress disorder. *American Journal of Health-System Pharmacy, 65*(8), 716–722. http://dx.doi.org/10.2146/ajhp070124, [Review].

Taylor, F. B., & Russo, J. (2001). Comparing guanfacine and dextroamphetamine for the treatment of adult attention-deficit/hyperactivity disorder. *Journal of Clinical Psychopharmacology, 21*(2), 223–228.

Thanos, P. K., Michaelides, M., Benveniste, H., Wang, G. J., & Volkow, N. D. (2008). The effects of cocaine on regional brain glucose metabolism is attenuated in dopamine transporter knockout mice. *Synapse, 62*(5), 319–324. http://dx.doi.org/10.1002/syn.20503, [Research Support, N.I.H., Extramural Research Support, U.S. Gov't, Non-P.H.S.].

Thanos, P. K., Taintor, N. B., Rivera, S. N., Umegaki, H., Ikari, H., Roth, G., et al. (2004). DRD2 gene transfer into the nucleus accumbens core of the alcohol preferring and non-preferring rats attenuates alcohol drinking. *Alcoholism, Clinical and Experimental Research, 28*(5), 720–728, [Comparative Study Research Support, U.S. Gov't, Non-P.H.S. Research Support, U.S. Gov't, P.H.S.].

Tice, D. M., Bratslavsky, E., & Baumeister, R. F. (2001). Emotional distress regulation takes precedence over impulse control: If you feel bad, do it!. *Journal of Personality and Social Psychology, 80*(1), 53–67, [Clinical Trial Randomized Controlled Trial Research Support, U.S. Gov't, P.H.S.].

Tzschentke, T. M. (2001). Pharmacology and behavioral pharmacology of the mesocortical dopamine system. *Progress in Neurobiology, 63*(3), 241–320.

Ungless, M. A., Whistler, J. L., Malenka, R. C., & Bonci, A. (2001). Single cocaine exposure in vivo induces long-term potentiation in dopamine neurons. *Nature, 411*(6837), 583–587. http://dx.doi.org/10.1038/35079077, [In Vitro Research Support, Non-U.S. Gov't Research Support, U.S. Gov't, P.H.S.].

van Zwieten, P. A. (1999). The renaissance of centrally acting antihypertensive drugs. *Journal of Hypertension Supplement, 17*(3), S15–S21, [Review].

Verdejo-Garcia, A., & Perez-Garcia, M. (2007). Ecological assessment of executive functions in substance dependent individuals. *Drug and Alcohol Dependence, 90*(1), 48–55. http://dx.doi.org/10.1016/j.drugalcdep.2007.02.010, [Research Support, Non-U.S. Gov't].

Verrico, C. D., Haile, C. N., Newton, T. F., Kosten, T. R., & De La Garza, R. (2013). Pharmacotherapeutics for substance-use disorders: A focus on dopaminergic medications. *Expert Opinion on Investigational Drugs, 22*, 1549–1568. http://dx.doi.org/10.1517/13543784.2013.836488.

Viola, T. W., Tractenberg, S. G., Pezzi, J. C., Kristensen, C. H., & Grassi-Oliveira, R. (2013). Childhood physical neglect associated with executive functions impairments in crack cocaine-dependent women. *Drug and Alcohol Dependence, 132*(1–2), 271–276. http://dx.doi.org/10.1016/j.drugalcdep.2013.02.014.

Vocci, F., & Ling, W. (2005). Medications development: Successes and challenges. *Pharmacology & Therapeutics, 108*(1), 94–108. http://dx.doi.org/10.1016/j.pharmthera.2005.06.010, [Research Support, N.I.H., Extramural Research Support, U.S. Gov't, P.H.S. Review].

Volkow, N. D., Fowler, J. S., Wang, G. J., & Goldstein, R. Z. (2002). Role of dopamine, the frontal cortex and memory circuits in drug addiction: Insight from imaging studies. *Neurobiology of Learning and Memory, 78*(3), 610–624, [Research Support, U.S. Gov't, Non-P.H.S. Research Support, U.S. Gov't, P.H.S.].

Volkow, N. D., Fowler, J. S., Wang, G. J., & Swanson, J. M. (2004). Dopamine in drug abuse and addiction: Results from imaging studies and treatment implications. *Molecular Psychiatry, 9*(6), 557–569. http://dx.doi.org/10.1038/sj.mp.4001507, [Research Support, U.S. Gov't, Non-P.H.S. Research Support, U.S. Gov't, P.H.S. Review].

Vranjkovic, O., Hang, S., Baker, D. A., & Mantsch, J. R. (2012). Beta-adrenergic receptor mediation of stress-induced reinstatement of extinguished cocaine-induced conditioned place preference in mice: Roles for beta1 and beta2 adrenergic receptors. *The Journal of Pharmacology and Experimental Therapeutics, 342*(2), 541–551. http://dx.doi.org/10.1124/jpet.112.193615, [Research Support, N.I.H., Extramural].

Waldrop, A. E., Back, S. E., Verduin, M. L., & Brady, K. T. (2007). Triggers for cocaine and alcohol use in the presence and absence of posttraumatic stress disorder. *Addictive Behaviors, 32*(3), 634–639. http://dx.doi.org/10.1016/j.addbeh.2006.06.001, [Comparative Study Research Support, N.I.H., Extramural].

Waldrop, A. E., Price, K. L., Desantis, S. M., Simpson, A. N., Back, S. E., McRae, A. L., et al. (2010). Community-dwelling cocaine-dependent men and women respond differently to social stressors versus cocaine cues. *Psychoneuroendocrinology, 35*(6), 798–806. http://dx.doi.org/10.1016/j.psyneuen.2009.11.005, [Comparative Study Research Support, N.I.H., Extramural Research Support, Non-U.S. Gov't].

Wang, M., Ji, J. Z., & Li, B. M. (2004). The alpha(2A)-adrenergic agonist guanfacine improves visuomotor associative learning in monkeys. *Neuropsychopharmacology, 29*(1), 86–92. http://dx.doi.org/10.1038/sj.npp.1300278, [Comparative Study Research Support, Non-U.S. Gov't].

Wang, M., Ramos, B. P., Paspalas, C. D., Shu, Y., Simen, A., Duque, A., et al. (2007). Alpha2A-adrenoceptors strengthen working memory networks by inhibiting cAMP-HCN channel signaling in prefrontal cortex. *Cell, 129*(2), 397–410. http://dx.doi.org/10.1016/j.cell.2007.03.015, [Research Support, N.I.H., Extramural Research Support, Non-U.S. Gov't].

Wang, B., Shaham, Y., Zitzman, D., Azari, S., Wise, R. A., & You, Z. B. (2005). Cocaine experience establishes control of midbrain glutamate and dopamine by corticotropin-releasing factor: A role in stress-induced relapse to drug seeking. *The Journal of Neuroscience, 25*(22), 5389–5396. http://dx.doi.org/10.1523/JNEUROSCI.0955-05.2005.

Washton, A. M., & Resnick, R. B. (1981). The clinical use of clonidine in outpatient detoxification from opiates. *Progress in Clinical and Biological Research*, 71, 277–284, [Research Support, Non-U.S. Gov't Research Support, U.S. Gov't, P.H.S.].

Williams, N., Simpson, A. N., Simpson, K., & Nahas, Z. (2009). Relapse rates with long-term antidepressant drug therapy: A meta-analysis. *Human Psychopharmacology*, 24(5), 401–408. http://dx.doi.org/10.1002/hup.1033, [Meta-Analysis Research Support, N.I.H., Extramural Research Support, Non-U.S. Gov't].

Wiseman, E. J., & McMillan, D. E. (1998). Relationship of cessation of cocaine use to cigarette smoking in cocaine-dependent outpatients. *The American Journal of Drug and Alcohol Abuse*, 24(4), 617–625.

Witkiewitz, K., & Marlatt, G. A. (2005). Emphasis on interpersonal factors in a dynamic model of relapse. *The American Psychologist*, 60(4), 341–342. http://dx.doi.org/10.1037/0003-066X.60.4.341, [Comment].

Wong, Y. N., Simcoe, D., Hartman, L. N., Laughton, W. B., King, S. P., McCormick, G. C., et al. (1999). A double-blind, placebo-controlled, ascending-dose evaluation of the pharmacokinetics and tolerability of modafinil tablets in healthy male volunteers. *Journal of Clinical Pharmacology*, 39(1), 30–40, [Clinical Trial Randomized Controlled Trial].

Woodward, J. J., Mansbach, R., Carroll, F. I., & Balster, R. L. (1991). Cocaethylene inhibits dopamine uptake and produces cocaine-like actions in drug discrimination studies. *European Journal of Pharmacology*, 197(2–3), 235–236, [Comparative Study Research Support, Non-U.S. Gov't Research Support, U.S. Gov't, P.H.S.].

Yamada, H., & Bruijnzeel, A. W. (2011). Stimulation of alpha2-adrenergic receptors in the central nucleus of the amygdala attenuates stress-induced reinstatement of nicotine seeking in rats. *Neuropharmacology*, 60(2–3), 303–311. http://dx.doi.org/10.1016/j.neuropharm.2010.09.013, [Comparative Study Research Support, N.I.H., Extramural].

Zahrt, J., Taylor, J. R., Mathew, R. G., & Arnsten, A. F. (1997). Supranormal stimulation of D1 dopamine receptors in the rodent prefrontal cortex impairs spatial working memory performance. *The Journal of Neuroscience*, 17(21), 8528–8535, [Research Support, U.S. Gov't, P.H.S.].

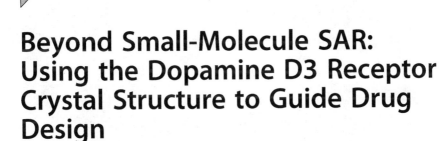

CHAPTER SEVEN

Beyond Small-Molecule SAR: Using the Dopamine D3 Receptor Crystal Structure to Guide Drug Design

Thomas M. Keck[*], Caitlin Burzynski[*], Lei Shi[†], Amy Hauck Newman[*,1]
[*]Medicinal Chemistry Section, Molecular Targets and Medications Discovery Branch, National Institute on Drug Abuse—Intramural Research Program, Baltimore, Maryland, USA
[†]Department of Physiology and Biophysics and Institute for Computational Biomedicine, Weill Cornell Medical College, New York, USA
[1]Corresponding author: e-mail address: anewman@intra.nida.nih.gov

Contents

Abstract

The dopamine D3 receptor is a target of pharmacotherapeutic interest in a variety of neurological disorders including schizophrenia, restless leg syndrome, and drug addiction. The high protein sequence homology between the D3 and D2 receptors has posed a challenge to developing D3 receptor-selective ligands whose behavioral actions can be attributed to D3 receptor engagement, *in vivo*. However, through primarily small-molecule structure–activity relationship (SAR) studies, a variety of chemical scaffolds have been discovered over the past two decades that have resulted in several D3 receptor-selective ligands with high affinity and *in vivo* activity. Nevertheless, viable clinical candidates remain limited. The recent determination of the high-resolution crystal structure of the D3 receptor has invigorated structure-based drug design, providing refinements to the molecular dynamic models and testable predictions about receptor–ligand interactions. This chapter will highlight recent preclinical and clinical studies demonstrating potential utility of D3 receptor-selective ligands in the treatment of addiction. In addition, new structure-based rational drug design strategies for D3 receptor-selective ligands that complement traditional small-molecule SAR to improve the selectivity and directed efficacy profiles are examined.

ABBREVIATIONS

AC adenylyl cyclase
ADMET absorption, distribution, metabolism, excretion, and toxicity
BBB blood–brain barrier
cAMP cyclic adenosine monophosphate
CNS central nervous system
CPP conditioned place preference
DA dopamine
ECL extracellular loop
FR fixed-ratio
GPCR G protein-coupled receptor
hERG human ether-à-go-go-related gene
ICL intracellular loop
log *P* logarithmic partition coefficient
MW molecular weight
OBS orthosteric binding site
PET positron emission tomography
PP primary pharmacophore
PR progressive ratio
QSAR quantitative structure–activity relationships
SAR structure–activity relationships
SBP secondary binding pocket
SP secondary pharmacophore
SUDs substance use disorders
TM transmembrane domain

1. INTRODUCTION

The neurotransmitter dopamine (DA) exerts its effects via DA receptors with varied signaling transduction mechanisms and expression patterns in the brain. DA receptors belong to the G protein-coupled receptor (GPCR) superfamily and are divided into two subfamilies. The D1-like DA receptors (D1 and D5) couple to stimulatory G_s proteins and enhance adenylyl cyclase

(AC) activity and increase cytosolic cyclic adenosine monophosphate (cAMP) levels. D2-like DA receptors (D2, D3, and D4) couple to inhibitory $G_{i/o}$ proteins that suppress AC activity and decrease cAMP. Within the D2-like receptor subfamily, the D2 and D3 receptors are the most homologous pair, sharing extensive sequence identity in the transmembrane domain and the putative ligand binding site (Chien et al., 2010).

First cloned and characterized in 1990 (Sokoloff, Giros, Martres, Bouthenet, & Schwartz, 1990), DA D3 receptors are expressed as postsynaptic receptors as well as autoreceptors (Diaz et al., 2000), providing inhibitory control on neuronal firing rates. The D3 receptor has a higher affinity for DA than the other receptor subtypes and may therefore be sensitive to tonic stimulation (Levesque et al., 1992). However, since D3 receptor antagonists fail to increase locomotor activity or elevate extracellular levels of DA in the nucleus accumbens or striatum, it appears that D3 autoreceptors exert primarily phasic rather than tonic control of DA neurons (Millan et al., 2000; Sokoloff et al., 2006).

The expression of D3 receptors in the human brain is primarily limited to mesolimbic regions, including particularly the ventral striatum, pallidum, nucleus accumbens, islands of Calleja, olfactory tubercle, and lateral septum (Cho, Zheng, & Kim, 2010; Gurevich & Joyce, 1999; Searle et al., 2010). This relatively focal expression of D3 receptors in brain regions that govern motivational behaviors and the reward properties of addictive drugs make the D3 receptor an enticing target for addiction pharmacotherapies. D3 receptors localized in the basolateral nucleus of the amygdala appear to regulate stimulus–reward associations that mediate reinstatement of drug-seeking behavior (Di Ciano, 2008). In the hippocampus, a modest density of D3 receptors have been found that regulate CREB signaling and could produce long-lasting effects on cognition and relapse behavior (Basile et al., 2006). In contrast, D2 receptors feature a broader distribution at higher concentrations, particularly in the dorsal striatum (Gurevich & Joyce, 1999); alteration of D2 receptor signaling is more commonly associated with side effects that influence locomotor activity, motor coordination, prolactin secretion, and catalepsy (Cho et al., 2010; Millan et al., 1995). Hence, selective targeting of D3 receptor signaling has the potential to provide a more focused therapeutic effect while limiting potential side effects believed to be mediated primarily through D2 receptors.

D3 receptors have additionally been shown to form heteromers with D1 receptors in the striatum. In these D1–D3 interactions, D3 receptor stimulation potentiates the effects of D1 signaling on neuronal and behavioral processes, including AC activation and locomotor activity (Fiorentini et al., 2008; Marcellino et al., 2008). Additional evidence exists for the functional coupling of D2 and D3 receptors, which may alter the apparent potency of some D2-like agonists (reviewed in Maggio, Aloisi, Silvano, Rossi, & Millan, 2009). It is tempting to consider future directions for the development of pharmacotherapeutics targeting these heteromeric complexes. However, it is too soon to know whether these complexes can be accessed by heteromer-selective drugs, *in vivo*.

The DA D3 receptor has been investigated as a potential target for medication development to treat substance use disorders (SUDs) with a particular focus on cocaine and methamphetamine. In addition to the expression and signaling patterns described earlier, alterations in D3 receptor expression patterns following drug exposure suggest an important role for D3 signaling in the development of addiction. Enhanced expression of D3 receptors has been shown following acute or chronic exposure to drugs of abuse in human postmortem studies (Mash & Staley, 1999; Segal, Moraes, & Mash, 1997; Staley & Mash, 1996). Increased expression of D3 receptors in polydrug users is correlated with self-reported drug craving (Boileau et al., 2012). This upregulation of D3 receptors may therefore contribute to the reinforcing effects of drugs of abuse and drug dependence (Le Foll, Diaz, & Sokoloff, 2003; Segal et al., 1997).

Currently, there are no approved medications to treat cocaine and methamphetamine addiction, and thus, developing pharmacotherapeutics to complement existing behavioral strategies is a fundamental goal. A commentary highlighting the D3 receptor as a viable target for the development of SUDs, with an emphasis on psychostimulants, has recently appeared (Newman, Blaylock, et al., 2012).

2. D3-SELECTIVE DRUG DESIGN USING SMALL-MOLECULE SAR

2.1. Brief review of the D3 receptor pharmacophore template and examples of promising D3-selective agents for preclinical evaluation

Several comprehensive reviews describing dozens of D3-selective agents and derived structure–activity relationships (SAR) have been published recently (Heidbreder & Newman, 2010; Micheli, 2011; Ye, Neumeyer, Baldessarini, Zhen, & Zhang, 2013). Despite fertile ground for modification of the classic D3 pharmacophore template, several challenges remain in identifying D3-selective ligands with efficacies that can be translated into *in vivo* models and ultimately therapeutic agents to treat human addiction.

In general, chemical modification, initially using readily available starting materials and simple, high-yielding synthetic strategies, results in libraries of compounds that are tested in *in vitro* binding and functional assays to develop SAR. Increasing the affinity and selectivity of these molecules toward the target of interest is typically the first goal. Classical medicinal chemistry, quantitative SAR (QSAR) and other computational methods, based on small-molecule structures, have been used to guide subsequent rational drug design to achieve this goal as efficiently as possible. Once molecules have been identified that show high affinity and selectivity for the target, lead optimization proceeds. Used by most labs to modify lead compounds into tools that can be used for *in vivo* studies, the now-classic Lipinski rule of 5 (Lipinski, 2000; Lipinski, Lombardo, Dominy, & Feeney, 1997) defined four parameters to aim for when designing molecules with drug-like physicochemical properties: a molecular weight (MW) <500, calculated logarithmic partition coefficient (log P) in the range of 2–5, <5 H-bond donors (OH, NH), and <10 H-bond acceptors (N, O). These criteria have been used to maximize blood–brain barrier (BBB) penetration and optimize other pharmacokinetic parameters. However, these specifications are often too strict to comply with the highly "decorated" and potent compounds that are discovered through target-based SAR. This has resulted in an abundance of compounds with high affinity and/or selectivity for their biological target but that are hopelessly large and lipophilic, resulting in poor absorption, distribution, metabolism, excretion, and toxicity (ADMET) profiles and ultimate failure in the clinic (Hann & Keseru, 2012).

"Fat and flat—the enemies of drug discovery" was recently coined (Robert J. Young, 2013; 31st Camerino-Cyprus-Noordwijkerhout Symposium), and clues as to how to achieve molecules that are more likely to be drug-like, but still have the pharmacological specificity required, remain one of the biggest challenges to medicinal chemists, especially for central nervous system (CNS)-active drugs (Hill & Young, 2010; Wager, Hou, Verhoest, & Villalobos, 2010). Hann and Keseru (2012) further elaborated on the risks of "molecular obesity" and advised that a "sweet spot" between molecular mass and log P values exists that narrows the Lipinski parameters even further to compounds with MWs in the range of 250–500 and log P values in the 2–4 range (Hann & Keseru, 2012). They refer to a set of ADMET "rules of thumb" published in 2008 (Gleeson, 2008) that provides further data to support aiming for molecules with log P values <4 and MW < 400, keeping in mind ionization at physiological pH, especially for CNS-penetrant drugs, where this is particularly important. High MWs not only preclude BBB penetration but also increase plasma protein binding and are associated with inhibition of voltage-gated potassium ion channels that control electrical activity within the heart, commonly known as hERG (named from the human ether-à-go-go-related gene that encodes the $K_v11.1$ protein). hERG channel inhibition is associated with cardiac arrhythmia and QT interval prolongation; therefore, hERG binding is an early eliminator of an otherwise potential drug candidate (Gleeson, 2008). Unfortunately, high affinity for the hERG channel is associated with basic molecules, especially lipophilic amines, and for most GPCRs, this provides an early roadblock between the biological target and the off-target drug design (Wager et al., 2010).

The classic template of the 4-phenylpiperazines, exemplified by the early D3-selective ligands BP 897 (Fig. 7.1; Pilla et al., 1999) and NGB 2904 (Fig. 7.1; Yuan et al., 1998), has undergone significant modification to yield some very interesting D3-selective compounds, some of which have reached the clinical trial stage and are discussed in Section 3. The primary goal has been to achieve high-affinity binding to the D3 receptor and to limit or design out "off-target" actions, especially at the other D2 family of receptors and also at 5-HT receptors that share common pharmacophoric elements (e.g., 5-HT_{1A}, 5-HT_{2A}, or β-adrenergic). Nevertheless, in some cases, multifunctional compounds that target serotonin 5-HT_{1A} and 5-HT_{2A} receptors have been designed to capitalize on the overlapping SAR and to identify ligands that have potential as treatments for other CNS disorders such as schizophrenia (Butini et al., 2010). In addition, as the template is long to begin with, and addition of molecular "decoration" has added MW and lipophilicity, confounding activity at hERG channels, for example, has precluded further development of otherwise selective and promising agents due to predicted cardiotoxicity. Significant effort has been made in recent years (Bonanomi et al., 2010; Butini et al., 2010; Micheli et al., 2007; Micheli & Heidbreder, 2013) to address this persistent challenge with this class of drugs.

The early prototypic D3-selective ligands were characterized as antagonists or partial agonists, primarily in cell-based functional assays. It has been noted that the efficacies derived from these D3 functional assays have not always been translated into distinct behavioral actions (Newman, Grundt, & Nader, 2005). Indeed, compounds that have been described as partial agonists or antagonists often show similar behavioral effects in the

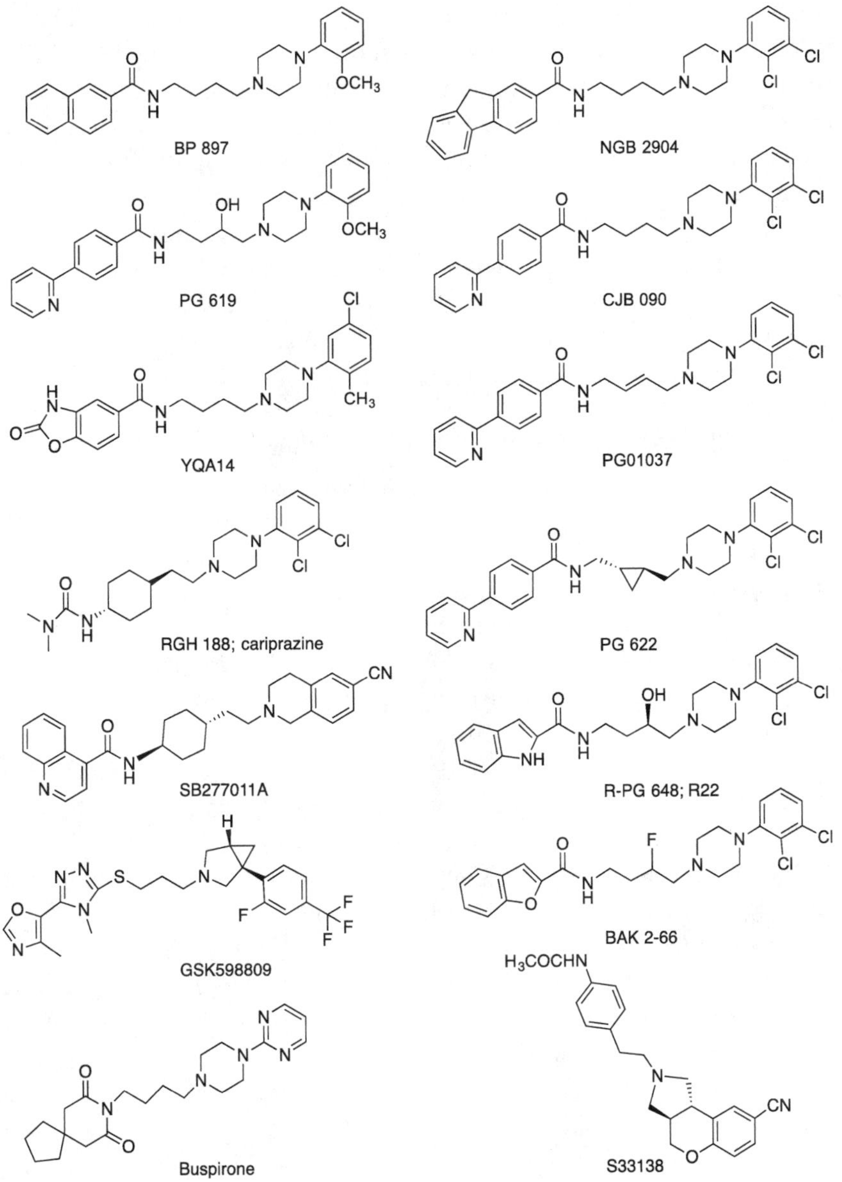

Figure 7.1 Chemical structures of D3 receptor antagonists/partial agonists used in preclinical and clinical studies.

preclinical models of addiction (see Heidbreder & Newman, 2010, for further discussion). In addition, the functional potencies in the *in vitro* assays are often not well correlated to binding affinities at D3 versus D2. To further complicate interpretation of behavioral results, many D3-selective compounds have less-than-optimal physicochemical properties, solubility, BBB permeability, and pharmacokinetics likely due to their high MWs and lipophilicities. These properties may also contribute to the need to use higher doses of drug to observe activity *in vivo* than might have been predicted from their low nanomolar D3 receptor binding affinities. Several examples of these early preclinical candidates have been compared (Heidbreder & Newman, 2010; Micheli, 2011). The early 2-OMe or 2,3-diCl-4-phenylpiperazine fragment has been substituted with many different substituents, and even the phenyl ring has been elaborated on with various heteroaryl ring systems. In the GSK analogs, for example, the 4-phenylpiperazine was first replaced with a tetrahydroisoquinoline in the prototypic SB277011A and later with several atypical bicyclic moieties, including the azabicyclo[3.1.0] hexane moiety found in their clinical candidate GSK598809 (Fig. 7.1), to be discussed in Section 3.

The requisite linker equivalent to a 4-methylene group chain (as seen in BP 897 and NGB 2904) remains in most D3-selective compounds, but the linker has appeared in many functionalized forms including transcyclohexyl (e.g., SB277011A), trans-olefin (e.g., PG01037), and transcyclopropyl (e.g., PG 622) (Fig. 7.1; for review, see Micheli, 2011). In all of these conformational isomers, the *trans* isomer is typically more D3-selective than the *cis*, due to higher affinity at D3 (Grundt et al., 2005, 2007; Newman et al., 2003; Ye et al., 2013, for review). In addition, modification to this linking chain has uncovered enantioselectivity and a point of separation between D3 and D2 (Newman et al., 2009). For example, with PG 648 (Fig. 7.1), significant enantioselectivity at D3 ($R > S \sim 15$-fold) was not observed for D2 binding (<2-fold difference between enantiomers).

The amide linker has also been replaced with either oxazoles or thiatriazoles that retain the desired pharmacological profile and may provide additional benefits over the amide group *in vivo* (Micheli et al., 2007). Although an extended aryl amide was thought to be required for high-affinity binding at D3, and also for selectivity over D2 and 5-HT$_{1A}$, there are several recent examples—especially with the triazole analogs—in which much smaller aryl ring systems provided comparable D3 selectivity and affinity profiles with reduced lipophilicity and MWs, which is more favorable for successful drug development (Bonanomi et al., 2010; Micheli, Arista, Bertani, et al., 2010; Micheli, Arista, Bonanomi, et al., 2010; and others highlighted in Micheli & Heidbreder, 2013). The sulfoxide moiety was also used in other analogs reported in the patent literature to be D3-selective

(Micheli & Heidbreder, 2013). Others have also reported successful replacement of the amide function of BP 897 (Jean et al., 2010). It should be noted, however, that reducing the amide linker to a secondary or tertiary amine severely decreases D3 receptor affinity and renders the resulting molecules nonselective over D2 receptors (Banala et al., 2011).

A recent review of the patent literature has appeared that describes the formidable contribution, primarily from pharmaceutical companies since 2007 (Micheli & Heidbreder, 2013). In this review, the authors also caution the field to recognize that potency and selectivity ratios can vary across labs and across *in vitro* assays, making direct comparisons of compounds impossible unless they are evaluated side by side. What is not clear from the patent literature is how these novel molecules were designed, especially those that are at substantial variance from the classic pharmacophoric template.

Small-molecule comparative molecular field analysis (CoMFA) or comparative molecular similarity index analysis (CoMSIA) and 3D-QSAR studies have been employed in the past (Boeckler et al., 2005; Liu, Li, Zhang, Xiao, & Ai, 2011; Lopez et al., 2010; Salama et al., 2007; Wang, Mach, Luedtke, & Reichert, 2010); however, the advent of GPCR homology modeling has opened additional platforms from which to design molecules with theoretically optimized interactions in the targeted receptor binding pocket(s) at the molecular level. As the high-resolution crystal structure of the D3 receptor was recently solved with the D2/D3 antagonist/inverse agonist eticlopride (Chien et al., 2010), a new opportunity for structure-based drug design is available and is being used for the design of novel compounds. Indeed, before the crystal structure of the D3 receptor was published, homology models developed using the structure of bacteriorhodopsin, and later using bovine rhodopsin and the β_2-adrenergic receptor structures, provided an excellent basis for D3 receptor homology models (e.g., Hobrath & Wang, 2006; Wang et al., 2010). One example of this strategy is work published by the Gmeiner group in which the crystal structure of the β_2-adrenergic receptor was used to derive models for the D2, D3, and D4 receptor subtypes (Ehrlich et al., 2009). Docking analyses led the authors to perform site-directed mutagenesis studies that examined amino acid residues in transmembrane segments (TMs) 2 and 3. By incorporating SAR from their library of small molecules, the individual contributions to D2-subtype selectivity were identified. Importantly, these studies recognized the 4-phenylpiperazine as being the primary recognition moiety for the orthosteric binding site (OBS) for all three members of the D2 family of receptors (Ehrlich et al., 2009).

Other groups have compared homology models for the D3 receptor with homology models for the hERG channel in an attempt to optimize their molecules for high-affinity binding to the D3 receptor while reducing affinity for the hERG channel (Bonanomi et al., 2010; Micheli, Arista, Bonanomi, et al., 2010; Micheli et al., 2007). This effort has resulted in the discovery of D3-selective antagonists without predicted QT interval prolongation, a very important finding for drug development.

2.2. The design of D3-selective agonists, partial agonists, and antagonists

Highly D3 receptor-selective agonists have been elusive until recently and are only now beginning to be tested preclinically (Chen et al., 2011; Johnson, Antonio, Reith, & Dutta, 2012). These compounds have been designed with a hybrid approach, using a classic D2/D3 agonist (e.g., pramipexole) as the primary pharmacophore (PP) and then elaborating with extended linkers attached via either piperazinylaryl amides or aryl amides to give fully efficacious, D3-selective agonists *in vitro* (Fig. 7.2). An additional report (Tschammer et al., 2011) used a similar template to discover compounds with enantioselectivity as well as functional selectivities, another very hot topic for drug discovery, with great interest to relate functional selectivity to behavioral activity in the future. Further characterization of

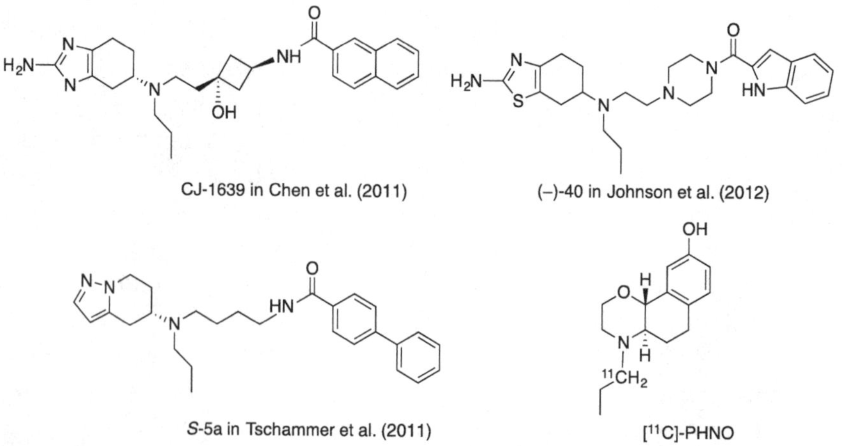

CJ-1639 in Chen et al. (2011)

(–)-40 in Johnson et al. (2012)

S-5a in Tschammer et al. (2011)

[^{11}C]-PHNO

Figure 7.2 Chemical structures of recently described D3 receptor agonists.

these molecules *in vivo* will provide critical data to assess the translation of cell-based functional assay results to D3 agonist-mediated behaviors.

D3-selective antagonists and partial agonists have been more easily designed as they typically share the classic pharmacophore. Nevertheless, modification of these molecules has thus far not led to tractable SAR regarding efficacies. This pursuit has been partially confounded by the paucity of functional assays that gave consistent efficacy predictions in the first few years of D3 receptor research (Levant, 1997), resulting in a diversity of assays used across labs, producing different measured potencies and efficacies for the same compounds (e.g., BP 897; for review, see Newman et al., 2005). To further confound the field, behavioral actions produced by partial agonists versus antagonists have not been well defined. Numerous studies suggest that these D3-selective compounds prevent extracellular DA from binding to the receptor and that this action leads to decreased self-administration and reinstatement to drug-seeking behaviors. However, it is still unclear whether or not an antagonist or partial agonist would be the preferred pharmacotherapy to treat SUDs. This has been debated in the literature (e.g., Newman, Blaylock, et al., 2012) and goes beyond the scope of this chapter. However, we describe recent examples of preclinical evaluation of D3 receptor antagonists and/or partial agonists in models of addiction to provide evidence that the D3 receptor is a promising target for drug development.

2.3. Recent examples of D3 receptor-selective compounds in preclinical models of addiction

Several classes of chemical structures have been explored in the search for D3-selective ligands. In this section, we discuss some of the major chemical classes that have been explored in SAR studies and tested in animal models of addiction. Because this chapter is not meant to be a comprehensive evaluation of the preclinical literature, we will focus on reports published since 2008 and recommend to the reader these reviews for earlier work (Heidbreder et al., 2005; Heidbreder & Newman, 2010; Joyce & Millan, 2005; Micheli, 2011; Micheli & Heidbreder, 2013; Newman, Blaylock, et al., 2012; Newman et al., 2005; Xi & Gardner, 2007).

Effective preclinical models are essential for identifying the *in vivo* profile of novel D3 receptor partial agonists and antagonists as well as advancing the field's understanding of the role of D3 receptor signaling in drug addiction. Since the cloning of the D3 receptor gene in 1990, animal studies have been crucial to elucidate the *in situ* functions of D3 receptors. Over the past

15 years, a variety of factors influencing the *in vivo* selectivity and efficacy of D3 receptor-selective compounds have been identified through behavioral evaluation in a variety of preclinical models, in rodents and nonhuman primates.

A common finding with D3-selective antagonists in behavioral models of addiction is that these compounds are typically ineffective in reducing drug self-administration under low fixed-ratio (FR) schedules, in which typically one (FR1) or two (FR2) lever presses in an operant chamber result in the delivery of the reinforcer (e.g., intravenous cocaine or methamphetamine). These low FR schedules of reinforcement are useful for exploring drug intake patterns, but are not well suited to measure the reinforcing effects of drugs of abuse (Heidbreder & Newman, 2010; O'Brien & Gardner, 2005). Similarly, D3-selective antagonists are often ineffective in second-order reinforcement schedules, in which a subject responds according to a unit schedule (such as FR10) for a brief stimulus presentation (such as a light) and the unit schedule is then reinforced according to a separate schedule of reinforcement (such as a fixed time interval) via drug delivery. In contrast, progressive ratio (PR) schedules of drug reinforcement—believed to be more sensitive to a drug's reinforcing effectiveness and motivational effects (Arnold & Roberts, 1997; O'Brien & Gardner, 2005; Richardson & Roberts, 1996)—are sensitive to D3 antagonism.

Other models of addiction are more sensitive to modulation of D3 receptor signaling. Drug-seeking behavior can be attenuated in several models of relapse-like behavior, such as drug-, cue-, or stress-induced reinstatement. In these models, animals are trained to self-administer methamphetamine (or another reinforcer) until stable behavior is established. Following this training, the reinforcer is removed from future training sessions, extinguishing the drug-seeking behavior. Robust drug-seeking behavior (i.e., active lever pressing) can be induced by noncontingent exposure to the drug, drug-associated cues, stress, or a stress-like trigger such as yohimbine (Shaham, Shalev, Lu, De Wit, & Stewart, 2003). Several studies have reported that D3 antagonism attenuates reinstated drug-seeking behavior.

The subjective, rewarding properties of addictive drugs are also commonly evaluated using conditioned place preference (CPP) tests in which the positive incentive salience of a drug can be measured using a fairly simple Pavlovian learning paradigm (O'Brien & Gardner, 2005; Tzschentke, 2007). D3 receptor antagonists have been reported to block the expression of CPP but less consistently to attenuate the acquisition of CPP (Beninger & Banasikowski, 2008).

2.3.1 4-Phenylpiperazines

A large library now exists of D3-selective or D3-preferential antagonists and partial agonists in which the 4-phenylpiperazine is the core structure, as illustrated in Fig. 7.1. This general molecular template has been explored in multiple SAR studies, and several "hits" from this class have shown efficacy in preclinical models of addiction.

2.3.1.1 BP 897

First reported in 1999 to attenuate cocaine-taking and cocaine-seeking behavior in rats (Pilla et al., 1999), BP 897 was one of the first D3-selective phenylpiperazines widely researched in addiction models. Since then, BP 897 has been reported to inhibit cocaine-seeking behavior, morphine CPP, and conditioned activity associated with amphetamine, nicotine, and cocaine (Garcia-Ladona & Cox, 2003; Le Foll, Goldberg, & Sokoloff, 2005). Recent work has shown that BP 897 did not reduce nicotine self-administration or cue-induced reinstatement to nicotine-seeking behavior (Khaled et al., 2010). BP 897 can attenuate methamphetamine-enhanced brain stimulation but produces an aversive effect at high doses (Spiller et al., 2008).

BP 897 entered early-phase clinical trials for the treatment of addictions to cocaine, nicotine, and alcohol as well as for treatments for schizophrenia and Parkinson's disease (Garcia-Ladona & Cox, 2003). Approximately 70-fold selective for human D3 receptors versus D2 receptors, with apparent partial agonist signaling properties, BP 897 was not successful as a clinical treatment. This may have been due to side effects arising from BP 897's insufficient selectivity for D3 over D2, 5-HT$_{1A}$, and α1- and α2-adrenoceptors (Garcia-Ladona & Cox, 2003; Xi & Gardner, 2007).

2.3.1.2 NGB 2904

Compared to BP 897, NGB 2904 has substantially improved D3 selectivity over D2, HT$_{1A}$, and α1- and α2-adrenoceptors (Xi & Gardner, 2007). NGB 2904 has been reported to reduce cocaine self-administration under a PR schedule and block reinstatement to cocaine-seeking behavior (Xi & Gardner, 2007). Pretreatment with NGB 2904 attenuated methamphetamine-enhanced brain stimulation reward in rats (Spiller et al., 2008). However, NGB 2904 is poorly water-soluble and is highly lipophilic, which likely precluded it from investigation as a clinical candidate (Mason et al., 2010).

2.3.1.3 PG01037

More than 100-fold selective for D3 over D2, PG01037 was initially reported in 2005 (Grundt et al., 2005). Since then, PG01037 has been investigated in a wide variety of addiction models. PG01037 did not alter methamphetamine or sucrose self-administration under low FR schedules of reinforcement in mice or rats (Caine et al., 2012; Higley, Spiller, et al., 2011; Orio, Wee, Newman, Pulvirenti, & Koob, 2010). However, PG01037 significantly lowered the breakpoint for methamphetamine and sucrose self-administration under PR reinforcement, attenuated methamphetamine-enhanced brain stimulation, and blocked cue-induced reinstatement of methamphetamine seeking (Higley, Spiller, et al., 2011; Orio et al., 2010). Similarly, low FR schedule cocaine and food self-administration were not altered by PG01037 administration in squirrel monkeys, but it significantly attenuated cocaine's discriminative stimulus effects and cocaine-induced reinstatement (Achat-Mendes et al., 2010). In an effect similar to genetic knockout of the D3 receptor, treatment with PG01037 in wild-type mice disrupted reconsolidation of cocaine-induced CPP memory (Yan, Kong, Wu, Newman, & Xu, 2013).

PG01037 has improved water solubility over NGB 2904 (Mason et al., 2010). However, it is also a substrate for P-glycoprotein, an ATP-dependent drug efflux pump found at the BBB, which likely limits its potential for translation to the clinic (Mason et al., 2010).

2.3.1.4 CJB 090

CJB 090 (Fig. 7.1) is the saturated analog of PG01037 and somewhat less D3-preferential (50- vs. 133-fold) in binding over D2 receptors (Newman et al., 2005). This compound attenuated methamphetamine self-administration under FR1 reinforcement in rats with long access (6 h sessions, 6 days per week) but not short access (1 h sessions, 3 days per week). Additionally, under a PR schedule of reinforcement, CJB 090 attenuated self-administration in both the short- and long-access groups (Orio et al., 2010). Pretreatment with CJB 090 significantly decreased cocaine's discriminative stimulus effects in squirrel monkeys. However, CJB 090 failed to inhibit either self-administration of cocaine or cocaine-induced reinstatement of drug seeking (Achat-Mendes, Platt, Newman, & Spealman, 2009).

2.3.1.5 PG 619

PG 619 (Fig. 7.1) was synthesized and characterized while looking for improvements to the PG01037 structure (Grundt et al., 2005, 2007). Cocaine self-administration by male rhesus monkeys under an FR30 schedule of reinforcement was not altered by PG 619. However, PG 619 significantly attenuated cocaine-induced reinstatement (Blaylock et al., 2011). Nevertheless, in a subsequent testing in a rhesus monkey food/drug choice paradigm, PG 619 failed to demonstrate any efficacy in attenuating self-administration of either cocaine or methamphetamine (Dr. Michael Nader, Wake Forest University Medical School, personal communication). In addition, a poor ADME profile in rats (Dr. Hazem Hassan, unpublished data) dampened enthusiasm for further development of this agent.

2.3.1.6 YQA14

Administration of YQA14 (Fig. 7.1) attenuated cocaine self-administration under PR reinforcement in rats without altering oral sucrose self-administration or locomotor activity at the same tested doses (Song et al., 2012). YQA14 decreased cocaine self-administration under FR1 and PR reinforcement schedules in wild-type mice but had no effect on D3 receptor knockout mice (Song et al., 2012), supporting a D3 receptor-mediated effect. Similarly, YQA14 attenuated acquisition and expression of cocaine-induced CPP in WT mice but not D3 receptor knockout mice (Song et al., 2013).

2.3.1.7 Cariprazine (RGH 188)

Cariprazine (RGH 188; Fig. 7.1) is a D3-preferring D3/D2 partial agonist in clinical development as an atypical antipsychotic for the treatment of schizophrenia and bipolar mania/mixed episodes (Agai-Csongor et al., 2012; Citrome, 2013). To date, only one study has been published evaluating cariprazine in addiction models. Román, Gyertyan, Saghy, Kiss, and Szombathelyi (2013) found that oral administration of cariprazine significantly increased cocaine self-administration in rats but inhibited cue-induced reinstatement of cocaine-seeking behavior. The enhanced self-administration effect may be due to a cariprazine-mediated reduction in the rewarding effects of cocaine, necessitating more cocaine infusions to achieve the same reward (Román et al., 2013).

2.3.2 Additional structural templates
2.3.2.1 SB277011A

One of the D3-selective ligands most extensively studied in addiction models over the past 5 years, SB277011A was initially described in 2000 (Reavill et al., 2000; Stemp et al., 2000). Previous reviews have covered the effects of SB277011A in preclinical addiction models (Heidbreder et al., 2005; Xi & Gardner, 2007). Since 2008, SB277011A has been tested in multiple models against a variety of different addictive drugs.

SB277011A blocked cue-induced reinstatement of nicotine seeking in rats (Khaled et al., 2010). Pretreatment with SB277011A did not alter methamphetamine self-administration under FR2 schedule of reinforcement but did significantly lower PR breakpoints and inhibit methamphetamine-induced reinstatement (Higley, Kiefer, et al., 2011). SB277011A significantly attenuated methamphetamine-enhanced brain stimulation reward in rats (Spiller et al., 2008). Cue-induced cocaine seeking and incubation of cocaine craving was attenuated by SB277011A administered either systemically or locally into nucleus accumbens or central amygdala in rats (Xi et al., 2013). Administration of SB277011A attenuated morphine-triggered reactivation of cocaine-induced CPP in adult male rats (Rice, Heidbreder, Gardner, Schonhar, & Ashby, 2013) and decreased the conditioned place aversion following naloxone-induced withdrawal from acute morphine administration (Rice, Gardner, Heidbreder, & Ashby, 2012). Infusion of SB277011A into the nucleus accumbens significantly inhibited the expression of morphine-induced context-specific locomotor sensitization (Liang et al., 2011).

GlaxoSmithKline halted clinical development of SB277011A (Xi & Gardner, 2007) after it was determined that the drug has a short half-life and poor oral bioavailability in primates (Austin et al., 2001) despite having favorable pharmacokinetics in the rat (Stemp et al., 2000).

2.3.2.2 S33138

The hexahydrochromeno[3,4-c]pyrrole, S33138 (Fig. 7.1), was reported in 2008 in an in-depth series of *in vitro* and *in vivo* pharmacological characterizations aimed at assessing its effects as an antipsychotic (Millan, Loiseau, et al., 2008; Millan, Mannoury la Cour, et al., 2008; Millan, Svenningsson, et al., 2008). Since then, it has been explored to a limited extent in models of addiction. In rats, pretreatment with low doses of S33138 attenuated cocaine-enhanced brain stimulation reward and cocaine-induced reinstatement of drug-seeking behavior. However, at higher doses, FR2 cocaine and sucrose self-administration behavior was altered, locomotion in a rotarod task was impaired, and an aversive-like rightward shift in brain stimulation rate-frequency reward functions was reported (Peng et al., 2009). Ethanol consumption in mice was significantly inhibited by S33138 administration, but only at doses that also decreased water consumption (Rice, Patrick, Schonhar, Ning, & Ashby, 2012).

2.3.2.3 Buspirone

Buspirone (Fig. 7.1) has received extensive recent interest as a clinically available drug that may be repurposed for addiction treatment (Le Foll & Boileau, 2013). An atypical anxiolytic, buspirone is a partial agonist at the 5-HT_{1A} receptor but is also a high-affinity antagonist of DA D3 and D4 receptors (Bergman et al., 2013). In adult male rhesus monkeys, buspirone pretreatment attenuated cocaine self-administration at doses that did not reliably alter food-maintained responding (Bergman et al., 2013; Mello, Fivel, Kohut, & Bergman, 2013). Chronic buspirone treatment was also effective in reducing cocaine, nicotine, or combined cocaine + nicotine self-administration in rhesus monkeys (Mello, Fivel, & Kohut, 2013; Mello, Fivel, Kohut, & Bergman, 2013). In rats, buspirone reduced anxiety from cocaine withdrawal (de Oliveira Citó et al., 2012).

2.3.3 Preclinical support and caveats for translation of the D3 hypothesis to the clinic

D3-selective ligands have been widely studied in addiction models. Among the patterns that emerge, D3 antagonism is clearly most effective in self-administration under a PR schedule of reinforcement and in reinstatement paradigms while generally ineffective in FR studies. This suggests that D3 antagonism reduces the rewarding efficacy and motivation to self-administer the drug of abuse, without substantially disrupting general behavior. However, studies that compare D3 antagonist effects on drug taking to effects on food or sucrose rewards have not been fully explored. In developing potential medications, it is important to ascertain whether or not these behavioral effects are specific to drug-induced reward-seeking behaviors or general to natural rewards as well.

Developing behavioral models in animals that translate to human behavior is a continual challenge in psychiatric drug development and may be especially challenging in the psychostimulant drug-abusing population. Moreover, many of the compounds tested in preclinical models have specific drawbacks that have halted or precluded translation to the clinic. The chemical structures of these compounds are commonly large and lipophilic, which can be problematic in terms of solubility and drug ADMET properties (see Section 2.1 for further discussion). Also, very few studies have detailed the metabolic profiles of these compounds.

Finally, it is not currently clear from preclinical studies whether antagonist or partial agonist effects on D3 receptors are preferable for treatment. More detailed study is needed of *in vivo* D3 signaling to determine whether there is a functional difference between D3 antagonists or partial agonists in drug-taking or drug-seeking animals; given the D3 receptor's high affinity for DA, partial agonism may be effectively indistinguishable from antagonism when DA levels are very high, as they are well known to be during drug-taking and drug-seeking behaviors. It is anticipated that many of these questions and caveats will be addressable with better drug molecules.

3. CLINICAL STUDIES TARGETING THE D3 RECEPTOR IN THE TREATMENT OF ADDICTION

A critical consideration for clinical trial success is the demonstration that the new drug engages its biological target (e.g., central D3 receptors) at doses that are related to its pharmacological action (e.g., drug craving cessation). Hence, the discovery of a D3-preferential positron emission tomography (PET) ligand to monitor drug occupancy and selectivity at D3 receptors was essential. As described earlier, selective D3 receptor ligands that are active *in vivo* have remained a challenge. The further requirements for a PET ligand including (1) high affinity ($K_i < 1$ nM), (2) >30-fold selectivity for the target, (3) rapid BBB penetration, and (4) limited metabolism have provided significant challenge to identifying a D3-preferntial PET ligand.

3.1. [^{11}C]PHNO

Currently, [^{11}C]PHNO (Fig. 7.2), a D3-prefential agonist, has been used in this capacity, although it is perhaps not ideal. First introduced as a nonselective D2/D3 receptor agonist (Horn et al., 1984; Martin et al., 1985), PHNO was developed as a potential agonist treatment for Parkinson's disease (Koller, Herbster, & Gordon, 1987; Rose & Nashef, 1987). Subsequently, [^{11}C]PHNO was first characterized as binding to high-affinity states of the D2/D3 receptor in human subjects (Willeit et al., 2006) and later as a D3 receptor agonist (Narendran et al., 2006). It has subsequently been further characterized (Ginovart et al., 2007) and more recently used to demonstrate D3 receptor involvement (Graff-Guerrero, Mamo, et al., 2009; Graff-Guerrero, Mizrahi, et al., 2009; Graff-Guerrero et al., 2008; Willeit et al., 2008) and upregulation in methamphetamine abusers (Boileau et al., 2012). In addition, [^{11}C]PHNO has been used to validate D3 receptor occupancy for the D3 antagonist ABT 925 (Graff-Guerrero et al., 2010). A [^{11}C]PHNO PET study is planned to evaluate whether D3 receptor expression is elevated in smokers versus nonsmokers and whether correlations exist between D3 receptor binding and the reactivity to smoking cues as measured by functional MRI (ClinicalTrials.gov Identifier: NCT01784016). Another planned [¹¹C]PHNO PET study seeks to determine whether the smoking cessation drug varenicline alters D2/D3 receptor binding in tobacco smokers (ClinicalTrials.gov Identifier: NCT01632189).

3.2. GSK598809

To date, only a few D3-selective antagonists have progressed to human clinical testing. The first compound from GlaxoSmithKline, GSK598809 (Fig. 7.1), entered phase 1 clinical trials in 2007 and phase 2 trials for smoking cessation and compulsive overeating (e.g., ClinicalTrials.gov Identifiers: NCT00437632, NCT01188967, NCT00793468, NCT00605241, NCT01039454). Cognate analog GSK618334 also entered phase 1 clinical trials in 2007 (ClinicalTrials.gov Identifiers: NCT00513279, NCT00814957, NCT01036061). To date, nine trials have been completed with GSK598809, and this compound was deemed to be safe and well tolerated in healthy volunteers (Mugnaini et al., 2013; Searle et al., 2010). Importantly, studies using the D3-preferential PET ligand [¹¹C]PHNO in human volunteers demonstrated that GSK598809 engages with D3 receptor-rich regions of the human brain, upon oral administration, in the substantia nigra but not in the dorsal regions of the striatum (Searle et al., 2010). Boileau et al. (2012) determined that methamphetamine polydrug users had higher [¹¹C]PHNO binding in the D3 receptor-rich substantia nigra, globus pallidus, and ventral pallidum and lower binding in the D2 receptor-rich dorsal striatum compared to healthy controls. [¹¹C]PHNO binding within the substantia nigra correlated with self-reported drug craving (Boileau et al., 2012).

A recent study using GSK598809 and [¹¹C]PHNO sought to predict the ability of GSK598809 to reduce nicotine-seeking/craving behavior in human cigarette smokers and the relationship to D3 occupancy by this D3 antagonist. These results were compared with an *ex vivo* autoradiography study in rats and the demonstration that GSK598809 dose-dependently reduced the expression of nicotine-induced CPP. Although an absolute translation of these findings was not achieved in this preliminary study, the results suggest that GSK598809 binds to D3 receptors in a dose-dependent manner and support further investigation of GSK598809 for smoking cessation in human subjects. Further translation of preclinical findings that GSK598809 and other D3 antagonists and partial agonists may be effective in reducing methamphetamine and/or cocaine craving in humans has yet to be evaluated. In order to advance to phase 2 clinical trials for cocaine or methamphetamine abuse, further drug-interaction studies must be conducted. In addition, as the D3 antagonists appear to be more effective in reducing drug and/or cue-induced reinstatement to drug seeking in laboratory animals than blocking self-administration of cocaine or methamphetamine, the design of clinical trials must take this into account.

3.3. BP1.4979

Bioprojet recently disclosed their novel D3 antagonist BP1.4979, and recruitment for a clinical trial on smoking cessation has begun (ClinicalTrials.gov Identifier: NCT01785147).

3.4. Buspirone

Finally, as noted earlier, the clinically available atypical anxiolytic drug buspirone (Fig. 7.1) has recently shown promise in preclinical studies (Bergman et al., 2013; Mello, Fivel, & Kohut, 2013; Mello, Fivel, Kohut, & Bergman, 2013; Newman, Blaylock, et al., 2012; Shelton, Hendrick, & Beardsley, 2013) for the treatment of psychostimulant abuse. Although buspirone is not a D3-selective antagonist, its metabolic profile suggests primary metabolites bind to D3 (and D4) receptors (Bergman et al., 2013). Target engagement using PET imaging and clinical studies is in progress (ClinicalTrials.gov Identifier: NCT01699828) that will inform future exploration of this repurposed drug for treatment of SUDs.

4. THE STRUCTURAL BASIS OF D3 OVER D2 RECEPTOR SELECTIVITY AND THE FUTURE OF RATIONAL DRUG DESIGN FOR D3 RECEPTOR-SELECTIVE LIGANDS

Despite a number of preclinical candidates and a handful of D3-selective antagonists or partial agonists in clinical trials for smoking cessation, the need to identify novel templates and better drug molecules to target the D3 receptor still exists. It is important to note, for example, that in treating SUDs, toxicology and safety studies must be done with the new medication candidate and in the presence of the abused drug, for example, cocaine. Drug combinations can produce untoward side effects that could not be predicted by the drug interacting with its primary target (e.g., D3 receptor) and may be related to off-target actions or metabolic vulnerability of a particular structural template. Hence, using all the available structural information to identify new leads remains important in the pursuit of medication candidates. Small-molecule drug discovery usually begins with identifying lead compounds that recognize the biological target of interest. The advancement of high-throughput screens (Macarron et al., 2011) and rational lead design and optimization with *in silico* models (Jorgensen, 2009) have been a more recent source of novel leads.

Common structural features of GPCRs include the 7 TMs and extracellular and intracellular loops (ECLs and ICLs) (Rosenbaum, Rasmussen, & Kobilka, 2009). Specifically for class A rhodopsin-like GPCRs, to which DA receptors belong, a conserved "toggle switch" in TM6 is involved in receptor activation—the impact of the reconfiguration of this switch upon agonist binding is propagated to the intracellular side and triggers the release of a conserved ionic lock between TM3 and TM6, which has been found to stabilize the receptor in an inactive state (Ballesteros, Jensen, et al., 2001; Shi et al., 2002). Such transitions between active and inactive states have significant impact on the shape and size of the orthosteric ligand binding site; it is computationally complex to design and optimize antagonists or agonists for a particular receptor with desired affinity and efficacy in a structure-based manner.

Due to the high homology among GPCRs especially within the same family (e.g., between rhodopsin and aminergic receptors), computational models of the D3 receptor were previously built based on the crystal structure of rhodopsin (Hobrath & Wang, 2006; Varady et al., 2003). These resulting homology models were then used to characterize points of interaction of small molecules at the binding site, through medicinal chemistry, chimera studies, and single point mutations on the receptor (e.g., Ehrlich et al., 2009). Before the crystallographic coordinates of the D3 crystal structure were published, a competition was held to determine how well various GPCR modeling and docking procedures performed in identifying key ligand–receptor interactions, comparing these results to the crystal structure of the D3 receptor. The best-performing complex models approached the accuracy of the crystallographically determined details, especially in revealing those in the conserved OBS (Kufareva et al., 2011).

Several groups have used homology models of the D3 receptor to design libraries of D3-selective ligands. For example, Levoin and colleagues recently demonstrated that the binding site in their "historical" rhodopsin-based D3 receptor homology model was as well suited for lead optimization as the crystal structure of the D3 receptor, which explained the successful utilization of the model in their drug discovery processes

(Levoin et al., 2011). Similarly, the β-adrenergic receptor-based D3 homology model appeared to perform as well as the D3 receptor crystal structure in retrieving known hit compounds in *in silico* high-throughput screening trials with a library of 3 million commercially available molecules. Interestingly, the homology model and the crystal structure have different enrichments of the chemical scaffolds, as the OBS in the homology model is slightly more open (Carlsson et al., 2011). In that study, because the compounds were screened against the OBS, none of the hit compounds showed appreciable selectivity for D3 over D2 receptor; nevertheless, novel scaffolds that can be modified to enhance selectivity were uncovered (Carlsson et al., 2011).

Interestingly, all of the novel hits identified by Carlsson et al. (2011) were found to be antagonists, which raises the question of how we may be able to rationally introduce efficacy into our D3 receptor-selective agents using computational modeling techniques. A recent review evaluating the progress in the structure-based drug design for GPCRs highlighted the advances that are being made with the availability of many high-resolution GPCR structures in both active and inactive states; thus far, the most successful investigations have improved ligand binding affinities toward individual receptors but, in most cases, without addressing selectivity or efficacy issues (Congreve, Langmead, Mason, & Marshall, 2011). Thus, in comparison, the novelty of our approach is to reveal molecular determinants of D3 over D2 receptor selectivity as well as D3 receptor efficacy. To this end, we have built and refined D3 and D2 receptor models in both inactive and active states. In addition to the D3 receptor structure, stabilized in an inactive conformation by eticlopride, a D3/D2 receptor-selective inverse agonist (Chien et al., 2010), we used the differences in the inactive and active structures of β_1- and β_2-adrenergic receptors (Cherezov et al., 2007; Rasmussen et al., 2011; Warne et al., 2011) to guide the construction of a D3 receptor model with the OBS in the active conformation. For comparative investigations of D3 versus D2 receptor, we also correspondingly built and refined D3 receptor-based homology models of the D2 receptor (Chien et al., 2010; Newman, Beuming, et al., 2012). Using these models, the results of our molecular docking and dynamics studies suggested that the PP of D3 receptor-selective compounds is bound in the OBS, while the arylamide secondary pharmacophore (SP) is accommodated in a secondary binding pocket (SBP) formed by residues from TMs 1, 2, 3, 7, and divergent ECL1 and ECL2 (Chien et al., 2010; Newman, Beuming, et al., 2012).

   To further dissect the contributions of individual pharmacophore components of D3 receptor-selective compounds to the selectivity and efficacy,
we incrementally deconstructed our D3 receptor-selective antagonist R22
(R-PG 648; Figs. 7.1 and 7.3) into "synthons". Starting with the PP, 2,3-
diCl-phenylpiperazine, we added N-alkyl substituents one methylene group
at a time toward the amide functional group. We also synthesized the SP,
N-n-butyl-indole-2-amide. These synthons were tested for receptor
binding affinities and functional efficacies at the D3 and D2 receptors. This
study confirmed that the 2,3-diCl-4-phenylpiperazine or its cognate
2-OMe-4-phenylpiperazine served as the PP and that addition of the
N-n-butyl linking chain resulted in increased binding affinities at both
the D2 and D3 receptors, with essentially no change in selectivity, until
the indole amide was added to make the full D3 receptor-selective ligands.
Given the near identity of the D3 and D2 receptor residues in the OBS that
bind the PP and the linker region, it is expected that the synthons lacking the
SP would have little or no selectivity for these two receptors (Newman,
Beuming, et al., 2012).
   Moreover, we also found the N-n-butyl-indole-2-amide had very
low affinities for both the D2 and D3 receptors and was functionally
inactive, suggesting that the SP alone does not confer D3 receptor selectivity. The question thus became: how does D3 selectivity arise in these

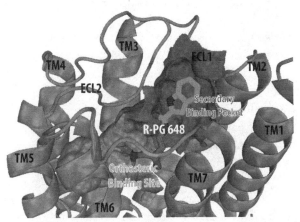

Figure 7.3 Predicted binding mode of R-PG 648 in the dopamine D3 receptor. The primary and secondary pharmacophores of R-PG 648 occupy the orthosteric binding site
(OBS) and the secondary binding pocket (SBP), respectively. The OBS and SBP are in surface representation. (For color version of this figure, the reader is referred to the online
version of this chapter.)

molecules? Our computational modeling and analysis indicated that substitutions on the terminal 4-phenylpiperazine ring, in combination with the linker, affect the orientation of the PP in the OBS, which consequently influences the exact orientation of the SP. Thus, we proposed that D3 receptor selectivity arises from divergent interactions of the SP within the SBP, separate but affected by the PP in the OBS (Newman, Beuming, et al., 2012).

Our study also demonstrated that depending on the 4-phenylpiperazine substitution pattern, efficacies could range from a nearly full agonist (2,3-diCl-4-phenylpiperazine) to a very low efficacy partial agonist (e.g., N-n-butyl-2,3-diCl-4-phenylpiperazine or the 2-OMe-4-phenylpiperazine). In the context of accumulated understanding of aminergic receptor activation (Ballesteros, Shi, & Javitch, 2001; Shi & Javitch, 2002), our modeling results indicated that efficacy depends on the binding mode in the OBS and suggested that the efficacy of D3 receptor-selective ligands could be manipulated by modifying the PP that binds to the OBS (Newman, Beuming, et al., 2012).

As noted earlier, the SBP diverges significantly between the D3 and D2 receptors. Initial chimera studies using R-PG 648 (R22) pointed to a role of the extracellular loops in receptor subtype selectivity (Newman et al., 2009). A more complete study, using eight D2/D3 chimeras and our most D3-selective compound to date (BAK 2-66; Fig. 7.1), suggested an appreciable role for the ECL2 in ligand binding: replacing this loop in the D2 receptor with the D3 receptor ECL2 sequence improved binding affinity by 37-fold. However, a more dramatic improvement was seen in chimeras of the D2 receptor that included TMs 1 and 2 and ECL1 of the D3 receptor, resulting in a dramatic 441-fold improvement in binding over the D2 wild-type receptor (Banala et al., 2011). Indeed, the binding affinity for BAK 2-66 at this chimera was nearly fourfold higher than at the wild-type D3 receptor (Banala et al., 2011). Follow-up studies have specifically characterized the divergence in the shape, size, and dynamics of the SBP of D3 and D2 receptors (Michino et al., 2013). The combined computational and experimental results indicated that ECL1 plays a key role in determining the D3 receptor over D2 receptor selectivity of R-PG 648. In particular, a single Gly residue in the EL1 was found to be able to interconvert the binding selectivity of R-PG 648 in D3 and D2, and suggest the non-conserved ECL1 can influence the orientation of conserved TM2, and thus render different shapes and sizes of the SBP in both D3 and D2 receptors (Michino et al., 2013).

5. CONCLUSION

The DA D3 receptor remains an enticing target for addiction pharmacotherapy. A panoply of D3-selective compounds have been tested *in vivo*, producing promising results in addiction models and supporting the hypothesis that D3 receptor signaling is an important component of the reinforcing aspects of addictive drugs. Promising recent clinical trial results suggest that the D3 receptor remains a viable clinical target, but data are still limited in this regard. Continued development of novel D3-selective compounds is necessary as there are currently no FDA-approved treatments for psychostimulant addiction and no current candidates in phase 3 clinical trials, to our knowledge. The new molecular tools discussed in this review hold great promise in identifying new D3-preferential ligands for clinical development.

This is a very exciting time in GPCR research and structure-based drug design. Many crystal structures of both active and inactive receptor states are now available, providing important clues to address the drug discovery issues that were difficult to tackle without high-resolution structural information, such as selectivity and efficacy. The efforts of medicinal chemists have already optimized many lead molecules, but there is still a need for "molecular tweaking" to convert research tools into viable medications. Combining crystal structure-informed computational models with, for example, the hERG channel model (Micheli, Arista, Bertani, et al., 2010; Micheli, Arista, Bonanomi, et al., 2010) will further refine small-molecule medicinal chemistry and enhance the likelihood of designing viable clinical candidates. Models of increasing complexity can be combined with molecular pharmacology techniques and may be able to identify unexplored (allosteric?) binding sites that will ultimately provide improved drug-like molecule design for the future.

CONFLICT OF INTEREST

The authors have no conflicts of interest to declare.

ACKNOWLEDGEMENTS

This work was supported in part by the NIDA Intramural Research Program (A. H. N.) and DA023694 (L. S.). T. M. K. is supported by an NIH IRTA postdoctoral fellowship and C. B. is supported by an NIH postbaccalaureate fellowship. A. H. N. and L. S. would like to acknowledge the members of our labs, past and present, and our wonderful collaborators who have helped move our D3 receptor program forward.

REFERENCES

Achat-Mendes, C., Grundt, P., Cao, J., Platt, D. M., Newman, A. H., & Spealman, R. D. (2010). Dopamine D3 and D2 receptor mechanisms in the abuse-related behavioral effects of cocaine: Studies with preferential antagonists in squirrel monkeys. *Journal of Pharmacology and Experimental Therapeutics, 334*, 556–565.

Achat-Mendes, C., Platt, D. M., Newman, A. H., & Spealman, R. D. (2009). The dopamine D3 receptor partial agonist CJB 090 inhibits the discriminative stimulus but not the reinforcing or priming effects of cocaine in squirrel monkeys. *Psychopharmacology, 206*, 73–84.

Agai-Csongor, E., Domany, G., Nogradi, K., Galambos, J., Vago, I., Keseru, G. M., et al. (2012). Discovery of cariprazine (RGH-188): A novel antipsychotic acting on dopamine D3/D2 receptors. *Bioorganic and Medicinal Chemistry Letters, 22*, 3437–3440.

Arnold, J. M., & Roberts, D. C. (1997). A critique of fixed and progressive ratio schedules used to examine the neural substrates of drug reinforcement. *Pharmacology, Biochemistry, and Behavior, 57*, 441–447.

Austin, N. E., Baldwin, S. J., Cutler, L., Deeks, N., Kelly, P. J., Nash, M., et al. (2001). Pharmacokinetics of the novel, high-affinity and selective dopamine D3 receptor antagonist SB-277011 in rat, dog and monkey: In vitro/in vivo correlation and the role of aldehyde oxidase. *Xenobiotica, 31*, 677–686.

Ballesteros, J. A., Jensen, A. D., Liapakis, G., Rasmussen, S. G., Shi, L., Gether, U., et al. (2001). Activation of the beta 2-adrenergic receptor involves disruption of an ionic lock between the cytoplasmic ends of transmembrane segments 3 and 6. *Journal of Biological Chemistry, 276*, 29171–29177.

Ballesteros, J. A., Shi, L., & Javitch, J. A. (2001). Structural mimicry in G protein-coupled receptors: Implications of the high-resolution structure of rhodopsin for structure-function analysis of rhodopsin-like receptors. *Molecular Pharmacology, 60*, 1–19.

Banala, A. K., Levy, B. A., Khatri, S. S., Furman, C. A., Roof, R. A., Mishra, Y., et al. (2011). N-(3-fluoro-4-(4-(2-methoxy or 2,3-dichlorophenyl)piperazine-1-yl)butyl) arylcarboxamides as selective dopamine D3 receptor ligands: Critical role of the carboxamide linker for D3 receptor selectivity. *Journal of Medicinal Chemistry, 54*, 3581–3594.

Basile, M., Lin, R., Kabbani, N., Karpa, K., Kilimann, M., Simpson, I., et al. (2006). Paralemmin interacts with D3 dopamine receptors: Implications for membrane localization and cAMP signaling. *Archives of Biochemistry and Biophysics, 446*, 60–68.

Beninger, R. J., & Banasikowski, T. J. (2008). Dopaminergic mechanism of reward-related incentive learning: Focus on the dopamine D(3) receptor. *Neurotoxicity Research, 14*, 57–70.

Bergman, J., Roof, R. A., Furman, C. A., Conroy, J. L., Mello, N. K., Sibley, D. R., et al. (2013). Modification of cocaine self-administration by buspirone (buspar®): Potential involvement of D3 and D4 dopamine receptors. *International Journal of Neuropsychopharmacology, 16*, 445–458.

Blaylock, B. L., Gould, R. W., Banala, A., Grundt, P., Luedtke, R. R., Newman, A. H., et al. (2011). Influence of cocaine history on the behavioral effects of dopamine D(3) receptor-selective compounds in monkeys. *Neuropsychopharmacology, 36*, 1104–1113.

Boeckler, F., Ohnmacht, U., Lehmann, T., Utz, W., Hubner, H., & Gmeiner, P. (2005). CoMFA and CoMSIA investigations revealing novel insights into the binding modes of dopamine D3 receptor agonists. *Journal of Medicinal Chemistry, 48*, 2493–2508.

Boileau, I., Payer, D., Houle, S., Behzadi, A., Rusjan, P. M., Tong, J., et al. (2012). Higher binding of the dopamine D3 receptor-preferring ligand [11C]-(+)-propyl-hexahydro-naphtho-oxazin in methamphetamine polydrug users: A positron emission tomography study. *Journal of Neuroscience, 32*, 1353–1359.

Bonanomi, G., Braggio, S., Capelli, A. M., Checchia, A., Di Fabio, R., Marchioro, C., et al. (2010). Triazolyl azabicyclo[3.1.0]hexanes: A class of potent and selective dopamine D (3) receptor antagonists. *ChemMedChem*, *5*, 705–715.

Butini, S., Campiani, G., Franceschini, S., Trotta, F., Kumar, V., Guarino, E., et al. (2010). Discovery of bishomo(hetero)arylpiperazines as novel multifunctional ligands targeting dopamine D(3) and serotonin 5-HT(1A) and 5-HT(2A) receptors. *Journal of Medicinal Chemistry*, *53*, 4803–4807.

Caine, S. B., Thomsen, M., Barrett, A. C., Collins, G. T., Grundt, P., Newman, A. H., et al. (2012). Cocaine self-administration in dopamine D(3) receptor knockout mice. *Experimental and Clinical Psychopharmacology*, *20*, 352–363.

Carlsson, J., Coleman, R. G., Setola, V., Irwin, J. J., Fan, H., Schlessinger, A., et al. (2011). Ligand discovery from a dopamine D3 receptor homology model and crystal structure. *Nature Chemical Biology*, *7*, 769–778.

Chen, J., Collins, G. T., Levant, B., Woods, J., Deschamps, J. R., & Wang, S. (2011). CJ-1639: A potent and highly selective dopamine D3 receptor full agonist. *ACS Medicinal Chemistry Letters*, *2*, 620–625.

Cherezov, V., Rosenbaum, D. M., Hanson, M. A., Rasmussen, S. G., Thian, F. S., Kobilka, T. S., et al. (2007). High-resolution crystal structure of an engineered human beta2-adrenergic G protein-coupled receptor. *Science*, *318*, 1258–1265.

Chien, E. Y., Liu, W., Zhao, Q., Katritch, V., Han, G. W., Hanson, M. A., et al. (2010). Structure of the human dopamine D3 receptor in complex with a D2/D3 selective antagonist. *Science*, *330*, 1091–1095.

Cho, D. I., Zheng, M., & Kim, K. M. (2010). Current perspectives on the selective regulation of dopamine D(2) and D(3) receptors. *Archives of Pharmacal Research*, *33*, 1521–1538.

Citrome, L. (2013). Cariprazine: Chemistry, pharmacodynamics, pharmacokinetics, and metabolism, clinical efficacy, safety, and tolerability. *Expert Opinion on Drug Metabolism & Toxicology*, *9*, 193–206.

Congreve, M., Langmead, C. J., Mason, J. S., & Marshall, F. H. (2011). Progress in structure based drug design for G protein-coupled receptors. *Journal of Medicinal Chemistry*, *54*, 4283–4311.

de Oliveira Citó, M. D. C., da Silva, F. C., Silva, M. I., Moura, B. A., Macedo, D. S., Woods, D. J., et al. (2012). Reversal of cocaine withdrawal-induced anxiety by ondansetron, buspirone and propranolol. *Behavioural Brain Research*, *231*, 116–123.

Diaz, J., Pilon, C., Le Foll, B., Gros, C., Triller, A., Schwartz, J. C., et al. (2000). Dopamine D3 receptors expressed by all mesencephalic dopamine neurons. *Journal of Neuroscience*, *20*, 8677–8684.

Di Ciano, P. (2008). Drug seeking under a second-order schedule of reinforcement depends on dopamine D3 receptors in the basolateral amygdala. *Behavioral Neuroscience*, *122*, 129–139.

Ehrlich, K., Gotz, A., Bollinger, S., Tschammer, N., Bettinetti, L., Harterich, S., et al. (2009). Dopamine D2, D3, and D4 selective phenylpiperazines as molecular probes to explore the origins of subtype specific receptor binding. *Journal of Medicinal Chemistry*, *52*, 4923–4935.

Fiorentini, C., Busi, C., Gorruso, E., Gotti, C., Spano, P., & Missale, C. (2008). Reciprocal regulation of dopamine D1 and D3 receptor function and trafficking by heterodimerization. *Molecular Pharmacology*, *74*, 59–69.

Garcia-Ladona, F. J., & Cox, B. F. (2003). BP 897, a selective dopamine D3 receptor ligand with therapeutic potential for the treatment of cocaine-addiction. *CNS Drug Reviews*, *9*, 141–158.

Ginovart, N., Willeit, M., Rusjan, P., Graff, A., Bloomfield, P. M., Houle, S., et al. (2007). Positron emission tomography quantification of [11C]-(+)-PHNO binding in the human brain. *Journal of Cerebral Blood Flow and Metabolism*, *27*, 857–871.

Gleeson, M. P. (2008). Generation of a set of simple, interpretable ADMET rules of thumb. *Journal of Medicinal Chemistry*, *51*, 817–834.

Graff-Guerrero, A., Mamo, D., Shammi, C. M., Mizrahi, R., Marcon, H., Barsoum, P., et al. (2009). The effect of antipsychotics on the high-affinity state of D2 and D3 receptors: A positron emission tomography study with [11C]-(+)-PHNO. *Archives of General Psychiatry*, *66*, 606–615.

Graff-Guerrero, A., Mizrahi, R., Agid, O., Marcon, H., Barsoum, P., Rusjan, P., et al. (2009). The dopamine D2 receptors in high-affinity state and D3 receptors in schizophrenia: A clinical [11C]-(+)-PHNO PET study. *Neuropsychopharmacology*, *34*, 1078–1086.

Graff-Guerrero, A., Redden, L., Abi-Saab, W., Katz, D. A., Houle, S., Barsoum, P., et al. (2010). Blockade of [11C](+)-PHNO binding in human subjects by the dopamine D3 receptor antagonist ABT-925. *International Journal of Neuropsychopharmacology*, *13*, 273–287.

Graff-Guerrero, A., Willeit, M., Ginovart, N., Mamo, D., Mizrahi, R., Rusjan, P., et al. (2008). Brain region binding of the D2/3 agonist [11C]-(+)-PHNO and the D2/3 antagonist [11C]raclopride in healthy humans. *Human Brain Mapping*, *29*, 400–410.

Grundt, P., Carlson, E. E., Cao, J., Bennett, C. J., McElveen, E., Taylor, M., et al. (2005). Novel heterocyclic trans olefin analogues of N-{4-[4-(2,3-dichlorophenyl)piperazin-1-yl]butyl}arylcarboxamides as selective probes with high affinity for the dopamine D3 receptor. *Journal of Medicinal Chemistry*, *48*, 839–848.

Grundt, P., Prevatt, K. M., Cao, J., Taylor, M., Floresca, C. Z., Choi, J. K., et al. (2007). Heterocyclic analogues of N-(4-(4-(2,3-dichlorophenyl)piperazin-1-yl)butyl)arylcarboxamides with functionalized linking chains as novel dopamine D3 receptor ligands: Potential substance abuse therapeutic agents. *Journal of Medicinal Chemistry*, *50*, 4135–4146.

Gurevich, E. V., & Joyce, J. N. (1999). Distribution of dopamine D3 receptor expressing neurons in the human forebrain: Comparison with D2 receptor expressing neurons. *Neuropsychopharmacology*, *20*, 60–80.

Hann, M. M., & Keseru, G. M. (2012). Finding the sweet spot: The role of nature and nurture in medicinal chemistry. *Nature Reviews Drug Discovery*, *11*, 355–365.

Heidbreder, C. A., Gardner, E. L., Xi, Z. X., Thanos, P. K., Mugnaini, M., Hagan, J. J., et al. (2005). The role of central dopamine D3 receptors in drug addiction: A review of pharmacological evidence. *Brain Research Brain Research Reviews*, *49*, 77–105.

Heidbreder, C. A., & Newman, A. H. (2010). Current perspectives on selective dopamine D (3) receptor antagonists as pharmacotherapeutics for addictions and related disorders. *Annals of the New York Academy of Sciences*, *1187*, 4–34.

Higley, A. E., Kiefer, S. W., Li, X., Gaal, J., Xi, Z. X., & Gardner, E. L. (2011). Dopamine D (3) receptor antagonist SB277011A inhibits methamphetamine self-administration and methamphetamine-induced reinstatement of drug-seeking in rats. *European Journal of Pharmacology*, *659*, 187–192.

Higley, A. E., Spiller, K., Grundt, P., Newman, A. H., Kiefer, S. W., Xi, Z. X., et al. (2011). PG01037, a novel dopamine D3 receptor antagonist, inhibits the effects of methamphetamine in rats. *Journal of Psychopharmacology*, *25*, 263–273.

Hill, A. P., & Young, R. J. (2010). Getting physical in drug discovery: A contemporary perspective on solubility and hydrophobicity. *Drug Discovery Today*, *15*, 648–655.

Hobrath, J. V., & Wang, S. (2006). Computational elucidation of the structural basis of ligand binding to the dopamine 3 receptor through docking and homology modeling. *Journal of Medicinal Chemistry*, *49*, 4470–4476.

Horn, A. S., Hazelhoff, B., Dijkstra, D., de Vries, J. B., Mulder, T. B., Timmermans, P., et al. (1984). The hydroxy-hexanydronaphthoxazines: A new group of very potent and selective dopamine agonists. *Journal of Pharmacy and Pharmacology*, *36*, 639–640.

Jean, M., Renault, J., Levoin, N., Danvy, D., Calmels, T., Berrebi-Bertrand, I., et al. (2010). Synthesis and evaluation of amides surrogates of dopamine D3 receptor ligands. *Bioorganic and Medicinal Chemistry Letters*, *20*, 5376–5379.

Johnson, M., Antonio, T., Reith, M. E., & Dutta, A. K. (2012). Structure-activity relationship study of N(6)-(2-(4-(1H-Indol-5-yl)piperazin-1-yl)ethyl)-N(6)-propyl-4,5,6,7-tetrahydroben zo[d]thiazole-2,6-diamine analogues: Development of highly selective D3 dopamine receptor agonists along with a highly potent D2/D3 agonist and their pharmacological characterization. *Journal of Medicinal Chemistry*, *55*, 5826–5840.

Jorgensen, W. L. (2009). Efficient drug lead discovery and optimization. *Accounts of Chemical Research*, *42*, 724–733.

Joyce, J. N., & Millan, M. J. (2005). Dopamine D3 receptor antagonists as therapeutic agents. *Drug Discovery Today*, *10*, 917–925.

Khaled, M. A., Farid Araki, K., Li, B., Coen, K. M., Marinelli, P. W., Varga, J., et al. (2010). The selective dopamine D3 receptor antagonist SB 277011-A, but not the partial agonist BP 897, blocks cue-induced reinstatement of nicotine-seeking. *International Journal of Neuropsychopharmacology*, *13*, 181–190.

Koller, W., Herbster, G., & Gordon, J. (1987). PHNO, a novel dopamine agonist, in animal models of parkinsonism. *Movement Disorders*, *2*, 193–199.

Kufareva, I., Rueda, M., Katritch, V., Stevens, R. C., Abagyan, R., & GPCR Dock 2010 participants (2011). Status of GPCR modeling and docking as reflected by community-wide GPCR Dock 2010 assessment. *Structure*, *19*, 1108–1126.

Le Foll, B., & Boileau, I. (2013). Repurposing buspirone for drug addiction treatment. *International Journal of Neuropsychopharmacology*, *16*, 251–253.

Le Foll, B., Diaz, J., & Sokoloff, P. (2003). Increased dopamine D3 receptor expression accompanying behavioral sensitization to nicotine in rats. *Synapse*, *47*, 176–183.

Le Foll, B., Goldberg, S. R., & Sokoloff, P. (2005). The dopamine D3 receptor and drug dependence: Effects on reward or beyond? *Neuropharmacology*, *49*, 525–541.

Levant, B. (1997). The D3 dopamine receptor: Neurobiology and potential clinical relevance. *Pharmacological Reviews*, *49*, 231–252.

Levesque, D., Diaz, J., Pilon, C., Martres, M. P., Giros, B., Souil, E., et al. (1992). Identification, characterization, and localization of the dopamine D3 receptor in rat brain using 7-[3H]hydroxy-N, N-di-n-propyl-2-aminotetralin. *Proceedings of the National Academy of Sciences of the United States of America*, *89*, 8155–8159.

Levoin, N., Calmels, T., Krief, S., Danvy, D., Berrebi-Bertrand, I., Lecomte, J. M., et al. (2011). Homology model versus X-ray structure in receptor-based drug design: A retrospective analysis with the dopamine D3 receptor. *ACS Medicinal Chemistry Letters*, *2*, 293–297.

Liang, J., Zheng, X., Chen, J., Li, Y., Xing, X., Bai, Y., et al. (2011). Roles of BDNF, dopamine D(3) receptors, and their interactions in the expression of morphine-induced context-specific locomotor sensitization. *European Neuropsychopharmacology*, *21*, 825–834.

Lipinski, C. A. (2000). Drug-like properties and the causes of poor solubility and poor permeability. *Journal of Pharmacological and Toxicological Methods*, *44*, 235–249.

Lipinski, C. A., Lombardo, F., Dominy, B. W., & Feeney, P. J. (1997). Experimental and computational approaches to estimate solubility and permeability in drug discovery and development settings. *Advanced Drug Delivery Reviews*, *23*, 3–25.

Liu, J., Li, Y., Zhang, S., Xiao, Z., & Ai, C. (2011). Studies of new fused benzazepine as selective dopamine D3 receptor antagonists using 3D-QSAR, molecular docking and molecular dynamics. *International Journal of Molecular Sciences*, *12*, 1196–1221.

Lopez, L., Selent, J., Ortega, R., Masaguer, C. F., Dominguez, E., Areias, F., et al. (2010). Synthesis, 3D-QSAR, and structural modeling of benzolactam derivatives with binding affinity for the D(2) and D(3) receptors. *ChemMedChem*, *5*, 1300–1317.

Macarron, R., Banks, M. N., Bojanic, D., Burns, D. J., Cirovic, D. A., Garyantes, T., et al. (2011). Impact of high-throughput screening in biomedical research. *Nature Reviews. Drug Discovery*, *10*, 188–195.

Maggio, R., Aloisi, G., Silvano, E., Rossi, M., & Millan, M. J. (2009). Heterodimerization of dopamine receptors: New insights into functional and therapeutic significance. *Parkinsonism & Related Disorders*, *15*(Suppl. 4), S2–S7.

Marcellino, D., Ferre, S., Casado, V., Cortes, A., Le Foll, B., Mazzola, C., et al. (2008). Identification of dopamine D1-D3 receptor heteromers. Indications for a role of synergistic D1-D3 receptor interactions in the striatum. *Journal of Biological Chemistry*, *283*, 26016–26025.

Martin, G. E., Williams, M., Pettibone, D. J., Zrada, M. M., Lotti, V. J., Taylor, D. A., et al. (1985). Selectivity of (+)-4-propyl-9-hydroxynaphthoxazine [(+)-PHNO] for dopamine receptors in vitro and in vivo. *Journal of Pharmacology and Experimental Therapeutics*, *233*, 395–401.

Mash, D. C., & Staley, J. K. (1999). D3 dopamine and kappa opioid receptor alterations in human brain of cocaine-overdose victims. *Annals of the New York Academy of Sciences*, *877*, 507–522.

Mason, C. W., Hassan, H. E., Kim, K. P., Cao, J., Eddington, N. D., Newman, A. H., et al. (2010). Characterization of the transport, metabolism, and pharmacokinetics of the dopamine D3 receptor-selective fluorenyl- and 2-pyridylphenyl amides developed for treatment of psychostimulant abuse. *Journal of Pharmacology and Experimental Therapeutics*, *333*, 854–864.

Mello, N. K., Fivel, P. A., & Kohut, S. J. (2013). Effects of chronic buspirone treatment on nicotine and concurrent nicotine + cocaine self-administration. *Neuropsychopharmacology*, *38*, 1264–1275.

Mello, N. K., Fivel, P. A., Kohut, S. J., & Bergman, J. (2013). Effects of chronic buspirone treatment on cocaine self-administration. *Neuropsychopharmacology*, *38*, 455–467.

Micheli, F. (2011). Recent advances in the development of dopamine D3 receptor antagonists: A medicinal chemistry perspective. *ChemMedChem*, *6*, 1152–1162.

Micheli, F., Arista, L., Bertani, B., Braggio, S., Capelli, A. M., Cremonesi, S., et al. (2010). Exploration of the amine terminus in a novel series of 1,2,4-triazolo-3-yl-azabicyclo [3.1.0]hexanes as selective dopamine D3 receptor antagonists. *Journal of Medicinal Chemistry*, *53*, 7129–7139.

Micheli, F., Arista, L., Bonanomi, G., Blaney, F. E., Braggio, S., Capelli, A. M., et al. (2010). 1,2,4-Triazolyl azabicyclo[3.1.0]hexanes: A new series of potent and selective dopamine D(3) receptor antagonists. *Journal of Medicinal Chemistry*, *53*, 374–391.

Micheli, F., Bonanomi, G., Blaney, F. E., Braggio, S., Capelli, A. M., Checchia, A., et al. (2007). 1,2,4-Triazol-3-yl-thiopropyl-tetrahydrobenzazepines: A series of potent and selective dopamine D(3) receptor antagonists. *Journal of Medicinal Chemistry*, *50*, 5076–5089.

Micheli, F., & Heidbreder, C. (2013). Dopamine D3 receptor antagonists: A patent review (2007–2012). *Expert Opinion on Therapeutic Patents*, *23*, 363–381.

Michino, M., Donthamsetti, P., Beuming, T., Banala, A., Duan, L., Roux, T., et al. (2013). A single glycine in extracellular loop 1 is the critical determinant for pharmacological specificity of dopamine D2 and D3 receptors. *Molecular Pharmacology*, *84*, 854–864.

Millan, M. J., Gobert, A., Newman-Tancredi, A., Lejeune, F., Cussac, D., Rivet, J. M., et al. (2000). S33084, a novel, potent, selective, and competitive antagonist at dopamine D(3)-receptors: I. Receptorial, electrophysiological and neurochemical profile compared with

GR218,231 and L741,626. *Journal of Pharmacology and Experimental Therapeutics, 293,* 1048–1062.

Millan, M. J., Loiseau, F., Dekeyne, A., Gobert, A., Flik, G., Cremers, T. I., et al. (2008). S33138 (N-[4-[2-[(3aS,9bR)-8-cyano-1,3a,4,9b-tetrahydro[1] benzopyrano[3,4-c]pyrrol-2(3H)-yl)-ethyl]phenyl-acetamide), a preferential dopamine D3 versus D2 receptor antagonist and potential antipsychotic agent: III. Actions in models of therapeutic activity and induction of side effects. *Journal of Pharmacology and Experimental Therapeutics, 324,* 1212–1226.

Millan, M. J., Mannoury la Cour, C., Novi, F., Maggio, R., Audinot, V., Newman-Tancredi, A., et al. (2008). S33138 [N-[4-[2-[(3aS,9bR)-8-cyano-1,3a,4,9b-tetrahydro[1]-benzopyrano [3,4-c]pyrrol-2(3H)-yl)-ethyl]phenylacetamide], a preferential dopamine D3 versus D2 receptor antagonist and potential antipsychotic agent: I. Receptor-binding profile and functional actions at G-protein-coupled receptors. *Journal of Pharmacology and Experimental Therapeutics, 324,* 587–599.

Millan, M. J., Peglion, J. L., Vian, J., Rivet, J. M., Brocco, M., Gobert, A., et al. (1995). Functional correlates of dopamine D3 receptor activation in the rat in vivo and their modulation by the selective antagonist, (+)-S 14297: 1. Activation of postsynaptic D3 receptors mediates hypothermia, whereas blockade of D2 receptors elicits prolactin secretion and catalepsy. *Journal of Pharmacology and Experimental Therapeutics, 275,* 885–898.

Millan, M. J., Svenningsson, P., Ashby, C. R., Jr., Hill, M., Egeland, M., Dekeyne, A., et al. (2008). S33138 [N-[4-[2-[(3aS,9bR)-8-cyano-1,3a,4,9b-tetrahydro[1]-benzopyrano [3,4-c]pyrrol-2(3H)-yl)-ethyl]phenylacetamide], a preferential dopamine D3 versus D2 receptor antagonist and potential antipsychotic agent. II. A neurochemical, electrophysiological and behavioral characterization in vivo. *Journal of Pharmacology and Experimental Therapeutics, 324,* 600–611.

Mugnaini, M., Iavarone, L., Cavallini, P., Griffante, C., Oliosi, B., Savoia, C., et al. (2013). Occupancy of brain dopamine D3 receptors and drug craving: A translational approach. *Neuropsychopharmacology, 38,* 302–312.

Narendran, R., Slifstein, M., Guillin, O., Hwang, Y., Hwang, D. R., Scher, E., et al. (2006). Dopamine (D2/3) receptor agonist positron emission tomography radiotracer [11C]-(+)-PHNO is a D3 receptor preferring agonist in vivo. *Synapse, 60,* 485–495.

Newman, A. H., Beuming, T., Banala, A. K., Donthamsetti, P., Pongetti, K., LaBounty, A., et al. (2012). Molecular determinants of selectivity and efficacy at the dopamine D3 receptor. *Journal of Medicinal Chemistry, 55,* 6689–6699.

Newman, A. H., Blaylock, B. L., Nader, M. A., Bergman, J., Sibley, D. R., & Skolnick, P. (2012). Medication discovery for addiction: Translating the dopamine D3 receptor hypothesis. *Biochemical Pharmacology, 84,* 882–890.

Newman, A. H., Cao, J., Bennett, C. J., Robarge, M. J., Freeman, R. A., & Luedtke, R. R. (2003). N-(4-[4-(2,3-dichlorophenyl)piperazin-1-yl]butyl, butenyl and butynyl)arylcarboxamides as novel dopamine D(3) receptor antagonists. *Bioorganic and Medicinal Chemistry Letters, 13,* 2179–2183.

Newman, A. H., Grundt, P., Cyriac, G., Deschamps, J. R., Taylor, M., Kumar, R., et al. (2009). N-(4-(4-(2,3-dichloro- or 2-methoxyphenyl)piperazin-1-yl)butyl)heterobiarylcarboxamides with functionalized linking chains as high affinity and enantioselective D3 receptor antagonists. *Journal of Medicinal Chemistry, 52,* 2559–2570.

Newman, A. H., Grundt, P., & Nader, M. A. (2005). Dopamine D3 receptor partial agonists and antagonists as potential drug abuse therapeutic agents. *Journal of Medicinal Chemistry, 48,* 3663–3679.

O'Brien, C. P., & Gardner, E. L. (2005). Critical assessment of how to study addiction and its treatment: Human and non-human animal models. *Pharmacology & Therapeutics, 108,* 18–58.

Orio, L., Wee, S., Newman, A. H., Pulvirenti, L., & Koob, G. F. (2010). The dopamine D3 receptor partial agonist CJB090 and antagonist PG01037 decrease progressive ratio responding for methamphetamine in rats with extended-access. *Addiction Biology*, *15*, 312–323.

Peng, X. Q., Ashby, C. R., Jr., Spiller, K., Li, X., Li, J., Thomasson, N., et al. (2009). The preferential dopamine D3 receptor antagonist S33138 inhibits cocaine reward and cocaine-triggered relapse to drug-seeking behavior in rats. *Neuropharmacology*, *56*, 752–760.

Pilla, M., Perachon, S., Sautel, F., Garrido, F., Mann, A., Wermuth, C. G., et al. (1999). Selective inhibition of cocaine-seeking behaviour by a partial dopamine D3 receptor agonist. *Nature*, *400*, 371–375.

Rasmussen, S. G., DeVree, B. T., Zou, Y., Kruse, A. C., Chung, K. Y., Kobilka, T. S., et al. (2011). Crystal structure of the beta2 adrenergic receptor-Gs protein complex. *Nature*, *477*, 549–555.

Reavill, C., Taylor, S. G., Wood, M. D., Ashmeade, T., Austin, N. E., Avenell, K. Y., et al. (2000). Pharmacological actions of a novel, high-affinity, and selective human dopamine D(3) receptor antagonist, SB-277011-A. *Journal of Pharmacology and Experimental Therapeutics*, *294*, 1154–1165.

Rice, O. V., Gardner, E. L., Heidbreder, C. A., & Ashby, C. R., Jr. (2012). The acute administration of the selective dopamine D(3) receptor antagonist SB277011A reverses conditioned place aversion produced by naloxone precipitated withdrawal from acute morphine administration in rats. *Synapse*, *66*, 85–87.

Rice, O. V., Heidbreder, C. A., Gardner, E. L., Schonhar, C. D., & Ashby, C. R., Jr. (2013). The selective D3 receptor antagonist SB277011A attenuates morphine-triggered reactivation of expression of cocaine-induced conditioned place preference. *Synapse*, *67*, 469–475.

Rice, O. V., Patrick, J., Schonhar, C. D., Ning, H., & Ashby, C. R., Jr. (2012). The effects of the preferential dopamine D(3) receptor antagonist S33138 on ethanol binge drinking in C57BL/6J mice. *Synapse*, *66*, 975–978.

Richardson, N. R., & Roberts, D. C. (1996). Progressive ratio schedules in drug self-administration studies in rats: A method to evaluate reinforcing efficacy. *Journal of Neuroscience Methods*, *66*, 1–11.

Román, V., Gyertyan, I., Saghy, K., Kiss, B., & Szombathelyi, Z. (2013). Cariprazine (RGH-188), a D(3)-preferring dopamine D(3)/D(2) receptor partial agonist antipsychotic candidate demonstrates anti-abuse potential in rats. *Psychopharmacology*, *226*, 285–293.

Rose, F. C., & Nashef, L. (1987). Parkinson's disease: Further steps forward. *Gerontology*, *33*, 369–373.

Rosenbaum, D. M., Rasmussen, S. G., & Kobilka, B. K. (2009). The structure and function of G-protein-coupled receptors. *Nature*, *459*, 356–363.

Salama, I., Hocke, C., Utz, W., Prante, O., Boeckler, F., Hubner, H., et al. (2007). Structure-selectivity investigations of D2-like receptor ligands by CoMFA and CoMSIA guiding the discovery of D3 selective PET radioligands. *Journal of Medicinal Chemistry*, *50*, 489–500.

Searle, G., Beaver, J. D., Comley, R. A., Bani, M., Tziortzi, A., Slifstein, M., et al. (2010). Imaging dopamine D3 receptors in the human brain with positron emission tomography, [11C]PHNO, and a selective D3 receptor antagonist. *Biological Psychiatry*, *68*, 392–399.

Segal, D. M., Moraes, C. T., & Mash, D. C. (1997). Up-regulation of D3 dopamine receptor mRNA in the nucleus accumbens of human cocaine fatalities. *Brain Research Molecular Brain Research*, *45*, 335–339.

Shaham, Y., Shalev, U., Lu, L., De Wit, H., & Stewart, J. (2003). The reinstatement model of drug relapse: History, methodology and major findings. *Psychopharmacology*, *168*, 3–20.

Shelton, K. L., Hendrick, E. S., & Beardsley, P. M. (2013). Efficacy of buspirone for attenuating cocaine and methamphetamine reinstatement in rats. *Drug and Alcohol Dependence*,
129, 210–216.

Shi, L., & Javitch, J. A. (2002). The binding site of aminergic G protein-coupled receptors:
The transmembrane segments and second extracellular loop. *Annual Review of Pharmacology and Toxicology*, *42*, 437–467.

Shi, L., Liapakis, G., Xu, R., Guarnieri, F., Ballesteros, J. A., & Javitch, J. A. (2002). Beta2
adrenergic receptor activation. Modulation of the proline kink in transmembrane 6 by a
rotamer toggle switch. *Journal of Biological Chemistry*, *277*, 40989–40996.

Sokoloff, P., Diaz, J., Le Foll, B., Guillin, O., Leriche, L., Bezard, E., et al. (2006). The dopamine D3 receptor: A therapeutic target for the treatment of neuropsychiatric disorders.
CNS & Neurological Disorders: Drug Targets, *5*, 25–43.

Sokoloff, P., Giros, B., Martres, M. P., Bouthenet, M. L., & Schwartz, J. C. (1990). Molecular cloning and characterization of a novel dopamine receptor (D3) as a target for neuroleptics. *Nature*, *347*, 146–151.

Song, R., Yang, R. F., Wu, N., Su, R. B., Li, J., Peng, X. Q., et al. (2012). YQA14: A novel
dopamine D3 receptor antagonist that inhibits cocaine self-administration in rats and
mice, but not in D3 receptor-knockout mice. *Addiction Biology*, *17*, 259–273.

Song, R., Zhang, H. Y., Peng, X. Q., Su, R. B., Yang, R. F., Li, J., et al. (2013). Dopamine
D3 receptor deletion or blockade attenuates cocaine-induced conditioned place preference in mice. *Neuropharmacology*, *72*, 82–87.

Spiller, K., Xi, Z. X., Peng, X. Q., Newman, A. H., Ashby, C. R., Jr., Heidbreder, C., et al.
(2008). The selective dopamine D3 receptor antagonists SB277011A and NGB 2904 and
the putative partial D3 receptor agonist BP-897 attenuate methamphetamine-enhanced
brain stimulation reward in rats. *Psychopharmacology*, *196*, 533–542.

Staley, J. K., & Mash, D. C. (1996). Adaptive increase in D3 dopamine receptors in the brain
reward circuits of human cocaine fatalities. *Journal of Neuroscience*, *16*, 6100–6106.

Stemp, G., Ashmeade, T., Branch, C. L., Hadley, M. S., Hunter, A. J., Johnson, C. N., et al. (2000).
Design and synthesis of trans-N-[4-[2-(6-cyano-1,2,3, 4-tetrahydroisoquinolin-2-yl)ethyl]
cyclohexyl]-4-quinolinecarboxamide (SB-277011): A potent and selective dopamine D(3)
receptor antagonist with high oral bioavailability and CNS penetration in the rat. *Journal of
Medicinal Chemistry*, *43*, 1878–1885.

Tschammer, N., Elsner, J., Goetz, A., Ehrlich, K., Schuster, S., Ruberg, M., et al. (2011).
Highly potent 5-aminotetrahydropyrazolopyridines: Enantioselective dopamine D3
receptor binding, functional selectivity, and analysis of receptor-ligand interactions.
Journal of Medicinal Chemistry, *54*, 2477–2491.

Tzschentke, T. M. (2007). Measuring reward with the conditioned place preference (CPP)
paradigm: Update of the last decade. *Addiction Biology*, *12*, 227–462.

Varady, J., Wu, X., Fang, X., Min, J., Hu, Z., Levant, B., et al. (2003). Molecular modeling
of the three-dimensional structure of dopamine 3 (D3) subtype receptor: Discovery of
novel and potent D3 ligands through a hybrid pharmacophore- and structure-based
database searching approach. *Journal of Medicinal Chemistry*, *46*, 4377–4392.

Wager, T. T., Hou, X., Verhoest, P. R., & Villalobos, A. (2010). Moving beyond rules: The
development of a central nervous system multiparameter optimization (CNS MPO)
approach to enable alignment of druglike properties. *ACS Chemical Neuroscience*, *1*,
435–449.

Wang, Q., Mach, R. H., Luedtke, R. R., & Reichert, D. E. (2010). Subtype selectivity of
dopamine receptor ligands: Insights from structure and ligand-based methods. *Journal of
Chemical Information and Modeling*, *50*, 1970–1985.

Warne, T., Moukhametzianov, R., Baker, J. G., Nehme, R., Edwards, P. C., Leslie, A. G.,
et al. (2011). The structural basis for agonist and partial agonist action on a beta(1)-
adrenergic receptor. *Nature*, *469*, 241–244.

Willeit, M., Ginovart, N., Graff, A., Rusjan, P., Vitcu, I., Houle, S., et al. (2008). First human evidence of d-amphetamine induced displacement of a D2/3 agonist radioligand: A [11C]-(+)-PHNO positron emission tomography study. *Neuropsychopharmacology, 33,* 279–289.

Willeit, M., Ginovart, N., Kapur, S., Houle, S., Hussey, D., Seeman, P., et al. (2006). High-affinity states of human brain dopamine D2/3 receptors imaged by the agonist [11C]-(+)-PHNO. *Biological Psychiatry, 59,* 389–394.

Xi, Z. X., & Gardner, E. L. (2007). Pharmacological actions of NGB 2904, a selective dopamine D3 receptor antagonist, in animal models of drug addiction. *CNS Drug Reviews, 13,* 240–259.

Xi, Z. X., Li, X., Li, J., Peng, X. Q., Song, R., Gaal, J., et al. (2013). Blockade of dopamine D3 receptors in the nucleus accumbens and central amygdala inhibits incubation of cocaine craving in rats. *Addiction Biology, 18,* 665–677.

Yan, Y., Kong, H., Wu, E. J., Newman, A. H., & Xu, M. (2013). Dopamine D3 receptors regulate reconsolidation of cocaine memory. *Neuroscience, 241,* 32–40.

Ye, N., Neumeyer, J. L., Baldessarini, R. J., Zhen, X., & Zhang, A. (2013). Update 1 of: Recent progress in development of dopamine receptor subtype-selective agents: Potential therapeutics for neurological and psychiatric disorders. *Chemical Reviews, 113,* R123–R178.

Yuan, J., Chen, X., Brodbeck, R., Primus, R., Braun, J., Wasley, J. W., et al. (1998). NGB 2904 and NGB 2849: Two highly selective dopamine D3 receptor antagonists. *Bioorganic and Medicinal Chemistry Letters, 8,* 2715–2718.

CHAPTER EIGHT

Dopamine D4 Receptors in Psychostimulant Addiction

Patricia Di Ciano[*], David K. Grandy[†], Bernard Le Foll[*,‡,§,¶,||,#,**,1]

[*]Translational Addiction Research Laboratory, Centre for Addiction and Mental Health, University of Toronto, Toronto, Canada
[†]Department of Physiology & Pharmacology, School of Medicine, Oregon Health & Science University, Portland, Oregon, USA
[‡]Alcohol Research and Treatment Clinic, Addiction Medicine Services, Ambulatory Care and Structured Treatments, Centre for Addiction and Mental Health, Toronto, Ontario, Canada
[§]Campbell Family Mental Health Research Institute, Centre for Addiction and Mental Health, Toronto, Ontario, Canada
[¶]Department of Family and Community Medicine, University of Toronto, Toronto, Ontario, Canada
[||]Department of Pharmacology, University of Toronto, Toronto, Ontario, Canada
[#]Department of Psychiatry, Division of Brain and Therapeutics, University of Toronto, Toronto, Ontario, Canada
[**]Institute of Medical Sciences, University of Toronto, Toronto, Ontario, Canada
[1]Corresponding author: e-mail address: bernard.lefoll@camh.ca

Contents

Abstract

Since the cloning of the D4 receptor in the 1990s, interest has been building in the role of this receptor in drug addiction, given the importance of dopamine in addiction. Like the D3 receptor, the D4 receptor has limited distribution within the brain, suggesting it may have a unique role in drug abuse. However, compared to the D3 receptor, few studies have evaluated the importance of the D4 receptor.

Advances in Pharmacology, Volume 69
ISSN 1054-3589
http://dx.doi.org/10.1016/B978-0-12-420118-7.00008-1

This may be due, in part, to the relative lack of compounds selective for the D4 receptor; the early studies were mainly conducted in mice lacking the D4 receptor. In this review, we summarize the literature on the structure and localization of the D4 receptor before reviewing the data from D4 knockout mice that used behavioral models relevant to the understanding of stimulant use. We also present evidence from more recent pharmacological studies using selective D4 agonists and antagonists and animal models of drug-seeking and drug-taking. The data summarized here suggest a role for D4 receptors in relapse to stimulant use. Therefore, treatments based on antagonism of the D4 receptor may be useful treatments for relapse to nicotine, cocaine, and amphetamine use.

ABBREVIATIONS

DA dopamine
DRD1 dopamine type 1 receptor
DRD2 dopamine type 2 receptor
DRD3 dopamine type 3 receptor
DRD4 dopamine type 4 receptor
DRD5 dopamine type 5 receptor
L long alleles
METH methamphetamine
S short alleles
VNTR variable number of tandem repeats

1. INTRODUCTION

Dopamine (DA) is an important neurotransmitter in the brain. For more than 25 years, it has been suggested that DA systems in the brain are involved in critical functions such as the primary motivation for natural stimuli such as food, water, and sex (Koob, 1992; Wise & Bozarth, 1987). DA primarily exerts its influence by interacting with, and activating, a family of G protein-coupled DA receptors. Between 1988 and 1991, five genes were identified that code for multiple DA receptor subtypes. The DA D_2 receptor gene (DRD2) was the first to be cloned (Bunzow et al., 1988; Giros et al., 1989; Grandy et al., 1989), followed by the DA D_1 receptor gene (DRD1) (Dearry et al., 1990; Monsma, Mahan, McVittie, Gerfen, & Sibley, 1991; Sunahara et al., 1990; Zhou et al., 1990), the DA D_3 (DRD3) gene (Sokoloff, Giros, Martres, Bouthenet, & Schwartz, 1990), the DA D_4 (DRD4) gene (Van Tol et al., 1991), and finally the DA D_5 (DRD5) gene (Grandy et al., 1991; Sunahara et al., 1991). Not only did it represent a new member of a growing family of unanticipated DA receptors, the high affinity of the antipsychotic clozapine for the DRD4 was intriguing from the standpoint of understanding this important drug's mechanism of action. Clozapine, being an antipsychotic, led to a flurry of interest in developing DRD4 agents for the treatment of schizophrenia. However, it is the highly polymorphic nature of DRD4, the large number of receptor protein variants predicted—each potentially with its own unique pharmacological and second messenger/signaling profiles (Seeman & Van Tol, 1994)—that put it among the most favorite neuropsychiatric candidate gene, a position strengthened by the repeated finding of associations between particular DRD4 VNTRs and a diagnosis of attention deficit hyperactivity disorder (reviewed in Kuntsi, McLoughlin, & Asherson, 2006).

The focus of this review will be on the putative role of the DRD4 in stimulant abuse, with a focus on the aspects of this receptor that make it a suitable target for treatment approaches for addiction to stimulants, in particular cocaine, amphetamine, and nicotine. The stimulants have in common the fact that they all produce behavioral arousal, with the ability to improve cognition, a property that may confer action on the DRD4, as discussed in the succeeding text. The properties of the DRD4 that make it unique will be summarized, followed by a description of the localization of the DRD4. Studies linking the DRD4 to addictions, in particular smoking, will be reviewed. Finally, the studies with knockout mice and preclinical pharmacological studies will be reviewed with an aim to determining the role of the DRD4 in stimulant abuse.

1.1. The DRD4

Interest in DRD4 was heightened with the 1992 report (Van Tol et al., 1992) of considerable variation in the human gene, DRD4, and subsequent studies documenting its being among the most highly polymorphic genes in the human genome (Chang, Kidd, Livak, Pakstis, & Kidd, 1996; Lichter et al., 1993). Arguably, the single most compelling feature of DRD4 that distinguishes it from almost every other gene in the human genome is its unusual polymorphism in exon 3. This polymorphism consists of an imperfect 48 bp open reading frame that is tandemly repeated 2–10 times per allele (Lichter et al., 1993; Van Tol et al., 1992). The most prevalent DRD4 VNTR alleles are those consisting of 4-, 7-, and 2-repeat alleles, with global mean allele frequencies of 64.3%, 20.6%, and 8.2%, respectively (Chang et al., 1996). Alleles with less than seven repeats are generally referred to as "short alleles" (S) while those having more than seven repeats are referred to as "long alleles" (L). When these polymorphisms are translated, the resulting receptor protein domains responsible for G protein-coupling are predicted to differ by as much as 128 amino acids. Naturally, this observation resulted in several early studies designed to understand what functional consequences, if any, are associated with each VNTR—a question still to be definitively answered. It should also be noted that there is good evidence to support the interpretation that this intracellular domain of the receptor protein not only interacts with G proteins but also binds nuclear factors with potential consequences for gene expression (Schoots & Van Tol, 2003).

Of course, two important aspects of deorphanizing a putative G protein-coupled receptor, which the DRD4 was initially, are characterizing its pharmacological profile and defining its second messenger coupling. Although initially the *in vitro* heterologous expression of DRD4 was difficult, enough protein was made so that its pharmacological profile and G protein coupling could be demonstrated. However, the tendency for heterologous D4 receptor expression to be low hampered *in vitro* efforts to broaden our understanding of the cellular processes influenced by activated D4 receptors. Once this impediment was overcome, it was reported that activation of the DRD4 receptor not only inhibits cAMP production but also opens the kir3 potassium channel, activates extracellular signal-regulated kinases (ERK1 and 2), and decreases functional γ-aminobutyric acid type A receptor levels (reviewed by Rondou, Haegeman, & Van Craenenbroeck, 2010), responses that may involve receptor oligomerization (Van Craenenbroeck et al., 2011). What remains considerably more elusive is convincingly demonstrating the contribution(s) that DRD4-mediated signaling makes to human health. Over the years, several approaches have been taken to this end with one of the most promising being the anatomical mapping of the receptor's mRNA and protein distribution in healthy and pathological human tissues with an emphasis on the brain because of its affinity for the atypical antipsychotic clozapine.

1.2. DRD4 distribution

DRD4 mRNA is found in various brain regions at low density compared with DRD1 or DRD2. It is most abundant in retina (Cohen, Todd, Harmon, & O' Malley, 1992), cerebral cortex, amygdala, hypothalamus, and pituitary, but sparse in the basal ganglia, as assessed by RT-PCR and Northern blot (Valerio et al., 1994), *in situ* hybridization (O'Malley,

Harmon, Tang, & Todd, 1992; Meador-Woodruff et al., 1994, 1997), and immunohistochemistry (Mrzljak et al., 1996). These studies also found DRD4 in both pyramidal and nonpyramidal cells of the cerebral cortex, particularly layer V, and in the hippocampus. Localization of DRD4 to mainly the cerebral cortex, amygdala, and hippocampus has functional implications for the role of DRD4. The amygdala and hippocampus are areas that have been implicated in learning and memory (Ito, Robbins, McNaughton, & Everitt, 2006), and, in particular, the amygdala is thought to be important in the learning of associations with emotional stimuli (Schultz, 2006). In this regard, the L-alleles have been associated with attention for emotional stimuli (Wells, Beevers, Knopik, & McGeary, 2013), and DRD4 agonists have been shown to improve performance in cognitive tasks that are memory-dependent (Bernaerts & Tirelli, 2003; Powell, Paulus, Hartman, Godel, & Geyer, 2003; Woolley et al., 2008). These are important considerations for the study of addiction, as "craving" and drug-seeking can be powerfully elicited by environmental stimuli that have been previously paired with drug use, and thus, the DRD4 may be important in this regard.

1.3. Beyond imaging: Genetic association studies

The anatomical mapping approach has resulted in important fundamental knowledge; however, considerable advances were obtained from genetic association studies, in particular the initial findings that a subset of DRD4 VNTRs were found associated with personality traits including excessive impulsivity, novelty-seeking, and risk-taking behavior (Benjamin et al., 1996; Ebstein et al., 1996; Frank & Fossella, 2011; Malhotra et al., 1996; Ptacek, Kuzelova, & Stefano, 2011). Given that associations were found between DRD4 VNTRs, impulsivity, novelty-seeking, and risk-taking behavior, it comes as no surprise there has been considerable interest in the receptor's potential role in drug-taking behavior and as a target for novel abstinence medications. However, both positive and negative associations have been reported between various DRD4 alleles and methamphetamine (METH) abuse. METH abusers had a significantly higher prevalence of the 7-repeat alleles than controls, while there were no significant differences in the DRD2 or DRD3 alleles between the METH abusers and controls (Chen et al., 2004), highlighting the importance specifically of the DRD4 receptor for drug abuse. In another study, however, no differences were found for DRD4 gene exon III polymorphisms (Tsai et al., 2002). In an attempt to reconcile these disparate findings, an intriguing new approach to assessing the contribution of the VNTR to drug-taking behaviors has been proposed (McGeary, 2009).

Although the studies of the relationship between alleles and DRD4 are somewhat compelling, the possible involvement of DRD4 variants in nicotine use provides the most comprehensive information. One study reports an association between DRD4 genotype and smoking in African-Americans but not Caucasians (Shields et al., 1998). Comparison of male carriers of an L-allele to those with the S-allele revealed that those with the L-allele started smoking earlier, had a higher rate of lifetime smoking, and smoked more cigarettes per day (Laucht, Becker, El-Faddagh, Hohm, & Schmidt, 2005). Interestingly, significantly less binding potential was detected using PET imaging of DRD2 receptors in carriers of DRD4 alleles with more than seven repeats (Brody et al., 2006); decreased binding potential of (^{11}C)-raclopride is an indirect measure of DA release and implies that DA release was increased. By categorizing participants as either DRD4 S or DRD4 L, other studies have found differences between those carrying the L- and S-alleles on smoking cue reactivity (Hutchison, LaChance, Niaura, Bryan, & Smolen, 2002; McClernon, Hutchison, Rose, & Kozink, 2007; Munafo & Johnstone, 2008) and some suggest the L-alleles are a risk factor for heavy smoking and may influence smoking cessation outcome (David et al., 2008; Ton et al., 2007; Vandenbergh et al., 2007); however, the authors indicate their findings are preliminary and need to be replicated in a controlled study with a larger sample size.

Even though the findings of genetic association studies are provocative and in some cases compelling, additional complementary approaches—including the development and use of animal models—will be required to provide a molecular explanation that connects a particular personality trait or mental health condition with one or more DRD4 VNTRs. Next, we will provide a short summary of the information that has been collected using knockout and pharmacological approaches to determine the role(s) its variants play in psychostimulant drug abuse (i.e., cocaine, METH, and nicotine).

2. DRD4 AND PSYCHOSTIMULANT ADDICTION

Although genetic association studies have provided compelling results, advances in the understanding of the role of DRD4 came about from studies with genetically modified mice (Rubinstein et al., 1997; Waddington et al., 2005) and, more recently, pharmacological studies with selective DRD4 agents. At the time that the use of genetically modified mice was first proposed (1995–1996), there were no selective antagonists available, and early studies into the role of the DRD4 were provided by findings with these mutants. In addition, the KO background would provide the perfect means of evaluating *in vivo* the selectivity of any emerging DRD4-selective compounds and any immunologic reagents. In genetically modified mice, one strategy is to "knockout" all expression of a functional DRD4 by completely eliminating the receptor protein. The strategy for targeting the *drd4* gene was accomplished relatively quickly and has been described in detail (Rubinstein et al., 1997).

Early findings with knockout mice have confirmed the pharmacological and electrophysiological consequences of altering the number of functional *drd4* alleles, but not all of the behavioral findings have. For example, whereas the findings of Ralph et al. (1999) indicated a role for the *drd4* gene product in mediating amphetamine's disruption of prepulse inhibition of the startle response (Ralph et al., 1999), a finding that is widely accepted, the findings reported by Dulawa, Grandy, Low, Paulus, and Geyer (1999) claiming a role for *drd4* in novelty-seeking behavior (Dulawa et al., 1999) have been challenged by the results of at least two independent studies (Keck, Suchland, Jimenez, & Grandy, 2013; Powell et al., 2003). Of relevance to the focus of this review is the observation that mice completely lacking functional *drd4* are dose-dependently hypersensitive to the locomotor-stimulating effect of METH (Katz et al., 2003; Rubinstein et al., 1997) and methylphenidate (Keck et al., 2013). Locomotor activity is believed to be related to addictive potential (Wise & Bozarth, 1987), and thus, the findings that D4 knockout mice are hypersensitive to locomotion suggest that DRD4 may mediate propensity to addiction. However, it has been found that *drd4* knockout mice show a decreased DA response to an amphetamine challenge (Thomas et al., 2007), a finding that is not in keeping with the locomotor hypersensitivity observed, given that increased locomotion is associated with increased DA release (Kuczenski & Segal, 1989). Thus, the findings with the *drd4* knockout mice are inconclusive and it may be best to look at behavioral measures more directly related to drug addiction and to consider the findings with knockout mice together with the more recent antagonist studies. These findings are provided in the following text and organized by animal model. Each section begins with a description of the animal model to frame the results with knockout mice and antagonists.

2.1. Drug self-administration

In preclinical studies of drug addiction, drug self-administration has become the "gold standard" for studying drugs of abuse. Once acquired, self-administration behavior remains stable over days; animals "titrate" their intake of drug to maintain constant blood levels of the drug (Yokel & Pickens, 1974) and brain levels of DA (Di Ciano et al., 1995; Pettit & Justice, 1991). In one study by Thanos, Habibi, et al. (2010), it was found that mice lacking the *drd4* were similar to controls in their response to cocaine. Consistent with the findings from knockout mice, it has been found that administration of L-745,870 has no effect on self-administration of nicotine (Yan, Pushparaj, Le Strat, et al., 2012). L-745,870 is a DRD4 antagonist with a K_i of 0.43, 960, and 2300 for DRD4, DRD2, and DRD3, respectively. It also has no appreciable binding to DRD1 or DRD5 ($K_i > 10,000$) (Kulagowski et al., 1996). Although this finding may suggest that DRD4 are not involved in drug addiction, it is important to consider these findings within a larger context. That is, it is known that when the dose of drug available is decreased, rats may increase their rate of responding to compensate for the decreased dose received (Pickens & Thompson, 1968). This is a problem with antagonists at the DRD2 (Woolverton, 1986; Yokel & Wise, 1975), but not those that target the DRD3 (Andreoli et al., 2003; Di Ciano, Underwood, Hagan, & Everitt, 2003; Gal & Gyertyan, 2003; Le Foll & Goldberg, 2006; Xi et al., 2005), as revealed in studies with rats. This suggests that DA DRD2 antagonists would not be ideal treatments for substance abuse, as they may increase drug intake. Thus, what the findings with the D4 knockout mice and DRD4 antagonists reveal is that DRD4 antagonists do not increase drug self-administration, a finding that is promising for the development of D4 antagonists as treatment for drug addiction, provided that D4 antagonists influence other models of drug addiction.

2.2. Reinstatement

Drug abuse is a chronic relapsing disorder and an understanding of the role of DRD4 in stimulant addiction can be obtained from a focus on the effects of interventions on relapse to drug-seeking. The main animal models of relapse are the reinstatement models that have evolved from studies with drugs that modeled the ability of environmental stimuli (de Wit & Stewart, 1981) and drugs (Gerber & Stretch, 1975; Stretch & Gerber, 1973) to induce relapse to drug-seeking. Reinstatement is an animal model with high predictive validity (Epstein & Preston, 2003) that has been studied in rats (Chiamulera, Borgo, Falchetto, Valerio, & Tessari, 1996; Forget, Coen, & Le Foll, 2009; Khaled et al., 2010; Pushparaj et al., 2013; Shaham,

Adamson, Grocki, & Corrigall, 1997), mice (Yan, Pushparaj, Gamaleddin, et al., 2012), nonhuman primates (Mascia et al., 2011), and humans (McKee, 2009). In this model, the animal is first trained to self-administer drug, and then the response is extinguished by removing the associated drug that was self-administered; responses have no consequences during extinction. Following extinction of the response, a condition such as stress, cues, or drug, is introduced that reinstates extinguished responding. It has been shown that a DA D4 antagonist, L-745,870, can block the reinstatement of nicotine-seeking induced by either cues paired with the drug or reexposure to nicotine itself (Yan, Pushparaj, Le Strat, et al., 2012). As seen in Fig. 8.1, administration of nicotine reinstated responding to above extinguished levels, and several doses of L-745,870 reduced this reinstatement. Similarly, cues previously paired with each self-administered nicotine infusion also reinstated extinguished responding, and L-745,870 also attenuated this. An effect on both types of reinstatement suggests that the effects of D4 antagonists may be related to an effect on relapse *per se*

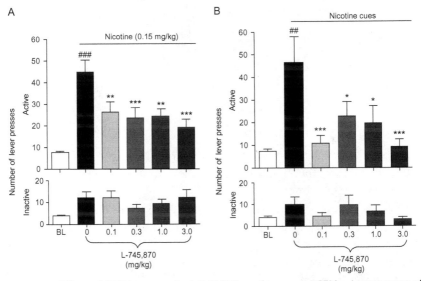

Figure 8.1 Effect of DRD4 antagonist L-745,870 on the mean ± SEM reinstatement of nicotine-seeking behavior in rats. (A) Pretreatment of L-745,870 significantly reduced the number of active (upper) but not inactive (lower) lever presses triggered by priming injection of nicotine (0.15 mg/kg s.c.; $n = 23$). (B) Pretreatment of L-745,870 significantly attenuated the number of active (upper) but not inactive (lower) lever presses induced by nicotine-associated cues ($n = 13$). $^*p < 0.05$; $^{**}p < 0.01$, $^{***}p < 0.001$ versus vehicle pre-treatment. Student's paired t-test $^{##}p < 0.01$; $^{###}p < 0.001$ versus the baseline (BL). *Taken from Yan, Pushparaj, Le Strat, et al. (2012) with permission.*

and not the ability of, for example, cues to maintain behavior or of nicotine to influence behavior. In sum, these findings suggest that DA DRD4 are involved in the relapse to drug-seeking. Although promising, the findings with nicotine should be generalized to other drugs of abuse to reveal the generality of the effect.

Together, the findings thus far suggest that DRD4 antagonists would be viable targets for treatments for stimulant abuse as they prolong abstinence while not increasing drug self-administration. This position is highlighted by further findings that L-745,870 did not affect reinstatement of food-seeking induced by either presentation of food or presentation of food-associated cues (Yan, Pushparaj, Le Strat, et al., 2012). Thus, the effects of DA D4 antagonists seem selective to stimulants and do not generalize to natural rewards, meaning that their use as treatments may not impact on general motivation, a problem with DA antagonists that are used in the clinic. This is encouraging as administration of the DRD4 agonist A-412997 increased locomotor activity (Woolley et al., 2008), implicating DRD4 in general activity levels, but the lack of effect of food is informative in that the role of DRD4 in general activity levels may not play a role in behaviors motivated for drug. This hypothesis warrants further testing by examining whether DRD4 antagonists have similar effects on other types of stimulants, such as cocaine or amphetamine, or whether their effects are only on nicotine.

2.3. Drug discrimination

All drugs of abuse have interoceptive properties, and in the drug discrimination procedure, the ability of rats to distinguish different interoceptive properties is tested. In the drug discrimination procedure, rats are trained, for example, to respond on a lever located on the left side of a test chamber when given a certain drug of abuse and to respond on the right-side lever when they are given saline. Over time, animals will learn to make differential responses on the two levers. The effects of drug challenges on drug-appropriate versus saline-appropriate responding can then be determined. As illustrated in Fig. 8.2, the amount of nicotine-appropriate responding increases with dose of a challenge dose of nicotine; nicotine feels "more like" nicotine as the dose is increased. Once discriminative responding has been established, a test compound can then be administered, and if the animal responds on the nicotine-appropriate lever, then this suggests that the test compound has similar interoceptive properties to the drug of abuse. Alternatively, a test compound can be administered with the drug of abuse and

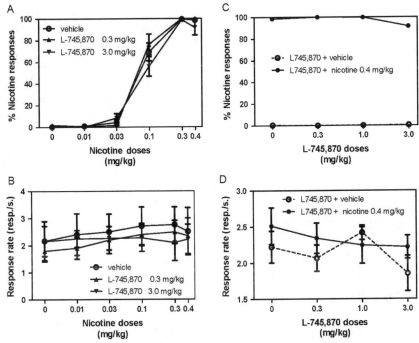

Figure 8.2 (A) Dose effect functions for the discriminative-stimulus effects of nicotine in rats trained to discriminate 0.4 mg/kg nicotine from saline. The percentage of responses on the lever associated with nicotine administration is shown as a function of dose (mg/kg) during tests with various doses of nicotine. The DRD4 antagonist L-745,870 administered acutely 30 min before the sessions did not modify discriminative-stimulus effects of nicotine (no curve shift). (B) L-745,870 also did not significantly affect rates of lever-press responding when administered together with different doses of nicotine or with vehicle. (C) Effects of different doses of L-745,870 on discriminative-stimulus effects of the training dose of nicotine when L-745,870 was administered with vehicle. (D) Effects of different doses of L-745,870 on rates of lever-press responding when administered together with the training dose of nicotine or with vehicle ($n = 9$–12). Data are expressed as means ($\pm$SEM) of the percentage of responses on the nicotine lever. *Taken from Yan, Pushparaj, Le Strat, et al. (2012), with permission.*

the effects on discrimination of responding for the drug of abuse as compared to that for saline can be determined. If the test compound decreases drug-appropriate responding, then the discriminative properties of the drug of abuse have been disrupted. This is important because the discriminative properties of drugs may maintain responding for drug, and thus, compounds that disrupt the discriminative properties of drugs of abuse may serve as potential treatments, especially if the animal has learned to discriminate drug from saline. As can be seen in Fig. 8.2, the D4 antagonist L-745,870 had no effect on discriminative responding for nicotine. At both doses of

L-745,870, the dose–response function for nicotine-appropriate responding after various doses of nicotine was similar to that observed after coadministration of nicotine with vehicle (Yan, Pushparaj, Le Strat, et al., 2012). Similarly, L-745,870 also did not affect cocaine-appropriate responding when coadministered with cocaine (Costanza & Terry, 1998); in this study, L-745,870 also did not produce cocaine-appropriate responding when administered on its own. In contrast, blockade of DRD4 did block the discriminative-stimulus properties of METH in mice (Yan et al., 2006). In sum, DRD4 does not appear to be involved in discriminative properties of nicotine and cocaine, but may participate to those of METH. Taken together, it appears that D4 antagonists do not have interoceptive properties that are similar to those of stimulants, and they disrupt drug-seeking through mechanisms that are not related to the discriminative properties of the drug. Similarly, a D4 agonist, ABT-724 was self-administered in only one of five monkeys tested and at levels lower than that for cocaine (Koffarnus et al., 2012), consistent with the lack of discriminative properties with cocaine.

2.4. Conditioned place preference

Another frequently used model of drug addiction is the conditioned place preference model (Liu, Le Foll, Wang, & Lu, 2008). Place preference is a well-established animal model of addiction in which two sides of a test chamber are uniquely identifiable to an animal and one side is paired with a rewarding substance while the other with vehicle. At test, the animal is placed in between the two sides and allowed to explore free of drugs. It is has been reported many times that, after administration of stimulants, the time spent on the drug-paired side is increased relative that paired with vehicle (Carr, Fibiger, & Phillips, 1989). Place preference is believed to be a measure of the rewarding aspects of drugs, especially those maintained by conditioned aspects of stimuli previously paired with drugs. In a report by Thanos, Bermeo, et al. (2010), it was found that *drd4* knockout mice were not impaired in conditioned place preference to methylphenidate, amphetamine, and cocaine relative to controls. Thus, DRD4 are not involved in this measure of drug addiction. Further insights may be gained from pharmacological interventions conducted in animal studies.

2.5. Sensitization

Sensitization is a model of drug addiction based on observations that a behavioral response to drugs of abuse can increase over time with repeated exposure to the drug. In the most frequently used model of sensitization, locomotor activity counts to a stimulant challenge are obtained at baseline and again after a course of treatment with the drug. When administered intermittently (as opposed to continually) (Robinson & Becker, 1986), repeated administration of a drug can potentiate the locomotor-activating effects of the drug. When administered the D4 antagonist PNU-101387G prior to the pretreatments with amphetamine, behavioral sensitization to a subsequent amphetamine challenge was blocked (Feldpausch et al., 1998). PNU-101387G has high selectivity for the DRD4 (K_i=3.6) as opposed to other DA receptor subtypes (DRD1 K_i > 8000; DRD2 K_i=5147; DRD3 K_i > 2778) (Merchant et al., 1996). It has been posited that the role of sensitization in addiction is to increase drug wanting over time, thus rendering the user addicted to a drug (Robinson & Berridge, 1993). Thus, DA DRD4 may be important in the development of sensitization to drugs of abuse and thereby be important in the establishment of an addiction. Again, these findings need to be replicated with other stimulants such as cocaine or nicotine to determine whether the stimulatory role of DRD4 is simply on the effects of amphetamine or whether they mediate some common aspect that underlies the sensitization process.

2.6. Rewarding properties of DRD4 agents

Consistent with their lack of discriminative properties similar to stimulants, a number of findings suggest that DA DRD4 may not have rewarding properties on their own. For example, as mentioned earlier, monkeys did not self-administer the D4 agonist ABT-724 (Koffarnus et al., 2012), and thus, DA D4 agonists may not have reinforcing effects on their own. Similarly, administration of A-412997, a D4 agonist, did not induce a conditioned place preference (Woolley et al., 2008). Thus, based on the findings of Woolley et al. (2008) that a D4 agonist did not induce place preference on its own, it is possible to conclude that stimulation of DRD4 is not rewarding on its own. Thus, DRD4 agents may not have addiction potential and may be viable treatments for addiction.

3. CONCLUSION

Since the cloning of the DRD4 in the 1990s, this receptor has received growing attention. Although genetic association studies have been compelling in implicating a role of the DRD4 in stimulant use, the real advances in understanding of this receptor emerged with the advent of knockout mice and, more recently, selective pharmacological agents. When interpreting the role of DRD4 in stimulant use, the findings from the knockout mice and pharmacological interventions tell a coherent story. From the literature, it is clear that DRD4 affect the reinstatement of nicotine-seeking and thus may be potential treatments for relapse, especially since DRD4 antagonists were without nonspecific effects on responding for food and DRD4 agonists were not self-administered themselves (therefore, they have no addictive potential). This is further supported by findings that DRD4 antagonists blocked the development of sensitization to stimulants. This finding must be taken into context with those that found no effect of D4 knockout or D4 antagonists on a place preference; perhaps DRD4 is not involved in the conditioned rewarding properties of drugs, but may, instead, mediate the relapse or other aspects of seeking. Issues that remain to be resolved are the findings of a blockade of discriminative properties of METH but not cocaine by DRD4 antagonists; further studies will need to determine whether DRD4 is involved in this function. Also, it remains to be determined whether the promising findings on reinstatement will generalize to other stimulant drugs, as the findings so far are only with nicotine. In sum, D4 antagonists may provide a means by which novel treatments for stimulant-seeking may be targeted. The fact that ligands that are available in clinic such as buspirone are also effective DRD4 antagonists (Bergman et al., 2013) could represent a translational opportunity for future work (Le Foll & Boileau, 2013). Indeed, recent findings implicate DRD4 in gambling, which is an addictive behavior (Cocker, Le Foll, Rogers, & Winstanley, 2013).

CONFLICT OF INTEREST
The authors have no conflicts of interest to declare.

ACKNOWLEDGMENTS
Some descriptions of the distribution of the dopamine receptors have been reproduced with permission from Behavioral Pharmacology (Le Foll, Gallo, Le Strat, Lu, & Gorwood, 2009).

REFERENCES
Andreoli, M., Tessari, M., Pilla, M., Valerio, E., Hagan, J. J., & Heidbreder, C. A. (2003). Selective antagonism at dopamine D3 receptors prevents nicotine-triggered relapse to nicotine-seeking behavior. Neuropsychopharmacology, 28(7), 1272–1280.
Benjamin, J., Li, L., Patterson, C., Greenberg, B. D., Murphy, D. L., & Hamer, D. H. (1996). Population and familial association between the D4 dopamine receptor gene and measures of Novelty Seeking. Nature Genetics, 12(1), 81–84. http://dx.doi.org/10.1038/ng0196-81.

Bergman, J., Roof, R. A., Furman, C. A., Conroy, J. L., Mello, N. K., Sibley, D. R., et al. (2013). Modification of cocaine self-administration by buspirone (buspar(R)): Potential involvement of D3 and D4 dopamine receptors. *The International Journal of Neuropsychopharmacology*, *16*(2), 445–458. http://dx.doi.org/10.1017/S1461145712 000661.

Bernaerts, P., & Tirelli, E. (2003). Facilitatory effect of the dopamine D4 receptor agonist PD168,077 on memory consolidation of an inhibitory avoidance learned response in C57BL/6J mice. *Behavioural Brain Research*, *142*(1–2), 41–52, S0166432802003716 [pii].

Brody, A. L., Mandelkern, M. A., Olmstead, R. E., Scheibal, D., Hahn, E., Shiraga, S., et al. (2006). Gene variants of brain dopamine pathways and smoking-induced dopamine release in the ventral caudate/nucleus accumbens. *Archives of General Psychiatry*, *63*(7), 808–816. http://dx.doi.org/10.1001/archpsyc.63.7.808, 63/7/808 [pii].

Bunzow, J. R., Van Tol, H. H. M., Grandy, D. K., Albert, P., Salon, J., Christie, M., et al. (1988). Cloning and expression of a rat D_2 receptor cDNA. *Nature*, *336*, 783–787.

Carr, G. D., Fibiger, H. C., & Phillips, A. G. (1989). Conditioned place preference as a measure of drug reward. In J. M. Liebman & S. J. Cooper (Eds.), *Neuropharmacological basis of reward* (pp. 264–319). New York: Oxford.

Chang, F. M., Kidd, J. R., Livak, K. J., Pakstis, A. J., & Kidd, K. K. (1996). The world-wide distribution of allele frequencies at the human dopamine D4 receptor locus. *Human Genetics*, *98*(1), 91–101.

Chen, C. K., Hu, X., Lin, S. K., Sham, P. C., Loh el, W., Li, T., et al. (2004). Association analysis of dopamine D2-like receptor genes and methamphetamine abuse. *Psychiatric Genetics*, *14*(4), 223–226, 00041444-200412000-00011 [pii].

Chiamulera, C., Borgo, C., Falchetto, S., Valerio, E., & Tessari, M. (1996). Nicotine reinstatement of nicotine self-administration after long-term extinction. *Psychopharmacology*, *127*(2), 102–107.

Cocker, P. J., Le Foll, B., Rogers, R. D., & Winstanley, C. A. (2013). A selective role for dopamine D receptors in modulating reward expectancy in a rodent slot machine task. *Biological Psychiatry*. (in press). http://dx.doi.org/10.1016/j.biopsych.2013.08.026.

Cohen, A. I., Todd, R. D., Harmon, S., & O'Malley, K. L. (1992). Photoreceptors of mouse retinas possess D_4 receptors coupled to adenylate cyclase. *Proceedings of the National Academy of Sciences of the United States of America*, *89*, 12093–12097.

Costanza, R. M., & Terry, P. (1998). The dopamine D4 receptor antagonist L-745,870: Effects in rats discriminating cocaine from saline. *European Journal of Pharmacology*, *345*(2), 129–132.

David, S. P., Munafo, M. R., Murphy, M. F., Proctor, M., Walton, R. T., & Johnstone, E. C. (2008). Genetic variation in the dopamine D4 receptor (DRD4) gene and smoking cessation: Follow-up of a randomised clinical trial of transdermal nicotine patch. *The Pharmacogenomics Journal*, *8*, 122–128. http://dx.doi.org/10.1038/sj.tpj.6500447, 6500447 [pii].

de Wit, H., & Stewart, J. (1981). Reinstatement of cocaine-reinforced responding in the rat. *Psychopharmacology*, *75*, 134–143.

Dearry, A., Gringrich, J. A., Falardeau, P., Fremeau, R. T., Bates, M. D., & Caron, M. G. (1990). Molecular cloning and expression of the gene for a human D_1 dopamine receptor. *Nature*, *347*, 72–76.

Di Ciano, P., Coury, A., Depoortere, R. Y., Egilmez, Y., Lane, J. D., Emmett-Oglesby, M. W., et al. (1995). Comparison of changes in extracellular dopamine concentrations in the nucleus accumbens during intravenous self-administration of cocaine or d-amphetamine. *Behavioural Pharmacology*, *6*(4), 311–322.

Di Ciano, P., Underwood, R. J., Hagan, J. J., & Everitt, B. J. (2003). Attenuation of cue-controlled cocaine-seeking by a selective D3 dopamine receptor antagonist SB-277011-A. *Neuropsychopharmacology*, *28*(2), 329–338.

Dulawa, S. C., Grandy, D. K., Low, M. J., Paulus, M. P., & Geyer, M. A. (1999). Dopamine D4 receptor-knock-out mice exhibit reduced exploration of novel stimuli. *The Journal of Neuroscience, 19*(21), 9550–9556.

Ebstein, R. P., Novick, O., Umansky, R., Priel, B., Osher, Y., Blaine, D., et al. (1996). Dopamine D4 receptor (D4DR) exon III polymorphism associated with the human personality trait of Novelty Seeking. *Nature Genetics, 12*(1), 78–80.

Epstein, D. H., & Preston, K. L. (2003). The reinstatement model and relapse prevention: A clinical perspective. *Psychopharmacology, 168*(1–2), 31–41.

Feldpausch, D. L., Needham, L. M., Stone, M. P., Althaus, J. S., Yamamoto, B. K., Svensson, K. A., et al. (1998). The role of dopamine D4 receptor in the induction of behavioral sensitization to amphetamine and accompanying biochemical and molecular adaptations. *The Journal of Pharmacology and Experimental Therapeutics, 286*(1), 497–508.

Forget, B., Coen, K. M., & Le Foll, B. (2009). Inhibition of fatty acid amide hydrolase reduces reinstatement of nicotine seeking but not break point for nicotine self-administration—Comparison with CB(1) receptor blockade. *Psychopharmacology, 205*(4), 613–624. http://dx.doi.org/10.1007/s00213-009-1569-5.

Frank, M. J., & Fossella, J. A. (2011). Neurogenetics and pharmacology of learning, motivation, and cognition. *Neuropsychopharmacology, 36*(1), 133–152. http://dx.doi.org/10.1038/npp.2010.96.

Gal, K., & Gyertyan, I. (2003). Targeting the dopamine D3 receptor cannot influence continuous reinforcement cocaine self-administration in rats. *Brain Research Bulletin, 61*(6), 595–601.

Gerber, G. J., & Stretch, R. (1975). Drug-induced reinstatement of extinguished self-administration behavior in monkeys. *Pharmacology, Biochemistry, and Behavior, 3*(6), 1055–1061.

Giros, B., Sokoloff, P., Martres, M.-P., Riou, J.-F., Emorine, L. J., & Schwartz, J.-C. (1989). Alternative splicing directs the expression of two D_2 dopamine receptor isoforms. *Nature, 342*, 923–926.

Grandy, D. K., Marchionni, M. A., Makan, H., Stofko, R. E., Alfano, M., Frothingham, L., et al. (1989). Cloning of the cDNA and gene for a human D_2 dopamine receptor. *Proceedings of the National Academy of Sciences of the United States of America, 84*, 9762–9766.

Grandy, D. K., Zhang, Y. A., Bouvier, C., Zhou, Q. Y., Johnson, R. A., Allen, L., et al. (1991). Multiple human D5 dopamine receptor genes: A functional receptor and two pseudogenes. *Proceedings of the National Academy of Sciences of the United States of America, 88*(20), 9175–9179.

Hutchison, K. E., LaChance, H., Niaura, R., Bryan, A., & Smolen, A. (2002). The DRD4 VNTR polymorphism influences reactivity to smoking cues. *Journal of Abnormal Psychology, 111*(1), 134–143.

Ito, R., Robbins, T. W., McNaughton, B. L., & Everitt, B. J. (2006). Selective excitotoxic lesions of the hippocampus and basolateral amygdala have dissociable effects on appetitive cue and place conditioning based on path integration in a novel Y-maze procedure. *The European Journal of Neuroscience, 23*(11), 3071–3080.

Katz, J. L., Chausmer, A. L., Elmer, G. I., Rubinstein, M., Low, M. J., & Grandy, D. K. (2003). Cocaine-induced locomotor activity and cocaine discrimination in dopamine D4 receptor mutant mice. *Psychopharmacology, 170*(1), 108–114.

Keck, T. M., Suchland, K. L., Jimenez, C. C., & Grandy, D. K. (2013). Dopamine D4 receptor deficiency in mice alters behavioral responses to anxiogenic stimuli and the psychostimulant methylphenidate. *Pharmacology, Biochemistry, and Behavior, 103*(4), 831–841. http://dx.doi.org/10.1016/j.pbb.2012.12.006.

Khaled, M. A., Farid Araki, K., Li, B., Coen, K. M., Marinelli, P. W., Varga, J., et al. (2010). The selective dopamine D3 receptor antagonist SB 277011-A, but not the partial agonist BP 897, blocks cue-induced reinstatement of nicotine-seeking. *The International Journal of Neuropsychopharmacology/Official Scientific Journal of the Collegium*

Internationale Neuropsychopharmacologicum, 13(2), 181–190. http://dx.doi.org/10.1017/S1461145709991064, S1461145709991064 [pii].

Koffarnus, M. N., Collins, G. T., Rice, K. C., Chen, J., Woods, J. H., & Winger, G. (2012). Self-administration of agonists selective for dopamine D2, D3, and D4 receptors by rhesus monkeys. *Behavioural Pharmacology, 23*(4), 331–338. http://dx.doi.org/10.1097/FBP.0b013e3283564dbb.

Koob, G. F. (1992). Neural mechanisms of drug reinforcement. *Annals of the New York Academy of Sciences, 654,* 171–191.

Kuczenski, R., & Segal, D. (1989). Concomitant characterization of behavioral and striatal neurotransmitter response to amphetamine using in vivo microdialysis. *The Journal of Neuroscience, 9*(6), 2051–2065.

Kulagowski, J. J., Broughton, H. B., Curtis, N. R., Mawer, I. M., Ridgill, M. P., Baker, R., et al. (1996). 3-((4-(4-Chlorophenyl)piperazin-1-yl)-methyl)-1H-pyrrolo-2,3-b-pyridine: An antagonist with high affinity and selectivity for the human dopamine D4 receptor. *Journal of Medicinal Chemistry, 39*(10), 1941–1942. http://dx.doi.org/10.1021/jm9600712.

Kuntsi, J., McLoughlin, G., & Asherson, P. (2006). Attention deficit hyperactivity disorder. *Neuromolecular Medicine, 8*(4), 461–484. http://dx.doi.org/10.1385/NMM:8:4:461.

Laucht, M., Becker, K., El-Faddagh, M., Hohm, E., & Schmidt, M. H. (2005). Association of the DRD4 exon III polymorphism with smoking in fifteen-year-olds: A mediating role for novelty seeking? *Journal of the American Academy of Child and Adolescent Psychiatry, 44*(5), 477–484.

Le Foll, B., & Boileau, I. (2013). Repurposing buspirone for drug addiction treatment. *The International Journal of Neuropsychopharmacology, 16*(2), 251–253. http://dx.doi.org/10.1017/S1461145712000995.

Le Foll, B., Gallo, A., Le Strat, Y., Lu, L., & Gorwood, P. (2009). Genetics of dopamine receptors and drug addiction: A comprehensive review. *Behavioural Pharmacology, 20*(1), 1–17. http://dx.doi.org/10.1097/FBP.0b013e3283242f05.

Le Foll, B., & Goldberg, S. R. (2006). Targeting the dopamine D3 receptor for treatment of tobacco dependence. In T. P. George (Ed.), *Medication treatments for nicotine dependence.* London: Taylor and Francis.

Lichter, J. B., Barr, C. L., Kenney, J. L., Van Tol, H. H. M., Kidd, K. K., & Livak, K. J. (1993). A hypervariable segment in the human dopamine D4 (DRD4) gene. *Human Molecular Genetics, 2,* 767–773.

Liu, Y., Le Foll, B., Wang, X., & Lu, L. (2008). Conditioned place preference induced by licit drugs: Establishment, extinction, and reinstatement. *Scientific World Journal, 8,* 1228–1245. http://dx.doi.org/10.1100/tsw.2008.154.

Malhotra, A. K., Virkkunen, M., Rooney, W., Eggert, M., Linnoila, M., & Goldman, D. (1996). The association between the dopamine D4 receptor (D4DR) 16 amino acid repeat polymorphism and novelty seeking. *Molecular Psychiatry, 1*(5), 388–391.

Mascia, P., Pistis, M., Justinova, Z., Panlilio, L. V., Luchicchi, A., Lecca, S., et al. (2011). Blockade of nicotine reward and reinstatement by activation of alpha-type peroxisome proliferator-activated receptors. *Biological Psychiatry, 69*(7), 633–641. http://dx.doi.org/10.1016/j.biopsych.2010.07.009, S0006-3223(10)00716-X [pii].

McClernon, F. J., Hutchison, K. E., Rose, J. E., & Kozink, R. V. (2007). DRD4 VNTR polymorphism is associated with transient fMRI-BOLD responses to smoking cues. *Psychopharmacology, 194*(4), 433–441. http://dx.doi.org/10.1007/s00213-007-0860-6.

McGeary, J. (2009). The DRD4 exon 3 VNTR polymorphism and addiction-related phenotypes: A review. *Pharmacology, Biochemistry, and Behavior, 93*(3), 222–229. http://dx.doi.org/10.1016/j.pbb.2009.03.010.

McKee, S. A. (2009). Developing human laboratory models of smoking lapse behavior for medication screening. *Addiction Biology, 14*(1), 99–107. http://dx.doi.org/10.1111/j.1369-1600.2008.00135.x.

Meador-Woodruff, J. H., Grandy, D. K., Van Tol, H. H. M., Damask, S. P., Little, K. Y., Civelli, O., et al. (1994). Dopamine receptor gene expression in the human medial temporal lobe. *Neuropsychopharmacology, 10*, 239–248.

Meador-Woodruff, J. H., Haroutunian, V., Powchik, P., Davidson, M., Davis, K. L., & Watson, S. J. (1997). Dopamine receptor transcript expression in striatum and prefrontal and occipital cortex. *Archives of General Psychiatry, 54*, 1089–1095.

Merchant, K. M., Gill, G. S., Harris, D. W., Huff, R. M., Eaton, M. J., Lookingland, K., et al. (1996). Pharmacological characterization of U-101387, a dopamine D4 receptor selective antagonist. *The Journal of Pharmacology and Experimental Therapeutics, 279*(3), 1392–1403.

Monsma, F. J., Mahan, L. C., McVittie, L. D., Gerfen, C. R., & Sibley, D. R. (1991). Molecular cloning and expression of a D_1 dopamine receptor linked to adenylyl cyclase activation. *Proceedings of the National Academy of Sciences of the United States of America, 87*, 6723–6727.

Mrzljak, L., Bergson, C., Pappy, M., Huff, R., Levenson, R., & Goldman-Rakic, P. S. (1996). Localization of dopamine D4 receptors in GABAergic neurons of the primate brain. *Nature, 381*(6579), 245–248. http://dx.doi.org/10.1038/381245a0.

Munafo, M. R., & Johnstone, E. C. (2008). Smoking status moderates the association of the dopamine D4 receptor (DRD4) gene VNTR polymorphism with selective processing of smoking-related cues. *Addiction Biology, 13*(3–4), 435–439. http://dx.doi.org/10.1111/j.1369-1600.2008.00098.x, ADB098 [pii].

O'Malley, K. L., Harmon, S., Tang, L., & Todd, R. D. (1992). The rat dopamine D_4 receptor sequence, gene structure, and demonstration of expression in the cardiovascular system. *The New Biologist, 2*, 137–146.

Pettit, H. O., & Justice, J. B., Jr. (1991). Effect of dose on cocaine self-administration behavior and dopamine levels in the nucleus accumbens. *Brain Research, 539*(1), 94–102.

Pickens, R., & Thompson, T. (1968). Cocaine-reinforced behavior in rats: Effects of reinforcement magnitude and fixed-ratio size. *The Journal of Pharmacology and Experimental Therapeutics, 161*(1), 122–129.

Powell, S. B., Paulus, M. P., Hartman, D. S., Godel, T., & Geyer, M. A. (2003). RO-10-5824 is a selective dopamine D4 receptor agonist that increases novel object exploration in C57 mice. *Neuropharmacology, 44*(4), 473–481.

Ptacek, R., Kuzelova, H., & Stefano, G. B. (2011). Dopamine D4 receptor gene DRD4 and its association with psychiatric disorders. [Review]. *Medical Science Monitor, 17*(9), RA215–RA220.

Pushparaj, A., Hamani, C., Yu, W., Shin, D. S., Kang, B., Nobrega, J. N., et al. (2013). Electrical stimulation of the insular region attenuates nicotine-taking and nicotine-seeking behaviors. *Neuropsychopharmacology, 38*(4), 690–698. http://dx.doi.org/10.1038/npp.2012.235, npp2012235 [pii].

Ralph, R. J., Varty, G. B., Kelly, M. A., Wang, Y. M., Caron, M. G., Rubinstein, M., et al. (1999). The dopamine D2, but not D3 or D4, receptor subtype is essential for the disruption of prepulse inhibition produced by amphetamine in mice. *The Journal of Neuroscience, 19*(11), 4627–4633.

Robinson, T. E., & Becker, J. B. (1986). Enduring changes in brain and behavior produced by chronic amphetamine administration: A review and evaluation of animal models of amphetamine psychosis. *Brain Research Reviews, 11*, 157–198.

Robinson, T. E., & Berridge, K. C. (1993). The neural basis of drug craving: An incentive-sensitization theory of addiction. *Brain Research Reviews, 18*, 247–291.

Rondou, P., Haegeman, G., & Van Craenenbroeck, K. (2010). The dopamine D4 receptor: Biochemical and signalling properties. *Cellular and Molecular Life Sciences, 67*(12), 1971–1986. http://dx.doi.org/10.1007/s00018-010-0293-y.

Rubinstein, M., Phillips, T. J., Bunzow, J. R., Falzone, T. L., Dziewczapolski, G., Zhang, G., et al. (1997). Mice lacking dopamine D4 receptors are supersensitive to ethanol, cocaine, and methamphetamine. *Cell, 90*(6), 991–1001.

Schoots, O., & Van Tol, H. H. (2003). The human dopamine D4 receptor repeat sequences modulate expression. *The Pharmacogenomics Journal, 3*(6), 343–348. http://dx.doi.org/10.1038/sj.tpj.6500208, 6500208 [pii].

Schultz, W. (2006). Behavioral theories and the neurophysiology of reward. *Annual Review of Psychology, 57,* 87–115.

Seeman, P., & Van Tol, H. H. (1994). Dopamine receptor pharmacology. *Trends in Pharmacological Sciences, 15*(7), 264–270.

Shaham, Y., Adamson, L. K., Grocki, S., & Corrigall, W. A. (1997). Reinstatement and spontaneous recovery of nicotine seeking in rats. *Psychopharmacology, 130*(4), 396–403.

Shields, P. G., Lerman, C., Audrain, J., Bowman, E. D., Main, D., Boyd, N. R., et al. (1998). Dopamine D4 receptors and the risk of cigarette smoking in African-Americans and Caucasians. *Cancer Epidemiology, Biomarkers and Prevention, 7,* 453–458.

Sokoloff, P., Giros, B., Martres, M.-P., Bouthenet, M.-L., & Schwartz, J.-C. (1990). Molecular cloning and characterization of a novel dopamine receptor (D_3) as a target for neuroleptics. *Nature, 347*(6289), 146–151.

Stretch, R., & Gerber, G. J. (1973). Drug-induced reinstatement of amphetamine self-administration behaviour in monkeys. *Canadian Journal of Psychology, 27*(2), 168–177.

Sunahara, R. K., Guan, H. C., O'Dowd, B. F., Seeman, P., Laurier, L. G., Ng, G., et al. (1991). Cloning of the gene for a human dopamine D_5 receptor with higher affinity for dopamine than D_1. *Nature, 350,* 614–619.

Sunahara, R. K., Niznik, H. B., Weiner, D. M., Stormann, T. M., Brann, M. R., Kennedy, J. L., et al. (1990). Human dopamine D_1 receptor encoded by an intronless gene on chromosome 5. *Nature, 347,* 80–83.

Thanos, P., Bermeo, C., Rubinstein,M., Suchland, K.,Wang, G., Grandy, D., et al. (2010). Conditioned place preference and locomotor activity in response to methylphenidate, amphetamine and cocaine in mice lacking dopamine D4 receptors. *Journal of Psychopharmacology, 24,* 897–904. http://dx.doi.org/10.1177/0269881109102613, 0269881109102613 [pii].

Thanos, P. K., Habibi, R., Michaelides, M., Patel, U. B., Suchland, K., Anderson, B. J., et al. (2010). Dopamine D4 receptor (D4R) deletion in mice does not affect operant responding for food or cocaine. *Behavioral Brain Research, 207*(2), 508–511. http://dx.doi.org/10.1016/j.bbr.2009.10.020, S0166-4328(09)00628-7 [pii].

Thomas, T. C., Kruzich, P. J., Joyce, B. M., Gash, C. R., Suchland, K., Surgener, S. P., et al. (2007). Dopamine D4 receptor knockout mice exhibit neurochemical changes consistent with decreased dopamine release. *Journal of Neuroscience Methods, 166*(2), 306–314. http://dx.doi.org/10.1016/j.jneumeth.2007.03.009.

Ton, T. G., Rossing, M. A., Bowen, D. J., Srinouanprachan, S., Wicklund, K., & Farin, F. M. (2007). Genetic polymorphisms in dopamine-related genes and smoking cessation in women: A prospective cohort study. *Behavioral and Brain Functions, 3,* 22.

Tsai, S. J., Cheng, C. Y., Shu, L. R., Yang, C. Y., Pan, C. W., Liou, Y. J., et al. (2002). No association for D2 and D4 dopamine receptor polymorphisms and methamphetamine abuse in Chinese males. *Psychiatric Genetics, 12*(1), 29–33.

Valerio, A., Belloni, M., Gorno, M. L., Tinti, C., Memo, M., & Spano, P. (1994). Dopamine D2, D3, and D4 receptor mRNA levels in rat brain and pituitary during aging. *Neurobiology of Aging, 15*(6), 713–719.

Van Craenenbroeck, K., Borroto-Escuela, D. O., Romero-Fernandez, W., Skieterska, K., Rondou, P., Lintermans, B., et al. (2011). Dopamine D4 receptor oligomerization—

Contribution to receptor biogenesis. *The FEBS Journal*, *278*(8), 1333–1344. http://dx. doi.org/10.1111/j.1742-4658.2011.08052.x.

Van Tol, H. H., Bunzow, J. R., Guan, H. C., Sunahara, R. K., Seeman, P., Niznik, H. B., et al. (1991). Cloning of the gene for a human dopamine D4 receptor with high affinity for the antipsychotic clozapine. *Nature*, *350*(6319), 610–614. http://dx.doi.org/ 10.1038/350610a0.

Van Tol, H. H. M., Wu, C. M., Guan, H. C., O'Hara, K., Bunzow, J. R., Civelli, O., et al. (1992). Multiple dopamine D_4 receptor variants in the human population. *Nature*, *358*, 149–152.

Vandenbergh, D. J., O'Connor, R. J., Grant, M. D., Jefferson, A. L., Vogler, G. P., Strasser, A. A., et al. (2007). Dopamine receptor genes (DRD2, DRD3 and DRD4) and gene–gene interactions associated with smoking-related behaviors. *Addiction Biology*, *12*(1), 106–116.

Waddington, J. L., O'Tuathaigh, C., O'Sullivan, G., Tomiyama, K., Koshikawa, N., & Croke, D. T. (2005). Phenotypic studies on dopamine receptor subtype and associated signal transduction mutants: Insights and challenges from 10 years at the psychopharmacology-molecular biology interface. *Psychopharmacology*, *181*(4), 611–638. http://dx.doi.org/10.1007/s00213-005-0058-8.

Wells, T. T., Beevers, C. G., Knopik, V. S., & McGeary, J. E. (2013). Dopamine D4 receptor gene variation is associated with context-dependent attention for emotion stimuli. *The International Journal of Neuropsychopharmacology/Official Scientific Journal of the Collegium Internationale Neuropsychopharmacologicum*, *16*(3), 525–534. http://dx.doi.org/10.1017/ S1461145712000478.

Wise, R. A., & Bozarth, M. A. (1987). A psychomotor stimulant theory of addiction. *Psychological Review*, *94*, 469–492.

Woolley, M. L., Waters, K. A., Reavill, C., Bull, S., Lacroix, L. P., Martyn, A. J., et al. (2008). Selective dopamine D4 receptor agonist (A-412997) improves cognitive performance and stimulates motor activity without influencing reward-related behaviour in rat. *Behavioural Pharmacology*, *19*(8), 765–776. http://dx.doi.org/10.1097/FBP.0b013e32831c3b06, 00008877-200812000-00002 [pii].

Woolverton, W. L. (1986). Effects of a D1 and a D2 dopamine antagonist on the self-administration of cocaine and piribedil by rhesus monkeys. *Pharmacology, Biochemistry, and Behavior*, *24*(3), 531–535, 0091-3057(86)90553-8 [pii].

Xi, Z. X., Gilbert, J. G., Pak, A. C., Ashby, C. R., Jr., Heidbreder, C. A., & Gardner, E. L. (2005). Selective dopamine D3 receptor antagonism by SB-277011A attenuates cocaine reinforcement as assessed by progressive-ratio and variable-cost-variable-payoff fixed-ratio cocaine self-administration in rats. *The European Journal of Neuroscience*, *21*(12), 3427–3438.

Yan, Y., Nitta, A., Mizuno, T., Nakajima, A., Yamada, K., & Nabeshima, T. (2006). Discriminative-stimulus effects of methamphetamine and morphine in rats are attenuated by cAMP-related compounds. *Behavioural Brain Research*, *173*(1), 39–46. http://dx.doi. org/10.1016/j.bbr.2006.05.029.

Yan, Y., Pushparaj, A., Gamaleddin, I., Steiner, R. C., Picciotto, M. R., Roder, J., et al. (2012). Nicotine-taking and nicotine-seeking in C57Bl/6J mice without prior operant training or food restriction. *Behavioural Brain Research*, *230*(1), 34–39. http://dx.doi.org/ 10.1016/j.bbr.2012.01.042.

Yan, Y., Pushparaj, A., Le Strat, Y., Gamaleddin, I., Barnes, C., Justinova, Z., et al. (2012). Blockade of dopamine d4 receptors attenuates reinstatement of extinguished nicotine-seeking behavior in rats. *Neuropsychopharmacology*, *37*(3), 685–696. http://dx.doi.org/ 10.1038/npp.2011.245.

Yokel, R. A., & Pickens, R. (1974). Drug level of d- and l-amphetamine during intravenous self-administration. *Psychopharmacologia, 34*(3), 255–264.

Yokel, R. A., & Wise, R. A. (1975). Increased lever pressing for amphetamine after pimozide in rats: Implications for a dopamine theory of reward. *Science, 187*(4176), 547–549.

Zhou, Q. Z., Grandy, D. K., Thambi, L., Kushner, J. A., Van Tol, H. H. M., Cone, R., et al. (1990). Cloning and expression of human and rat D$_1$ dopamine receptors. *Nature, 347*, 76–86.

CHAPTER NINE

Sigma (σ) Receptors as Potential Therapeutic Targets to Mitigate Psychostimulant Effects

Rae R. Matsumoto[1], Linda Nguyen, Nidhi Kaushal[2], Matthew J. Robson[3]

West Virginia University, One Medical Center Drive, Morgantown, West Virginia, USA
[1]Corresponding author: e-mail address: rmatsumoto@hsc.wvu.edu
[2]Current address: Takeda Pharmaceuticals, San Diego, California, USA
[3]Current address: Department of Pharmacology, Vanderbilt University, Nashville, Tennessee, USA

Contents

Advances in Pharmacology, Volume 69
ISSN 1054-3589
http://dx.doi.org/10.1016/B978-0-12-420118-7.00009-3

Abstract

Many psychostimulants, including cocaine and methamphetamine, interact with sigma (σ) receptors at physiologically relevant concentrations. The potential therapeutic relevance of this interaction is underscored by the ability to selectively target σ receptors to mitigate many behavioral and physiological effects of psychostimulants in animal and cell-based model systems. This chapter begins with an overview of these enigmatic proteins. Provocative preclinical data showing that σ ligands modulate an array of cocaine and methamphetamine effects are summarized, along with emerging areas of research. Together, the literature suggests targeting of σ receptors as an innovative option for combating undesired actions of psychostimulants through both neuronal and glial mechanisms.

ABBREVIATIONS

AC927 1-(2-phenethyl)piperidine
ALCAM activated leukocyte cell-adhesion molecule
AZ66 3-(4-(4-cyclohexylpiperazin-1-yl)pentyl)-6-fluorobenzo[d]thiazol-2(3H)-one
BBB blood–brain barrier
BD1047 N-[2-(3,4-dichlorophenyl)ethyl]-N-methyl-2-(dimethylamino)ethylamine
BD1063 1-[2-(3,4,-dichlorophenyl)ethyl]-4-methylpiperazine
BMY14802 1-(4-fluorophenyl)-4-[4-(5-fluoropyrimidin-2-yl)piperazin-1-yl]butan-1-ol
BPRS Brief Psychiatric Rating Scale
CD68 cluster of differentiation 68
CM156 3-(4-(4-cyclohexylpiperazin-1-yl)butyl)benzo[d]thiazole-2(3H)-thione
CNS central nervous system
DAT dopamine transporter
DHEA dehydroepiandrosterone
DMT N,N-dimethyltryptamine
DTG 1,3-di-(2-tolyl)guanidine
ER endoplasmic reticulum
ERK extracellular signal-regulated kinase
FDA Food and Drug Administration
FPS 1-(3-fluoropropyl)-4-(4-cyanophenoxymethyl)piperidine
GFAP glial fibrillary acidic protein
gp130 glycoprotein 130
GPCR G protein-coupled receptor
HBMEC human brain microvascular endothelial cell
HIV human immunodeficiency virus
IBA-1 ionized calcium-binding adapter molecule 1
IL-6 interleukin 6
IP$_3$ inositol trisphosphate
JAK2 Janus kinase 2
JNK c-Jun N-terminal kinase
LIF leukemia inhibitory factor
MCP-1 monocyte chemoattractant protein-1
MS377 (R)-(+)-1-(4-chlorophenyl)-3-[4-(2-methoxyethyl)piperazin-1-yl] methyl-2-pyrrolidinone

NE-100 4-methoxy-3-(2-phenylethoxy)-*N*,*N*-di-propylbenzeneethanamine
NF-κB nuclear factor-kappa B
NMDA *N*-methyl-D-aspartate
OSM oncostatin M
PCP phencyclidine
PDGF platelet-derived growth factor
PERK PKR-like ER kinase
PGRMC1 progesterone receptor membrane component 1
PKA protein kinase A
RNS reactive nitrogen species
ROS reactive oxygen species
SA4503 1-(3,4-dimethoxyphenethyl)-4-(3-phenylpropyl)piperazine
SERT serotonin transporter
SFE 1-(2-fluoropropyl)-4-(4-cyanophenoxymethyl)piperidine
SKF10,047 *N*-allylnormetazocine
SN79 6-acetyl-3-(4-(4-(4-fluorophenyl)piperazin-1-yl)butyl)benzo[d]oxazol-2(3H)-one
STAT3 signal transducer and activator of transcription factor 3
TPCNE 1(*trans*-[123I]iodopropen-2-yl)-4-[(4-cyanophenoxy)methyl] piperidine

1. INTRODUCTION

Sigma (σ) receptors have been proposed as therapeutic targets for many central nervous system (CNS) disorders, consistent with their high concentrations in the brain and spinal cord (Fishback, Robson, Xu, & Matsumoto, 2010; Hayashi, Tsai, Mori, Fujimoto, & Su, 2011; Kourrich, Su, Fujimoto, & Bonci, 2012; Zamanillo, Romero, Merlos, & Vela, 2013). It has been recognized since the 1980s that many classes of CNS medications such as antipsychotics, antidepressants, and dissociative anesthetics interact with these proteins (Su, 1982; Tam, 1983; Tam & Cook, 1984), although the cellular mechanisms and pathways through which σ ligands convey therapeutic benefits are only now beginning to be illuminated.

The significant affinity of many drugs of abuse, including cocaine, methamphetamine, 3,4-methylenedioxymethamphetamine, phencyclidine (PCP), and some opiates for σ receptors, raises the intriguing possibility that interactions with these proteins may serve as common targets for abused substances (Brammer, Gilmore, & Matsumoto, 2006; Matsumoto, 2009; Sharkey, Glen, Wolfe, & Kuhar, 1988; Weber et al., 1986). Through these interactions, σ receptors are believed to convey and modulate some of the physiological and behavioral effects of abused substances and serve as potential therapeutic targets for mitigating their effects. This chapter focuses on the psychostimulants cocaine and methamphetamine, which are among the best studied drugs of abuse with regard to interactions with σ receptors.

The chapter begins with an overview of σ receptors, from a historical perspective to our contemporary understanding of these enigmatic proteins. Then, preclinical data with regard to their implications for cocaine and methamphetamine are addressed, and the chapter concludes with our clinical knowledge of this class of compounds.

2. BACKGROUND ON σ RECEPTORS

2.1. Historical perspective

σ Receptors were first proposed as a type of opiate receptor based on the actions of (±)-SKF10,047 (N-allylnormetazocine) and related benzomorphans, with the name originating from the first letter "S" in SKF10,047, which was thought to be the prototypic ligand for this subtype (Martin, Eades, Thompson, Huppler, & Gilbert, 1976). Studies since then have shown that SKF10,047 interacts with at least three distinct binding sites: the kappa opioid receptor, the PCP binding site within the ionophore of the N-methyl-D-aspartate (NMDA) receptor, and the proteins that today retain the designation of the σ receptor (Matsumoto, Liu, Lerner, Howard, & Brackett, 2003). σ Receptors can be distinguished from kappa and NMDA receptors based on their distinct drug selectivity patterns, structures, and molecular biological profiles (Table 9.1). Moreover, it is essential to emphasize that while σ receptors are ligand-activated, they are structurally distinct from classical G protein-coupled receptors (GPCRs) (like kappa opioid receptors) or ligand-gated ionotropic receptors (like NMDA receptors). Thus, many of the signaling motifs and patterns of activity that are commonly associated with these classical CNS receptor families do not apply to σ receptors.

2.2. σ Receptor subtypes

There are two established subtypes of σ receptors, which were initially proposed based on distinct pharmacological profiles and subsequently supported by differing molecular biological properties. The two subtypes have been designated σ_1 and σ_2. Selected features of the two subtypes including their structures, functions, pharmacology, and distribution are summarized in Table 9.2.

2.2.1 σ_1 Receptors

σ_1 Receptors are ligand-activated chaperone proteins that can modulate an array of cellular functions. They are composed of 223 amino acids that share >90% identity across rodents and humans and no significant homology (<30%) with other mammalian proteins (Hanner et al., 1996; Mei &

Table 9.1 Comparison of (±)-SKF10,047 binding sites

	Kappa opioid receptor	NMDA receptor (PCP site)	Sigma receptor
Binding of SKF10,047	(−)-Isomer	(+)-Isomer	(+)-Isomer
	(−)-Isomer, naloxone-sensitive		(−)-Isomer, naloxone-insensitive
Selective ligands[a]	U69593	MK-801	DTG
	Nor-BNI	Tenocyclidine	BD1047
Size	43 kDa	Approx. 500 kDa	18–29 kDa
Structure	7TM G protein-coupled receptor	Heterotetrameric, ionotropic glutamate receptor	Nonopioid, non-PCP binding site
Sequence[b]	NM_000912 (human)	NM_000832 (NR1, human)	U75282 (human)
	NM_017167 (rat)	NM_001270602 (NR1, rat)	AF004218 (rat)
	NM_001204371 (mouse)	NM_008169 (NR1, mouse)	AF030100 (mouse)

[a]Selectivity defined as >100-fold higher binding affinities over the other two receptors.
[b]Accession numbers for representative sequences. For the σ receptor, the accession numbers refer to the σ₁ subtype.

Pasternak, 2001; Prasad et al., 1998). They are predicted to have two transmembrane (TM)-spanning regions, with an additional C-terminal region enriched in alpha helices and beta sheets, which are classic structural features that participate in protein–protein interactions (Hayashi & Su, 2007; Ortega-Roldan, Ossa, & Schnell, 2013; Pal et al., 2008). They thus appear to represent a unique structural class of proteins, distinct from GPCRs and ionotropic receptors.

σ_1 Receptors exist in numerous cell types including both neurons and glia in the brain (Bouchard & Quirion, 1997; Palacios et al., 2003). Within cells, they have been reported in the following intracellular locations: endoplasmic reticulum (ER), mitochondria, nuclear membrane envelope, and plasma membrane (Alonso et al., 2000). Under basal conditions, σ_1 receptors are believed to reside at the ER and mitochondrial interface where they can modulate cellular bioenergetics by affecting calcium flux through inositol trisphosphate (IP_3) receptors (Hayashi & Su, 2007).

Table 9.2 Comparison of the two σ receptor subtypes

	σ_1	σ_2
Size	25–29 kDa (223 amino acids)[a]	18–22 kDa[b]
Putative structure	2TM chaperone protein[c]	PGRMC1-like[d]
Affinity for benzomorphan and morphinan isomers[b, e]	$(+) > (-)$	$(-) < (+)$
Putative endogenous ligands	DMT[f] Neurosteroids (DHEA, pregnenolone sulfate, and progesterone)[g] Sphingosine[h]	Zn^{2+i}
Cellular localization	• Exist on lipid rafts at mitochondrion-associated ER[j] • Translocate between ER, mitochondria, plasma membrane, and nuclear membrane[i, k]	• Enriched in lipid rafts[l] • Reside in ER, mitochondria, plasma membrane, and lysosomes[m]
Tissue expression[e]		
Brain	High	High
Heart	High	Low
Liver	High	High
Spleen	High	Low
GI tract	High	High
Physiological functions	• Modulate activity of GPCRs, ion channels, and signaling molecules[k] • Promote cell growth and inhibit apoptosis[n] • Protect against oxidative stress[o] • Regulate synaptogenesis and neuroplasticity[p] • Modulate cardiac contractility and arterial vasomotor tone[q]	• Modulate calcium signaling[r] • Induce growth arrest and cell death[s] • Regulate CYP450 proteins[t]

Table 9.2 Comparison of the two σ receptor subtypes—cont'd

	σ_1	σ_2
Clinical implications	• CNS disorders (depression, anxiety, schizophrenia, psychosis, drug addiction, pain, Alzheimer's disease, Parkinson's disease, ALS, retinal diseases, and stroke)[u] • Cardiovascular diseases[v] • Cancer[w] • Inflammatory and autoimmune conditions[x] • GI diseases (gastric/duodenal ulcer and diarrhea)[y]	• CNS disorders (depression and drug addiction)[z] • Cancer[m, s, w] Inflammatory and autoimmune conditions[x]

[a]Hanner et al. (1996), Mei and Pasternak (2001), Prasad et al. (1998).
[b]Hellewell and Bowen (1990), Hellewell et al. (1994), Xu et al. (2011).
[c]Aydar, Palmer, Klyachko, and Jackson (2002).
[d]Xu et al. (2011).
[e]Matsumoto, Bowen, and Su (2007).
[f]Fontanilla et al. (2009).
[g]Maurice, Roman, and Privat (1996), McCann and Su (1991), Monnet and Maurice (2006), Su, London, and Jaffe (1988).
[h]Ramachandran et al. (2009).
[i]Connor and Chavkin (1992).
[j]Hayashi and Su (2007).
[k]Su, Hayashi, Maurice, Buch, and Ruoho (2010).
[l]Gebreselassie and Bowen (2004).
[m]Zeng et al. (2007).
[n]Spruce et al. (2004).
[o]Pal et al. (2012).
[p]Kourrich et al. (2012), Lucas, Rymar, Sadikot, and Debonnel (2008), Moriguchi et al. (2013), Sha et al. (2013), Takebayashi, Hayashi, and Su (2002).
[q]Ela, Barg, Vogel, Hasin, and Eilam (1994), Novakova et al. (1995).
[r]Vilner and Bowen (2000).
[s]Crawford and Bowen (2002), van Waarde et al. (2010).
[t]Ahmed, Chamberlain, and Craven (2012), Basile, Paul, and de Costa (1992).
[u]Hayashi and Su (2004), Hayashi et al. (2011), Kourrich et al. (2013), Maurice and Su (2009).
[v]Monassier and Bousquet (2002).
[w]Aydar, Palmer, and Djamgoz (2004), van Waarde et al. (2010), Vilner, John, and Bowen (1995), Wang et al. (2004).
[x]Bourrie, Bribes, Derocq, Vidal, and Casellas (2004), Bourrie et al. (2002), Su et al. (1988), Wolfe, Kulsakdinun, Battaglia, Jaffe, and De Souza (1988).
[y]Pascaud et al. (1993), Roze, Bruley Des Varannes, Shi, Geneve, and Galmiche (1998), Theodorou et al. (2002).
[z]Kaushal and Matsumoto (2011), Nuwayhid and Werling (2006), Sanchez and Papp (2000).

As chaperone proteins, σ_1 receptors do not have their own intrinsic signaling machinery. Instead, upon ligand activation, they participate in protein–protein interactions to modulate the activity of GPCRs (e.g., μ opioid and dopamine D_1), ion channels (e.g., potassium, sodium, and NMDA), or signaling molecules (e.g., inositol phosphates, protein kinases, and calcium) through a mechanism involving translocation between different cellular compartments (Aydar et al., 2002; Balasuriya et al., 2012; Kinoshita, Matsuoka, Suzuki, Mirrielees, & Yang, 2012; Kourrich et al., 2013; Navarro et al., 2010, 2013; Su et al., 2010). σ_1 Receptors can also modulate cellular functions through protein trafficking and alterations in transcriptional and posttranslational processes (Crottes et al., 2011).

The physiological relevance of σ_1 receptors is supported by knockdown studies in which antisense oligonucleotides or siRNAs targeting them interfere with receptor functions under both *in vitro* and *in vivo* conditions. These types of studies indicate that σ_1 receptors have implications not only for drug abuse but also for numerous other CNS functions and conditions including learning and memory (Kitaichi et al., 2000), depression (Takebayashi et al., 2002), pain (Mei & Pasternak, 2002), and stroke (Ruscher et al., 2011).

2.2.2 σ_2 Receptors

σ_2 Receptors were first proposed based on their overlapping but distinct pharmacological profile compared to σ_1 receptors. Although many compounds including 1,3-di-o-tolylguanidine (DTG) and SKF10,047 interact with both σ_1 and σ_2 receptors, the differing stereoselectivity of benzomorphans and morphinans at the two subtypes is the hallmark distinguishing feature. The (+)-isomers of benzomorphans and morphinans often have similar affinity for both σ_1 and σ_2 receptors. However, the subtypes differ in their affinities for the (−)-isomers, with the σ_2 subtype exhibiting preferential affinity for the (−)-isomer compared to the (+)-isomer; the opposite pattern is exhibited by the σ_1 subtype that has preferential affinity for the (+)-isomer compared to the (−)-isomer.

Early photoaffinity-labeling studies also demonstrate that the σ_2 receptor (18–22 kDa) is smaller in size than the σ_1 subtype (25–29 kDa), a pattern that has been confirmed by a number of investigators (Hellewell & Bowen, 1990; Hellewell et al., 1994; Xu et al., 2011). A recent study has proposed that σ_2 receptors may be identical to the progesterone receptor membrane component 1 (PGRMC1) (Xu et al., 2011). However, since this discovery is dependent on the use of novel ligands and the early history of σ receptors is plagued with confusion due to the use of nonselective compounds, it will be important to have this finding independently confirmed by other groups. Confirmation that the σ_2 receptor is identical to PGRMC1 will open up new perspectives and opportunities for research through the availability of existing research tools and information. Alternately, it is possible that some ligands bind both σ_2 receptors and PGRMC1 and possibly that PGRMC1 represents a distinct protein closely associated with the σ_2 subtype.

Nevertheless, there is consensus in the literature that σ_2 receptors are enriched in lipid rafts and are involved in cholesterol synthesis and calcium signaling through sphingolipid products (Ahmed et al., 2012; Crawford, Coop, & Bowen, 2002; Gebreselassie & Bowen, 2004; van Waarde et al., 2010). σ_2 Receptors are also found in a variety of locations within cells including the ER, mitochondria, lysosomes, and plasma membrane (Zeng et al., 2007). They also associate with select cytochrome P450 (CYP450) proteins, with the functional consequences of these interactions under active investigation (Ahmed et al., 2012; Basile et al., 1992).

Functionally, σ_2 receptors have been the most studied in the context of cancer research where they appear to have important roles in cell-cycle functions and cell survival and death pathways (van Waarde et al., 2010). In tumor cells, σ_2 receptors can be targeted to inhibit proliferation and induce apoptosis through both p53 and caspase-dependent and caspase-independent pathways (van Waarde et al., 2010). There is also evidence for the involvement of this subtype in the effects of drugs of abuse, including cocaine and methamphetamine, although much less is known about their role compared to the σ_1 subtype (Kaushal & Matsumoto, 2011; Nuwayhid & Werling, 2006).

2.3. Expression across species and cell types

σ Receptors appear highly conserved across species and have been reported in some invertebrates and vertebrates including rodents and humans (Kekuda, Prasad, Fei, Leibach, & Ganapathy, 1996; Matsumoto, Bowen, de Costa, & Houk, 1999; Mei & Pasternak, 2001; Prasad et al., 1998; Vu, Weissman, & London, 1990). Both subtypes are found in many organ systems and cell types in the body, as well as in derived cell lines used in research (Matsumoto et al., 2007). However, select cell lines and organ systems are enriched in a particular subtype such as the preponderance of σ_1 receptors in the heart and spleen (Matsumoto et al., 2007). For the purposes of this chapter, studies implicating a particular subtype of σ receptor will be specified when known; otherwise, the use of the general designation of σ receptor will be used.

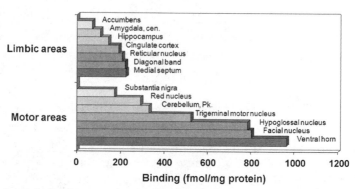

Figure 9.1 Relative expression levels of σ receptors in various CNS regions. σ Receptors, labeled with [³H](+)3PPP in the guinea pig CNS, were quantified using standard auto-radiography methods (Gundlach et al., 1986). The highest concentrations are found in motor regions of the CNS, with significant levels also found in limbic areas. (For color version of this figure, the reader is referred to the online version of this chapter.)

With regard to psychostimulant effects, σ receptors are found in organ systems such as the brain and heart. In the brain, σ receptors are found in highest concentrations in brainstem motor areas, with significant expression in limbic regions (Bouchard & Quirion, 1997; Gundlach, Largent, & Snyder, 1986; Largent, Gundlach, & Snyder, 1986; McLean & Weber, 1988) (Fig. 9.1). Within the brain, they are expressed in a variety of cell types including both neurons and glia (Gekker et al., 2006; Gundlach et al., 1986; Jansen, Faull, Dragunow, & Leslie, 1991; Palacios et al., 2003; Palacios, Muro, Verdu, Pumarola, & Vela, 2004). Given the historical importance of the dopamine system in mediating psychostimulant effects, it is important to note that σ receptors are found on dopaminergic neurons (Graybiel, Besson, & Weber, 1989; Gundlach et al., 1986). Also, in light of the inter-play between the nervous and immune systems, it is noteworthy that σ receptors are expressed in the spleen and other immune cells, including peripheral blood leukocytes and lymphocytes (Carr, De Costa, Radesca, & Blalock, 1991; Liu, Whitlock, Pultz, & Wolfe, 1995; Paul et al., 1994; Wolfe et al., 1988). They are also found on endothelial cells, which could have implications for blood–brain barrier (BBB) functions and/or vascular events related to cocaine exposure (Wilbert-Lampen, Seliger, Zilker, & Arendt, 1998).

2.4. Endogenous ligand(s)

Numerous lines of evidence support the existence of endogenous ligands for σ receptors, with potential candidates including some neuroactive steroids and trace amines (Table 9.2). Although no consensus has yet been reached as to the endogenous ligand(s) for these proteins, the following types of evidence strongly support the existence of physiologically relevant entities that bind to and have functional consequences at σ receptors.

Initial efforts to identify endogenous ligand(s) for σ receptors involved serial fractionation of extracts from tissues containing the receptors (i.e., brain and liver) in an effort to identify constituents that displace binding to σ receptors. Numerous extracts were found by several groups to bind to σ receptors (Contreras, DiMaggio, & O'Donohue, 1987; Nagornaia, Samovilova, Korobov, & Vinogradov, 1988; Su, Weissman, & Yeh, 1986). Although none of the investigations achieved purification of a single chemical entity, these studies suggest multiple endogenous ligands for σ receptors from different chemical classes since active constituents from some groups were peptides (e.g., susceptible to trypsin digestion or proteolysis) (Contreras et al., 1987; Su et al., 1986), while the extracts from other groups appeared nonpeptidic (e.g., resistant to pronase digestion) (Nagornaia et al., 1988).

Using physiological approaches, early efforts also demonstrate the release of substances that displace binding to σ receptors under conditions known to cause neurotransmitter release. Depolarization of hippocampal brain slices preloaded with a radioligand to occupy σ receptors causes a displacement of radioligand binding, suggesting the release of endogenous ligands that compete for binding to σ receptors (Connor & Chavkin, 1991; Neumaier & Chavkin, 1989). This is observed after depolarization with potassium chloride (Neumaier & Chavkin, 1989), as well as with electrical stimulation (Connor & Chavkin, 1991). Interestingly, electrical stimulation patterns that have previously been associated with neurotransmitter release are more effective in causing displacement of the σ radioligand, and this is only seen when certain hippocampal regions are stimulated (perforant path and mossy fibers) and not others (Connor & Chavkin, 1991). Together, the data provide a compelling picture that under physiologically relevant conditions, there is release of endogenous substances from defined brain circuits that bind to σ receptors.

Profiling of known substances for binding to σ receptors led to the initial identification of progesterone and some other neuroactive steroids as potential endogenous ligands (Su et al., 1988). Since then, numerous laboratories have confirmed progesterone binding to σ receptors, and this interaction is with the σ_1 subtype (Fishback, Rosen, Bhat, McCurdy, & Matsumoto, 2012; Ganapathy et al., 1999; Hanner et al., 1996; Klein, Cooper, & Musacchio, 1994; Ramachandran, Lu, Prabhu, & Ruoho, 2007). Moreover, progesterone attenuates the effects of selective σ receptor ligands *in vitro* and *in vivo*, confirming its ability to mediate functional effects through these proteins (Monnet & Maurice, 2006). More recently, trace amines such as *N,N*-dimethyltryptamine (DMT) have been proposed as endogenous ligands for σ receptors (Fontanilla et al., 2009). Although DMT has micromolar affinity for σ receptors, this interaction appears functionally relevant since mice lacking these receptors lose their response to the DMT-induced effects tested (Fontanilla et al., 2009). This latter observation suggests that there may be a need to revisit the assumption that endogenous ligands for σ receptors must bind with robust nanomolar affinity.

2.5. Pharmacology: Agonists and antagonists

The assignment of agonist and antagonist designations of ligands at σ receptors follows classical pharmacological definitions. Agonists are compounds that produce effects on their own in a dose-dependent manner; they also produce a leftward shift in the dose–response curve when combined with another agonist. Antagonists are compounds that have no effects on their own, but block the action of agonists; they elicit a rightward or downward shift in the agonist dose–response curve. These pharmacological designations have often been supported by complementary molecular biological approaches where overexpression of the receptors produces agonist-like actions, whereas knockdown of the receptors elicits antagonist-like effects.

Although it could be argued that these may not be the most appropriate/accurate nomenclature to use for σ receptor ligands, they are well-established terms that predict certain dose-dependent patterns that have more often than not been observed in the data. However, there are anomalies such as inverted U-shaped dose–response curves for agonists often reported. Also, unlike classical GPCRs where agonist/antagonist binding to the receptor activates/blocks specific signaling pathways, the functional readout for σ receptor ligands may vary and conceptually operate more like modulators of GPCRs or for evaluating protein–protein interactions. At σ_1 receptors, there appears to be multiple regions for ligand interactions with the receptor protein, some of which have functional implications for agonist versus antagonist activity (Cobos, Baeyens, & Del Pozo, 2005; Pal et al., 2008; Wu & Bowen, 2008; Yamamoto et al., 1999). The interaction of agonists versus antagonists at σ_2 receptors is less clear as truly selective ligands for this subtype have only recently been developed.

Table 9.3 summarizes σ receptor agonists that are described in this chapter. All of these compounds can produce effects on their own and/or

Table 9.3 Representative list of σ receptor putative agonists and antagonists

Compound	σ₁ Affinity (K_i, nM)	σ₂ Affinity (K_i, nM)	σ_1/σ_2	Structure and chemical name
Agonists				
Nonselective				
BD1031[a]	1 ± 0.2	80 ± 9	0.01	3(R)-1-[2-(3,4-dichlorophenyl)ethyl]-1,4-diazabicyclo[4.3.0]nonane
BD1052[b]	2 ± 0.5	60 ± 3	0.03	N-[2-(3,4-dichlorophenyl)ethyl]-N-allyl-2-(1-pyrrolidinyl)ethylamine
DTG[c]	74.3 ± 13.9	61.2 ± 13.4	1.2	1,3-Di-(2-tolyl)guanidine

Continued

Table 9.3 Representative list of σ receptor putative agonists and antagonists—cont'd

Compound	σ₁ Affinity (Kᵢ, nM)	σ₂ Affinity (Kᵢ, nM)	σ₁/σ₂	Structure and chemical name
σ₁-preferring				
(+)-Pentazocine[c]	6.7 ± 1.2	1361 ± 134	0.005	(+)-[2S-(2a,6a,11R*)]-1,2,3,4,5,6-hexahydro-6,11-dimethyl-3-(3-methyl-2-butenyl)-2,6-methano-3-benzazocin-8-ol
(+)-SKF10,047[c]	28.7 ± 2.8	33654 ± 409	0.0009	[2S-(2α,6α,11R*)]-1,2,3,4,5,6-hexahydro-6,11-dimethyl-3-(2-propenyl)-2,6-methano-3-benzazocin-8-ol
SA4503[d]	4.6 ± 0.2	63.1 ± 4.3	0.07	1-[2-(3,4-Dimethoxyphenyl)ethyl]-4-(3-phenylpropyl)piperazine

σ₂-preferring

CM699[e] 16.6 ± 1.1 0.014 ± 0.0003 1186

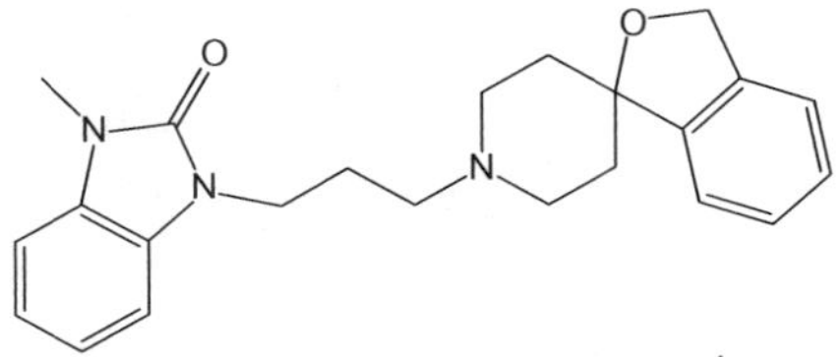

1-(3-(3H-spiro[isobenzofuran-1,4'-piperidine]-1'-yl)propyl)-3-methyl-1H-benzo[d]imidazol-2(3H)-one

Antagonists

Nonselective

AC927[f] 30 ± 2 138 ± 18 0.2

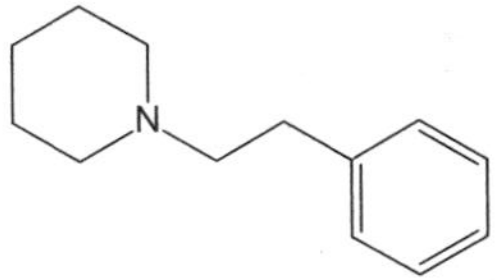

1-(2-Phenethyl)piperidine oxalate

AZ66[g] 2.4 ± 0.63 0.51 ± 0.15 4.7

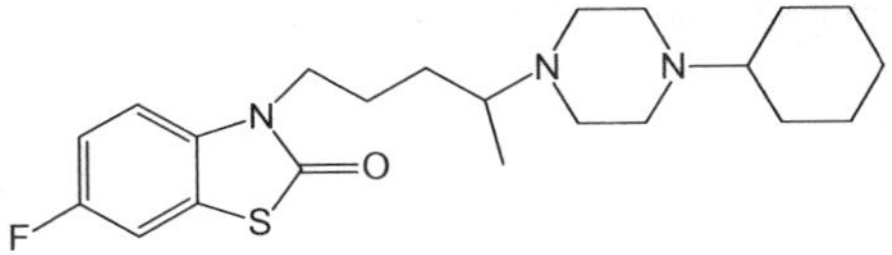

3-(4-(4-Cyclohexylpiperazin-1-yl)pentyl)-6-fluorobenzo[d]thiazol-2(3H)-one

Continued

Table 9.3 Representative list of σ receptor putative agonists and antagonists—cont'd

Compound	σ₁ Affinity (K_i, nM)	σ₂ Affinity (K_i, nM)	σ_1/σ_2	Structure and chemical name
BD1008[h]	2 ± 1	8 ± 2	0.2	*N*-[2-(3,4-dichlorophenyl)ethyl]-*N*-methyl-1-pyrrolidineethanamine
BD1018[a]	5 ± 0.7	49 ± 4	0.1	3(*S*)-1-[2-(3,4-dichlorophenyl)ethyl]-1,4-diazabicyclo[4.3.0]nonane
BMY14802[i]	60	230	0.3	1-(4-Fluorophenyl)-4-[4-(5-fluoropyrimidin-2-yl)piperazin-1-yl] butan-1-ol
CM156[j]	1.3 ± 0.4	0.6 ± 0.1	2.2	3-(4-(4-Cyclohexylpiperazin-1-yl)butyl)benzo[d]thiazole-2(3*H*)-thione

SN79[k]	27±2	7±0.09	3.9

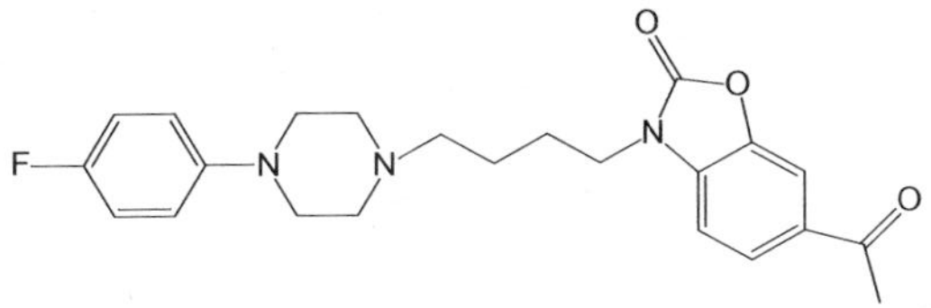

6-Acetyl-3-(4-(4-(4-fluorophenyl)piperazin-1-yl)butyl)benzo[d]oxazol-2(3H)-one

σ_1-preferring

BD1047[l]	0.93±0.14	47±0.60	0.02

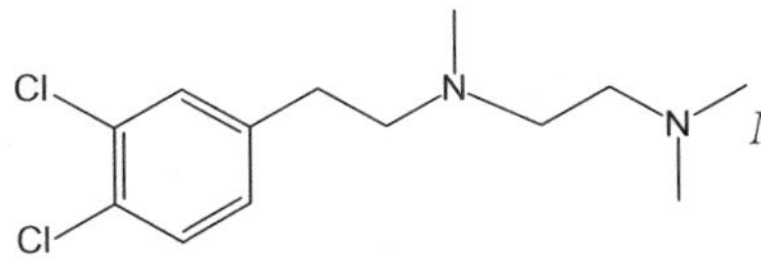

N,N,N'-trimethyl-N'-[2-(3,4-dichlorophenyl)ethyl]ethane-1,2-diamine

N,N,N'-trimethylethane-1,2-diamine

BD1063[l]	9.15±1.28	449±11	0.02

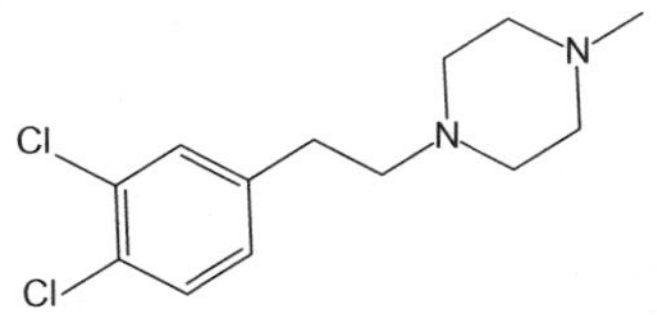

1-[2-(3,4-dichlorophenyl)ethyl]-4-methylpiperazine

Continued

Table 9.3 Representative list of σ receptor putative agonists and antagonists—cont'd

Compound	σ_1 Affinity (K_i, nM)	σ_2 Affinity (K_i, nM)	σ_1/σ_2	Structure and chemical name
LR132[a]	2 ± 0.1	701 ± 375	0.003	1R,2S-(+)-*cis*-N-[2,(3,4-dichlorophenyl)ethyl]-2-(1-pyrrolidinyl) cyclohexylamine
NE100[m]	2.8 ± 0.5	95.5 ± 1.0	0.03	4-Methoxy-3-(2-phenylethoxy)-*N,N*-dipropylbenzeneethanamine
σ_2-preferring				
CM398[c]	560.4 ± 8.7	0.43 ± 0.02	1303	1-(4-(6,7-Dimethoxy-3,4-dihydroisoquinoline-2(1*H*)-yl)butyl)-3-methyl-1*H*-benzol[*d*]imidazol-2(3*H*)-one

CM775[e]	2274 ± 187	4.27 ± 0.29	533

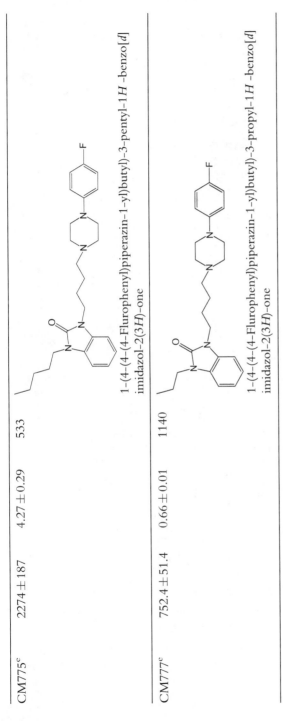

1-(4-(4-(4-Flurophenyl)piperazin-1-yl)butyl)-3-pentyl-1*H*-benzo[*d*]imidazol-2(3*H*)-one

CM777[e]	752.4 ± 51.4	0.66 ± 0.01	1140

1-(4-(4-(4-Flurophenyl)piperazin-1-yl)butyl)-3-propyl-1*H*-benzo[*d*]imidazol-2(3*H*)-one

[a]Matsumoto, McCracken, Friedman, et al. (2001).
[b]Matsumoto, McCracken, Pouw, et al. (2001).
[c]Bowen, de Costa, Hellewell, Walker, and Rice (1993).
[d]Lever, Gustafson, Xu, Allmon, and Lever (2006).
[e]Noorbakhsh et al. (2011).
[f]Matsumoto, Shaikh, Wilson, Vedam, and Coop (2008).
[g]Seminerio, Robson, Abdelazeem, et al. (2012).
[h]McCracken, Bowen, and Matsumoto (1999).
[i]Reported value is IC$_{50}$; Perregaard, Moltzen, Meier, and Sanchez (1995).
[j]Xu et al. (2010).
[k]Kaushal, Robson, et al. (2011).
[l]Matsumoto et al. (1995).
[m]Fishback et al. (2012).

enhance the effects of psychostimulants, although the specific downstream cellular mediators through which these changes are achieved may differ across experimental conditions. Agonists for σ receptors are hypothesized to elicit functional changes in cells by affecting an array of potential targets downstream from the receptor. σ_1 Receptor agonists may promote certain types of protein–protein interactions to modulate the activity of known GPCRs or ion channels (Aydar et al., 2002; Ha et al., 2011). Agonists for both σ receptor subtypes could modulate known signaling pathways, particularly through enhancement of intracellular calcium (Kourrich et al., 2012; Su & Hayashi, 2003). There is also evidence that σ receptor agonists can produce changes in gene and protein expression, which alter cellular functions and behavior (Sabino et al., 2011). In addition, σ receptor agonists are capable of eliciting morphological and structural changes in existing cells that can support neuroplasticity and synaptogenesis and also promote the formation of new cells through neurogenesis (Lucas et al., 2008; Moriguchi et al., 2013; Sha et al., 2013; Takebayashi et al., 2002).

Similarly, antagonists for σ receptors may inhibit the actions of agonists through a variety of hypothesized mechanisms. The binding of σ_1 receptor antagonists may inhibit the ability of agonists to form proper protein–protein interactions with targets (Aydar et al., 2002). σ Receptor antagonism has also been reported to inhibit agonist-stimulated increases in intracellular calcium and changes in gene and protein expression, neurogenesis, and neurite formation (Hayashi, Maurice, & Su, 2000; Hayashi & Su, 2007; Moriguchi et al., 2013; Takebayashi et al., 2002). Select σ receptor antagonists that are described in this chapter are shown in Table 9.3.

3. COCAINE AND σ RECEPTORS

3.1. Background

Cocaine continues to be among the most abused illicit substances. It is responsible for more serious intoxications and emergency room mentions than any other illicit drug (Substance Abuse & Health Services Administration, 2008). In the United States, it is estimated that over 36 million Americans have used cocaine at least once and that nearly 2 million individuals consider themselves current users of the drug (Substance Abuse & Health Services Administration, 2009).

Cocaine interacts with multiple protein targets and is best known as an indirect dopamine agonist through its interaction with dopamine transporters (DATs). However, medication development efforts spanning over

20 years that target dopaminergic mechanisms have yet to result in a US Food and Drug Administration (FDA)-approved drug to treat cocaine-related disorders, underscoring the need to consider alternative approaches for mitigating the effects of this psychostimulant. Several early observations that spurred investigations of σ receptors as potential medication development targets for cocaine include the following: (i) σ Receptors are found on dopaminergic neurons and in brain regions associated with cocaine effects (Gundlach et al., 1986); (ii) σ Receptors are also found in peripheral organs that are affected by the toxic effects of cocaine including the heart, lung, and gastrointestinal tract (Matsumoto et al., 2007); (iii) Cocaine interacts with σ receptors at physiologically relevant concentrations (Sharkey et al., 1988).

Cocaine appears to act as an agonist at σ receptors. It produces effects on its own, which can be attenuated with antagonists for each of the σ receptor subtypes; the actions at σ_1 receptors have been further confirmed by molecular knockdown of this subtype. In contrast, selective σ receptor agonists often mimic the actions of cocaine or shift the dose–response curve for cocaine to the left.

Among the two σ receptor subtypes, cocaine has about a 10-fold higher affinity for σ_1 receptors (2–7 µM) compared to σ_2 receptors (29–31 µM) in the brain (Matsumoto et al., 2007; Matsumoto, McCracken, Pouw, Zhang, & Bowen, 2002), with select biologically active metabolites also interacting with σ receptors (Table 9.4). Both subtypes appear to modulate the actions of cocaine, although most studies to date have focused on the σ_1 receptor due to the availability of experimental tools to manipulate receptor function. Over the years, σ receptors have emerged as promising drug discovery targets for their ability to mitigate a diverse array of effects and pathologies elicited by cocaine, which are summarized in the sections that follow.

Table 9.4 Affinity of cocaine and metabolites for σ receptors

Compound	σ_1 Receptor	σ_2 Receptor
Cocaine	2.9 ± 1.9	29.2 ± 12.9
Benzoylecgonine	>100	>100
Norcocaine	2.4 ± 0.2	33.1 ± 9.5
Cocaethylene	7.8 ± 0.6	20.5 ± 0.5

Affinities (K_i in µM) were determined in competition assays in rat brain using 5 nM [^{3}H](+)-pentazocine to label σ_1 receptors and 3 nM [^{3}H]DTG in the presence of 300 nM (+)-pentazocine to label σ_2 receptors using methods previously published (Matsumoto et al., 2002). The values in the table represent the mean ± SEM from two to three experiments, each performed in duplicate. Values of >100 µM in the table signify that there was less than 30% displacement of radioligand at this concentration.

3.2. Behavioral effects

Table 9.5 summarizes the effects of σ receptor ligands against a variety of cocaine-induced behaviors in preclinical studies. In general, pretreatment with σ receptor antagonists attenuates most behavioral effects of cocaine, with the exception of self-administration. For self-administration, it appears that agonists at σ receptors may convey therapeutic benefit as replacement/ substitution therapies. Interestingly, σ receptor ligands mitigate both acute and subchronic effects of cocaine. Targeting the σ_1 subtype alone appears sufficient for attenuating many behavioral effects of cocaine, although mixed $\sigma_{1/2}$ compounds appear to produce more robust effects. These effects are hypothesized to involve modulation of classical neurotransmitter systems such as dopamine and glutamate and alterations in drug-induced neuroadaptations including changes in gene and protein expression. Figure 9.2 summarizes some key mechanisms that have been reported thus far and hypothesized to occur.

3.2.1 Cocaine-induced Convulsions

One symptom of the behavioral toxicity of cocaine is the onset of convulsions. Cocaine-induced convulsions do not often respond well to conventional antiepileptic medications and can be problematic to treat in overdose situations (Derlet & Albertson, 1990). Thus, it is noteworthy that the attenuation of σ receptors significantly reduces the convulsive effects of cocaine in preclinical rodent models (Kaushal, McCurdy, & Matsumoto, 2011, Kaushal, Robson, et al., 2011; Matsumoto, Gilmore, et al., 2004; Matsumoto, Li, Katz, Fantegrossi, & Coop, 2011; Matsumoto, McCracken, Friedman, et al., 2001; Matsumoto, McCracken, Pouw, et al., 2001; Matsumoto et al., 2002; Matsumoto, Potelleret, et al., 2004; Xu et al., 2010), with pharmacological antagonism or molecular knockdown of the σ_1 subtype sufficient to mitigate these effects (Matsumoto, McCracken, Friedman, et al., 2001; Matsumoto et al., 2002). Recent studies also suggest that selective antagonism of the σ_2 subtype, utilizing recently developed subtype-selective ligands, also reduces the convulsive effects of cocaine (Noorbakhsh et al., 2011).

In contrast, σ receptor agonists worsen the convulsive effects of cocaine, with a shift to the left in the cocaine dose–response curve, although the agonists themselves do not induce convulsions at the doses tested (Matsumoto, McCracken, Friedman, et al., 2001; Matsumoto, McCracken, Pouw, et al., 2001; Matsumoto et al., 2002). The shift to

Table 9.5 Summary of effects of σ ligands on cocaine-induced behaviors

Behavior	Antagonist effects	Agonist effects
Convulsions	Attenuate cocaine effect: • AC927[a] • BD1008, BD1060, BD1067[b] • BD1018, BD1063, LR132[c] • BD1047, LR172[d] • BMY14802[b] • CM156[e] • CM398, CM775, CM777[f] • NPC16377[g] • SN79[h] • UMB100, UMB101, UMB103[i] • YZ011, YZ016, YZ018[j] • YZ027, YZ028, YZ029[j] • YZ030, YZ032, YZ033[j] • YZ069, YZ184[k] • Antisense confirmation[c, j]	Shift cocaine dose–response curve to the left: • BD1031[c] • BD1052[b] • DTG[b, c, d, j] No effect on cocaine dose–response curve: • CM699[l] • (+)-Pentazocine[b]
Lethality	Attenuate cocaine effect: • AC927[a] • BD1008, BD1060, BD1067[b] • BD1018, BD1063, LR132[c] • BD1047, LR172[d] • BMY14802[b] • LR132 (also effective posttreatment)[c] • UMB100, UMB101, UMB103[i] • YZ011 (also effective posttreatment)[j] • YZ027, YZ032 [j]	Shift cocaine dose–response curve to the left: • DTG[c]

Continued

Table 9.5 Summary of effects of σ ligands on cocaine-induced behaviors—cont'd

Behavior	Antagonist effects	Agonist effects
Locomotor activity	Attenuate cocaine effect: • AC927[a] • BD1008[m] • BD1018, BD1063, LR132[c] • BD1047, LR172[d] • CM156[e] • NPC 16377[g] • SN79[h] • YZ011, YZ027, YZ032[j] • Antisense confirmation[c, j]	Mimic cocaine effect (i.e., increases locomotor activity following intracerebral injection):[n]
Locomotor sensitization	Attenuate development of cocaine effect: • BD1063[o] • BMY14802[p] • NPC 16377[g] • SN79[h] Attenuate expression of cocaine effect: • CM156[e] • SN79[h]	
Place conditioning	Attenuate development of cocaine effect: • AC927[a] • BD1047[q, r, s] • NE-100[q, s] • Progesterone[r] • Antisense confirmation[q] Attenuate expression or reactivation of cocaine effect:	Potentiate cocaine effect: • DHEA[r] • Pregnenolone[r] • Igmesine[r] No change in cocaine effect: • (+)-Pentazocine[u] Attenuate cocaine effect: • SA4503[u]

Table 9.5 Summary of effects of σ ligands on cocaine-induced behaviors—cont'd

Behavior	Antagonist effects	Agonist effects
	• BD1047[q, s] • CM156[e, t] • NE-100[q, s]	
Self-administration	No change in cocaine effect:	Mimic cocaine effect (i.e., self-administered):
	• AC927[v] • BD1047, BD1063[w] • NE-100[v]	• DTG[w] • PRE-084[w] • (+)-SKF10,047[x] Substitute for cocaine: • PRE-084[w]

[a]Matsumoto, Li, Katz, Fantegrossi, and Coop (2011).
[b]Matsumoto, McCracken, Pouw, et al. (2001).
[c]Matsumoto, McCracken, Friedman, et al. (2001).
[d]McCracken et al. (1999).
[e]Xu et al. (2010).
[f]Noorbakhsh et al. (2011).
[g]Witkin et al. (1993).
[h]Kaushal, Robson, et al. (2011).
[i]Matsumoto, Gilmore, et al. (2004).
[j]Matsumoto et al. (2002).
[k]Matsumoto, Potelleret, et al. (2004).
[l]Matsumoto (unpublished data).
[m]McCracken et al. (1999).
[n]Bastianetto, Rouquier, Perrault, and Sanger (1995), Goldstein et al. (1989).
[o]Liu and Matsumoto (2008).
[p]Ujike, Kuroda, and Otsuki (1996).
[q]Romieu, Martin-Fardon, and Maurice (2000).
[r]Romieu, Martin-Fardon, Bowen, and Maurice (2003).
[s]Romieu, Phan, Martin-Fardon, and Maurice (2002).
[t]Xu et al. (2012).
[u]Mori et al. (2012).
[v]Hiranita, Soto, Kohut, et al., 2011; Hiranita, Soto, Tanda, and Katz (2011).
[w]Hiranita, Soto, Tanda, and Katz (2010).
[x]Slifer and Balster (1983).

the left in the dose–response curve is not parallel, suggesting noncompetitive interactions between cocaine and the σ receptor agonists (Matsumoto, McCracken, Friedman, et al., 2001; Matsumoto, McCracken, Pouw, et al., 2001; Matsumoto et al., 2002). Moreover, all of the σ ligands tested that shift the cocaine dose–response curve for convulsions are mixed $\sigma_{1/2}$ agonists. The σ_1-preferring agonist (+)-pentazocine and the σ_2-preferring agonist CM398 do not significantly shift the cocaine dose–response curve for convulsions (Matsumoto, McCracken, Pouw, et al., 2001; unpublished

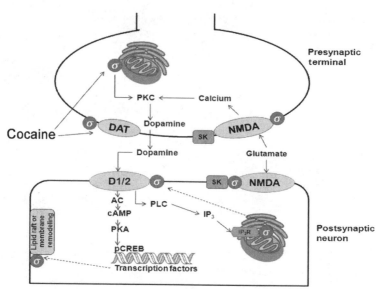

Figure 9.2 Hypothesized mechanisms through which σ receptors modulate pathways implicated in cocaine-induced behavioral actions. Cocaine interacts with σ receptors in addition to serving as an indirect dopamine agonist by blocking dopamine transporters. The release of dopamine from the presynaptic terminal can activate dopamine (D1 and D2) receptors in the midbrain, which subserve locomotor stimulation and self-administration behaviors. In addition, the activation of dopamine signaling pathways can lead to the phosphorylation of CREB and changes in gene and protein expression, including a variety of transcription factors (e.g., c-Fos, c-Jun, and ΔFosB) and σ receptors, which can lead to alterations in the morphology and structure of cells in the nervous system. Cocaine administration is also associated with increases in glutamatergic activity, and the activation of NMDA receptors is implicated in the convulsive effects of cocaine. NMDA receptors also play an important role in neuroadaptations that result upon repeated exposure to cocaine and have relevance for behaviors such as sensitization, place conditioning, and self-administration. AC, adenylyl cyclase; cAMP, cyclic AMP; CREB, cyclic AMP response element binding; D1/2, dopamine D1 and D2 receptor; DAT, dopamine transporters; IP$_3$, inositol trisphosphate; NMDA, N-methyl-D-aspartate; PKA, protein kinase A; PKC, protein kinase C; SK, small conductance calcium-activated potassium channel. (For color version of this figure, the reader is referred to the online version of this chapter.)

data), indicating that the activation of each of the subtypes alone is not sufficient to alter the cocaine response. Since σ$_{1/2}$ receptor agonists themselves do not elicit convulsions, the data suggest that the activation of σ receptors *per se* is not the primary cause of the cocaine–induced convulsions and that the modulation by σ ligands may be occurring downstream from cellular activation by cocaine of its initial target proteins.

Since glutamatergic systems are important in convulsive effects, including those produced by cocaine (Brackett, Pouw, Blyden, Nour, & Matsumoto, 2000; Rockhold, 1998), it is hypothesized that the effects of σ receptor ligands on cocaine-induced convulsions involve modulation of glutamatergic function. Selective σ receptor agonists enhance NMDA receptor function in a number of *in vitro* and *in vivo* models, which can be attenuated by σ receptor antagonists (Bermack & Debonnel, 2005; Maurice & Su, 2009; Monnet, Debonnel, & de Montigny, 1992). In addition, 5-HT$_2$ receptor antagonists can mitigate cocaine-induced convulsions (O'Dell, Kreifeldt, George, & Ritz, 2000), and there is evidence for σ receptor-mediated modulation of serotonergic function (Bermack & Debonnel, 2005).

3.2.2 Cocaine-induced lethality

Death is the ultimate toxic end point in overdose situations and can occur rapidly in humans. Therefore, it is noteworthy that σ receptor antagonists can significantly reduce the incidence of death in rodents receiving a lethal overdose of cocaine (Matsumoto, Gilmore, et al., 2004; Matsumoto et al., 2002, 2011; Matsumoto, McCracken, Friedman, et al., 2001; Matsumoto, McCracken, Pouw, et al., 2001). Most reported studies involve pretreatment of the animals to ensure that the σ receptors are occupied at the time of the cocaine overdose to establish the involvement of these proteins. Of note are the limited studies introducing σ receptor antagonists following exposure to a lethal dose of cocaine, which show that posttreatment can also significantly mitigate death. For the posttreatment dosing, the administration of σ receptor antagonists was delayed until the animals start convulsing, giving about a 2–4 min window in which death could be prevented. Even with intraperitoneal administration, the select σ receptor antagonists reported could prevent death in a significant proportion of animals (Matsumoto, McCracken, Friedman, et al., 2001; Matsumoto et al., 2002), supporting the translational potential of these types of ligands especially when other supportive measures are available in emergency situations.

In contrast to the protective effects of the antagonists, administration of the σ receptor agonist DTG shifts the dose–response curve for the lethal effects of cocaine to the left (Matsumoto, McCracken, Friedman, et al., 2001). The potential contribution of each of the σ receptor subtypes has not been investigated in this paradigm to date.

Most cocaine deaths from overdose result from respiratory depression and cardiovascular collapse. Thus, the presence of σ receptors in the lungs and heart, in addition to the brain, provides strategically placed targets for pharmacotherapeutic intervention. Very little is currently known about the function of σ receptors in the lungs, although their localization there has been confirmed by multiple research groups (Kawamura et al., 2000; Moebius et al., 1993). In the heart, σ receptors are primarily of the σ_1 subtype and are located on both parasympathetic neurons that innervate the heart and cardiac myocytes (Novakova et al., 1995; Zhang & Cuevas, 2002, 2005). σ Receptor ligands alter contractility, calcium influx, beating rate of cardiac myocytes (Ela et al., 1994; Novakova et al., 1995), and neuronal excitability through calcium (σ_1) and potassium (σ_2) channels in intracardiac neurons (Zhang & Cuevas, 2002, 2005). The multifaceted actions of σ receptors thus provide numerous modes and sites of action through which pharmacotherapeutic intervention may occur.

3.2.3 Cocaine-induced locomotor stimulation

Locomotor activity is a useful experimental measure of the stimulant actions of cocaine. Numerous σ receptor antagonists attenuate the acute locomotor-stimulant effects of cocaine, with both subtypes capable of mediating these effects (Kaushal, Robson, et al., 2011; Matsumoto et al., 2002, 2011; Matsumoto, McCracken, Friedman, et al., 2001; Noorbakhsh et al., 2011; Xu et al., 2010). σ_1-Preferring antagonists and knockdown of this subtype significantly reduce the locomotor-stimulant effects of cocaine (Matsumoto, McCracken, Friedman, et al., 2001; Matsumoto et al., 2002). Alone, antagonism of σ_1 receptors using pharmacological or molecular biological manipulations does not affect basal locomotor activity (Matsumoto et al., 2002), indicating that the treatments are preferentially targeting and normalizing dysfunctional systems rather than being crucial to normal physiological function. Similarly, antagonists for σ_2 receptors significantly attenuate the locomotor hyperactivity produced by cocaine, at doses that alone do not affect basal locomotor activity (Noorbakhsh et al., 2011).

Selective agonists for σ receptors, on the other hand, can increase locomotor behavior on their own, although these effects are most pronounced after intracerebral administration as compared to systemic injections (Bastianetto et al., 1995; Goldstein et al., 1989). With systemic injections, the actions of σ receptor agonists are mixed, with most reports indicating no significant effects on behavior at the doses tested or DTG producing a reduction in activity (Maj, Rogoz, & Skuza, 1996). The effects of σ receptor agonists on locomotor activity have yet to be tested in combination with cocaine.

The locomotor stimulation produced by cocaine is primarily mediated through the activation of dopaminergic systems in the midbrain. Thus, it is noteworthy that σ receptors are located on nigrostriatal dopamine neurons and experimental lesions of this pathway can prevent locomotor activation by selective σ receptor agonists (Goldstein et al., 1989). Moreover, the administration of selective σ receptor agonists causes the release of dopamine in the striatum (Bastianetto et al., 1995), which is thought to underlie the locomotor-activating effects of the drugs. Early pharmacological studies implicate σ_2 receptors as having an important role in motor function (Walker et al., 1993), with recent studies also confirming a role for σ_1 receptors (Mavlyutov et al., 2013). At the cellular level, it is noteworthy that σ_1 receptors form heteromers with dopamine receptors (D_1 and D_2) to modulate the function of classical dopaminergic signaling mechanisms (Navarro et al., 2010, 2013).

3.2.4 Cocaine-induced locomotor sensitization

Repeated administration of cocaine leads to increases in the behavioral response to the same dose of drug; this phenomenon is known as behavioral sensitization or reverse tolerance. It can be used as a behavioral measure of neuroadaptations that occur in the brain as a result of repeated exposure to cocaine.

The development of cocaine-induced locomotor sensitization is accompanied by a concomitant increase in the expression of σ_1 receptors in the striatum and cortex, but not the cerebellum (Liu & Matsumoto, 2008). The striatum and cortex are brain regions that are implicated in the effects of cocaine, while the cerebellum contains high concentrations of σ receptors, but is not typically associated with the actions of cocaine. This suggests that σ_1 receptors in brain regions known to mediate cocaine effects are involved in the altered behavioral response to repeated cocaine exposures. The specific role of the σ_2 subtype has not yet been studied in locomotor sensitization models.

Administration of σ receptor antagonists, including σ_1-preferring antagonists, can attenuate the development of cocaine-induced locomotor sensitization (Kaushal, Robson, et al., 2011; Liu & Matsumoto, 2008). Moreover, antagonist treatment also prevents the expected cocaine-induced increases in σ_1 receptor gene and protein expression in the striatum and cortex (Liu & Matsumoto, 2008). These data thus support the importance of alterations in σ_1 receptor expression on the behavioral consequences of cocaine.

Of the many changes in gene and protein expression that occur after cocaine exposure, a σ_1 receptor-dependent upregulation of D-type potassium (Kv1.2) currents in the nucleus accumbens also appears particularly relevant for the sensitized response to cocaine (Kourrich et al., 2013). Repeated exposure to cocaine results in persistent protein–protein interactions between σ_1 receptors and Kv1.2 channels, which results in neuronal hypoactivity in the nucleus accumbens and behavioral sensitization (Kourrich et al., 2013). Inhibition of σ_1 receptor function using either pharmacological antagonists or adeno-associated viral vectors into the nucleus accumbens attenuates these responses (Kourrich et al., 2013).

Even after the behavioral sensitization to repeated cocaine exposures is allowed to occur, introduction of a σ receptor antagonist can eliminate the expression of the sensitized response (Kaushal, Robson, et al., 2011; Xu et al., 2010). This is observed after a single dose of antagonist suggesting that a sufficiently high dose of antagonist can mask the functional ramifications of the increased expression of σ_1 receptors. The translational implications of the expression of sensitization experiments are noteworthy since they suggest that introduction of σ receptor ligands to individuals who are already exposed to cocaine and subject to resulting neuroadaptations can produce significant changes in behavior.

3.2.5 Cocaine-induced place conditioning

Place conditioning is an experimental measure of the rewarding effects of drugs; it has also been proposed as a model of drug seeking. When animals are repeatedly exposed to drugs that are rewarding in a particular environment, they form an association with environmental cues such that they demonstrate a preference for that environment even in the absence of drug.

Cocaine produces robust place conditioning. Administration of σ receptor antagonists significantly attenuates the development of cocaine-induced place conditioning (Matsumoto et al., 2011; Romieu et al., 2000, 2002). The σ_1 subtype is implicated in this effect, as σ_1-preferring antagonists and antisense knockdown prevent the development of cocaine-induced place conditioning (Romieu et al., 2000). Moreover, progesterone, a neurosteroid that acts as a σ_1 receptor antagonist under a variety of conditions, produces similar effects as other σ_1 receptor antagonists and antisense knockdown (Romieu et al., 2003). In contrast, dehydroepiandrosterone (DHEA) and pregnenolone, neurosteroids that act as putative σ_1 agonists, enhance cocaine-induced place conditioning similar to the σ receptor agonist igmesine (Romieu et al., 2003). Reminiscent of the pattern observed with behavioral sensitization, repeated exposure to cocaine in the place conditioning paradigm is accompanied by an increase in σ_1 receptor gene expression in the nucleus accumbens (Romieu et al., 2002). Although the body of data indicates that σ_1 receptor antagonists attenuate place conditioning to cocaine while agonists enhance it, there are some exceptions. One research group has reported that the σ_1 receptor agonist (+)-pentazocine has no significant effects on the development of cocaine-induced place conditioning, while 1-(3,4-dimethoxyphenethyl)-4-(3-phenylpropyl)piperazine (SA4503) attenuates it (Mori et al., 2012); the reason(s) these particular ligands produce different effects from the other agonists remains unknown. The specific role of σ_2 receptors in cocaine-induced place conditioning has not yet been investigated.

When place conditioning to cocaine is allowed to occur before intervention with σ receptor antagonists, the expression of cocaine-induced place conditioning is being tested. This posttreatment experimental paradigm (expression of place conditioning) is of particular translational relevance as addicts will already have been exposed to cocaine with the resulting neuroadaptations in place before pharmacotherapies are introduced. σ Receptor antagonists, including σ_1-preferring antagonists, can mask the expression of the conditioned response to cocaine (Romieu et al., 2002; Xu et al., 2010). Moreover, σ receptor antagonists and antisense targeting σ_1 can inhibit reactivation of the conditioned response to cocaine following a period of abstinence from cocaine in animals who have previously acquired the conditioned response (Romieu et al., 2004). In contrast, σ_1 receptor agonists themselves can precipitate the reactivation of the conditioned response in a σ receptor antagonist-sensitive manner (Romieu et al., 2004). Similar to other behavioral studies involving repeated cocaine exposure, *in vivo* administration of $[^3H](+)$-SKF10,047 to mice at various stages of the reactivation experiments reveals sustained, elevated binding in numerous brain regions in animals exposed to cocaine (Romieu et al., 2004), suggesting that cocaine exposure causes upregulation of σ_1 receptors. Thus, it is anticipated that treatment with σ receptor antagonists has the potential to reduce cocaine-seeking behaviors.

Microarray profiling of gene expression in the whole brain following place conditioning with cocaine reveals that even after a single treatment with a σ receptor antagonist in the expression of place conditioning experiment, there is significant reversal of cocaine-induced alterations in numerous genes (Xu et al., 2012). The ability of σ receptor antagonism to mitigate the cocaine-induced expression of select genes is particularly robust as they appear in all analysis methods: metastasis-associated lung adenocarcinoma transcript 1, tyrosine 3-monooxygenase/tryptophan 5-monooxygenase activation protein, and transthyretin (Xu et al., 2012). A common theme is the involvement of these genes in processes related to neuroplasticity and RNA editing (Xu et al., 2012).

3.2.6 Cocaine-induced self-administration

Similar to humans, laboratory animals will self-administer cocaine. σ Receptor antagonists do not prevent self-administration of cocaine (Hiranita, Soto, Kohut, et al., 2011, Hiranita, Soto, Tanda, & Katz, 2011; Hiranita et al., 2010). However, animals can be taught to self-administer σ receptor agonists, and σ receptor agonists will substitute for cocaine indicating that they have the potential to be used as replacement therapies (Hiranita et al., 2010). The substitution of cocaine with σ receptor agonists in self-administration paradigms appears to be mediated through σ receptors because this effect is attenuated by σ receptor antagonists (Hiranita et al., 2010).

This substitution mechanism is somewhat complex because σ receptor agonists lack cocaine-like discriminative stimulus effects (Hiranita, Soto, Tanda, & Katz, 2011). However, animals acquire self-administration to σ receptor agonists more readily if they have previously self-administered cocaine (Hiranita, Mereu, Soto, Tanda, & Katz, 2013), suggesting that cocaine induces neuroadaptations that facilitate self-administration of σ receptor agonists. Interesting, in both cocaine-experienced and naïve rats, the administration of doses of σ receptor agonists that are self-administered is not accompanied by increases in dopamine release from the nucleus accumbens, suggesting that the σ receptor agonists are substituting for cocaine through a dopamine-independent mechanism (Hiranita et al., 2013). Additional studies are warranted to identify the unique mechanisms that support this effect as they could serve as novel targets for the development of new therapies for the treatment of cocaine addiction.

3.3. Effects of cocaine on nonneuronal cells

σ Receptors also modulate the actions of cocaine on cells other than neurons: endothelial cells, microglia, and leukocytes. All of these effects have implications for BBB function, which are summarized in the succeeding text.

3.3.1 Endothelial cells

Human brain microvascular endothelial cells (HBMECs) are a major cell type of the BBB. Cocaine upregulates an isoform of platelet-derived growth factor (PDGF) in these cells, which is associated with the disruption of the BBB (Yao, Duan, & Buch, 2011). The increased expression of PDGF appears mediated through extracellular signal-regulated kinase (ERK)1/2 and c-Jun N-terminal kinase (JNK) signaling and subsequent activation of the transcription factor EGR-1 (Yao, Duan, et al., 2011). Pretreatment of HBMECs with the σ receptor antagonist N-[2-(3,4-dichlorophenyl) ethyl]-N-methyl-2-(dimethylamino)ethylamine (BD1047) or knockdown of σ_1 receptors attenuates EGR-1 expression, with a subsequent decrease in PDGF expression (Yao, Duan, et al., 2011). These studies provide the first evidence that σ_1 receptors mediate effects of cocaine on the BBB.

3.3.2 Microglia
Cocaine abuse by individuals infected with human immunodeficiency virus (HIV) is associated with increased BBB permeability and monocyte migration into the CNS, which is believed to contribute to enhanced cognitive impairments in this cohort (Eugenin et al., 2006; Fiala et al., 1998). A major determinant of increased monocyte migration is monocyte chemoattractant protein 1 (MCP-1). In BV-2 microglial cells, the induction of MCP-1 by cocaine is dependent on σ_1 receptor translocation to lipid raft microdomains along with the activation of ERK and Akt signaling pathways (Yao et al., 2010). The σ receptor antagonist BD1047 or knockdown of σ_1 receptors has been shown to prevent the cocaine-induced activation of ERK and Akt signaling, as well as induction of MCP-1 expression (Yao et al., 2010). Moreover, BD1047 also attenuates monocyte transmigration in a BBB model *in vitro* and *in vivo* (Yao et al., 2010).

3.3.3 Leukocytes
The transport of leukocytes, and to a lesser extent other immune cells, across the BBB is facilitated in HIV-infected individuals who also abuse cocaine due to increased activated leukocyte cell-adhesion molecule (ALCAM) in the endothelium (Yao, Duan, et al., 2011, Yao, Kim, et al., 2011). Recent studies show that cocaine causes the translocation of σ_1 receptors to the plasma membrane, resulting in the phosphorylation of platelet-derived growth factor β receptors through a direct interaction with σ receptors (Yao, Kim, et al., 2011). This phosphorylation induces ERK, JNK, p38, and Akt signaling, resulting in the activation of the transcription factor nuclear factor-kappa B (NF-κB) and a corresponding increase in ALCAM expression (Yao, Kim, et al., 2011). The σ receptor antagonist BD1047 attenuates cocaine-induced activation of ERK, JNK, p38, and Akt signaling,

with a reduction in ALCAM expression (Yao, Kim, et al., 2011). Knock-down of σ_1 receptors also mitigates cocaine-induced activation of NF-κB (Yao, Kim, et al., 2011). Together, the studies demonstrate that σ_1 receptors influence BBB function through a variety of mechanisms and cell types.

4. METHAMPHETAMINE AND σ RECEPTORS

4.1. Background

Among the psychostimulants, methamphetamine distinguishes itself as one of the most abused substances worldwide (United Nations Office on Drugs, 2010). In the United States, over 12 million Americans have used metham-phetamine at least once in their life (Substance Abuse & Health Services Administration, 2009), and there are roughly 16 million users of metham-phetamine worldwide, a number which exceeds that of combined heroin and cocaine users (United Nations Office on Drugs, 2010). In 2005, an esti-mated 20–40 billion dollars was spent on methamphetamine-related com-plications stemming from addiction, premature death, and psychosocial treatment (Nicosia, Pacula, Kilmer, Lundberg, & Chiesa, 2009).

Similar to cocaine, no FDA-approved medications exist to assist with treating the negative health consequences resulting from methamphetamine abuse (Jupp & Lawrence, 2010). Methamphetamine interacts with brain σ receptors at physiologically relevant concentrations and exhibits a slight preference for the σ_1 (2 μM) compared to the σ_2 (47 μM) subtype (Nguyen, McCracken, Liu, Pouw, & Matsumoto, 2005). Methamphet-amine appears to act as an agonist at σ receptors. It has competitive inter-actions with the σ_1 binding site (labeled with [^{3}H](+)-pentazocine) (Nguyen et al., 2005), but the nature with which it interacts with protein partners such as glucose-regulated protein BiP can be atypical compared to other σ receptor agonists (Hayashi & Su, 2007).

Both σ receptor subtypes appear to mediate the actions of methamphet-amine (Kaushal & Matsumoto, 2011). Selectively manipulating the σ_1 sub-type can produce changes in methamphetamine effects (Nguyen et al., 2005; Rodvelt et al., 2011), although the effects are modest compared to when mixed $\sigma_{1/2}$ ligands are used. Based on the literature, σ_2 receptors are hypothesized to mediate many actions of methamphetamine (Kaushal & Matsumoto, 2011), but direct testing has been delayed due to the dearth of truly selective ligands for this subtype, which are suitable for use *in vivo*; the recent development of such tools will enable such studies in the future.

4.2. Behavioral and physiological effects of methamphetamine *in vivo*

Table 9.6 summarizes the actions of σ receptor ligands against a variety of behavioral and physiological effects of methamphetamine in preclinical studies. Similar to cocaine, methamphetamine produces acute stimulant effects, which can be measured experimentally as alterations in locomotor activity. In addition, repeated exposure to methamphetamine can cause neuroadaptations in the brain that manifest behaviorally as sensitization and self-administration. The involvement of σ receptors in these effects has only just begun to be evaluated and is summarized in the succeeding text.

4.2.1 Locomotor activity and sensitization

Acute stimulant effects: Methamphetamine causes biphasic effects on locomotor activity, which manifest as locomotor-stimulant effects at lower doses and a diminution of this effect at higher doses presumably due to the onset of competing stereotyped behaviors. Similar to the pattern of data observed against the stimulant effects of cocaine, σ receptor antagonists attenuate locomotor hyperactivity produced by methamphetamine (Kaushal, Seminerio, et al., 2011; Nguyen et al., 2005; Seminerio, Robson, Abdelazeem, et al., 2012). This attenuation involves a reduction in the maximal effect of methamphetamine, which may or may not also be accompanied by a shift to the right in the dose–response curve (Kaushal, Seminerio, et al., 2011; Nguyen et al., 2005). It is hypothesized that the reduction in maximal effect is associated with antagonism of σ_1 receptors, while the shift to the right is mediated through σ_2 receptors (Kaushal, Seminerio, et al., 2011). The involvement of the σ_1 subtype is suggested by the ability of antisense knockdown to attenuate the locomotor-stimulant effects of methamphetamine (Nguyen et al., 2005). However, it should be noted that methamphetamine can still produce locomotor-stimulant effects in σ_1 knockout mice (Fontanilla et al., 2009). It is hypothesized that in the σ_1 knockout mice, there may be compensatory effects through σ_2 receptors, which have a known role in motor functions.

The effects of σ receptor agonists on the locomotor-stimulant effects of methamphetamine appear complex, and more work is needed in this area. Thus far, only the σ_1 receptor agonist SA4503 has been tested, and depending on dose, it can both enhance and attenuate the locomotor-stimulant effects of methamphetamine. Low-dose (1 mg/kg) SA4503 potentiates the methamphetamine effect (Rodvelt et al., 2011), as may be

Table 9.6 Summary of effects of σ ligands on methamphetamine (METH) effects *in vivo*

Behavior	Antagonist effects	Agonist effects
Locomotor activity	Attenuate METH effect: • AC927[a] • AZ66[b] • BD1047[c] • BD1063[c] • CM156[d] • Antisense confirmation[c]	Potentiate and attenuate METH effect: • SA4503[e]
Locomotor sensitization	Attenuate development of METH effect: • AZ66[b] • BMY14802[f] • MS377[g] Attenuate expression of METH effect: • AZ66[b]	Not tested
Drug discrimination	• Not tested	Enhance METH effect: • SA4503[e]
Hyperthermia	Attenuate METH effect: • AC927[a] • AZ66[h] • CM156[d] • SN79[i]	Mimic METH effect (i.e., increases body temperature): • DTG[i]
Neurotoxicity (dopamine)	Attenuate METH effect: • AC927[a] • AZ66[h] • BMY14802[j] • CM156[d] • SN79[i]	Not tested—caused lethality in combination with METH
Neurotoxicity (serotonin)	Attenuate METH effect: • AC927[k] • CM156[d] • SN79[i]	Not tested—caused lethality in combination with METH

Table 9.6 Summary of effects of σ ligands on methamphetamine (METH) effects *in vivo*—cont'd

Behavior	Antagonist effects	Agonist effects
Neurotoxicity (cognition)	Attenuate METH effect: • AZ66[h]	Not tested

[a]Matsumoto et al. (2008).
[b]Seminerio, Robson, Abdelazeem, et al. (2012).
[c]Nguyen et al. (2005).
[d]Kaushal, Seminerio, et al., 2011.
[e]Rodvelt et al. (2011).
[f]Ujike, Kanazaki, Okumura, Akiyama, and Otsuki (1992).
[g]Takahashi, Miwa, and Horikomi (2000).
[h]Seminerio et al. (2013).
[i]Kaushal, Seminerio, Robson, McCurdy, and Matsumoto (2013).
[j]Terleckyj and Sonsalla (1994).
[k]Seminerio et al. (2011).

expected of an agonist. However, higher doses (10 and 30 mg/kg) of SA4503 elicit a paradoxical attenuation of the stimulant effects of methamphetamine, with the highest dose also producing sedation on its own (Rodvelt et al., 2011). It is unclear whether this biphasic pattern of response is typical of σ receptor agonists or specific to SA4503; testing of additional σ receptor agonists, including σ_2-selective ligands, is still needed.

Behavioral sensitization: Repeated dosing with methamphetamine elicits locomotor sensitization. Recent and early studies concur that σ receptor antagonists prevent the development of locomotor sensitization to methamphetamine (Seminerio, Robson, Abdelazeem, et al., 2012; Takahashi et al., 2000; Ujike et al., 1992). Moreover, the expression of methamphetamine-induced locomotor sensitization can be masked by administration of a σ receptor antagonist (Seminerio, Robson, Abdelazeem, et al., 2012). Although additional studies are needed to determine the involvement of each of the σ receptor subtypes in these effects, the data suggest that similar to the pattern seen with cocaine, σ receptor antagonists have the ability to mitigate neuroadaptations that result from repeated exposures to methamphetamine. The effects of selective σ receptor agonists on methamphetamine-induced locomotor sensitization remain unknown. Although not studied specifically in the context of behavioral sensitization, repeated dosing with methamphetamine also increases σ_1 receptor expression in several brain regions, including the substantia nigra (Itzhak, 1993), which is an important neurobiological substrate for mediating motor effects.

4.2.2 Self-administration

Similar to humans, laboratory animals self-administer methamphetamine, which can cause neuroadaptations that are believed to sustain addiction-related behaviors. Although the effects of σ receptor antagonists and agonists on methamphetamine self-administration remain unreported, there is evidence that $σ_1$ receptors are upregulated in several brain regions in rodents that self-administer methamphetamine (Hayashi et al., 2010; Stefanski et al., 2004). Moreover, some of these changes are specific to self-administering animals, as compared to yoked controls who passively receive the same amount of methamphetamine (Hayashi et al., 2010; Stefanski et al., 2004).

The upregulation of $σ_1$ receptors in methamphetamine self-administering animals is further accompanied by a concomitant increase in ERK and a decrease in protein kinase A (PKA) (Hayashi et al., 2010). This decrease in PKA expression coupled with the ability of $σ_1$ receptors to modulate cAMP signaling upstream of PKA through its interactions with dopamine D_1 receptors (Navarro et al., 2010) may be one molecular mechanism by which σ receptors can mediate neuronal signaling believed to be crucial in psychostimulant-mediated neuroplastic changes that manifest as addictive behaviors (Chen, Chen, & Chiang, 2009). The evidence in further support of this hypothesis is studies where σ receptor activation results in CREB phosphorylation in a PKA-dependent manner (Yang, Alkayed, Hurn, & Kirsch, 2009), an effect believed to be involved in the neuroadaptations associated with repeated psychostimulant exposure (Chen et al., 2009). Additionally, it has been shown that $σ_1$ receptors also colocalize with dopamine D_2 receptors where they can modulate dopamine D_2-mediated ERK signaling (Navarro et al., 2013). Although many of these studies used cocaine to elicit dopamine receptor activation, it is believed that these signaling pathways are ubiquitous in mediating addictive behaviors (Chen et al., 2009; Hyman & Malenka, 2001) and may be relevant to the actions of σ receptors in the self-administration of psychostimulants, including methamphetamine. Additionally, they show that alterations in $σ_1$ receptor expression are linked to repeated psychostimulant exposure under various conditions and that these changes may confer a functional component that has yet to be fully elucidated.

4.2.3 Hyperthermia

Exposure to high doses of methamphetamine elicits hyperthermia, which is a principal cause of death resulting from methamphetamine overdose (Bowyer et al., 1994). Methamphetamine also elevates body temperature in laboratory animals in a dose-dependent manner to lethal levels (Bowyer et al., 1994). In preclinical studies, numerous σ receptor antagonists attenuate the hyperthermic effects of methamphetamine (Kaushal et al., 2013; Kaushal, Seminerio, et al., 2011; Matsumoto et al., 2008; Seminerio, Robson, McCurdy, et al., 2012). At higher doses, some of the antagonists also reduce basal body temperature (Kaushal et al., 2013; Seminerio et al., 2013). All of the compounds tested thus far are mixed $\sigma_{1/2}$ antagonists, and studies have yet to determine the contribution of each of the σ receptor subtypes. Administration of the σ receptor agonist DTG alone increases body temperature, but does not further exacerbate methamphetamine hyperthermia (Kaushal et al., 2013).

The mechanisms underlying the effects of the σ receptor ligands on body temperature remain unknown. Potential σ-mediated modulation of hypothalamic mechanisms is possible since σ receptors are localized in this and related brain regions with thermoregulatory functions (Bouchard & Quirion, 1997; McLean & Weber, 1988). Although the specific mechanisms have yet to be determined, they do not appear to involve modulation of interleukin-1β (Seminerio, Robson, McCurdy, et al., 2012). There is a clinical need to better understand this phenomenon because elevations in body temperature not only increase the risk of death in overdose situations but also are associated with increased neurotoxicity (Bowyer et al., 1994; Kaushal et al., 2013; Robson, Seminerio, McCurdy, Coop, & Matsumoto, 2013).

4.2.4 Neurotoxicity

Methamphetamine can cause neurotoxicity, with damage to the striatum as a predominant feature (Krasnova & Cadet, 2009). In humans, significant reductions in DATs and serotonin transporters (SERTs) in the striatum and cortex result in functional deficits in cognition, attention, and motor control with an increased risk for developing Parkinson's disease (Callaghan, Cunningham, Sykes, & Kish, 2012; Gonzalez, Bechara, & Martin, 2007; Hart, Marvin, Silver, & Smith, 2012; Sekine et al., 2001, 2003, 2006; Volkow, Chang, Wang, Fowler, Franceschi, et al. et al., 2001; Volkow, Chang, Wang, Fowler, Leonido-Yee, et al., 2001; Woods et al., 2005).

Dopamine deficits: Experimental animals also exhibit reductions in striatal dopamine and DAT following neurotoxic dosing with methamphetamine (Krasnova & Cadet, 2009). σ Receptor antagonists, which attenuate the hyperthermic effects of methamphetamine, also mitigate dopaminergic neurotoxicity (Kaushal et al., 2013; Kaushal, Seminerio, et al., 2011; Matsumoto et al., 2008; Seminerio et al., 2013). Pretreatment with the compounds can achieve nearly complete protection at the most effective doses. The protective effects when administered as a posttreatment following neurotoxic dosing with methamphetamine are modest (about 25%) (Kaushal et al., 2013) but are likely sufficient to convey therapeutic benefits under clinically relevant conditions (e.g., keep patients asymptomatic of Parkinson's disease).

Serotonin deficits: Similarly, methamphetamine-induced deficits in serotonin levels and SERT expression in the striatum occur following neurotoxic exposures (Krasnova & Cadet, 2009). Compared to the dopamine deficits, higher doses of methamphetamine are needed to produce serotonin neurotoxicity, which is consistent with the higher affinity of methamphetamine for DAT compared to SERT (Han & Gu, 2006), as well as its greater release of dopamine compared to serotonin in the striatum (Gough, Imam, Blough, Slikker, & Ali, 2002). The serotonergic neurotoxicity can be mitigated by pretreatment with σ receptor antagonists (Kaushal et al., 2013; Kaushal, Seminerio, et al., 2011; Seminerio et al., 2011). For both the serotonin and dopamine neurotoxicity studies, testing with σ receptor agonists in combination with methamphetamine is deterred by deaths, whereby there is a significant increase in lethality in the presence of σ receptor agonists compared to neurotoxic dosing with methamphetamine alone (Kaushal et al., 2013).

4.3. Neuroprotective mechanisms

The cellular mechanisms underlying the neuroprotective effects of σ receptor antagonists against methamphetamine deficits appear quite diverse (Fig. 9.3). *In vivo* and *in vitro* studies concur that methamphetamine triggers numerous cell death and damage pathways including ER stress and caspase activation through both Fas/FasL death receptor and mitochondrial death pathways (Krasnova & Cadet, 2009). In addition, reactive oxygen species (ROS) and reactive nitrogen species (RNS) are released and stimulate these various pathways (Krasnova & Cadet, 2009).

Recent studies have shown that σ receptor antagonists intervene at many of these known pathways. Using an NG108-15 model system, ROS/RNS generated by methamphetamine is mitigated by σ receptor antagonists (Kaushal, 2012; Kaushal et al., 2012). The antagonists appear to target caspase-dependent pathways as they can attenuate methamphetamine-induced increases in caspases 3, 8, and 9, suggesting the involvement of both extrinsic death receptors and intrinsic mitochondrial death pathways (Kaushal, 2012; Kaushal, McCurdy, & Matsumoto, 2011). Although

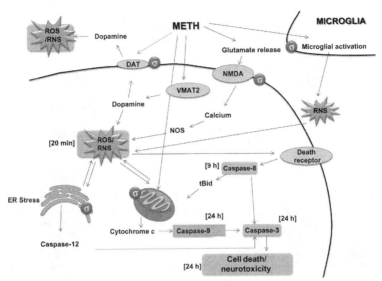

Figure 9.3 Hypothesized mechanisms through which σ receptors modulate the neurotoxic effects of methamphetamine. Methamphetamine (METH) stimulates dopamine and glutamate release, which can lead to the generation of reactive oxygen species (ROS) and reactive nitrogen species (RNS). Subsequently, the activation of caspases and onset of cytotoxicity, which have been reported to occur within 9–24 h of neurotoxic methamphetamine exposure *in vitro* and *in vivo*, may be triggered through (i) ER stress, (ii) cytochrome *c*, and (iii) Fas/FasL death receptor pathways, each of which can contribute to cell death and/or damage *in vitro* and *in vivo*. σ Receptors can intervene at a number of points in this process by modulating calcium-dependent mechanisms associated with the ER and mitochondria in neurons and/or activating microglia. σ Receptors may also form protein–protein interactions to modulate *N*-methyl-D-aspartate (NMDA) and dopamine transporter (DAT) function. (For color version of this figure, the reader is referred to the online version of this chapter.)

methamphetamine can also trigger ER stress in NG108-15 cells, with the PKR-like ER kinase (PERK) pathway significantly stimulated, σ receptor antagonism does not appear to mitigate these changes (Robson, 2013; Robson, McCurdy, & Matsumoto, 2012), demonstrating that there is some mechanistic selectivity to the ability of σ receptor antagonists to convey neuroprotective actions. Additional studies to validate the proposed σ-mediated mechanisms, especially *in vivo*, are needed, as well as additional studies to delineate the σ receptor subtypes involved.

4.4. Methamphetamine and glia

In addition to their localization in neurons, σ receptors are found in a variety of glia, including microglia and astrocytes (Ruscher et al., 2011).

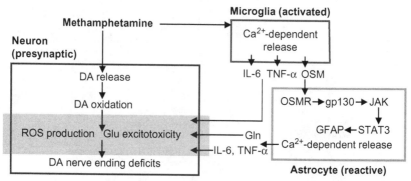

Figure 9.4 Hypothesized mechanisms through which glial cells modulate the neurotoxic effects of methamphetamine. The activation of microglia and astrocytes by methamphetamine is hypothesized to amplify cellular neuronal processes that contribute to dopaminergic neurotoxicity. In addition to its well-characterized effects on neurons, methamphetamine can cause the activation of microglia and subsequent release of proinflammatory cytokines. Along with damaging neurons, these inflammatory mediators can lead to the activation of astrocytes, which can then release additional proinflammatory cytokines and glutamine. These astrocytic molecules can then act on neurons to trigger excitotoxic cascades and reactive oxygen species to further amplify the oxidative stress burden on the presynaptic neuron to promote neurotoxicity. σ Receptor ligands are hypothesized to mitigate these responses by modulating intracellular calcium-dependent processes in each of the cell types. DA, dopamine; IL-6, interleukin 6; Gln, glutamine; Glu, glutamate; gp130, glycoprotein 130; JAK, Janus kinase; OSM, oncostatin M; OSMR, oncostatin M receptor; ROS, reactive oxygen species; STAT3, signal transducer and activator of transcription factor 3; TNF-α, tissue necrosis factor-α. (For color version of this figure, the reader is referred to the online version of this chapter.)

Accumulating evidence implicates the importance of glia, in addition to neurons, in understanding the effects of methamphetamine. Methamphetamine-induced activation of glial mechanisms may precede or occur in parallel to those affecting neurons and have implications for both the neurotoxic and stimulant effects of psychostimulant actions, which are discussed in the succeeding text. Potential mechanisms through which glia may influence the neurotoxic effects of methamphetamine are summarized in Fig. 9.4.

4.4.1 Microglia

Microglia are the resident macrophages in the CNS and become activated when they detect perturbations in their surrounding environment (Saijo & Glass, 2011). There are two classically defined types of microglia, denoted M1 (associated with inflammation and degeneration) and M2 (associated with regeneration and anti-inflammatory processes) (Perry, Nicoll, &

Holmes, 2010). Accumulating evidence indicates that methamphetamine causes rapid activation of microglia in both humans and experimental animals (Sekine et al., 2008; Thomas et al., 2004). This effect is believed to contribute to the neurotoxic effects of methamphetamine because it (i) occurs in regions of the brain susceptible to neurotoxicity, (ii) is persistent and long-lasting in affected brain regions even after extended abstinence from methamphetamine, and (iii) is accompanied by the upregulation of proinflammatory cytokines such as interleukin 6 (IL-6) in affected brain regions (Kelly, Miller, Bowyer, & O'Callaghan, 2012; Robson, Seminerio, et al., 2013, Robson, Turner, et al., 2013; Sekine et al., 2008).

6-Acetyl-3-(4-(4-(4-fluorophenyl)piperazin-1-yl)butyl)benzo[d]oxazol-2(3H)-one (SN79), a σ receptor antagonist, prevents methamphetamine-induced microglial activation and cytokine production *in vivo*, providing a novel mechanism for mitigating the neurotoxic effects of methamphetamine. Pretreatment with SN79 prior to neurotoxic dosing with methamphetamine in experimental animals prevents cluster of differentiation 68 (CD68) and ionized calcium-binding adapter molecule 1 (IBA-1) upregulation in the striatum, two classical markers of microglial activation (Robson, Turner, et al., 2013). In addition, SN79 attenuates methamphetamine-induced upregulation of several genes in the striatum that are members of the IL-6 family of cytokines: interleukin-6, oncostatin M, and leukemia inhibitory factor (Robson, Turner, et al., 2013). The therapeutic effects of SN79 appear to target M1 microglia, with M2 microglia showing no significant changes to methamphetamine and/or SN79 exposure under the experimental conditions (Robson, Turner, et al., 2013), indicating attenuation of the detrimental consequences of microglial activation rather than activation of regenerative processes.

σ Receptor ligands modulate microglial activation and migration through alterations in intracellular calcium levels (Cuevas, Rodriguez, Behensky, & Katnik, 2011; Hall, Herrera, Ajmo, Cuevas, & Pennypacker, 2009). Each of the σ receptor subtypes is involved in these responses and is recruited by an array of microglial activators, including adenosine triphosphate, uridine triphosphate, lipopolysaccharide, and monocyte chemoattractant protein-1 (MCP-1) (Cuevas et al., 2011; Hall et al., 2009; Yao et al., 2010). It is likely that methamphetamine and/or SN79 operates through similar mechanisms.

4.4.2 Astrocytes

Astrocytes are activated in response to a variety of CNS insults, including exposure to methamphetamine. The activation of astrocytes is characterized by morphological changes and increased expression of glial fibrillary acidic protein (GFAP), through a process known as astrogliosis (Raivich et al., 1999). Similar to many other neurotoxicants, neurotoxic dosing with methamphetamine induces astrogliosis by activating Janus kinase 2 (JAK2)/signal transducer and activator of transcription factor 3 (STAT3) signaling through glycoprotein 130 (gp130)-linked cytokine signaling (Hebert & O'Callaghan, 2000). The associated methamphetamine-induced increases in astrocytic oncostatin M receptor expression and the phosphorylation of STAT3 are prevented by pretreatment with SN79, a σ receptor antagonist (Robson, 2013). SN79 also prevents the resulting morphological changes and increased GFAP expression following JAK2/STAT3 activation caused by neurotoxic methamphetamine exposure (Robson, 2013). The involvement of each of the σ receptor subtypes in these effects remains to be determined, as well as the implications of these changes for both the neurotoxic and nontoxic effects of methamphetamine.

5. CLINICAL IMPLICATIONS

No selective σ receptor ligands are currently approved by the FDA for use in humans. Thus, this section summarizes efforts to repurpose non-selective medications with σ affinity for psychostimulant applications, efforts to develop more selective σ ligands for clinical use, and efforts to develop selective σ ligands as suitable CNS imaging agents.

5.1. Repurposing of medications with σ affinity for psychostimulant-related indications

Many marketed medications have significant affinity for σ receptors, and some have been tested for psychostimulant-related conditions: haloperidol, bupropion, donepezil, DHEA, and sertraline. Although it is difficult to ascertain whether the clinical results from the repurposed medications reflect actions through σ receptors, under preclinical conditions, there is evidence that each of these drugs can impart functional activity through σ receptors by altering receptor levels using pharmacological agents or molecular biological manipulations that selectively target σ receptors. Therefore, the observations summarized in the succeeding text should be confirmed through the testing of selective σ ligands in the future.

Haloperidol: Haloperidol is an antipsychotic generally classified as a dopamine D_2 antagonist. It has high affinity for both σ_1 and σ_2 receptors and has been reported to act as an antagonist or agonist at these receptors depending on the experimental conditions. In a small cohort of cocaine-dependent individuals, it reduced craving and anxiety following exposure to cocaine cues (Berger et al., 1996).

Bupropion: Bupropion is a smoking-cessation agent generally classified as a dopamine and norepinephrine reuptake inhibitor. It also appears to act as an agonist through σ receptors (Dhir & Kulkarni, 2008). Bupropion has been reported to decrease methamphetamine use in "light" users, although "heavy" users do not benefit (Shoptaw, Heinzerling, Rotheram-Fuller, Steward, et al., 2008). It also reduces smoking in these patients (Shoptaw, Heinzerling, Rotheram-Fuller, Steward, et al., 2008). However, bupropion appears ineffective at treating cocaine addicts when coupled with cognitive behavioral therapy, as evidenced by a lack of reduction in cocaine craving and usage (Shoptaw, Heinzerling, Rotheram-Fuller, Kao, et al., 2008).

Donepezil: Donepezil is a cognitive enhancer generally classified as an acetylcholinesterase inhibitor. It also binds to σ_1 receptors, where it acts as an agonist (Ishikawa et al., 2009; Maurice, Meunier, Feng, Ieni, & Monaghan, 2006). Donepezil has been reported to provide significant overall improvement in low-dose cocaine treatment but fails to produce effects against a higher dose of cocaine (Grasing, Mathur, Newton, & DeSouza, 2010). In a separate study, donepezil failed to decrease cocaine intake in outpatients (Winhusen et al., 2005). However, donepezil has been reported to improve cognitive performance in a severe and chronic methamphetamine abuser (Jovanovski & Zakzanis, 2003) and suggested to reduce craving (Kuehn, 2006).

DHEA: DHEA is generally considered a neurosteroid. It has also been proposed as an endogenous ligand for σ_1 receptors, where it has agonist actions (Monnet & Maurice, 2006). DHEA does not appear suitable for treating cocaine abuse and has in fact been reported to enhance cocaine use and decrease treatment retention (Shoptaw et al., 2004).

Sertraline: Sertraline is an antidepressant drug generally classified as a selective serotonin reuptake inhibitor. It also has significant affinity for σ receptors, particularly the σ_1 subtype where it is thought to act as an agonist (Fishback et al., 2010). Sertraline has been reported ineffective in treating cocaine addiction in an outpatient setting (Winhusen et al., 2005). It also appears ineffective against methamphetamine with or without contingency management, decreasing retention (without contingency management) and also failing to reduce craving or depressive symptoms (Shoptaw et al., 2006).

5.2. Clinical trials of σ ligands for CNS indications

No selective σ receptor ligands are yet undergoing human clinical trials for psychostimulant-related effects. However, it should be noted that a number of σ receptor ligands are currently being tested in clinical trials for an array of CNS-related disorders. They include the following: SA4503 (cutamesine) a σ_1 agonist for depression and neurodegeneration, S1RA (E-52862) a σ_1 antagonist for pain, and ANAVEX2-73 a mixed σ_1/muscarinic ligand for Alzheimer's disease.

In addition, several other σ ligands have earlier undergone human clinical trials for CNS-related conditions: igmesine for depression, panamesine for schizophrenia, and opipramol for anxiety. They vary in efficacy for their targeted indications and elicit few major side effects, suggesting that they may be amenable to repurposing or further investigation. Such efforts may facilitate future testing of σ ligands for psychostimulant-related conditions.

Igmesine: The σ_1 receptor agonist igmesine has been tested for major depression and shown to be as effective as fluoxetine with reduced side effects initially in an open-label trial, which was followed by a double-blind, placebo-controlled trial (Fishback et al., 2010). A subsequent clinical trial, however, was inconclusive due to a high placebo-response rate and equivocal outcomes in eastern European populations compared to the United Kingdom (Volz & Stoll, 2004).

Panamesine: Also known as EMD57445, panamesine has high affinity for both σ_1 and σ_2 receptors. It has been tested for schizophrenia in three open-label trials. No major side effects were observed, but it had limited efficacy in a small study involving 12 patients where only five responded (>50% improvement in Brief Psychiatric Rating Scale (BPRS)), six showed slight improvement, and one deteriorated (Frieboes, Murck, Wiedemann, Holsboer, & Steiger, 1997). In an independent study by another group, limited efficacy was also observed in 12 patients presenting with an acute episode of schizophrenia, with four responding (>50% improvement in BPRS) and two slightly improving; two patients also developed extrapyramidal side effects (Huber, Gotthardt, Schreiber, & Krieg, 1999). Using the same study design as the other two groups, a third group also evaluated the compound in 12 patients and reported limited efficacy against schizophrenia with moderate occurrence of side effects (Muller et al., 1999). One complication in the interpretation of these studies is that EMD59983, a major metabolite of EMD57445, has significant affinity for dopamine receptors (Grunder et al., 1999).

Opipramol: Opipramol has preferential affinity for σ_1 and σ_2 receptors, where it appears to act as an agonist (Rao et al., 1990). However, it also displays interactions with other neuroreceptors, notably 5-HT_2 and dopamine D_2 (Volz & Stoll, 2004). A meta-analysis of early clinical trials of opipramol in the 1960s and 1970s reveals efficacy for anxiety, depression, and menopausal symptoms (Volz & Stoll, 2004). More recent double-blind, placebo-controlled studies of opipramol for generalized anxiety disorder confirm efficacy and tolerability, with postmarket surveillance studies also confirming its anxiolytic effects (Moller, Volz, Reimann, & Stoll, 2001; Volz & Stoll, 2004).

5.3. σ Radioprobes for CNS imaging

Earlier investigations have led to the development and testing of σ_1 ligands as imaging agents, which can be used for CNS applications. Thus far, the only one that has been utilized in humans in both normal and CNS disease states is [^{11}C]SA4503 (Toyohara, Sakata, & Ishiwata, 2009). [^{11}C]SA4503 has high affinity and selectivity for σ_1 receptors and is suitable for brain imaging (Toyohara, Sakata, & Ishiwata, 2012). When used in humans, it has shown decreased levels of σ_1 receptors in the putamen of patients with Parkinson's disease (Mishina et al., 2005). There are also significant decreases in σ_1 receptors in patients with early Alzheimer's disease in the frontal, temporal, and occipital lobes, cerebellum, and thalamus (Mishina et al., 2008). In addition, [^{11}C]SA4503 labeling can be displaced by a number of known σ-active medications including haloperidol, donepezil, fluvoxamine, and progesterone (Ishikawa et al., 2009; Toyohara et al., 2009).

A fluorinated σ_1 imaging agent [^{18}F]1-(3-fluoropropyl)-4-(4-cyanophenoxymethyl)piperidine (FPS) has also been tested in humans. Although initial animal studies were promising, it did not display favorable kinetics in humans, and efforts to redesign a related lower-affinity probe, [^{18}F]1-(2-fluoroethyl)-4-[(4-cyanophenoxy)methyl]piperidine (SFE), have been undertaken with promising *in vivo* results in experimental animals (Waterhouse, Chang, Zhao, & Carambot, 2006).

The iodinated σ_1 imaging agent 1(*trans*-[^{123}I]iodopropen-2-yl)-4-[(4-cyanophenoxy)methyl] piperidine (TPCNE) has been reported in a small cohort of normal humans. Brain labeling was observed, with favorable kinetics and binding that could be displaced by haloperidol (Stone et al., 2006).

In addition to the aforementioned entities that have been tested in humans, many other fluorinated imaging agents have been reported for *in vivo* labeling of σ_1 receptors in the brains of nonhuman living subjects and may be amenable for translation to humans. Initial development of σ_2 probes has begun, mostly in the context of cancer research, and their potential for CNS applications remains untested (Mach & Wheeler, 2009). The availability of imaging agents for σ receptors will provide exciting new opportunities to facilitate our understanding of them under dynamic conditions, including psychostimulant abuse.

6. CONCLUSION

The ability of psychostimulants such as cocaine and methamphetamine to interact with σ receptors provides a viable target for the discovery and development of new therapeutic and diagnostic tools. Preclinical studies to date demonstrate that σ receptor antagonists can mitigate many psychostimulant-induced changes in behavior and gene and protein expression. On the other hand, σ receptor agonists may have potential as replacement therapies to reduce drug taking and craving and to improve cognition. Many σ-active compounds have been utilized clinically for various neuropsychiatric disorders and appear to have few notable side effects. The utilization of new compounds and repurposing of σ ligands that have already undergone small-scale clinical trials may provide future drug development opportunities for the treatment of addiction and side effects associated with psychostimulant abuse.

CONFLICT OF INTEREST

R. M. is a consultant and contract recipient for Avanir Pharmaceuticals for her expertise on σ receptors; none of the research related to her work for Avanir Pharmaceuticals is described in this chapter. N. K. is an employee of Takeda Pharmaceuticals. Her contribution to the work described herein represents her Ph.D. research on a topic distinct from her responsibilities at Takeda. The authors have no other potential conflicts of interest to declare.

ACKNOWLEDGMENTS

Some of the research described herein was supported by the National Institute on Drug Abuse (DA017756, DA011979, DA013978, and DA023205). We appreciate the expert technical assistance of Buddy Pouw and Joshua Blyden for generating the data on cocaine metabolites. We also appreciate the contributions of Ashley Brandebura in preparing the tables.

REFERENCES

Ahmed, I. S., Chamberlain, C., & Craven, R. J. (2012). S2R(Pgrmc1): The cytochrome-related sigma-2 receptor that regulates lipid and drug metabolism and hormone signaling. *Expert Opinion on Drug Metabolism & Toxicology*, 8(3), 361–370. http://dx.doi.org/10.1517/17425255.2012.658367.

Alonso, G., Phan, V., Guillemain, I., Saunier, M., Legrand, A., Anoal, M., et al. (2000). Immunocytochemical localization of the sigma₁ receptor in the adult rat central nervous system. *Neuroscience*, 97(1), 155–170, S0306452200000142 [pii].

Aydar, R., Palmer, C. P., & Djamgoz, M. B. (2004). Sigma receptors and cancer: Possible involvement of ion channels. *Cancer Research*, 64(15), 5029–5035.

Aydar, E., Palmer, C. P., Klyachko, V. A., & Jackson, M. B. (2002). The sigma receptor as a ligand-regulated auxiliary potassium channel subunit. *Neuron*, 34(3), 399–410, S0896627302006773 [pii].

Balasuriya, D., Stewart, A. P., Crottes, D., Borgese, F., Soriani, O., & Edwardson, J. M. (2012). The sigma-1 receptor binds to the Nav1.5 voltage-gated Na+ channel with 4-fold symmetry. *The Journal of Biological Chemistry*, 287(44), 37021–37029. http://dx.doi.org/10.1074/jbc.M112.382077, M112.382077 [pii].

Basile, A. S., Paul, I. A., & de Costa, B. (1992). Differential effects of cytochrome P-450 induction on ligand binding to sigma receptors. *European Journal of Pharmacology*, 227(1), 95–98.

Bastianetto, S., Rouquier, L., Perrault, G., & Sanger, D. J. (1995). DTG-induced circling behaviour in rats may involve the interaction between sigma sites and nigro-striatal dopaminergic pathways. *Neuropharmacology*, 34(3), 281–287, 002839089400156M [pii].

Berger, S. P., Hall, S., Mickalian, J. D., Reid, M. S., Crawford, C. A., Delucchi, K., et al. (1996). Haloperidol antagonism of cue-elicited cocaine craving. *Lancet*, 347(9000), 504–508.

Bermack, J. E., & Debonnel, G. (2005). The role of sigma receptors in depression. *Journal of Pharmacological Sciences*, 97(3), 317–336, JST.JSTAGE/jphs/CRJ04005X [pii].

Bouchard, P., & Quirion, R. (1997). [³H]1,3-di(2-tolyl)guanidine and [³H](+)pentazocine binding sites in the rat brain: Autoradiographic visualization of the putative sigma1 and sigma2 receptor subtypes. *Neuroscience*, 76(2), 467–477, S0306-4522(96)00221-7 [pii].

Bourrie, B., Bribes, E., De Nys, N., Esclangon, M., Garcia, L., Galiegue, S., et al. (2002). SSR125329A, a high affinity sigma receptor ligand with potent anti-inflammatory properties. *European Journal of Pharmacology*, 456(1–3), 123–131.

Bourrie, B., Bribes, E., Derocq, J. M., Vidal, H., & Casellas, P. (2004). Sigma receptor ligands: Applications in inflammation and oncology. *Current Opinion in Investigational Drugs*, 5(11), 1158–1163.

Bowen, W. D., de Costa, B. R., Hellewell, S. B., Walker, J. M., & Rice, K. C. (1993). [³H]-(+)-Pentazocine: a potent and highly selective benzomorphan-based probe for sigma-1 receptors. *Molecular Neuropharmacology*, 3, 117–126.

Bowyer, J. F., Davies, D. L., Schmued, L., Broening, H. W., Newport, G. D., Slikker, W., Jr., et al. (1994). Further studies of the role of hyperthermia in methamphetamine neurotoxicity. *The Journal of Pharmacology and Experimental Therapeutics*, 268(3), 1571–1580.

Brackett, R. L., Pouw, B., Blyden, J. F., Nour, M., & Matsumoto, R. R. (2000). Prevention of cocaine-induced convulsions and lethality in mice: Effectiveness of targeting different sites on the NMDA receptor complex. *Neuropharmacology*, 39(3), 407–418, S0028390899001513 [pii].

Brammer, M. K., Gilmore, D. L., & Matsumoto, R. R. (2006). Interactions between 3,4-methylenedioxymethamphetamine and sigma₁ receptors. *European Journal of Pharmacology*, 553(1–3), 141–145. http://dx.doi.org/10.1016/j.ejphar.2006.09.038, S0014-2999 (06)01070-3 [pii].

Callaghan, R. C., Cunningham, J. K., Sykes, J., & Kish, S. J. (2012). Increased risk of Parkinson's disease in individuals hospitalized with conditions related to the use of methamphetamine or other amphetamine-type drugs. *Drug and Alcohol Dependence*, *120*(1–3), 35–40. http://dx.doi.org/10.1016/j.drugalcdep.2011.06.013, S0376-8716 (11)00276-6 [pii].

Carr, D. J., De Costa, B. R., Radesca, L., & Blalock, J. E. (1991). Functional assessment and partial characterization of [³H](+)-pentazocine binding sites on cells of the immune system. *Journal of Neuroimmunology*, *35*(1–3), 153–166.

Chen, J. C., Chen, P. C., & Chiang, Y. C. (2009). Molecular mechanisms of psychostimulant addiction. *Chang Gung Medical Journal*, *32*(2), 148–154, 3202/320204 [pii].

Cobos, E. J., Baeyens, J. M., & Del Pozo, E. (2005). Phenytoin differentially modulates the affinity of agonist and antagonist ligands for sigma 1 receptors of guinea pig brain. *Synapse*, *55*(3), 192–195. http://dx.doi.org/10.1002/syn.20103.

Connor, M. A., & Chavkin, C. (1991). Focal stimulation of specific pathways in the rat hippocampus causes a reduction in radioligand binding to the haloperidol-sensitive sigma receptor. *Experimental Brain Research*, *85*(3), 528–536.

Connor, M. A., & Chavkin, C. (1992). Ionic zinc may function as a endogenous ligand for the haloperidol-sensitive sigma 2 receptor in rat brain. *Molecular Pharmacology*, *42*(3), 471–479.

Contreras, P. C., DiMaggio, D. A., & O'Donohue, T. L. (1987). An endogenous ligand for the sigma opioid binding site. *Synapse*, *1*(1), 57–61. http://dx.doi.org/10.1002/syn.890010108.

Crawford, K. W., & Bowen, W. D. (2002). Sigma-2 receptor agonists activate a novel apoptotic pathway and potentiate antineoplastic drugs in breast tumor cell lines. *Cancer Research*, *62*(1), 313–322.

Crawford, K. W., Coop, A., & Bowen, W. D. (2002). sigma2 Receptors regulate changes in sphingolipid levels in breast tumor cells. *European Journal of Pharmacology*, *443*(1–3), 207–209, S0014299902015819 [pii].

Crottes, D., Martial, S., Rapetti-Mauss, R., Pisani, D. F., Loriol, C., Pellissier, B., et al. (2011). Sig1R protein regulates hERG channel expression through a post-translational mechanism in leukemic cells. *The Journal of Biological Chemistry*, *286*(32), 27947–27958. http://dx.doi.org/10.1074/jbc.M111.226738, M111.226738 [pii].

Cuevas, J., Rodriguez, A., Behensky, A., & Katnik, C. (2011). Afobazole modulates microglial function via activation of both sigma-1 and sigma-2 receptors. *The Journal of Pharmacology and Experimental Therapeutics*, *339*(1), 161–172. http://dx.doi.org/10.1124/jpet.111.182816, jpet.111.182816 [pii].

Derlet, R. W., & Albertson, T. E. (1990). Anticonvulsant modification of cocaine-induced toxicity in the rat. *Neuropharmacology*, *29*(3), 255–259.

Dhir, A., & Kulkarni, S. K. (2008). Possible involvement of sigma-1 receptors in the anti-immobility action of bupropion, a dopamine reuptake inhibitor. *Fundamental & Clinical Pharmacology*, *22*(4), 387–394. http://dx.doi.org/10.1111/j.1472-8206.2008.00605.x, FCP605 [pii].

Ela, C., Barg, J., Vogel, Z., Hasin, Y., & Eilam, Y. (1994). Sigma receptor ligands modulate contractility, Ca^{++} influx and beating rate in cultured cardiac myocytes. *The Journal of Pharmacology and Experimental Therapeutics*, *269*(3), 1300–1309.

Eugenin, E. A., Osiecki, K., Lopez, L., Goldstein, H., Calderon, T. M., & Berman, J. W. (2006). CCL2/monocyte chemoattractant protein-1 mediates enhanced transmigration of human immunodeficiency virus (HIV)-infected leukocytes across the blood-brain barrier: A potential mechanism of HIV-CNS invasion and NeuroAIDS. *The Journal of Neuroscience*, *26*(4), 1098–1106. http://dx.doi.org/10.1523/JNEUROSCI.3863-05.2006, 26/4/1098 [pii].

Fiala, M., Gan, X. H., Zhang, L., House, S. D., Newton, T., Graves, M. C., et al. (1998). Cocaine enhances monocyte migration across the blood-brain barrier. Cocaine's connection to AIDS dementia and vasculitis? *Advances in Experimental Medicine and Biology*, *437*, 199–205.

Fishback, J. A., Robson, M. J., Xu, Y. T., & Matsumoto, R. R. (2010). Sigma receptors: Potential targets for a new class of antidepressant drug. *Pharmacology & Therapeutics*, *127*(3), 271–282. http://dx.doi.org/10.1016/j.pharmthera.2010.04.003, S0163-7258 (10)00077-X [pii].

Fishback, J. A., Rosen, A., Bhat, R., McCurdy, C. R., & Matsumoto, R. R. (2012). A 96-well filtration method for radioligand binding analysis of sigma receptor ligands. *Journal of Pharmaceutical and Biomedical Analysis*, *71*, 157–161. http://dx.doi.org/10.1016/j.jpba.2012.07.023, S0731-7085(12)00429-3 [pii].

Fontanilla, D., Johannessen, M., Hajipour, A. R., Cozzi, N. V., Jackson, M. B., & Ruoho, A. E. (2009). The hallucinogen N, N-dimethyltryptamine (DMT) is an endogenous sigma-1 receptor regulator. *Science*, *323*(5916), 934–937. http://dx.doi.org/10.1126/science.1166127, 323/5916/934 [pii].

Frieboes, R. M., Murck, H., Wiedemann, K., Holsboer, F., & Steiger, A. (1997). Open clinical trial on the sigma ligand panamesine in patients with schizophrenia. *Psychopharmacology*, *132*(1), 82–88.

Ganapathy, M. E., Prasad, P. D., Huang, W., Seth, P., Leibach, F. H., & Ganapathy, V. (1999). Molecular and ligand-binding characterization of the sigma-receptor in the Jurkat human T lymphocyte cell line. *The Journal of Pharmacology and Experimental Therapeutics*, *289*(1), 251–260.

Gebreselassie, D., & Bowen, W. D. (2004). Sigma-2 receptors are specifically localized to lipid rafts in rat liver membranes. *European Journal of Pharmacology*, *493*(1–3), 19–28. http://dx.doi.org/10.1016/j.ejphar.2004.04.005, S0014299904003802 [pii].

Gekker, G., Hu, S., Sheng, W. S., Rock, R. B., Lokensgard, J. R., & Peterson, P. K. (2006). Cocaine-induced HIV-1 expression in microglia involves sigma-1 receptors and transforming growth factor-beta1. *International Immunopharmacology*, *6*(6), 1029–1033. http://dx.doi.org/10.1016/j.intimp.2005.12.005, S1567-5769(05)00354-1 [pii].

Goldstein, S. R., Matsumoto, R. R., Thompson, T. L., Patrick, R. L., Bowen, W. D., & Walker, J. M. (1989). Motor effects of two sigma ligands mediated by nigrostriatal dopamine neurons. *Synapse*, *4*(3), 254–258. http://dx.doi.org/10.1002/syn.890040311.

Gonzalez, R., Bechara, A., & Martin, E. M. (2007). Executive functions among individuals with methamphetamine or alcohol as drugs of choice: Preliminary observations. *Journal of Clinical and Experimental Neuropsychology*, *29*(2), 155–159. http://dx.doi.org/10.1080/13803390600582446, 770388106 [pii].

Gough, B., Imam, S. Z., Blough, B., Slikker, W., Jr., & Ali, S. F. (2002). Comparative effects of substituted amphetamines (PMA, MDMA, and METH) on monoamines in rat caudate: A microdialysis study. *Annals of the New York Academy of Sciences*, *965*, 410–420.

Grasing, K., Mathur, D., Newton, T. F., & DeSouza, C. (2010). Donepezil treatment and the subjective effects of intravenous cocaine in dependent individuals. *Drug and Alcohol Dependence*, *107*(1), 69–75. http://dx.doi.org/10.1016/j.drugalcdep.2009.09.010, S0376-8716(09)00365-2 [pii].

Graybiel, A. M., Besson, M. J., & Weber, E. (1989). Neuroleptic-sensitive binding sites in the nigrostriatal system: Evidence for differential distribution of sigma sites in the substantia nigra, pars compacta of the cat. *The Journal of Neuroscience*, *9*(1), 326–338.

Grunder, G., Muller, M. J., Andreas, J., Heydari, N., Wetzel, H., Schlosser, R., et al. (1999). Occupancy of striatal D₂-like dopamine receptors after treatment with the sigma ligand EMD 57445, a putative atypical antipsychotic. *Psychopharmacology*, *146*(1), 81–86. 91460081.213 [pii].

Gundlach, A. L., Largent, B. L., & Snyder, S. H. (1986). Autoradiographic localization of sigma receptor binding sites in guinea pig and rat central nervous system with $(+)^3$H-3-(3-hydroxyphenyl)-N-(1-propyl)piperidine. *The Journal of Neuroscience, 6*(6), 1757–1770.

Ha, Y., Dun, Y., Thangaraju, M., Duplantier, J., Dong, Z., Liu, K., et al. (2011). Sigma receptor 1 modulates endoplasmic reticulum stress in retinal neurons. *Investigative Ophthalmology & Visual Science, 52*(1), 527–540. http://dx.doi.org/10.1167/iovs.10-5731, iovs.10-5731 [pii].

Hall, A. A., Herrera, Y., Ajmo, C. T., Jr., Cuevas, J., & Pennypacker, K. R. (2009). Sigma receptors suppress multiple aspects of microglial activation. *Glia, 57*(7), 744–754. http://dx.doi.org/10.1002/glia.20802.

Han, D. D., & Gu, H. H. (2006). Comparison of the monoamine transporters from human and mouse in their sensitivities to psychostimulant drugs. *BMC Pharmacology, 6*, 6. http://dx.doi.org/10.1186/1471-2210-6-6, 1471-2210-6-6 [pii].

Hanner, M., Moebius, F. F., Flandorfer, A., Knaus, H. G., Striessnig, J., Kempner, E., et al. (1996). Purification, molecular cloning, and expression of the mammalian sigma$_1$-binding site. *Proceedings of the National Academy of Sciences of the United States of America, 93*(15), 8072–8077.

Hart, C. L., Marvin, C. B., Silver, R., & Smith, E. E. (2012). Is cognitive functioning impaired in methamphetamine users? A critical review. *Neuropsychopharmacology, 37*(3), 586–608. http://dx.doi.org/10.1038/npp.2011.276, npp2011276 [pii].

Hayashi, T., Justinova, Z., Hayashi, E., Cormaci, G., Mori, T., Tsai, S. Y., et al. (2010). Regulation of sigma-1 receptors and endoplasmic reticulum chaperones in the brain of methamphetamine self-administering rats. *The Journal of Pharmacology and Experimental Therapeutics, 332*(3), 1054–1063. http://dx.doi.org/10.1124/jpet.109.159244, jpet.109.159244 [pii].

Hayashi, T., Maurice, T., & Su, T. P. (2000). Ca^{2+} signaling via sigma$_1$-receptors: Novel regulatory mechanism affecting intracellular Ca^{2+} concentration. *The Journal of Pharmacology and Experimental Therapeutics, 293*(3), 788–798.

Hayashi, T., & Su, T. P. (2004). Sigma-1 receptor ligands: Potential in the treatment of neuropsychiatric disorders. *CNS Drugs, 18*(5), 269–284.

Hayashi, T., & Su, T. P. (2007). Sigma-1 receptor chaperones at the ER-mitochondrion interface regulate Ca^{2+} signaling and cell survival. *Cell, 131*(3), 596–610. http://dx.doi.org/10.1016/j.cell.2007.08.036, S0092-8674(07)01099-9 [pii].

Hayashi, T., Tsai, S. Y., Mori, T., Fujimoto, M., & Su, T. P. (2011). Targeting ligand-operated chaperone sigma-1 receptors in the treatment of neuropsychiatric disorders. *Expert Opinion on Therapeutic Targets, 15*(5), 557–577. http://dx.doi.org/10.1517/14728222.2011.560837.

Hebert, M. A., & O'Callaghan, J. P. (2000). Protein phosphorylation cascades associated with methamphetamine-induced glial activation. *Annals of the New York Academy of Sciences, 914*, 238–262.

Hellewell, S. B., & Bowen, W. D. (1990). A sigma-like binding site in rat pheochromocytoma (PC12) cells: Decreased affinity for $(+)$-benzomorphans and lower molecular weight suggest a different sigma receptor form from that of guinea pig brain. *Brain Research, 527*(2), 244–253, 0006-8993(90)91143-5 [pii].

Hellewell, S. B., Bruce, A., Feinstein, G., Orringer, J., Williams, W., & Bowen, W. D. (1994). Rat liver and kidney contain high densities of sigma 1 and sigma 2 receptors: Characterization by ligand binding and photoaffinity labeling. *European Journal of Pharmacology, 268*(1), 9–18.

Hiranita, T., Mereu, M., Soto, P. L., Tanda, G., & Katz, J. L. (2013). Self-administration of cocaine induces dopamine-independent self-administration of sigma agonists. *Neuropsychopharmacology, 38*(4), 605–615. http://dx.doi.org/10.1038/npp.2012.224, npp2012224 [pii].

Hiranita, T., Soto, P. L., Kohut, S. J., Kopajtic, T., Cao, J., Newman, A. H., et al. (2011). Decreases in cocaine self-administration with dual inhibition of the dopamine transporter and sigma receptors. *The Journal of Pharmacology and Experimental Therapeutics*, *339*(2), 662–677. http://dx.doi.org/10.1124/jpet.111.185025, jpet.111.185025 [pii].

Hiranita, T., Soto, P. L., Tanda, G., & Katz, J. L. (2010). Reinforcing effects of sigma-receptor agonists in rats trained to self-administer cocaine. *The Journal of Pharmacology and Experimental Therapeutics*, *332*(2), 515–524. http://dx.doi.org/10.1124/jpet.109.159236, jpet.109.159236 [pii].

Hiranita, T., Soto, P. L., Tanda, G., & Katz, J. L. (2011). Lack of cocaine-like discriminative-stimulus effects of sigma-receptor agonists in rats. *Behavioural Pharmacology*, *22*(5–6), 525–530. http://dx.doi.org/10.1097/FBP.0b013e328349ab22.

Huber, M. T., Gotthardt, U., Schreiber, W., & Krieg, J. C. (1999). Efficacy and safety of the sigma receptor ligand EMD 57445 (panamesine) in patients with schizophrenia: An open clinical trial. *Pharmacopsychiatry*, *32*(2), 68–72. http://dx.doi.org/10.1055/s-2007-979194.

Hyman, S. E., & Malenka, R. C. (2001). Addiction and the brain: the neurobiology of compulsion and its persistence. *Nature Reviews Neuroscience*, *2*(10), 695–703.

Ishikawa, M., Sakata, M., Ishii, K., Kimura, Y., Oda, K., Toyohara, J., et al. (2009). High occupancy of sigma1 receptors in the human brain after single oral administration of donepezil: A positron emission tomography study using [^{11}C]SA4503. *The International Journal of Neuropsychopharmacology*, *12*(8), 1127–1131. http://dx.doi.org/10.1017/S1461145709990204, S1461145709990204 [pii].

Itzhak, Y. (1993). Repeated methamphetamine-treatment alters brain sigma receptors. *European Journal of Pharmacology*, *230*(2), 243–244.

Jansen, K. L., Faull, R. L., Dragunow, M., & Leslie, R. A. (1991). Autoradiographic distribution of sigma receptors in human neocortex, hippocampus, basal ganglia, cerebellum, pineal and pituitary glands. *Brain Research*, *559*(1), 172–177, 0006-8993(91)90303-D [pii].

Jovanovski, D., & Zakzanis, K. K. (2003). Donepezil in a chronic drug user—A potential treatment? *Human Psychopharmacology*, *18*(7), 561–564. http://dx.doi.org/10.1002/hup.530.

Jupp, B., & Lawrence, A. J. (2010). New horizons for therapeutics in drug and alcohol abuse. *Pharmacology & Therapeutics*, *125*(1), 138–168. http://dx.doi.org/10.1016/j.pharmthera.2009.11.002, S0163-7258(09)00212-5 [pii].

Kaushal, N. (2012). Evaluation of novel sigma receptor antagonists against methamphetamine-induced neurotoxicity: In vivo and in vitro studies. Ph.D., West Virginia University, Morgantown.

Kaushal, N., Elliott, M., Robson, M. J., Iyer, A. K., Rojanasakul, Y., Coop, A., et al. (2012). AC927, a sigma receptor ligand, blocks methamphetamine-induced release of dopamine and generation of reactive oxygen species in NG108-15 cells. *Molecular Pharmacology*, *81*(3), 299–308. http://dx.doi.org/10.1124/mol.111.074120, mol.111.074120 [pii].

Kaushal, N., & Matsumoto, R. R. (2011). Role of sigma receptors in methamphetamine-induced neurotoxicity. *Current Neuropharmacology*, *9*(1), 54–57. http://dx.doi.org/10.2174/157015911795016930, CN-9-54 [pii].

Kaushal, N., McCurdy, C. R., & Matsumoto, R. R. (2011). SN79 attenuates the neurotoxic effects of methamphetamine: In vivo and in vitro studies. Paper presented at the Society for Neuroscience.

Kaushal, N., Robson, M. J., Vinnakota, H., Narayanan, S., Avery, B. A., McCurdy, C. R., et al. (2011). Synthesis and pharmacological evaluation of 6-acetyl-3-(4-(4-(4-fluorophenyl)piperazin-1-yl)butyl)benzo[d]oxazol-2(3H)-one (SN79), a cocaine antagonist, in rodents. *The AAPS Journal*, *13*(3), 336–346. http://dx.doi.org/10.1208/s12248-011-9274-9.

Kaushal, N., Seminerio, M. J., Robson, M. J., McCurdy, C. R., & Matsumoto, R. R. (2013). Pharmacological evaluation of SN79, a sigma (σ) receptor ligand, against methamphetamine-induced neurotoxicity in vivo. *European Neuropsychopharmacology*, *23*, 960–971. http://dx.doi.org/10.1016/j.euroneuro.2012.08.005, S0924-977X(12) 00223-4 [pii].

Kaushal, N., Seminerio, M. J., Shaikh, J., Medina, M. A., Mesangeau, C., Wilson, L. L., et al. (2011). CM156, a high affinity sigma ligand, attenuates the stimulant and neurotoxic effects of methamphetamine in mice. *Neuropharmacology*, *61*(5–6), 992–1000. http:// dx.doi.org/10.1016/j.neuropharm.2011.06.028, S0028-3908(11)00275-9 [pii].

Kawamura, K., Ishiwata, K., Tajima, H., Ishii, S., Matsuno, K., Homma, Y., et al. (2000). In vivo evaluation of [^{11}C]SA4503 as a PET ligand for mapping CNS sigma$_1$ receptors. *Nuclear Medicine and Biology*, *27*(3), 255–261, S0969805100000810 [pii].

Kekuda, R., Prasad, P. D., Fei, Y. J., Leibach, F. H., & Ganapathy, V. (1996). Cloning and functional expression of the human type 1 sigma receptor (hSigmaR1). *Biochemical and Biophysical Research Communications*, *229*(2), 553–558. http://dx.doi.org/10.1006/ bbrc.1996.1842, S0006-291X(96)91842-2 [pii].

Kelly, K. A., Miller, D. B., Bowyer, J. F., & O'Callaghan, J. P. (2012). Chronic exposure to corticosterone enhances the neuroinflammatory and neurotoxic responses to metham- phetamine. *Journal of Neurochemistry*, *122*(5), 995–1009. http://dx.doi.org/10.1111/ j.1471-4159.2012.07864.x.

Kinoshita, M., Matsuoka, Y., Suzuki, T., Mirrielees, J., & Yang, J. (2012). Sigma-1 receptor alters the kinetics of Kv1.3 voltage gated potassium channels but not the sensitivity to receptor ligands. *Brain Research*, *1452*, 1–9. http://dx.doi.org/10.1016/j. brainres.2012.02.070, S0006-8993(12)00432-5 [pii].

Kitaichi, K., Chabot, J. G., Moebius, F. F., Flandorfer, A., Glossmann, H., & Quirion, R. (2000). Expression of the purported sigma (σ$_1$) receptor in the mammalian brain and its possible relevance in deficits induced by antagonism of the NMDA receptor complex as revealed using an antisense strategy. *Journal of Chemical Neuroanatomy*, *20*(3–4), 375–387, S0891-0618(00)00106-X [pii].

Klein, M., Cooper, T. B., & Musacchio, J. M. (1994). Effects of haloperidol and reduced haloperidol on binding to sigma sites. *European Journal of Pharmacology*, *254*(3), 239–248.

Kourrich, S., Hayashi, T., Chuang, J. Y., Tsai, S. Y., Su, T. P., & Bonci, A. (2013). Dynamic interaction between sigma-1 receptor and Kv1.2 shapes neuronal and behavioral responses to cocaine. *Cell*, *152*(1–2), 236–247. http://dx.doi.org/10.1016/j. cell.2012.12.004, S0092-8674(12)01491-2 [pii].

Kourrich, S., Su, T. P., Fujimoto, M., & Bonci, A. (2012). The sigma-1 receptor: Roles in neuronal plasticity and disease. *Trends in Neurosciences*, *35*(12), 762–771. http://dx.doi. org/10.1016/j.tins.2012.09.007, S0166-2236(12)00171-3 [pii].

Krasnova, I. N., & Cadet, J. L. (2009). Methamphetamine toxicity and messengers of death. *Brain Research Reviews*, *60*(2), 379–407. http://dx.doi.org/10.1016/j.brainresrev. 2009.03.002, S0165-0173(09)00034-4 [pii].

Kuehn, B. M. (2006). Nicotine, donepezil may dampen meth craving. *JAMA*, *296*(1), 31. http://dx.doi.org/10.1001/jama.296.1.31, 296/1/31 [pii].

Largent, B. L., Gundlach, A. L., & Snyder, S. H. (1986). Pharmacological and autoradio- graphic discrimination of sigma and phencyclidine receptor binding sites in brain with (+)-[^{3}H]SKF 10,047, (+)-[^{3}H]-3-[3-hydroxyphenyl]-N-(1-propyl)piperidine and [^{3}H]-1-[1-(2-thienyl)cyclohexyl]piperidine. *The Journal of Pharmacology and Experimental Therapeutics*, *238*(2), 739–748.

Lever, J. R., Gustafson, J. L., Xu, R., Allmon, R. L., & Lever, S. Z. (2006). Sigma-1 and sigma-2 receptor binding affinity and selectivity of SA4503 and fluoroethyl SA4503. *Synapse*, *59*(6), 350–358.

Liu, Y., & Matsumoto, R. R. (2008). Alterations in fos-related antigen 2 and sigma$_1$ receptor gene and protein expression are associated with the development of cocaine-induced behavioral sensitization: Time course and regional distribution studies. *The Journal of Pharmacology and Experimental Therapeutics, 327*(1), 187–195. http://dx.doi.org/10.1124/jpet.108.141051, jpet.108.141051 [pii].

Liu, Y., Whitlock, B. B., Pultz, J. A., & Wolfe, S. A., Jr. (1995). Sigma-1 receptors modulate functional activity of rat splenocytes. *Journal of Neuroimmunology, 59*(1–2), 143–154.

Lucas, G., Rymar, V. V., Sadikot, A. F., & Debonnel, G. (2008). Further evidence for an antidepressant potential of the selective sigma$_1$ agonist SA 4503: Electrophysiological, morphological and behavioural studies. *The International Journal of Neuropsychopharmacology, 11*(4), 485–495. http://dx.doi.org/10.1017/S1461145708008547, S1461145708008547 [pii].

Mach, R. H., & Wheeler, K. T. (2009). Development of molecular probes for imaging sigma-2 receptors in vitro and in vivo. *Central Nervous System Agents in Medicinal Chemistry, 9*(3), 230–245.

Maj, J., Rogoz, Z., & Skuza, G. (1996). Some behavioral effects of 1,3-di-o-tolylguanidine, opipramol and sertraline, the sigma site ligands. *Polish Journal of Pharmacology, 48*(4), 379–395.

Martin, W. R., Eades, C. G., Thompson, J. A., Huppler, R. E., & Gilbert, P. E. (1976). The effects of morphine- and nalorphine-like drugs in the nondependent and morphine-dependent chronic spinal dog. *The Journal of Pharmacology and Experimental Therapeutics, 197*(3), 517–532.

Matsumoto, R. R. (2009). Targeting sigma receptors: Novel medication development for drug abuse and addiction. *Expert Review of Clinical Pharmacology, 2*(4), 351–358. http://dx.doi.org/10.1586/ecp.09.18.

Matsumoto, R. R., Bowen, W. D., de Costa, B. R., & Houk, J. C. (1999). Relationship between modulation of the cerebellorubrospinal system in the in vitro turtle brain and changes in motor behavior in rats: Effects of novel sigma ligands. *Brain Research Bulletin, 48*(5), 497–508, S0361-9230(99)00029-5 [pii].

Matsumoto, R. R., Bowen, W. D., & Su, T.-P. (2007). *Sigma receptors: Chemistry, cell biology and clinical implications*. New York: Springer.

Matsumoto, R. R., Bowen, W. D., Tom, M. A., Vo, V. N., Truong, D. D., & De Costa, B. R. (1995). Characterization of two novel σ receptor ligands: antidystonic effects in rats suggest σ receptor antagonism. *European Journal of Pharmacology, 280*(3), 301–310.

Matsumoto, R. R., Gilmore, D. L., Pouw, B., Bowen, W. D., Williams, W., Kausar, A., et al. (2004). Novel analogs of the sigma receptor ligand BD1008 attenuate cocaine-induced toxicity in mice. *European Journal of Pharmacology, 492*(1), 21–26. http://dx.doi.org/10.1016/j.ejphar.2004.03.037, S0014299904002948 [pii].

Matsumoto, R. R., Li, S. M., Katz, J. L., Fantegrossi, W. E., & Coop, A. (2011). Effects of the selective sigma receptor ligand, 1-(2-phenethyl)piperidine oxalate (AC927), on the behavioral and toxic effects of cocaine. *Drug and Alcohol Dependence, 118*(1), 40–47. http://dx.doi.org/10.1016/j.drugalcdep.2011.02.017, S0376-8716(11)00117-7 [pii].

Matsumoto, R. R., Liu, Y., Lerner, M., Howard, E. W., & Brackett, D. J. (2003). Sigma receptors: Potential medications development target for anti-cocaine agents. *European Journal of Pharmacology, 469*(1–3), 1–12, S0014299903017230 [pii].

Matsumoto, R. R., McCracken, K. A., Friedman, M. J., Pouw, B., De Costa, B. R., & Bowen, W. D. (2001). Conformationally restricted analogs of BD1008 and an antisense oligodeoxynucleotide targeting sigma1 receptors produce anti-cocaine effects in mice. *European Journal of Pharmacology, 419*(2–3), 163–174.

Matsumoto, R. R., McCracken, K. A., Pouw, B., Miller, J., Bowen, W. D., Williams, W., et al. (2001). N-alkyl substituted analogs of the sigma receptor ligand BD1008 and traditional sigma receptor ligands affect cocaine-induced convulsions and lethality in mice. *European Journal of Pharmacology, 411*(3), 261–273, S0014299900009171 [pii].

Matsumoto, R. R., McCracken, K. A., Pouw, B., Zhang, Y., & Bowen, W. D. (2002). Involvement of sigma receptors in the behavioral effects of cocaine: Evidence from novel ligands and antisense oligodeoxynucleotides. *Neuropharmacology*, *42*(8), 1043–1055, S0028390802000564 [pii].

Matsumoto, R. R., Potelleret, F. H., Mack, A., Pouw, B., Zhang, Y., & Bowen, W. D. (2004). Structure-activity comparison of YZ-069, a novel sigma ligand, and four analogs in receptor binding and behavioral studies. *Pharmacology, Biochemistry and Behavior*, *77*(4), 775–781. http://dx.doi.org/10.1016/j.pbb.2004.01.014, S0091305704000322 [pii].

Matsumoto, R. R., Shaikh, J., Wilson, L. L., Vedam, S., & Coop, A. (2008). Attenuation of methamphetamine-induced effects through the antagonism of sigma (σ) receptors: Evidence from in vivo and in vitro studies. *European Neuropsychopharmacology*, *18*(12), 871–881. http://dx.doi.org/10.1016/j.euroneuro.2008.07.006, S0924-977X(08)00177-6 [pii].

Maurice, T., Meunier, J., Feng, B., Ieni, J., & Monaghan, D. T. (2006). Interaction with sigma$_1$ protein, but not N-methyl-D-aspartate receptor, is involved in the pharmacological activity of donepezil. *The Journal of Pharmacology and Experimental Therapeutics*, *317*(2), 606–614. http://dx.doi.org/10.1124/jpet.105.097394, jpet. 105.097394 [pii].

Maurice, T., Roman, F. J., & Privat, A. (1996). Modulation by neurosteroids of the in vivo (+)-[^{3}H]SKF-10,047 binding to sigma 1 receptors in the mouse forebrain. *Journal of Neuroscience Research*, *46*(6), 734–743.

Maurice, T., & Su, T. P. (2009). The pharmacology of sigma-1 receptors. *Pharmacology & Therapeutics*, *124*(2), 195–206. http://dx.doi.org/10.1016/j.pharmthera.2009.07.001, S0163-7258(09)00141-7 [pii].

Mavlyutov, T. A., Epstein, M. L., Verbny, Y. I., Huerta, M. S., Zaitoun, I., Ziskind-Conhaim, L., et al. (2013). Lack of sigma-1 receptor exacerbates ALS progression in mice. *Neuroscience*, *240*, 129–134. http://dx.doi.org/10.1016/j.neuroscience.2013.02.035, S0306-4522(13)00169-3 [pii].

McCann, D. J., & Su, T. P. (1991). Solubilization and characterization of haloperidol-sensitive (+)-[^{3}H]SKF-10,047 binding sites (sigma sites) from rat liver membranes. *The Journal of Pharmacology and Experimental Therapeutics*, *257*(2), 547–554.

McCracken, K. A., Bowen, W. D., & Matsumoto, R. R. (1999). Novel sigma receptor ligands attenuate the locomotor stimulatory effects of cocaine. *European Journal of Pharmacology*, *365*, 35–38.

McLean, S., & Weber, E. (1988). Autoradiographic visualization of haloperidol-sensitive sigma receptors in guinea-pig brain. *Neuroscience*, *25*(1), 259–269.

Mei, J., & Pasternak, G. W. (2001). Molecular cloning and pharmacological characterization of the rat sigma1 receptor. *Biochemical Pharmacology*, *62*(3), 349–355, S0006-2952(01) 00666-9 [pii].

Mei, J., & Pasternak, G. W. (2002). Sigma$_1$ receptor modulation of opioid analgesia in the mouse. *The Journal of Pharmacology and Experimental Therapeutics*, *300*(3), 1070–1074.

Mishina, M., Ishiwata, K., Ishii, K., Kitamura, S., Kimura, Y., Kawamura, K., et al. (2005). Function of sigma$_1$ receptors in Parkinson's disease. *Acta Neurologica Scandinavica*, *112*(2), 103–107. http://dx.doi.org/10.1111/j.1600-0404.2005.00432.x, ANE432 [pii].

Mishina, M., Ohyama, M., Ishii, K., Kitamura, S., Kimura, Y., Oda, K., et al. (2008). Low density of sigma$_1$ receptors in early Alzheimer's disease. *Annals of Nuclear Medicine*, *22*(3), 151–156. http://dx.doi.org/10.1007/s12149-007-0094-z.

Moebius, F. F., Burrows, G. G., Hanner, M., Schmid, E., Striessnig, J., & Glossmann, H. (1993). Identification of a 27-kDa high affinity phenylalkylamine-binding polypeptide as the sigma 1 binding site by photoaffinity labeling and ligand-directed antibodies. *Molecular Pharmacology*, *44*(5), 966–971.

Moller, H. J., Volz, H. P., Reimann, I. W., & Stoll, K. D. (2001). Opipramol for the treatment of generalized anxiety disorder: A placebo-controlled trial including an alprazolam-treated group. *Journal of Clinical Psychopharmacology, 21*(1), 59–65.

Monassier, L., & Bousquet, P. (2002). Sigma receptors: From discovery to highlights of their implications in the cardiovascular system. *Fundamental & Clinical Pharmacology, 16*(1), 1–8.

Monnet, F. P., Debonnel, G., & de Montigny, C. (1992). In vivo electrophysiological evidence for a selective modulation of N-methyl-D-aspartate-induced neuronal activation in rat CA3 dorsal hippocampus by sigma ligands. *The Journal of Pharmacology and Experimental Therapeutics, 261*(1), 123–130.

Monnet, F. P., & Maurice, T. (2006). The sigma1 protein as a target for the non-genomic effects of neuro(active)steroids: Molecular, physiological, and behavioral aspects. *Journal of Pharmacological Sciences, 100*(2), 93–118, JST.JSTAGE/jphs/CR0050032 [pii].

Mori, T., Rahmadi, M., Yoshizawa, K., Itoh, T., Shibasaki, M., & Suzuki, T. (2012). Inhibitory effects of SA4503 on the rewarding effects of abused drugs. *Addiction Biology* [Epub ahead of print]. http://dx.doi.org/10.1111/j.1369-1600.2012.00488.x.

Moriguchi, S., Shinoda, Y., Yamamoto, Y., Sasaki, Y., Miyajima, K., Tagashira, H., et al. (2013). Stimulation of the sigma-1 receptor by DHEA enhances synaptic efficacy and neurogenesis in the hippocampal dentate gyrus of olfactory bulbectomized mice. *PLoS One, 8*(4), e60863. http://dx.doi.org/10.1371/journal.pone.0060863, PONE-D-13-02750 [pii].

Muller, M. J., Grunder, G., Wetzel, H., Muller-Siecheneder, F., Marx-Dannigkeit, P., & Benkert, O. (1999). Antipsychotic effects and tolerability of the sigma ligand EMD 57445 (panamesine) and its metabolites in acute schizophrenia: An open clinical trial. *Psychiatry Research, 89*(3), 275–280, S0165178199001006 [pii].

Nagornaia, L. V., Samovilova, N. N., Korobov, N. V., & Vinogradov, V. A. (1988). Partial purification of endogenous inhibitors of (+)-[³H] SKF 10047 binding with sigma-opioid receptors of the liver. *Biulleten Eksperimentalnoi Biologii I Meditsiny, 106*(9), 314–317.

Navarro, G., Moreno, E., Aymerich, M., Marcellino, D., McCormick, P. J., Mallol, J., et al. (2010). Direct involvement of sigma-1 receptors in the dopamine D₁ receptor-mediated effects of cocaine. *Proceedings of the National Academy of Sciences of the United States of America, 107*(43), 18676–18681. http://dx.doi.org/10.1073/pnas.1008911107, 1008911107 [pii].

Navarro, G., Moreno, E., Bonaventura, J., Brugarolas, M., Farre, D., Aguinaga, D., et al. (2013). Cocaine inhibits dopamine D₂ receptor signaling via sigma-1-D₂ receptor heteromers. *PLoS One, 8*(4), e61245. http://dx.doi.org/10.1371/journal.pone.0061245, PONE-D-12-34649 [pii].

Neumaier, J. F., & Chavkin, C. (1989). Calcium-dependent displacement of haloperidol-sensitive sigma receptor binding in rat hippocampal slices following tissue depolarization. *Brain Research, 500*(1–2), 215–222.

Nguyen, E. C., McCracken, K. A., Liu, Y., Pouw, B., & Matsumoto, R. R. (2005). Involvement of sigma (sigma) receptors in the acute actions of methamphetamine: Receptor binding and behavioral studies. *Neuropharmacology, 49*(5), 638–645. http://dx.doi.org/10.1016/j.neuropharm.2005.04.016, S0028-3908(05)00165-6 [pii].

Nicosia, N., Pacula, R. L., Kilmer, B., Lundberg, R., & Chiesa, J. (2009). *The economic cost of methamphetamine use in the United States, 2005*. Santa Monica: RAND Drug Policy Research Center. www.rand.org.

Noorbakhsh, B., Seminerio, M. J., Xu, Y.-T., Beatty, C., Mesangeau, C., McCurdy, C. R., et al. (2011). Synthesis and pharmacological characterization of sigma-2 preferring compounds: Implications for cocaine-induced behaviors. *Society for Neuroscience Abstract*, #896.02.

Novakova, M., Ela, C., Barg, J., Vogel, Z., Hasin, Y., & Eilam, Y. (1995). Inotropic action of sigma receptor ligands in isolated cardiac myocytes from adult rats. *European Journal of Pharmacology*, 286(1), 19–30, 0014-2999(95)00424-J [pii].

Nuwayhid, S. J., & Werling, L. L. (2006). Sigma$_2$ (σ_2) receptors as a target for cocaine action in the rat striatum. *European Journal of Pharmacology*, 535(1–3), 98–103. http://dx.doi.org/10.1016/j.ejphar.2005.12.077, S0014-2999(05)01353-1 [pii].

O'Dell, L. E., Kreifeldt, M. J., George, F. R., & Ritz, M. C. (2000). The role of serotonin$_2$ receptors in mediating cocaine-induced convulsions. *Pharmacology, Biochemistry and Behavior*, 65(4), 677–681, S0091-3057(99)00253-1 [pii].

Ortega-Roldan, J. L., Ossa, F., & Schnell, J. R. (2013). Characterization of the human sigma-1 receptor chaperone domain structure and binding immunoglobulin protein (BiP) interactions. *The Journal of Biological Chemistry*, 288(29), 21448–21457. http://dx.doi.org/10.1074/jbc.M113.450379, M113.450379 [pii].

Pal, A., Chu, U. B., Ramachandran, S., Grawoig, D., Guo, L. W., Hajipour, A. R., et al. (2008). Juxtaposition of the steroid binding domain-like I and II regions constitutes a ligand binding site in the sigma-1 receptor. *The Journal of Biological Chemistry*, 283(28), 19646–19656. http://dx.doi.org/10.1074/jbc.M802192200, M802192200 [pii].

Pal, A., Fontanilla, D., Gopalakrishnan, A., Chae, Y. K., Markley, J. L., & Ruoho, A. E. (2012). The sigma-1 receptor protects against cellular oxidative stress and activates antioxidant response elements. *European Journal of Pharmacology*, 682(1–3), 12–20.

Palacios, G., Muro, A., Vela, J. M., Molina-Holgado, E., Guitart, X., Ovalle, S., et al. (2003). Immunohistochemical localization of the sigma1-receptor in oligodendrocytes in the rat central nervous system. *Brain Research*, 961(1), 92–99, S0006899302038921 [pii].

Palacios, G., Muro, A., Verdu, E., Pumarola, M., & Vela, J. M. (2004). Immunohistochemical localization of the sigma$_1$ receptor in Schwann cells of rat sciatic nerve. *Brain Research*, 1007(1–2), 65–70. http://dx.doi.org/10.1016/j.brainres.2004.02.013, S000689930400 2392 [pii].

Pascaud, X. B., Chovet, M., Soulard, P., Chevalier, E., Roze, C., & Junien, J. L. (1993). Effects of a new sigma ligand, JO 1784, on cysteamine ulcers and duodenal alkaline secretion in rats. *Gastroenterology*, 104(2), 427–434.

Paul, R., Lavastre, S., Floutard, D., Floutard, R., Canat, X., Casellas, P., et al. (1994). Allosteric modulation of peripheral sigma binding sites by a new selective ligand: SR 31747. *Journal of Neuroimmunology*, 52(2), 183–192.

Perregaard, J., Moltzen, E. K., Meier, E., & Sanchez, C. (1995). Sigma ligands with subnanomolar affinity and preference for the sigma 2 binding site. 1. 3-(omega-aminoalkyl)-1H-indoles. *Journal of Medicinal Chemistry*, 38(11), 1998–2008.

Perry, V. H., Nicoll, J. A., & Holmes, C. (2010). Microglia in neurodegenerative disease. *Nature Reviews Neurology*, 6(4), 193–201. http://dx.doi.org/10.1038/nrneurol.2010.17, nrneurol.2010.17 [pii].

Prasad, P. D., Li, H. W., Fei, Y. J., Ganapathy, M. E., Fujita, T., Plumley, L. H., et al. (1998). Exon-intron structure, analysis of promoter region, and chromosomal localization of the human type 1 sigma receptor gene. *Journal of Neurochemistry*, 70(2), 443–451.

Raivich, G., Bohatschek, M., Kloss, C. U., Werner, A., Jones, L. L., & Kreutzberg, G. W. (1999). Neuroglial activation repertoire in the injured brain: Graded response, molecular mechanisms and cues to physiological function. *Brain Research Brain Research Reviews*, 30(1), 77–105, S0165017399000077 [pii].

Ramachandran, S., Chu, U. B., Mavlyutov, T. A., Pal, A., Pyne, S., & Ruoho, A. E. (2009). The sigma$_1$ receptor interacts with N-alkyl amines and endogenous sphingolipids. *European Journal of Pharmacology*, 609(1–3), 19–26.

Ramachandran, S., Lu, H., Prabhu, U., & Ruoho, A. E. (2007). Purification and characterization of the guinea pig sigma-1 receptor functionally expressed in Escherichia coli.

Protein Expression and Purification, *51*(2), 283–292. http://dx.doi.org/10.1016/j.pep. 2006.07.019, S1046-5928(06)00231-2 [pii].

Rao, T. S., Cler, J. A., Mick, S. J., Dilworth, V. M., Contreras, P. C., Iyengar, S., et al. (1990). Neurochemical characterization of dopaminergic effects of opipramol, a potent sigma receptor ligand, in vivo. *Neuropharmacology*, *29*(12), 1191–1197.

Robson, M. J. (2013). The involvement of sigma receptor modulation in the antidepressant effects of ketamine and the neurotoxic actions of methamphetamine. Ph.D., West Virginia University, Morgantown.

Robson, M. J., McCurdy, C. R., & Matsumoto, R. R. (2012). Methamphetamine elicits PERK-mediated endoplasmic reticulum transcriptional responses in NG108-15 cells. *Society for Neuroscience*, Abstract, #360.12.

Robson, M. J., Seminerio, M. J., McCurdy, C. R., Coop, A., & Matsumoto, R. R. (2013). σ Receptor antagonist attenuation of methamphetamine-induced neurotoxicity is correlated to body temperature modulation. *Pharmacological Reports*, *65*(2), 343–349.

Robson, M. J., Turner, R. C., Naser, Z. J., McCurdy, C. R., Huber, J. D., & Matsumoto, R. R. (2013). SN79, a sigma receptor ligand, blocks methamphetamine-induced microglial activation and cytokine upregulation. *Experimental Neurology*, *247C*, 134–142. http://dx. doi.org/10.1016/j.expneurol.2013.04.009, S0014-4886(13)00137-4 [pii].

Rockhold, R. W. (1998). Glutamatergic involvement in psychomotor stimulant action. *Progress in Drug Research*, *50*, 155–192.

Rodvelt, K. R., Oelrichs, C. E., Blount, L. R., Fan, K. H., Lever, S. Z., Lever, J. R., et al. (2011). The sigma receptor agonist SA4503 both attenuates and enhances the effects of methamphetamine. *Drug and Alcohol Dependence*, *116*(1–3), 203–210. http://dx.doi.org/ 10.1016/j.drugalcdep.2010.12.018, S0376-8716(11)00040-8 [pii].

Romieu, P., Martin-Fardon, R., Bowen, W. D., & Maurice, T. (2003). Sigma1 receptor-related neuroactive steroids modulate cocaine-induced reward. *The Journal of Neuroscience*, *23*(9), 3572–3576, 23/9/3572 [pii].

Romieu, P., Martin-Fardon, R., & Maurice, T. (2000). Involvement of the sigma$_1$ receptor in the cocaine-induced conditioned place preference. *Neuroreport*, *11*(13), 2885–2888.

Romieu, P., Meunier, J., Garcia, D., Zozime, N., Martin-Fardon, R., Bowen, W. D., et al. (2004). The sigma$_1$ (σ$_1$) receptor activation is a key step for the reactivation of cocaine conditioned place preference by drug priming. *Psychopharmacology*, *175*(2), 154–162. http://dx.doi.org/10.1007/s00213-004-1814-x.

Romieu, P., Phan, V. L., Martin-Fardon, R., & Maurice, T. (2002). Involvement of the sigma$_1$ receptor in cocaine-induced conditioned place preference: Possible dependence on dopamine uptake blockade. *Neuropsychopharmacology*, *26*(4), 444–455. http://dx.doi. org/10.1016/S0893-133X(01)00391-8, S0893133X01003918 [pii].

Roze, C., Bruley Des Varannes, S., Shi, G., Geneve, J., & Galmiche, J. P. (1998). Inhibition of prostaglandin-induced intestinal secretion by igmesine in healthy volunteers. *Gastroenterology*, *115*(3), 591–596.

Ruscher, K., Shamloo, M., Rickhag, M., Ladunga, I., Soriano, L., Gisselsson, L., et al. (2011). The sigma-1 receptor enhances brain plasticity and functional recovery after experimental stroke. *Brain*, *134*(Pt. 3), 732–746. http://dx.doi.org/10.1093/brain/ awq367, awq367 [pii].

Sabino, V., Cottone, P., Blasio, A., Iyer, M. R., Steardo, L., Rice, K. C., et al. (2011). Activation of sigma-receptors induces binge-like drinking in Sardinian alcohol-preferring rats. *Neuropsychopharmacology*, *36*(6), 1207–1218. http://dx.doi.org/ 10.1038/npp.2011.5, npp20115 [pii].

Saijo, K., & Glass, C. K. (2011). Microglial cell origin and phenotypes in health and disease. *Nature Reviews Immunology*, *11*(11), 775–787. http://dx.doi.org/10.1038/nri3086, nri3086 [pii].

Sanchez, C., & Papp, M. (2000). The selective sigma$_2$ ligand Lu 28-179 has an antidepressant-like profile in the rat chronic mild stress model of depression. *Behavioural Pharmacology*, *11*(2), 117–124.

Sekine, Y., Iyo, M., Ouchi, Y., Matsunaga, T., Tsukada, H., Okada, H., et al. (2001). Methamphetamine-related psychiatric symptoms and reduced brain dopamine transporters studied with PET. *The American Journal of Psychiatry*, *158*(8), 1206–1214.

Sekine, Y., Minabe, Y., Ouchi, Y., Takei, N., Iyo, M., Nakamura, K., et al. (2003). Association of dopamine transporter loss in the orbitofrontal and dorsolateral prefrontal cortices with methamphetamine-related psychiatric symptoms. *The American Journal of Psychiatry*, *160*(9), 1699–1701.

Sekine, Y., Ouchi, Y., Sugihara, G., Takei, N., Yoshikawa, E., Nakamura, K., et al. (2008). Methamphetamine causes microglial activation in the brains of human abusers. *The Journal of Neuroscience*, *28*(22), 5756–5761. http://dx.doi.org/10.1523/JNEUROSCI.1179-08.2008, 28/22/5756 [pii].

Sekine, Y., Ouchi, Y., Takei, N., Yoshikawa, E., Nakamura, K., Futatsubashi, M., et al. (2006). Brain serotonin transporter density and aggression in abstinent methamphetamine abusers. *Archives of General Psychiatry*, *63*(1), 90–100. http://dx.doi.org/10.1001/archpsyc.63.1.90, 63/1/90 [pii].

Seminerio, M. J., Hansen, R., Kaushal, N., Zhang, H. T., McCurdy, C. R., & Matsumoto, R. R. (2013). The evaluation of AZ66, an optimized sigma receptor antagonist, against methamphetamine-induced dopaminergic neurotoxicity and memory impairment in mice. *The International Journal of Neuropsychopharmacology*, *16*(5), 1033–1044. http://dx.doi.org/10.1017/S1461145712000831, S1461145712000831 [pii].

Seminerio, M. J., Kaushal, N., Shaikh, J., Huber, J. D., Coop, A., & Matsumoto, R. R. (2011). Sigma (σ) receptor ligand, AC927 (N-phenethylpiperidine oxalate), attenuates methamphetamine-induced hyperthermia and serotonin damage in mice. *Pharmacology, Biochemistry and Behavior*, *98*(1), 12–20. http://dx.doi.org/10.1016/j.pbb.2010.11.023, S0091-3057(10)00361-8 [pii].

Seminerio, M. J., Robson, M. J., Abdelazeem, A. H., Mesangeau, C., Jamalapuram, S., Avery, B. A., et al. (2012). Synthesis and pharmacological characterization of a novel sigma receptor ligand with improved metabolic stability and antagonistic effects against methamphetamine. *The AAPS Journal*, *14*(1), 43–51. http://dx.doi.org/10.1208/s12248-011-9311-8.

Seminerio, M. J., Robson, M. J., McCurdy, C. R., & Matsumoto, R. R. (2012). Sigma receptor antagonists attenuate acute methamphetamine-induced hyperthermia by a mechanism independent of IL-1β mRNA expression in the hypothalamus. *European Journal of Pharmacology*, *691*(1–3), 103–109. http://dx.doi.org/10.1016/j.ejphar.2012.07.029, S0014-2999(12)00623-1 [pii].

Sha, S., Qu, W. J., Li, L., Lu, Z. H., Chen, L., & Yu, W. F. (2013). Sigma-1 receptor knockout impairs neurogenesis in dentate gyrus of adult hippocampus via down-regulation of NMDA receptors. *CNS Neuroscience & Therapeutics*, *19*, 705–713. http://dx.doi.org/10.1111/cns.12129.

Sharkey, J., Glen, K. A., Wolfe, S., & Kuhar, M. J. (1988). Cocaine binding at sigma receptors. *European Journal of Pharmacology*, *149*(1–2), 171–174, 0014-2999(88) 90058-1 [pii].

Shoptaw, S., Heinzerling, K. G., Rotheram-Fuller, E., Kao, U. H., Wang, P. C., Bholat, M. A., et al. (2008). Bupropion hydrochloride versus placebo, in combination with cognitive behavioral therapy, for the treatment of cocaine abuse/dependence. *Journal of Addictive Diseases*, *27*(1), 13–23. http://dx.doi.org/10.1300/J069v27n01_02.

Shoptaw, S., Heinzerling, K. G., Rotheram-Fuller, E., Steward, T., Wang, J., Swanson, A. N., et al. (2008). Randomized, placebo-controlled trial of bupropion for the treatment of methamphetamine dependence. *Drug and Alcohol Dependence*, *96*(3),

222–232. http://dx.doi.org/10.1016/j.drugalcdep.2008.03.010, S0376-8716(08) 00104-X [pii].

Shoptaw, S., Huber, A., Peck, J., Yang, X., Liu, J., Jeff, D., et al. (2006). Randomized, placebo-controlled trial of sertraline and contingency management for the treatment of methamphetamine dependence. *Drug and Alcohol Dependence*, *85*(1), 12–18. http://dx.doi.org/10.1016/j.drugalcdep.2006.03.005, S0376-8716(06)00075-5 [pii].

Shoptaw, S., Majewska, M. D., Wilkins, J., Twitchell, G., Yang, X., & Ling, W. (2004). Participants receiving dehydroepiandrosterone during treatment for cocaine dependence show high rates of cocaine use in a placebo-controlled pilot study. *Experimental and Clinical Psychopharmacology*, *12*(2), 126–135. http://dx.doi.org/10.1037/1064-1297.12.2.126, 2004-13592-005 [pii].

Slifer, B. L., & Balster, R. L. (1983). Reinforcing properties of stereoisomers of the putative sigma agonists N-allylnormetazocine and cyclazocine in rhesus monkeys. *The Journal of Pharmacology and Experimental Therapeutics*, *225*(3), 522–528.

Spruce, B. A., Campbell, L. A., McTavish, N., Cooper, M. A., Appleyard, M. V., O'Neill, M., et al. (2004). Small molecule antagonists of the sigma-1 receptor cause selective release of the death program in tumor and self-reliant cells and inhibit tumor growth in vitro and in vivo. *Cancer Research*, *64*(14), 4875–4886.

Stefanski, R., Justinova, Z., Hayashi, T., Takebayashi, M., Goldberg, S. R., & Su, T. P. (2004). Sigma$_1$ receptor upregulation after chronic methamphetamine self-administration in rats: A study with yoked controls. *Psychopharmacology*, *175*(1), 68–75. http://dx.doi.org/10.1007/s00213-004-1779-9.

Stone, J. M., Arstad, E., Erlandsson, K., Waterhouse, R. N., Ell, P. J., & Pilowsky, L. S. (2006). [123I]TPCNE–a novel SPET tracer for the sigma-1 receptor: First human studies and in vivo haloperidol challenge. *Synapse*, *60*(2), 109–117. http://dx.doi.org/10.1002/syn.20281.

Su, T. P. (1982). Evidence for sigma opioid receptor: Binding of [^{3}H]SKF-10047 to etorphine-inaccessible sites in guinea-pig brain. *The Journal of Pharmacology and Experimental Therapeutics*, *223*(2), 284–290.

Su, T. P., & Hayashi, T. (2003). Understanding the molecular mechanism of sigma-1 receptors: Towards a hypothesis that sigma-1 receptors are intracellular amplifiers for signal transduction. *Current Medicinal Chemistry*, *10*(20), 2073–2080.

Su, T. P., Hayashi, T., Maurice, T., Buch, S., & Ruoho, A. E. (2010). The sigma-1 receptor chaperone as an inter-organelle signaling modulator. *Trends in Pharmacological Sciences*, *31*(12), 557–566. http://dx.doi.org/10.1016/j.tips.2010.08.007, S0165-6147(10) 00153-7 [pii].

Su, T. P., London, E. D., & Jaffe, J. H. (1988). Steroid binding at sigma receptors suggests a link between endocrine, nervous, and immune systems. *Science*, *240*(4849), 219–221.

Su, T. P., Weissman, A. D., & Yeh, S. Y. (1986). Endogenous ligands for sigma opioid receptors in the brain ("sigmaphin"): Evidence from binding assays. *Life Sciences*, *38*(24), 2199–2210.

Substance Abuse and Mental Health Services Administration. (2008). Drug Abuse Warning Network, 2006: National Estimates of Drug-Related Emergency Visits.

Substance Abuse and Mental Health Services Administration. (2009). 2008 National Survey on Drug Use and Health.

Takahashi, S., Miwa, T., & Horikomi, K. (2000). Involvement of sigma$_1$ receptors in methamphetamine-induced behavioral sensitization in rats. *Neuroscience Letters*, *289*(1), 21–24, S0304-3940(00)01258-1 [pii].

Takebayashi, M., Hayashi, T., & Su, T. P. (2002). Nerve growth factor-induced neurite sprouting in PC12 cells involves sigma-1 receptors: Implications for antidepressants. *The Journal of Pharmacology and Experimental Therapeutics*, *303*(3), 1227–1237. http://dx.doi.org/10.1124/jpet.102.041970.

Tam, S. W. (1983). Naloxone-inaccessible sigma receptor in rat central nervous system. *Proceedings of the National Academy of Sciences of the United States of America*, *80*(21), 6703–6707.

Tam, S. W., & Cook, L. (1984). Sigma opiates and certain antipsychotic drugs mutually inhibit (+)-[^{3}H] SKF 10,047 and [^{3}H]haloperidol binding in guinea pig brain membranes. *Proceedings of the National Academy of Sciences of the United States of America*, *81*(17), 5618–5621.

Terleckyj, I., & Sonsalla, P. K. (1994). The sigma receptor ligand (+/-)-BMY 14802 prevents methamphetamine-induced dopaminergic neurotoxicity via interactions at dopamine receptors. *The Journal of Pharmacology and Experimental Therapeutics*, *269*(1), 44–50.

Theodorou, V., Chovet, M., Eutamene, H., Fargeau, H., Dassaud, M., Toulouse, M., et al. (2002). Antidiarrhoeal properties of a novel sigma ligand (JO 2871) on toxigenic diarrhoea in mice: Mechanisms of action. *Gut*, *51*(4), 522–528.

Thomas, D. M., Dowgiert, J., Geddes, T. J., Francescutti-Verbeem, D., Liu, X., & Kuhn, D. M. (2004). Microglial activation is a pharmacologically specific marker for the neurotoxic amphetamines. *Neuroscience Letters*, *367*(3), 349–354. http://dx.doi.org/10.1016/j.neulet.2004.06.065, S0304-3940(04)00767-0 [pii].

Toyohara, J., Sakata, M., & Ishiwata, K. (2009). Imaging of sigma$_1$ receptors in the human brain using PET and [^{11}C]SA4503. *Central Nervous System Agents in Medicinal Chemistry*, *9*(3), 190–196.

Toyohara, J., Sakata, M., & Ishiwata, K. (2012). Re-evaluation of in vivo selectivity of [^{11}C] SA4503 to sigma$_1$ receptors in the brain: Contributions of emopamil binding protein. *Nuclear Medicine and Biology*, *39*(7), 1049–1052. http://dx.doi.org/10.1016/j.nucmedbio.2012.03.002, S0969-8051(12)00053-4 [pii].

Ujike, H., Kanazaki, A., Okumura, K., Akiyama, K., & Otsuki, S. (1992). Sigma (σ) antagonist BMY 14802 prevents methamphetamine-induced sensitization. *Life Sciences*, *50*(16), L129–L134.

Ujike, H., Kuroda, S., & Otsuki, S. (1996). Sigma receptor antagonists block the development of sensitization to cocaine. *European Journal of Pharmacology*, *296*(2), 123–128.

United Nations Office on Drugs and Crime. (2010). World Drug Report 2010.

van Waarde, A., Rybczynska, A. A., Ramakrishnan, N., Ishiwata, K., Elsinga, P. H., & Dierckx, R. A. (2010). Sigma receptors in oncology: Therapeutic and diagnostic applications of sigma ligands. *Current Pharmaceutical Design*, *16*(31), 3519–3537, BSP/CPD/ E-Pub/000240 [pii].

Vilner, B. J., & Bowen, W. D. (2000). Modulation of cellular calcium by sigma-2 receptors: Release from intracellular stores in human SK-N-SH neuroblastoma cells. *The Journal of Pharmacology and Experimental Therapeutics*, *292*(3), 900–911.

Vilner, B. J., John, C. S., & Bowen, W. D. (1995). Sigma-1 and sigma-2 receptors are expressed in a wide variety of human and rodent tumor cell lines. *Cancer Research*, *55*(2), 408–413.

Volkow, N. D., Chang, L., Wang, G. J., Fowler, J. S., Franceschi, D., Sedler, M., et al. (2001). Loss of dopamine transporters in methamphetamine abusers recovers with protracted abstinence. *The Journal of Neuroscience*, *21*(23), 9414–9418, 21/23/9414 [pii].

Volkow, N. D., Chang, L., Wang, G. J., Fowler, J. S., Leonido-Yee, M., Franceschi, D., et al. (2001). Association of dopamine transporter reduction with psychomotor impairment in methamphetamine abusers. *The American Journal of Psychiatry*, *158*(3), 377–382.

Volz, H. P., & Stoll, K. D. (2004). Clinical trials with sigma ligands. *Pharmacopsychiatry*, *37*(Suppl. 3), S214–S220. http://dx.doi.org/10.1055/s-2004-832680.

Vu, T. H., Weissman, A. D., & London, E. D. (1990). Pharmacological characteristics and distributions of sigma- and phencyclidine receptors in the animal kingdom. *Journal of Neurochemistry*, *54*(2), 598–604.

Walker, J. M., Bowen, W. D., Patrick, S. L., Williams, W. E., Mascarella, S. W., Bai, X., et al. (1993). A comparison of (-)-deoxybenzomorphans devoid of opiate activity with their dextrorotatory phenolic counterparts suggests role of sigma₂ receptors in motor function. *European Journal of Pharmacology, 231*(1), 61–68.

Wang, B., Rouzier, R., Albarracin, C. T., Sahin, A., Wagner, P., Yang, Y., et al. (2004). Expression of sigma₁ receptor in human breast cancer. *Breast Cancer Research and Treatment, 87*(3), 205–214.

Waterhouse, R. N., Chang, R. C., Zhao, J., & Carambot, P. E. (2006). In vivo evaluation in rats of [^{18}F]1-(2-fluoroethyl)-4-[(4-cyanophenoxy)methyl]piperidine as a potential radiotracer for PET assessment of CNS sigma-1 receptors. *Nuclear Medicine and Biology, 33*(2), 211–215. http://dx.doi.org/10.1016/j.nucmedbio.2005.10.007, S0969-8051(05) 00270-2 [pii].

Weber, E., Sonders, M., Quarum, M., McLean, S., Pou, S., & Keana, J. F. (1986). 1,3-Di(2-[5-^{3}H]tolyl)guanidine: A selective ligand that labels sigma-type receptors for psychotomimetic opiates and antipsychotic drugs. *Proceedings of the National Academy of Sciences of the United States of America, 83*(22), 8784–8788.

Wilbert-Lampen, U., Seliger, C., Zilker, T., & Arendt, R. M. (1998). Cocaine increases the endothelial release of immunoreactive endothelin and its concentrations in human plasma and urine: Reversal by coincubation with sigma-receptor antagonists. *Circulation, 98*(5), 385–390.

Winhusen, T. M., Somoza, E. C., Harrer, J. M., Mezinskis, J. P., Montgomery, M. A., Goldsmith, R. J., et al. (2005). A placebo-controlled screening trial of tiagabine, sertraline and donepezil as cocaine dependence treatments. *Addiction, 100*(Suppl. 1), 68–77. http://dx.doi.org/10.1111/j.1360-0443.2005.00992.x, ADD992 [pii].

Witkin, J. M., Terry, P., Menkel, M., Hickey, P., Pontecorvo, M., Ferkany, J., et al. (1993). Effects of the selective sigma receptor ligand, 6-[6-(4-hydroxypiperidinyl)hexyloxy]-3-methylflavone (NPC 16377), on behavioral and toxic effects of cocaine. *The Journal of Pharmacology and Experimental Therapeutics, 266*(2), 473–482.

Wolfe, S. A., Jr., Kulsakdinun, C., Battaglia, G., Jaffe, J. H., & De Souza, E. B. (1988). Initial identification and characterization of sigma receptors on human peripheral blood leukocytes. *The Journal of Pharmacology and Experimental Therapeutics, 247*(3), 1114–1119.

Woods, S. P., Rippeth, J. D., Conover, E., Gongvatana, A., Gonzalez, R., Carey, C. L., et al. (2005). Deficient strategic control of verbal encoding and retrieval in individuals with methamphetamine dependence. *Neuropsychology, 19*(1), 35–43. http://dx.doi.org/ 10.1037/0894-4105.19.1.35, 2005-00128-005 [pii].

Wu, Z., & Bowen, W. D. (2008). Role of sigma-1 receptor C-terminal segment in inositol 1,4,5-trisphosphate receptor activation: Constitutive enhancement of calcium signaling in MCF-7 tumor cells. *The Journal of Biological Chemistry, 283*(42), 28198–28215. http:// dx.doi.org/10.1074/jbc.M802099200, M802099200 [pii].

Xu, Y. T., Kaushal, N., Shaikh, J., Wilson, L. L., Mesangeau, C., McCurdy, C. R., et al. (2010). A novel substituted piperazine, CM156, attenuates the stimulant and toxic effects of cocaine in mice. *The Journal of Pharmacology and Experimental Therapeutics, 333*(2), 491–500. http://dx.doi.org/10.1124/jpet.109.161398, jpet.109.161398 [pii].

Xu, Y. T., Robson, M. J., Szeszel-Fedorowicz, W., Patel, D., Rooney, R., McCurdy, C. R., et al. (2012). CM156, a sigma receptor ligand, reverses cocaine-induced place conditioning and transcriptional responses in the brain. *Pharmacology, Biochemistry and Behavior, 101*(1), 174–180. http://dx.doi.org/10.1016/j.pbb.2011.12.016, S0091-3057(11)00437-0 [pii].

Xu, J., Zeng, C., Chu, W., Pan, F., Rothfuss, J. M., Zhang, F., et al. (2011). Identification of the PGRMC1 protein complex as the putative sigma-2 receptor binding site. *Nature Communications, 2*, 380. http://dx.doi.org/10.1038/ncomms1386, ncomms1386 [pii].

Yamamoto, H., Miura, R., Yamamoto, T., Shinohara, K., Watanabe, M., Okuyama, S., et al. (1999). Amino acid residues in the transmembrane domain of the type 1 sigma receptor critical for ligand binding. *FEBS Letters*, *445*(1), 19–22, S0014-5793(99) 00084-8 [pii].

Yang, S., Alkayed, N. J., Hurn, P. D., & Kirsch, J. R. (2009). Cyclic adenosine monophosphate response element-binding protein phosphorylation and neuroprotection by 4-phenyl-1-(4-phenylbutyl) piperidine (PPBP). *Anesthesia and Analgesia*, *108*(3), 964–970. http://dx.doi.org/10.1213/ane.0b013e318192442c, 108/3/964 [pii].

Yao, H., Duan, M., & Buch, S. (2011). Cocaine-mediated induction of platelet-derived growth factor: Implication for increased vascular permeability. *Blood*, *117*(8), 2538–2547. http://dx. doi.org/10.1182/blood-2010-10-313593, blood-2010-10-313593 [pii].

Yao, H., Kim, K., Duan, M., Hayashi, T., Guo, M., Morgello, S., et al. (2011). Cocaine hijacks sigma$_1$ receptor to initiate induction of activated leukocyte cell adhesion molecule: Implication for increased monocyte adhesion and migration in the CNS. *The Journal of Neuroscience*, *31*(16), 5942–5955. http://dx.doi.org/10.1523/JNEUROSCI.5618-10.2011, 31/ 16/5942 [pii].

Yao, H., Yang, Y., Kim, K. J., Bethel-Brown, C., Gong, N., Funa, K., et al. (2010). Molecular mechanisms involving sigma receptor-mediated induction of MCP-1: Implication for increased monocyte transmigration. *Blood*, *115*(23), 4951–4962. http://dx.doi.org/ 10.1182/blood-2010-01-266221, blood-2010-01-266221 [pii].

Zamanillo, D., Romero, L., Merlos, M., & Vela, J. M. (2013). Sigma1 receptor: A new therapeutic target for pain. *European Journal of Pharmacology*, *716*, 78–93. http://dx.doi.org/ 10.1016/j.ejphar.2013.01.068, S0014-2999(13)00167-2 [pii].

Zeng, C., Vangveravong, S., Xu, J., Chang, K. C., Hotchkiss, R. S., Wheeler, K. T., et al. (2007). Subcellular localization of sigma-2 receptors in breast cancer cells using two-photon and confocal microscopy. *Cancer Research*, *67*(14), 6708–6716. http://dx.doi. org/10.1158/0008-5472.CAN-06-3803, 67/14/6708 [pii].

Zhang, H., & Cuevas, J. (2002). Sigma receptors inhibit high-voltage-activated calcium channels in rat sympathetic and parasympathetic neurons. *Journal of Neurophysiology*, *87*(6), 2867–2879.

Zhang, H., & Cuevas, J. (2005). Sigma receptor activation blocks potassium channels and depresses neuroexcitability in rat intracardiac neurons. *The Journal of Pharmacology and Experimental Therapeutics*, *313*(3), 1387–1396. http://dx.doi.org/10.1124/jpet.105.084152, jpet.105.084152 [pii].

CHAPTER TEN

Mixed Kappa/Mu Partial Opioid Agonists as Potential Treatments for Cocaine Dependence

Jean M. Bidlack[1]
School of Medicine and Dentistry, University of Rochester, Rochester, New York, USA
[1]Corresponding author: e-mail address: jean_bidlack@urmc.rochester.edu

Contents

Abstract

Cocaine use activates the dopamine reward pathway, leading to the reinforcing effects of dopamine. There is no FDA-approved medication for treating cocaine dependence. Opioid agonists and antagonists have been approved for treating opioid and alcohol dependence. Agonists that activate the μ opioid receptor increase dopamine levels in the nucleus accumbens, while μ receptor antagonists decrease dopamine levels by blocking the effects of endogenous opioid peptides. Activation of the κ opioid receptor decreases dopamine levels and leads to dysphoria. In contrast, inhibition of

Advances in Pharmacology, Volume 69
ISSN 1054-3589
http://dx.doi.org/10.1016/B978-0-12-420118-7.00010-X

the κ opioid receptor decreases dopamine levels in the nucleus accumbens. Antagonists acting at the κ receptor reduce stress-mediated behaviors and anxiety. Mixed partial μ/κ agonists have the potential of striking a balance between dopamine levels and attenuating relapse to cocaine. The pharmacological properties of mixed μ/κ opioid receptor agonists will be discussed and results from clinical and preclinical studies will be presented. Results from studies with some of the classical benzomorphans and morphinans will be presented as they lay the foundation for structure–activity relationships. Recent results with other partial opioid agonists, including buprenorphine derivatives and the mixed μ/κ peptide CJ-15,208, will be discussed. The behavioral effects of the mixed μ/κ MCL-741, an aminothiazolomorphinan, in attenuating cocaine-induced locomotor activity will be presented. While not a mixed μ/κ opioid, results obtained with GSK1521498, a μ receptor inverse agonist, will be discussed. Preclinical strategies and successes will lay the groundwork for the further development of mixed μ/κ opioid receptor agonists to treat cocaine dependence.

ABBREVIATIONS
8-CAC 8-carboxamidocyclazocine
Arodyn (Ac[Phe(1,2,3),Arg(4),D-Ala(8)]Dyn A-(1–11)NH$_2$)
ATPM (−)-3-amino-thiazolo-[5,4,b]-N-cyclopropylmethylmorphinan
CHO Chinese hamster ovary
CJ-15,208 *cyclo*[Phe-D-Pro-Phe-Trp]
EKC ethylketocyclazocine
MAPK mitogen-activated protein kinase
NOP nociceptin/orphanin FQ
nor-BNI nor-binaltorphimine
Zyklophin [N-benzylTyr1,cyclo(D-Asp5,Dap8)]Dyn A-(1–11)NH$_2$

1. INTRODUCTION

There is general acceptance that the abuse-related effects of cocaine and other drugs of abuse are mediated primarily by increases in extracellular dopamine levels in the mesolimbic dopamine system (Johanson & Fischman, 1989; Kuhar, Ritz, & Boja, 1991; Ritz, Lamb, Goldberg, & Kuhar, 1987). Cocaine directly activates the dopaminergic mesocortical/mesolimbic and nigrostriatal systems by binding to the dopamine reuptake transporter (Kreek et al., 2012; Maisonneuve, Ho, & Kreek, 1995; Pettit, Ettenberg, Bloom, & Koob, 1984; Zhang et al., 2013). Changes in dopamine levels are part of the addiction–abstinence cycle (Zhang et al., 2013). Accordingly, one treatment strategy has involved modulation of cocaine's dopaminergic effects (Mendelson & Mello, 1996). However, with dopamine antagonists, only a transient blockade of the abuse-related effects of cocaine was observed, and direct and indirect dopamine agonists may produce unacceptable side effects, including high abuse potential that may complicate pharmacotherapy (Kleven & Woolverton, 1990; Negus, Mello, Lamas, & Mendelson, 1996). Activation of the μ opioid receptor stimulates dopamine release, while κ opioid agonists decrease dopamine release (Di Chiara & Imperato, 1988; Koob et al., 2014; Spanagel, Herz, & Shippenberg, 1990). Both μ and κ opioids have been postulated to play a direct role in the reinforcing effects of cocaine (Koob et al., 2014; Kuzmin, Gerrits, Zvartau, & van Ree, 2000). The dynorphin/κ receptor system is upregulated following cocaine administration (Spangler, Unterwald, & Kreek, 1993).

Stimulation of the κ opioid receptor antagonizes the rewarding properties of cocaine (Wee & Koob, 2010). Blocking the κ receptor with the κ-selective antagonist nor-binaltorphimine did not attenuate cocaine self-administration in monkeys (Negus, Mello, Portoghese, & Lin, 1997) and rodent studies (Wee & Koob, 2010). However, in a cocaine-dependent state, κ antagonists have been effective in reducing cocaine use (Butelman, Yuferov, & Kreek, 2012; Shippenberg, Zapata, & Chefer, 2007; Wee & Koob, 2010). Antagonists acting at the κ receptor prevented stress-induced relapse in abstinent subjects (Beardsley, Howard, Shelton, & Carroll, 2005; Redila & Chavkin, 2008). Selective κ antagonists have been shown to decrease both compulsive cocaine-seeking behavior and intake in the absence of stress in rats (Wee, Orio, Ghirmai, Cashman, & Koob, 2009; Wee, Vendruscolo, Misra, Schlosburg, & Koob, 2012).

In addition to dopamine, serotonin plays a role in drug-seeking behaviors (Cunningham & Anastasio, 2014; Cunningham et al., 2013; Devroye, Filip, Przegalinski, McCreary, & Spampinato, 2013; Murnane et al., 2013; Picetti et al., 2013; Schindler et al., 2012). Activation of the κ opioid receptor leads to an increase in serotonin levels (Ruedi-Bettschen, Rowlett, Spealman, & Platt, 2010). Impulsivity and cue reactivity in rodents appears to be mediated by serotonin (Anastasio et al., 2013). Stress-induced activation of the dynorphin and κ opioid receptor system produces a transient increase in serotonin transport locally in the ventral striatum that may underlie some of the adverse consequences of stress exposure, including the potentiation of the rewarding effects of cocaine (Schindler et al., 2012).

By studying mixed μ/κ agonists with vary degrees of efficacy, it may be possible to identify compounds that attenuate cocaine dependence without producing opioid dependence or other adverse effects. Opioids used to treat addiction have some unwanted properties. Methadone can induce a prolonged QT interval in patients (Martin et al., 2011). Buprenorphine may be lead to dependence or cause relapse in abstinent heroin users (Kreek, LaForge, & Butelman, 2002). Opioid antagonists have fewer liabilities but can produce withdrawal in opioid-dependent subjects. By obtaining an optimal balance in dopamine and serotonin levels, mixed μ/κ agonists may be developed to treat cocaine dependence without unwanted side effects. An ideal medication would be orally bioavailable, have a half-life greater than 12 h, and would reduce cocaine cravings and relapse, while not producing unwanted effects, such as producing opioid dependence.

2. OPIOIDS USED TO TREAT DRUG AND ALCOHOL DEPENDENCE: PRECLINICAL AND CLINICAL EVIDENCE

Medications that bind to opioid receptors are used for the treatment of opioid and alcohol dependence. Figure 10.1 shows the opioid medications that have been approved in the United States or Europe for the treatment of

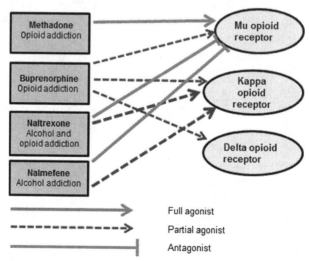

Figure 10.1 Opioids used to treat drugs of abuse and the opioid receptors involved in their mechanism of action. The mechanism of action is shown in the figure as follows: green arrow, full agonist; dashed blue arrow, partial agonist; and red line with a bar at end, antagonist. This figure only shows the interaction of the medications with the receptors that they bind to with high affinity. (For interpretation of the references to color in this figure legend, the reader is referred to the online version of this chapter.)

addictive disorders. Methadone and buprenorphine are used to treat opioid dependence. Naltrexone and nalmefene are used to treat alcohol dependence.

2.1. Methadone

Methadone is the first opioid-based medication developed for the treatment of opiate dependence. Methadone, a full opioid agonist, was developed in the 1960s for the long-term treatment of addiction to heroin and other opiates (Dole & Nyswander, 1965; Dole, Nyswander, & Kreek, 1966; Kreek, 1973, 2000; Kreek et al., 2012). Methadone produces its pharmacological effect by acting as a full agonist at the μ opioid receptor, increasing dopamine levels in a sustained manner due to its relatively long half-life (Eap, Buclin, & Baumann, 2002). Methadone produces physical dependence and that is why it is not used in opiate naïve patients. In patients taking both opiates and cocaine, high dosages of methadone reduced cocaine use (Peles, Kreek, Kellogg, & Adelson, 2006). In a rat model, methadone was effective in preventing cocaine-induced conditioned place preference and cocaine-induced neuroadaptations (Leri, Zhou, Goddard, Cummins, & Kreek, 2006; Leri et al., 2009).

2.2. Naltrexone

Naltrexone has been recognized as an efficacious treatment for alcohol dependence. Naltrexone is an antagonist at the μ receptor and a partial agonist at the κ receptor (Wentland, Lou, Lu, Bu, Denhardt, et al., 2009). By antagonizing the μ receptor and partially stimulating the κ receptor, naltrexone may balance dopamine levels and thereby reduce cravings. Recently, naltrexone has been reported to reduce opiate use in opiate-dependent patients (Sullivan et al., 2013) and to reduce cocaine craving in cocaine-dependent subjects (Comer et al., 2013; Sofuoglu et al., 2003). Differences have been observed between males and females. A high daily dose of naltrexone reduced both alcohol and cocaine use in dependent males, while an increase in alcohol and cocaine use was observed in females (Pettinati et al., 2008). Naltrexone and extended-release naltrexone are being evaluated alone and in combination with buprenorphine as a possible pharmacotherapeutic treatment for cocaine dependence.

A number of preclinical studies have evaluated naltrexone as a possible therapeutic for treating cocaine dependence. Naltrexone reduced cocaine self-administration in rats under both a fixed-ratio schedule and a progressive-ratio schedule (Wee et al., 2009) and in rats trained to seek cocaine under a second-order schedule of reinforcement (Giuliano, Robbins, Wille, Bullmore, & Everitt, 2013). Naltrexone reduced cocaine-induced reinstatement of drug-seeking behavior in abstinent rats (Burattini, Burbassi, Aicardi, & Cervo, 2008). Pretreatment with naltrexone blocked cue-induced cocaine reinstatement (Burattini et al., 2008) and progressively attenuated cocaine-induced reinstatement, with a significant reduction on days 3 and 5 of reinstatement testing in rats (Gerrits, Kuzmin, & van Ree, 2005). Chronic naltrexone treatment of rats along with chronic cocaine slightly attenuated cocaine-induced locomotor activity in rats (Kunko, French, & Izenwasser, 1998). Naltrexone reduced locomotor response to a priming dose of amphetamine without affecting general locomotor behavior (Haggkvist, Lindholm, & Franck, 2009). Cocaine-seeking was dose-dependently decreased following naltrexone treatment (Giuliano et al., 2013). However, the same treatment had no effect on cocaine self-administration under a continuous reinforcement schedule (Giuliano et al., 2013). Collectively, these preclinical findings strongly suggest that naltrexone may have a prominent role in treating cocaine dependence.

2.3. Buprenorphine and buprenorphine/naltrexone combination

Buprenorphine was developed as an opiate analgesic with lower abuse potential than morphine (Cowan, Lewis, & Macfarlane, 1977; Downing, Leary, & White, 1977). Buprenorphine has been successful in treating opioid dependence (Ling & Wesson, 2003; McCance-Katz, Sullivan, & Nallani, 2010). Patients in buprenorphine maintenance treatment used less cocaine than opioid-dependent cocaine use (Montoya et al., 2004). In rhesus monkeys, buprenorphine attenuated cocaine self-administration without affecting food intake (Mello, Lukas, Mendelson, & Drieze, 1993). In rats, buprenorphine enhanced the dopamine response to cocaine (Sorge & Stewart, 2006).

Buprenorphine together with naltrexone is being investigated as a potential combination treatment for cocaine abuse and polydrug abuse (McCann, 2008; Mooney et al., 2013). In humans, a functional κ antagonist, produced by the combination of buprenorphine and naltrexone, gave encouraging results with opioid-dependent patients (Gerra, Fantoma, & Zaimovic, 2006; Rothman et al., 2000). Patients treated with naltrexone and buprenorphine had lower positive urines for morphine and cocaine metabolites than patients treated with naltrexone alone (Gerra et al., 2006). The conceptual and practical issues in relation to the use of μ opioid agonists, partial agonists, and antagonists in the treatment of opiate addiction have been discussed (Nutt, 2010). Clinical trials are ongoing to determine if naltrexone together with buprenorphine will attenuate cocaine use and if extended-release naltrexone will block physiological dependence on buprenorphine (Mooney et al., 2013). The advantage of this combination besides the pharmacological properties that both compounds may contribute to reducing cocaine use is that inclusion of naltrexone will prevent any opioid dependence that may be produced by buprenorphine.

Animal studies strongly support the efficacy of a buprenorphine/naltrexone combination. In preclinical studies, the combination of naltrexone and buprenorphine blocked cocaine self-administration in rats that had extended access to cocaine, and did not produce opioid dependence (Wee et al., 2012). Also, the combination of buprenorphine and naltrexone blocked drug-primed reinstatement in cocaine-conditioned rats (Cordery et al., 2012). A number of novel orvinols structurally related to buprenorphine have been synthesized recently (Greedy et al., 2013; Husbands, 2013). These compounds are of interest to determine if they will be more efficacious than buprenorphine.

2.4. Nalmefene

Like naltrexone, nalmefene has been shown to reduce alcohol consumption (Soyka & Rosner, 2008). In March 2013, nalmefene was approved by the European Commission for the reduction of alcohol consumption by adult patients with alcohol dependence http://www.ema.europa.eu/ema/index.jsp?curl=pages/medicines/human/medicines/002583/human_med_001620.jsp&mid=WC0b01ac058001d124. Nalmefene was approved for use, as needed, to reduce cravings for alcohol. Similar to naltrexone, nalmefene is a μ opioid antagonist and a partial agonist at the κ receptor (Bart et al., 2005; Wentland, Lou, Lu, Bu, Denhardt, et al., 2009). Nalmefene increased serum prolactin levels in humans, indicating that it is producing a physiological κ agonist effect (Bart et al., 2005). There is a lack of preclinical studies on the effects of nalmefene on cocaine-mediated behaviors, possibly due to the high cost of obtaining nalmefene (Violin & Lefkowitz, 2007).

2.5. Nalbuphine and butorphanol

In rhesus monkeys on a second order of reinforcement, both nalbuphine and butorphanol produced the greatest decreases in cocaine self-administration and the smallest effects on food-maintained responding (Negus & Mello, 2002). However, nalbuphine and butorphanol did not block the discriminative stimulus effects of cocaine in monkeys trained to discriminate 0.4 mg/kg cocaine from saline in a food-reinforced drug discrimination procedure (Negus & Mello, 2002). Also, both nalbuphine and butorphanol reduced food intake and reduced cocaine intake in rhesus monkeys (Mello, Kamien, Lukas, Drieze, & Mendelson, 1993). In male Long–Evans rats, nalbuphine, butorphanol, buprenorphine, and (−) pentazocine dose-dependently enhanced the effects of cocaine at doses that did not alter locomotor activity when administered alone (Smith et al., 2003). This study concluded that low-efficacy μ opioids may potentiate the effects of cocaine similar to the effects observed with high-efficacy μ agonists. However, another interpretation of the data is that nalbuphine, butorphanol, buprenorphine, and (−)-pentazocine enhanced cocaine-induced locomotor activity because of their κ agonist properties. Rats treated with cocaine exhibited a progressive increase in locomotor activity over the 10-day treatment period, and this effect was significantly reduced in rats treated with cocaine plus nalbuphine (Smith et al., 2013). These authors suggest that nalbuphine attenuates the development of sensitization to the behavioral effects of cocaine (Smith et al., 2013).

Clinically, nalbuphine attenuated cocaine's effects on ACTH, cortisol, and luteinizing hormone in cocaine-dependent males (Goletiani, Mendelson, Sholar, Siegel, & Mello, 2009). Butorphanol failed to reduce cocaine subjective effects in humans and did not reduce cocaine self-administration in an 8-week inpatient study (Walsh, Geter-Douglas, Strain, & Bigelow, 2001).

2.6. Cyclazocine and pentazocine

Cyclazocine, a benzomorphan, was tested during the 1960s to determine if it would be a possible treatment for heroin addicts (Archer, Albertson, Harris, Pierson, & Bird, 1964; Archer, Glick, & Bidlack, 1996; Freedman, Fink, Sharoff, & Zaks, 1967; Harris & Pierson, 1964). Freedman and colleagues showed that 4–5 mg of cyclazocine daily blocked the effects of 15 mg of intravenous heroin. This report was one of the first reports of cyclazocine's antagonistic properties. Cyclazocine was investigated to determine if it would attenuate cigarette smoking in polydrug abusers (Pickworth, Lee, Abreu, Umbricht, & Preston, 2004) and in cocaine-dependent patients (Preston et al., 2004). Cyclazocine was not effective in blocking the craving for cigarettes or cocaine. This lack of effect may be due to the fact that cyclazocine is a full κ agonist in addition to being a μ partial agonist (Bidlack & Knapp, 2013). However, tolerance often develops to the κ agonist effects (Archer et al., 1996; Preston et al., 2004).

The next section of this chapter discusses the pharmacological properties of the classical opioids and opioids that are being developed as potential therapeutics for treating cocaine dependence.

 ## 3. MECHANISTIC AND *IN VITRO* CHARACTERIZATION OF MIXED μ/κ AGONISTS

Recently, studies have suggested unique mechanisms may account for physiological effects observed with opioid partial agonists. Biased ligand signaling involves phosphorylation of the receptor and recruitment of β-arrestin, leading to other signaling, and endocytosis of the receptor (Kenakin, 2007; Violin & Lefkowitz, 2007). Differences in receptor phosphorylation have been observed between a full agonist and a partial agonist (Lau et al., 2011). Differences in μ receptor regulation may be determined not only by net incorporation of phosphate into the receptor populations as a whole but also by individual receptors achieving a critical number of phosphorylated residues in a specific region of the C-tail (Lau et al., 2011).

Biased signaling has been observed with κ agonists and this signaling differed between the human and rat κreceptor. Pentazocine and butorphanol were significantly more potent at activating p38 MAPK mediated by the human κ receptor than the rat κ receptor expressed in HEK293 cells, but these two κ full agonists were equally potent at arrestin-independent activation of ERK1/2 mediated by human and rat κ receptors (Schattauer et al., 2012).

The binding of each full and partial agonist to a receptor will alter receptor conformation in a unique manner. Changes in receptor conformation will lead undoubtedly to differences in receptor phosphorylation, signaling, and, ultimately, behavioral effects. To start understanding unique properties of full and partial agonists, the affinity and selectivity of the compound for each opioid receptor should be known. Affinity and selectivity will determine if a compound is likely to signal and produce behavioral effects mediated by a specific opioid receptor. The $[^{35}S]GTP\gamma S$ binding assay is able to predict *in vivo* properties of compounds. This assay can effectively determine if a compound is a full agonist, partial agonist, or antagonist.

3.1. Affinity of classical opioids and some opioids in preclinical testing for the multiple opioid receptors

Figure 10.2 shows the structures of some opioids, both classical and novel, that are discussed in this chapter. In order to know which opioid receptor mediates a physiological response, it is important to understand the affinity that a compound has for the multiple opioid receptors. Table 10.1 shows the K_i values for the inhibition of binding to the μ, κ, and δ opioid receptors by medications used to treat opiate or alcohol dependence and by some novel mixed μ/κ opioids.

Methadone has a high affinity and selectivity for the μ opioid receptor, which is responsible for its pharmacological effects. Methadone had a 290-fold greater affinity for the μ receptor than the κ receptor and a 2200-fold greater affinity for the μ receptor than the δ receptor (Table 10.1). Buprenorphine had a threefold greater affinity for the μ receptor than the κ receptor and a 14-fold greater affinity for the μ receptor than the δ receptor (Wentland, Lou, Lu, Bu, VanAlstine, et al., 2009). Buprenorphine has been reported to bind to the NOP receptor, but with a considerably lower affinity for the NOP receptor ranging from 50-fold lower affinity (Spagnolo et al., 2008; Toll, Khroyan, Polgar, Husbands, & Zaveri, 2013) to 3500-fold lower affinity (Huang, Kehner, Cowan, & Liu-Chen, 2001) for the NOP receptor than the μ opioid receptor. Naltrexone had an almost twofold greater affinity for the μ than the κ receptor and a 500-fold greater affinity for the μ receptor than the δ opioid receptor (Wentland, Lou, Lu, Bu, Denhardt, et al., 2009; Wentland et al., 2005). Nalmefene had a K_i value of 0.083 nM at the κ receptor, which was threefold greater than at the μ receptor and 190-fold greater than at the δ receptor. The novel opioids are discussed in the sections in the succeeding text.

3.2. Pharmacological properties of classical and novel opioids for the μ and κ opioid receptors as measured by the [^{35}S]GTPγS binding assay

Table 10.2 shows the pharmacological properties at μ and κ receptors, as measured by [^{35}S]GTPγS binding, of the opioids listed in Table 10.1. The compounds had the lowest affinity for the δ receptor, and therefore, the pharmacological properties of the compound would not be mediated by the δ receptor. A partial agonist stimulates [^{35}S]GTPγS binding, but not to the same efficacy as a full agonist. Partial agonists will shift the concentration–response curve for a full agonist to the right. In other words, partial agonists will attenuate the potency, but not the efficacy of a full agonist.

Classical and novel opioids

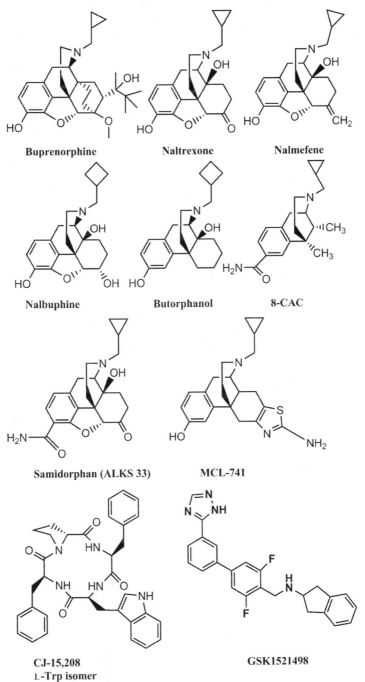

Figure 10.2 Chemical structures of some classical and novel μ/κ opioids discussed in this chapter.

Table 10.1 Affinity and selectivity of opioids for the multiple opioid receptors

Opioid	[³H]DAMGO (MOR)	[³H]U69,593 (KOR)	[³H] Naltrindole (DOR)	References
	K_i (nM) ± SEM			
Methadone	0.79 ± 0.07	230 ± 11	1700 ± 60	Bidlack, J.M. and Knapp, B.I. (unpublished)
Buprenorphine	0.21 ± 0.02	0.62 ± 0.07	2.9 ± 0.4	Wentland, Lou, Lu, Bu, VanAlstine, et al. (2009)
Naltrexone	0.11 ± 0.006	0.19 ± 0.005	60 ± 3	Wentland, Lou, Lu, Bu, Denhardt, et al. (2009), Wentland et al. (2005)
Nalmefene	0.24 ± 0.006	0.083 ± 0.0008	16 ± 1	Bart et al. (2005)
Nalbuphine	1.6 ± 0.3	3.0 ± 0.6	580 ± 80	Wentland, Lou, Lu, Bu, Denhardt, et al. (2009)
Butorphanol	0.22 ± 0.01	0.12 ± 0.01	12 ± 1	Fulton, Knapp, Bidlack, and Neumeyer (2008)
8-CAC	0.31 ± 0.03	0.060 ± 0.001	5.2 ± 0.3	Wentland et al. (2006)
Samidorphan (ALKS 33)	0.052 ± 0.004	0.23 ± 0.01	2.6 ± 0.2	Wentland, Lou, Lu, Bu, Denhardt, et al. (2009), Wentland et al. (2005)
MCL-741	6.7 ± 0.7	1.9 ± 0.1	13 ± 1	Provencher et al. (2013)
[L-Trp] CJ-15,208	619 ± 87	35.4 ± 3.6	4150 ± 3020	Ross, Reilley, Murray, Aldrich, and McLaughlin (2012)
[D-Trp] CJ-15,208	259 ± 29	30.6 ± 3.4	2910 ± 1350	Ross et al. (2012)
GSK1521498	1.5 ± 0.08	39 ± 5	670 ± 70	Bidlack, J.M. and Knapp, B.I. (unpublished)

Receptor-binding experiments were performed as described in the references. The mean K_i values ± SEM are reported.

Table 10.2 Pharmacological properties of classical and novel opioids as measured with [^{35}S]GTPγS binding

Compound	Mu receptor	Kappa receptor	References
Methadone	Full agonist	No effect measurable	Bidlack and Knapp (unpublished)
Buprenorphine	Partial agonist	Partial agonist	Huang et al. (2001), Wentland, Lou, Lu, Bu, VanAlstine, et al. (2009)
Naltrexone	Antagonist	Partial agonist	Wentland, Lou, Lu, Bu, Denhardt, et al. (2009)
Nalmefene	Antagonist	Partial agonist	Bart et al. (2005)
Nalbuphine	Partial agonist	Partial agonist	Wentland, Lou, Lu, Bu, Denhardt, et al. (2009)
Butorphanol	Partial agonist	Full agonist	Neumeyer et al. (2012)
8-CAC	Partial agonist	Full agonist	Wentland et al. (2006)
Samidorphan (ALKS 33)	Antagonist	Partial agonist	Wentland, Lou, Lu, Bu, Denhardt, et al. (2009)
MCL-741	Partial agonist	Full agonist	Provencher et al. (2013)
[L-Trp] CJ-15,208	Antagonist	Antagonist	Ross et al. (2012)
[D-Trp] CJ-15,208	No effect	Antagonist	Ross et al. (2012)
GSK1521498	Inverse agonist	Inverse agonist	Ignar et al. (2011)

[^{35}S]GTPγS binding was measured as described in the references.

Methadone is the only full μ agonist used to treat opioid dependence. Because of its high affinity and high selectivity for the μ receptor, its pharmacological properties are mediated solely by the μ receptor. Buprenorphine is a partial agonist at both the μ and κ receptors (Huang et al., 2001; Wentland, Lou, Lu, Bu, VanAlstine, et al., 2009). As shown in Table 10.1, buprenorphine has a threefold greater affinity for the μ receptor than the κ receptor. Because buprenorphine is not selective, its pharmacological properties are mediated by both the μ and κ receptors. Both naltrexone and nalmefene are μ antagonists and κ partial agonists.

3.2.1 Pharmacological properties of benzomorphans: Cyclazocine derivatives

The benzomorphans, such as cyclazocine, EKC, and (−)-pentazocine, have been studied for almost 50 years. Some benzomorphans, such as cyclazocine and pentazocine, and many morphinans were studied *in vivo* before the three types of opioid receptors had been cloned and then expressed in cell lines. At the same time, *in vitro* assays, such as $[^{35}S]GTP\gamma S$ binding, were developed and shown to accurately predict the *in vivo* pharmacological properties of the opioids. Structure–activity relationships show that all benzomorphans are full agonists at the κ opioid receptor with varying activity at the μ receptor (Bidlack & Knapp, 2013). Exploring the pharmacological effects of benzomorphans and morphinans gives us an understanding of how the effects of compounds that are full κ agonists combined with μ activity ranging from partial agonist activity to a pure antagonist at the μ receptor affect *in vivo* parameters of drug abuse.

After the finding that EKC reduced cocaine self-administration in monkeys without having a serious effect on food intake (Negus et al., 1997), there was a renewed interest in evaluating mixed κ/μ opioid agonists as possible therapeutics for cocaine abuse. Previous research suggested that at least two pharmacological characteristics may be important determinants of κ opioid effects. First, the magnitude of effect on cocaine self-administration was related to efficacy at κ receptors while still having μ activity (Mello & Negus, 1998, 2000; Negus et al., 1997). Second, the selectivity of the ligand for the κ and μ opioid receptors also influenced κ opioid effects on cocaine self-administration. EKC was the most effective κ agonist in decreasing cocaine self-administration in rhesus monkeys (Negus et al., 1997). The fact that EKC attenuated cocaine self-administration and produced fewer undesirable effects than the full, κ-selective agonist U50,488 leads to a renewed interest in studying benzomorphans and morphinans, with similar pharmacological properties, as possible treatments for cocaine dependence.

(−)-Pentazocine, another benzomorphan, which was developed as analgesic in the early 1960s, was a partial agonist at the μ receptor and a full agonist at κ receptors (Archer et al., 1964; Bidlack, McLaughlin, & Wentland, 2000). Subsequently, structure–activity relationship studies have shown that all benzomorphans are full κ agonists, but they have varying efficacy at the μ receptor (Bidlack & Knapp, 2013). Most benzomorphans have approximately 50-fold lower affinity for the δ opioid receptor than the μ and κ receptors, so most of the activity of the benzomorphans is mediated by the κ and μ opioid receptors (Bidlack & Knapp, 2013).

Derivatives of cyclazocine and other benzomorphans were prepared in the hope of obtaining a compound that had a longer duration of action than cyclazocine and EKC while maintaining pharmacological properties similar to EKC. 8-CAC, shown in Fig. 10.2, was synthesized by Dr. Wentland's group in 2001 (Wentland, Lou, Ye, et al., 2001). 8-CAC had high affinity for κ and μ receptors (Table 10.1). 8-CAC was a partial agonist at the μ receptor and a full κ agonist as shown in Table 10.2. 8-CAC produced antinociception in mice for up to 8 h in comparison to antinociception produced by cyclazocine that lasted for less than 90 min (Bidlack et al., 2002). This study showed that a carboxamide group could replace the phenolic group in C-8 in benzomorphans and the C-3 position in morphinans (Wentland, Lou, Dehnhardt, et al., 2001) and compounds retained high affinity for opioid receptors. 8-CAC attenuated cocaine self-administration in rhesus monkeys, but 8-CAC also reduced food intake at doses that reduced cocaine self-administration (Stevenson, Wentland, Bidlack, Mello, & Negus, 2004). Also, tolerance developed to the reduction of cocaine intake by 8-CAC (Stevenson et al., 2004). These results are probably due to 8-CAC being a full κ agonist.

3.2.2 Pharmacological properties of some classical Mu opioid antagonists: Naltrexone and nalmefene

Unlike benzomorphans that are partial agonists at μ receptors and full κ agonists, some morphinans, such as nalmefene and naltrexone, are μ antagonists and partial κ agonists (Bart et al., 2005; Bidlack & Knapp, 2013). Figure 10.3A shows that both nalmefene and naltrexone stimulate [^{35}S] GTPγS binding to membranes prepared from CHO cells expressing the human κ opioid receptor (Bart et al., 2005; Wentland, Lou, Lu, Bu, Denhardt, et al., 2009). Naltrexone and nalmefene also inhibited [^{35}S] GTPγS binding stimulated by the κ agonist U50,488 (Fig. 10.3B). These data demonstrate that both nalmefene and naltrexone are partial κ agonists with similar efficacy and potency. Likewise, in the [^{35}S]GTPγS binding assay, the short-acting μ antagonist naloxone is a partial agonist at the κ receptor (Bidlack & Knapp, 2013). Historically, naltrexone, nalmefene, naloxone, and diprenorphine have been regarded as opioid antagonists. Since the cloning of the three opioid receptors (Evans, Keith, Morrison, Magendzo, & Edwards, 1992; Kieffer, Befort, Gaveriaux-Ruff, & Hirth,

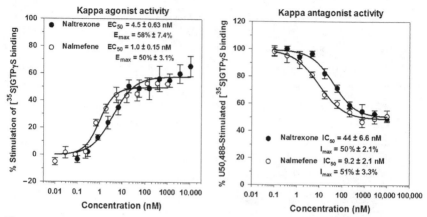

Figure 10.3 Naltrexone and nalmefene are partial agonists in the [^{35}S]GTPγS binding assay mediated by the κ opioid receptor. In membranes from CHO cells that expressed the human κ receptor, both nalmefene and naltrexone stimulated [^{35}S]GTPγS binding indicating that these compounds had agonist properties (A). Similarly, both nalmefene and naltrexone inhibited [^{35}S]GTPγS binding that was stimulated by the κ-selective agonist U50,488 (B).

1992; Simonin et al., 1994; Wang et al., 1994; Zhu et al., 1995) and advancements in *in vitro* techniques, such as the use of [^{35}S]GTPγS binding to characterize the pharmacological properties of compounds (Befort, Tabbara, & Kieffer, 1996; Selley, Sim, Xiao, Liu, & Childers, 1997; Sim, Selley, & Childers, 1995; Traynor & Nahorski, 1995), nalmefene, naltrexone, naloxone, and diprenorphine have been shown to be partial agonists at the κ receptor (Bart et al., 2005; Wentland, Lou, Lu, Bu, Denhardt, et al., 2009; Wentland, Lou, Lu, Bu, VanAlstine, et al., 2009).

There have been reports showing that naltrexone slightly stimulated [^{35}S]GTPγS binding mediated by the μ opioid receptor (Ignar et al., 2011; Wentland, Lou, Lu, Bu, Denhardt, et al., 2009). We have reported a 14% stimulation of [^{35}S]GTPγS binding mediated by the μ receptor. Whether such a small stimulation in [^{35}S]GTPγS has a physiological consequence is not known.

3.2.3 Pharmacological properties of samidorphan (ALKS 33): A naltrexone derivative

3-Carboxamide substitutions were made to naltrexone, nalmefene, buprenorphine, and other opiates (Wentland, Lou, Lu, Bu, Denhardt, et al., 2009; Wentland, Lou, Lu, Bu, VanAlstine, et al., 2009; Zhang, Xiong, Bidlack, et al., 2004). Samidorphan (ALKS 33), a derivative of naltrexone having a 3-carboxamide group, an open furan ring, and a 4-hydroxyl group (Fig. 10.2), was synthesized initially by Dr. Mark Wentland's laboratory (Wentland et al., 2005). As shown in Table 10.1, samidorphan (ALKS 33) has a twofold higher affinity for the μ receptor than naltrexone and an affinity similar to naltrexone for the κ receptor. Samidorphan (ALKS 33) is an antagonist at the μ receptor and a partial agonist at the κ receptor, retaining the pharmacological properties of naltrexone, as summarized in Table 10.2. Samidorphan (ALKS 33), alone and in combination with buprenorphine, is being evaluated as a possible treatment for cocaine dependence.

3.2.4 Pharmacological properties of nalbuphine, cyclorphan, butorphan, and butorphanol

Nalbuphine is a morphinan with high affinity for the μ and κ opioid receptors and a very low affinity for the δ receptor (Table 10.1). This very low affinity for the δ receptor is not shared by most other mixed μ/κ agonists. Nalbuphine is a partial agonist at both the μ and κ receptors (Table 10.2). Because nalbuphine is nonselective between the μ and κ receptors (Table 10.1), its pharmacological effects would be mediated by both receptors. However, nalbuphine has much higher affinity for the μ and κ receptors than the δ receptor (Table 10.1); therefore, all of pharmacological effects produced by nalbuphine are mediated by the μ and κ receptors, and not the δ receptor.

Open-ring morphinans such as cyclorphan (Gates, 1973) and butorphanol analogs were synthesized as mixed μ/κ opioids (Neumeyer et al., 2000). Cyclorphan has high affinity at κ and μ opioid receptors (Neumeyer et al., 2000, 2012). Cyclorphan has a 75-fold lower affinity for the δ receptor than the κ receptor (Neumeyer et al., 2012). Cyclorphan, which contains an N-cyclopropylmethyl group, and butorphan (MCL-101), which contains an N-cyclobutylmethyl group, were μ partial agonists, exhibiting agonist and antagonist properties both in vivo (Mathews et al., 2005) and in vitro (Neumeyer et al., 2012). Likewise, cyclorphan and butorphan (MCL-101) were κ full agonists (Neumeyer et al., 2000, 2012). Both cyclorphan and butorphan produced antinociception that was mediated by μ and κ receptors (Mathews et al., 2005). However, both compounds only antagonized antinociception mediated by the μ opioid receptor (Mathews et al., 2005).

Butorphanol is very similar to butorphan. The only difference is that butorphanol has a OH group in C-14. Butorphanol has high affinity for µ and κ receptors (Table 10.1). Butorphanol is a partial agonist at the µ receptor and a full agonist at the κ opioid receptor as shown in Table 10.2. The pharmacological properties of butorphanol are not changed when a $CONH_2$ group was added at C-3 position (Neumeyer et al., 2012). Like the benzomorphans, cyclorphan derivatives, like butorphan and butorphanol, are full agonists at the κ receptor. Bivalent ligands of butorphan were synthesized and characterized (Fulton, Knapp, Bidlack, & Neumeyer, 2010). They retained high affinity for µ and κ receptors. A hydrocarbon spacer of eight was optimal in producing a high-affinity bivalent ligand (Fulton et al., 2010).

3.2.5 Pharmacological properties of buprenorphine and buprenorphine derivatives

Buprenorphine has high affinity for the µ and κ opioid receptors and about a 10-fold lower affinity for the δ receptor as shown in Table 10.1. Buprenorphine has been postulated to attenuate alcohol abuse by acting at the NOP receptor (Ciccocioppo et al., 2007), but buprenorphine has a much lower affinity for the NOP receptor than it does for either the µ or κ opioid receptors (Huang et al., 2001). Because of its lower affinity for the NOP receptor, it is unlikely that most of buprenorphine's *in vivo* pharmacological effects are mediated by the NOP receptor. Buprenorphine is a partial agonist at µ and κ receptors and a very weak, low-efficacy partial agonist at δ receptors as measured by $[^{35}S]GTP\gamma S$ binding (Huang et al., 2001; Wentland, Lou, Lu, Bu, Denhardt, et al., 2009) and *in vivo* assays (Negus et al., 2002). Nalmefene and naltrexone are more efficacious in the $[^{35}S]$ GTPγS binding assay at the κ receptor than buprenorphine, but buprenorphine was more potent (Huang et al., 2001; Wentland, Lou, Lu, Bu, Denhardt, et al., 2009). Buprenorphine produces analgesia through the µ opioid receptor (Lutfy et al., 2003). Its primary metabolite norbuprenorphine, like buprenorphine, was a partial agonist at both the µ and κ opioid receptors (Huang et al., 2001).

Recently, an orvinol series of compounds related to buprenorphine was synthesized and characterized for pharmacological properties at κ and µ receptors (Greedy et al., 2013). This study showed that a predictive model for efficacy at the κ receptor can be derived, with efficacy in the orvinol series being controlled by the length of the group attached to C-20 and the introduction of branching into the side chain (Greedy et al., 2013). This series of buprenorphine derivatives has yielded a number of mixed µ/κ agonists for further study.

3.2.6 Aminothiazolomorphinans

Aminothiazolomorphinans represent a new class of compounds with high affinity for μ and κ opioid receptors (Zhang, Xiong, Hilbert, et al., 2004; Zhang et al., 2011). These compounds are full agonists at the κ receptor and have activities at the μ receptor ranging from a weak partial agonist to a full agonist (Zhang et al., 2011). The resulting compound ATPM is a partial μ agonist and a full κ agonist (Zhang et al., 2011). ATPM produced antinociception mediated by both μ and κ opioid receptors. This compound was reported to attenuate morphine antinociceptive tolerance and decrease heroin self-administration in mice (Wang et al., 2009).

Figure 10.2 shows the structure of MCL-741, an aminothiazole derivative of cyclorphan. Its parent compound, MCL-420, had a 3-hydroxyl group instead of the O-methyl group. With the hydroxyl group, MCL-420 was a partial agonist at both the μ and κ receptors (Neumeyer et al., 2012). To increase oral bioavailability, the hydroxyl group was replaced with an O-methyl group. This compound, MCL-741, shown in Fig. 10.2, is a full κ agonist and a partial μ agonist with slightly lower affinity than the parent compound MCL-420 (Provencher et al., 2013).

Recently, the effects of MCL-420 and MCL-741 on cocaine-induced locomotor activity in mice were determined (Bidlack, Sromek, & Neumeyer, 2013). After an i.p. administration, doses of MCL-420 between 10 and 30 mg/kg attenuated cocaine-induced locomotion with a maximal suppression of approximately 40%. MCL-420 did not have good oral bioavailability. MCL-741 was synthesized because like codeine, it was expected to have better oral bioavailability than MCL-420. Figure 10.4 shows that when mice were pretreated for 60 min with an oral administration of MCL-741, cocaine-induced ambulations were suppressed to the same level observed with a high dose of MCL-741 alone. These results are encouraging and demonstrate that it was possible to synthesize an aminothiazole-derived opioid that had oral bioavailability and reduced cocaine-induced activity.

3.2.7 Opioid peptides: Arodyn, zyklophin, and CJ-15,208

Arodyn is a peptidic derivative of the endogenous κ opioid peptide dynorphin (Bennett, Murray, & Aldrich, 2005). In receptor-binding experiments, arodyn had K_i values of 10, 1740, and 5830 nM for the κ, μ, and δ receptors, respectively (Bennett et al., 2005). In the adenylyl cyclase assay, arodyn blocked the agonist effect of Dyn A-(1–13)NH_2 (Bennett et al., 2005). After i.c.v. administration, arodyn antagonized antinociception mediated by the κ agonist U50,488 in the 55 °C warm-water tail flick

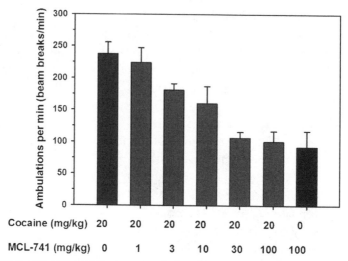

Figure 10.4 MCL-741 inhibited cocaine-induced locomotor activity in mice after oral administration. Increasing doses of MCL-471 were administered to mice by oral gavage. After 60 min, an i.p. injection of cocaine (20 mg/kg) was administered. Locomotor activity was monitored in an Accuscan fusion sensor for 120 min. Data are reported as ambulations per min ± SEM from 10 mice per dose. (For color version of this figure, the reader is referred to the online version of this chapter.)

(Carey, Borozny, Aldrich, & McLaughlin, 2007). Arodyn also blocks stress-induced reinstatement of cocaine-seeking behavior in a conditioned place preference model in mice, demonstrating that a peptide κ antagonist that had a short duration of action could have potential therapeutic application in treating cocaine dependence (Carey et al., 2007). However, arodyn is rapidly metabolized in blood, presumably by endopeptidases (Aldrich & McLaughlin, 2009), precluding its systemic administration.

The cyclic κ peptidic antagonist zyklophin (Patkar, Murray, & Aldrich, 2009) exhibits better metabolic stability than arodyn (Aldrich & McLaughlin, 2009). Zyklophin had K_i values of 30, 5880, and >10,000 nM for the inhibition of binding to the κ, μ, and δ receptors, respectively (Patkar, Yan, Murray, & Aldrich, 2005). Zyklophin antagonized dynorphin A-(1–3)NH_2-induced inhibition of adenylyl cyclase activity mediated by the rat κ receptor (Patkar et al., 2005). Systemically administered zyklophin attenuated the antinociceptive activity of centrally administered U50,488, suggesting that zyklophin crosses the blood–brain barrier (Aldrich, Patkar, & McLaughlin, 2009). Systemically administered zyklophin (3 mg/kg s.c.) also prevented stress-induced reinstatement of cocaine-seeking behavior in a conditioned place preference assay (Aldrich et al., 2009). Zyklophin antagonized κ-mediated antinociception for less than 12 h, which was shorter than the duration of action of κ-selective alkaloid antagonists, such as nor-BNI, which produced antagonism for weeks, probably due to nor-BNI remaining as a depot in brain (Patkar et al., 2013).

A novel κ opioid receptor-binding inhibitor CJ-15,208 (Fig. 10.2) was isolated from the fermentation broth of a fungus, Ctenomyces serratus ATCC15502 (Saito et al., 2002). CJ-15,208 had IC_{50} values for the inhibition of binding to κ, μ, and δ receptors of 47, 260, and 2600 nM, respectively (Saito et al., 2002). In the electrically stimulated twitch response assay of rabbit vas deferens, CJ-15,208 recovered the suppression by a κ agonist asimadoline with an ED_{50} value of 1.3 μM, indicating that CJ-15,208 is a κ antagonist (Saito et al., 2002). Using cloned rat (κ, μ) and mouse (δ) opioid receptors expressed in cell lines, the natural tryptophan isomer of CJ-15,208 (Ross, Kulkarni, McLaughlin, & Aldrich, 2010), the L-Trp isomer had a 17-fold greater affinity for the κ than the μ receptor and a 117-fold grater affinity for the κ than the δ receptor (Table 10.1). Also, the D-Trp isomer of CJ-15,208 was synthesized, and in receptor-binding experiments, the D-Trp isomer had an eightfold greater affinity for the κ than μ receptors and a 95-fold greater affinity for the κ than the δ receptor (Table 10.1). In the [^{35}S]GTPγS binding assay, both isomers of CJ-15,208 were antagonists at the κ receptor. The L-Trp isomer was an antagonist at the μ receptor, while the D-Trp isomer did not have measurable activity at the μ receptor (Table 10.2). This finding is surprising considering the D-Trp isomer had higher affinity for the μ receptor than the L-Trp isomer did in receptor-binding experiments (Ross et al., 2012).

In the mouse 55 ^{0}C warm-water tail flick test, the L-Trp isomer of CJ-15,208 produced antinociception that was antagonized by both μ- and κ-selective antagonists (Ross et al., 2012). This result is surprising considering that [L-Trp]CJ-15,208 did not stimulate [^{35}S]GTPγS binding (Ross et al., 2012) and inhibited electrically stimulated twitch response assay of rabbit vas deferens (Saito et al., 2002). In the same antinociceptive assay, the D-Trp isomer produced less than 25% antinociception after an i.c.v., s.c., or p.o. administration (Eans et al., 2013; Ross et al., 2012). This peptide was active after oral administration, probably because it is cyclic and therefore more resistant to proteases. Both L-Trp and D-Trp isomers antagonized antinociception induced by the κ-selective agonist U50,488 for less than 18 h after pretreatment, but did not antagonize antinociception mediated by either μ or δ receptor. Based on the antinociceptive studies, [D-Trp]

CJ-15,208 is a partial agonist at the κ receptor and a μ agonist with limited efficacy. [D-Trp]CJ-208 did not antagonize antinociception induced by morphine (Eans et al., 2013). Pretreatment with [D-Trp]CJ-15,208 prevented stress-induced, but not cocaine-induced, reinstatement of extinguished cocaine in conditioned place preference (Ross et al., 2012). These findings show that [D-Trp]CJ-15,208 is a κ partial agonist/μ agonist that blocks stress-induced reinstatement of extinguished cocaine-seeking behavior, suggesting that this peptide or derivatives may be useful therapeutically to maintain abstinence from cocaine abuse.

3.2.8 GSK1521498

While GSK1521498, shown in Fig. 10.2, is not a mixed μ/κ agonist, inclusion of GSK1521498 in this review is timely because this compound is unique by being an inverse agonist at μ and κ receptors (Ignar et al., 2011). Its affinity for the κ receptor is approximately 25 times lower than for the μ receptor (Table 10.1). GSK1521498 has poorer affinity for the δ receptor. GSK1521498 was also an inverse agonist at κ and δ opioid receptors (Ignar et al., 2011). In lean rats, GSK1521498 reduced the reinforcement efficacy of palatable food reward and enhance satiety (Ignar et al., 2011). GSK1521498 is being evaluated as a possible treatment for obesity and binge-eating (Cambridge et al., 2013). It should be noted that clinically, inverse agonists are often called antagonists because they function as antagonists.

In rats, under a second-order schedule of reinforcement, in which responding was maintained by contingent presentation of a drug-associated reinforcer, GSK1521498 dose-dependently decreased cocaine-seeking. However, under a continuous reinforcement schedule, GSK1521498 had no effect on cocaine self-administration. These initial experiments suggest that GSK1521498 may have therapeutic potential to attenuate cocaine-seeking (Giuliano et al., 2013).

4. CONCLUSION

Mixed μ/κ opioid agonists continue to be a primary target for treating cocaine and other stimulant dependence. Naltrexone, buprenorphine, and nalmefene are already used clinically to treat alcohol and opioid dependence. Full κ agonists produce strong dysphoria and potentiate the use of cocaine in animal models (Smith et al., 2003). The fact that benzomorphans are full κ agonists limits their use as a therapeutic to treat cocaine dependence. Partial κ agonists, either coupled with μ partial agonist activity such as seen with buprenorphine or coupled with μ antagonist properties such as naltrexone, have a role in suppression cocaine self-administration. Compounds with antagonistic effects at the κ receptor decrease cocaine-seeking behavior and intake in the absence (Wee et al., 2009, 2012) and presence of stress-induced drug relapse (Jackson, McLaughlin, Carroll, & Damaj, 2013; Ross et al., 2012; Wee et al., 2009). Currently, a number of mixed μ/κ partial agonists are being tested in preclinical and clinical studies. The next few years hold great excitement in the prospect of obtaining a medication approved for the treatment of cocaine dependence.

CONFLICT OF INTEREST
Dr. Jean Bidlack is a consultant for Alkermes, Inc.

ACKNOWLEDGMENTS
The Paul Stark Professorship at the University of Rochester and NIH/NIDA grant DA014251 partially supported this work. I thank my collaborators Drs. Mark P. Wentland and John L. Neumeyer for their insightful input into mixed μ/κ agonists and Dr. Jay P. McLaughlin for helpful comments on the chapter.

REFERENCES
Aldrich, J. V., & McLaughlin, J. P. (2009). Peptide kappa opioid receptor ligands: Potential for drug development. *The AAPS Journal, 11*(2), 312–322. http://dx.doi.org/10.1208/s12248-009-9105-4.
Aldrich, J. V., Patkar, K. A., & McLaughlin, J. P. (2009). Zyklophin, a systemically active selective kappa opioid receptor peptide antagonist with short duration of action. *Proceedings of the National Academy of Sciences of the United States of America, 106*(43), 18396–18401. http://dx.doi.org/10.1073/pnas.0910180106.
Anastasio, N. C., Stutz, S. J., Fox, R. G., Sears, R. M., Emeson, R. B., Dileone, R. J., et al. (2013). Functional status of the serotonin 5-ht2c receptor (5-ht2cr) drives interlocked phenotypes that precipitate relapse-like behaviors in cocaine dependence. *Neuropsychopharmacology, 39*, 370–382. http://dx.doi.org/10.1038/npp.2013.199.
Archer, S., Albertson, N. F., Harris, L. S., Pierson, A. K., & Bird, J. G. (1964). Pentazocine. Strong analgesics and analgesic antagonists in the benzomorphan series. *Journal of Medicinal Chemistry, 7*, 123–127.
Archer, S., Glick, S. D., & Bidlack, J. M. (1996). Cyclazocine revisited. *Neurochemical Research, 21*(11), 1369–1373. http://dx.doi.org/10.1007/bf02532378.
Bart, G., Schluger, J. H., Borg, L., Ho, A., Bidlack, J. M., & Kreek, M. J. (2005). Nalmefene induced elevation in serum prolactin in normal human volunteers: Partial kappa opioid agonist activity? *Neuropsychopharmacology, 30*(12), 2254–2262. http://dx.doi.org/10.1038/sj.npp.1300811.
Beardsley, P. M., Howard, J. L., Shelton, K. L., & Carroll, F. I. (2005). Differential effects of the novel kappa opioid receptor antagonist, JDTic, on reinstatement of cocaine-seeking induced by footshock stressors vs cocaine primes and its antidepressant-like effects in rats. *Psychopharmacology (Berlin), 183*(1), 118–126. http://dx.doi.org/10.1007/s00213-005-0167-4.

Befort, K., Tabbara, L., & Kieffer, B. L. (1996). [^{35}S]GTP gamma S binding: A tool to evaluate functional activity of a cloned opioid receptor transiently expressed in COS cells. *Neurochemical Research, 21*(11), 1301–1307.

Bennett, M. A., Murray, T. F., & Aldrich, J. V. (2005). Structure-activity relationships of arodyn, a novel acetylated kappa opioid receptor antagonist. *Journal of Peptide Research, 65*(3), 322–332. http://dx.doi.org/10.1111/j.1399-3011.2005.00216.x.

Bidlack, J. M., Cohen, D. J., McLaughlin, J. P., Lou, R. L., Ye, Y. C., & Wentland, M. P. (2002). 8-Carboxamidocyclazocine: A long-acting, novel benzomorphan. *Journal of Pharmacology and Experimental Therapeutics, 302*(1), 374–380. http://dx.doi.org/10.1124/jpet.302.1.374.

Bidlack, J. M., & Knapp, B. I. (2013). *Mixed mu/kappa opioid agonists research and development of opioid-related ligands* (Vol. 1131, pp. 257–272). Washington, DC: American Chemical Society.

Bidlack, J. M., McLaughlin, J. P., & Wentland, M. P. (2000). Partial opioids. Medications for the treatment of pain and drug abuse. *Annals of New York Academy of Sciences, 909*, 1–11.

Bidlack, J. M., Knapp, B. I., Sromek, A., & Neumeyer, J. L. (2013). A mixed kappa/mu partial opioid agonist attenuated cocaine-induced locomotion. In *College on problems of drug dependence meeting abstracts*. doi:http://www.cpdd.vcu.edu/Pages/Meetings/CPDD13AbstractBook.pdf.

Burattini, C., Burbassi, S., Aicardi, G., & Cervo, L. (2008). Effects of naltrexone on cocaine- and sucrose-seeking behaviour in response to associated stimuli in rats. *International Journal of Neuropsychopharmacology, 11*(1), 103–109. http://dx.doi.org/10.1017/s14611 45707007705.

Butelman, E. R., Yuferov, V., & Kreek, M. J. (2012). Kappa-opioid receptor/dynorphin system: Genetic and pharmacotherapeutic implications for addiction. *Trends in Neurosciences, 35*(10), 587–596. http://dx.doi.org/10.1016/j.tins.2012.05.005.

Cambridge, V. C., Ziauddeen, H., Nathan, P. J., Subramaniam, N., Dodds, C., Chamberlain, S. R., et al. (2013). Neural and behavioral effects of a novel mu opioid receptor antagonist in binge-eating obese people. *Biological Psychiatry, 73*(9), 887–894. http://dx.doi.org/10.1016/j.biopsych.2012.10.022.

Carey, A. N., Borozny, K., Aldrich, J. V., & McLaughlin, J. P. (2007). Reinstatement of cocaine place-conditioning prevented by the peptide kappa-opioid receptor antagonist arodyn. *European Journal of Pharmacology, 569*(1–2), 84–89. http://dx.doi.org/10.1016/j. ejphar.2007.05.007.

Ciccocioppo, R., Economidou, D., Rimondini, R., Sommer, W., Massi, M., & Heilig, M. (2007). Buprenorphine reduces alcohol drinking through activation of the nociceptin/ orphanin FQ-NOP receptor system. *Biological Psychiatry, 61*(1), 4–12. http://dx.doi.org/ 10.1016/j.biopsych.2006.01.006.

Comer, S. D., Mogali, S., Saccone, P. A., Askalsky, P., Martinez, D., Walker, E. A., et al. (2013). Effects of acute oral naltrexone on the subjective and physiological effects of oral d-amphetamine and smoked cocaine in cocaine abusers. *Neuropsychopharmacology, 38*, 2427–2438. http://dx.doi.org/10.1038/npp.2013.143.

Cordery, S. F., Taverner, A., Ridzwan, I. E., Guy, R. H., Delgado-Charro, M. B., Husbands, S. M., et al. (2012). A non-rewarding, non-aversive buprenorphine/naltrexone combination attenuates drug-primed reinstatement to cocaine and morphine in rats in a conditioned place preference paradigm. *Addiction Biology.* http://dx.doi.org/10.1111/ adb.12020.

Cowan, A., Lewis, J. W., & Macfarlane, I. R. (1977). Agonist and antagonist properties of buprenorphine, a new antinociceptive agent. *British Journal of Pharmacology, 60*(4), 537–545.

Cunningham, K. A., & Anastasio, N. C. (2014). Serotonin at the nexus of impulsivity and cue reactivity in cocaine addiction. *Neuropharmacology.* http://dx.doi.org/10.1016/j. neuropharm.2013.06.030.

Cunningham, K. A., Anastasio, N. C., Fox, R. G., Stutz, S. J., Bubar, M. J., Swinford, S. E., et al. (2013). Synergism between a serotonin 5-HT2A receptor (5-HT2AR) antagonist and 5-HT2CR agonist suggests new pharmacotherapeutics for cocaine addiction. *ACS Chemical Neuroscience, 4*(1), 110–121. http://dx.doi.org/10.1021/cn300072u.

Devroye, C., Filip, M., Przegalinski, E., McCreary, A. C., & Spampinato, U. (2013). Serotonin receptors and drug addiction: Focus on cocaine. *Experimental Brain Research, 230*, 537–545. http://dx.doi.org/10.1007/s00221-013-3593-2.

Di Chiara, G., & Imperato, A. (1988). Opposite effects of mu and kappa opiate agonists on dopamine release in the nucleus accumbens and in the dorsal caudate of freely moving rats. *Journal of Pharmacology and Experimental Therapeutics, 244*(3), 1067–1080.

Dole, V. P., & Nyswander, M. (1965). A medical treatment for diacetylmorphine (heroin) addiction. A clinical trial with methadone hydrochloride. *JAMA, 193*, 646–650.

Dole, V. P., Nyswander, M. E., & Kreek, M. J. (1966). Narcotic blockade. *Archives of Internal Medicine, 118*(4), 304–309.

Downing, J. W., Leary, W. P., & White, E. S. (1977). Buprenorphine: A new potent long-acting synthetic analgesic. Comparison with morphine. *British Journal of Anaesthesia, 49*(3), 251–255.

Eans, S. O., Ganno, M. L., Reilley, K. J., Patkar, K. A., Senadheera, S. N., Aldrich, J. V., et al. (2013). The macrocyclic tetrapeptide [D-Trp]CJ-15,208 produces short-acting kappa opioid receptor antagonism in the CNS after oral administration. *British Journal of Pharmacology, 169*(2), 426–436. http://dx.doi.org/10.1111/bph.12132.

Eap, C. B., Buclin, T., & Baumann, P. (2002). Interindividual variability of the clinical pharmacokinetics of methadone—Implications for the treatment of opioid dependence. *Clinical Pharmacokinetics, 41*(14), 1153–1193. http://dx.doi.org/10.2165/00003088-200 241140-00003.

Evans, C. J., Keith, D. E., Jr., Morrison, H., Magendzo, K., & Edwards, R. H. (1992). Cloning of a delta opioid receptor by functional expression. *Science, 258*(5090), 1952–1955.

Freedman, A. M., Fink, M., Sharoff, R., & Zaks, A. (1967). Cyclazocine and methadone in narcotic addiction. *JAMA, 202*(3), 191–194.

Fulton, B. S., Knapp, B. I., Bidlack, J. M., & Neumeyer, J. L. (2008). Synthesis and pharmacological evaluation of hydrophobic esters and ethers of butorphanol at opioid receptors. *Bioorganic & Medicinal Chemistry Letters, 18*(16), 4474–4476. http://dx.doi.org/10.1016/j.bmcl.2008.07.054.

Fulton, B. S., Knapp, B. L., Bidlack, J. M., & Neumeyer, J. L. (2010). Effect of linker substitution on the binding of butorphan univalent and bivalent ligands to opioid receptors. *Bioorganic & Medicinal Chemistry Letters, 20*(5), 1507–1509. http://dx.doi.org/10.1016/j.bmcl.2010.01.101.

Gates, M. (1973). Cyclorphan and related compounds. *Advances in Biochemical Psychopharmacology, 8*, 51–56.

Gerra, G., Fantoma, A., & Zaimovic, A. (2006). Naltrexone and buprenorphine combination in the treatment of opioid dependence. *Journal of Psychopharmacology, 20*(6), 806–814. http://dx.doi.org/10.1177/0269881106060835.

Gerrits, M. A., Kuzmin, A. V., & van Ree, J. M. (2005). Reinstatement of cocaine-seeking behavior in rats is attenuated following repeated treatment with the opioid receptor antagonist naltrexone. *European Neuropsychopharmacology, 15*(3), 297–303. http://dx.doi.org/10.1016/j.euroneuro.2004.11.004.

Giuliano, C., Robbins, T. W., Wille, D. R., Bullmore, E. T., & Everitt, B. J. (2013). Attenuation of cocaine and heroin seeking by mu-opioid receptor antagonism. *Psychopharmacology, 227*(1), 137–147. http://dx.doi.org/10.1007/s00213-012-2949-9.

Goletiani, N. V., Mendelson, J. H., Sholar, M. B., Siegel, A. J., & Mello, N. K. (2009). Opioid and cocaine combined effect on cocaine-induced changes in HPA and HPG axes hormones in men. *Pharmacology Biochemistry and Behavior, 91*(4), 526–536. http://dx.doi. org/10.1016/j.pbb.2008.09.007.

Greedy, B. M., Bradbury, F., Thomas, M. P., Grivas, K., Cami-Kobeci, G., Archambeau, A., et al. (2013). Orvinols with mixed kappa/mu opioid receptor agonist activity. *Journal of Medicinal Chemistry, 56*(8), 3207–3216. http://dx.doi.org/10.1021/jm301543e.

Haggkvist, J., Lindholm, S., & Franck, J. (2009). The effect of naltrexone on amphetamine-induced conditioned place preference and locomotor behaviour in the rat. *Addiction Biology, 14*(3), 260–269. http://dx.doi.org/10.1111/j.1369-1600.2009.00150.x.

Harris, L. S., & Pierson, A. K. (1964). Some narcotic antagonists in the benzomorphan series. *Journal of Pharmacology and Experimental Therapeutics, 143*, 141–148.

Huang, P., Kehner, G. B., Cowan, A., & Liu-Chen, L. Y. (2001). Comparison of pharmacological activities of buprenorphine and norbuprenorphine: Norbuprenorphine is a potent opioid agonist. *Journal of Pharmacology and Experimental Therapeutics, 297*(2), 688–695.

Husbands, S. M. (2013). Buprenorphine and related orvinols. *Research and development of opioid-related ligands* (Vol. 1131, pp. 127–144). Washington, DC: American Chemical Society.

Ignar, D. M., Goetz, A. S., Noble, K. N., Carballo, L. H., Stroup, A. E., Fisher, J. C., et al. (2011). Regulation of ingestive behaviors in the rat by GSK1521498, a novel mu-opioid receptor-selective inverse agonist. *Journal of Pharmacology and Experimental Therapeutics, 339*(1), 24–34. http://dx.doi.org/10.1124/jpet.111.180943.

Jackson, K. J., McLaughlin, J. P., Carroll, F. I., & Damaj, M. I. (2013). Effects of the kappa opioid receptor antagonist, norbinaltorphimine, on stress and drug-induced reinstatement of nicotine-conditioned place preference in mice. *Psychopharmacology, 226*(4), 763–768. http://dx.doi.org/10.1007/s00213-012-2716-y.

Johanson, C. E., & Fischman, M. W. (1989). The pharmacology of cocaine related to its abuse. *Pharmacological Reviews, 41*(1), 3–52.

Kenakin, T. (2007). Collateral efficacy in drug discovery: Taking advantage of the good (allo-steric) nature of 7TM receptors. *Trends in Pharmacological Sciences, 28*(8), 407–415. http:// dx.doi.org/10.1016/j.tips.2007.06.009.

Kieffer, B. L., Befort, K., Gaveriaux-Ruff, C., & Hirth, C. G. (1992). The delta-opioid receptor: Isolation of a cDNA by expression cloning and pharmacological characterization. *Proceedings of the National Academy of Sciences of the United States of America, 89*(24), 12048–12052.

Kleven, M. S., & Woolverton, W. L. (1990). Effects of continuous infusions of SCH 23390 on cocaine- or food-maintained behavior in rhesus monkeys. *Behavioural Pharmacology, 1*(4), 365–373.

Koob, G. F., Buck, C. L., Cohen, A., Edwards, S., Park, P. E., Schlosburg, J. E., et al. (2014). Addiction as a stress surfeit disorder. *Neuropharmacology, 76*(Pt B), 370–382. http://dx.doi.org/10.1016/j.neuropharm.2013.05.024.

Kreek, M. J. (1973). Medical safety and side effects of methadone in tolerant individuals. *JAMA, 223*(6), 665–668.

Kreek, M. J. (2000). Methadone-related opioid agonist pharmacotherapy for heroin addiction. History, recent molecular and neurochemical research and future in mainstream medicine. *Annals of New York Academy of Sciences, 909*, 186–216.

Kreek, M. J., LaForge, K. S., & Butelman, E. (2002). Pharmacotherapy of addictions. *Nature Reviews Drug Discovery, 1*(9), 710–726. http://dx.doi.org/10.1038/nrd897.

Kreek, M. J., Levran, O., Reed, B., Schlussman, S. D., Zhou, Y., & Butelman, E. R. (2012). Opiate addiction and cocaine addiction: Underlying molecular neurobiology and genetics. *Journal of Clinical Investigation, 122*(10), 3387–3393. http://dx.doi.org/10.1172/jci60390.

Kuhar, M. J., Ritz, M. C., & Boja, J. W. (1991). The dopamine hypothesis of the reinforcing properties of cocaine. *Trends in Neurosciences, 14*(7), 299–302.

Kunko, P. M., French, D., & Izenwasser, S. (1998). Alterations in locomotor activity during chronic cocaine administration: Effect on dopamine receptors and interaction with opioids. *Journal of Pharmacology and Experimental Therapeutics, 285*(1), 277–284.

Kuzmin, A. V., Gerrits, M. A., Zvartau, E. E., & van Ree, J. M. (2000). Influence of buprenorphine, butorphanol and nalbuphine on the initiation of intravenous cocaine self-administration in drug naive mice. *European Neuropsychopharmacology, 10*(6), 447–454.

Lau, E. K., Trester-Zedlitz, M., Trinidad, J. C., Kotowski, S. J., Krutchinsky, A. N., Burlingame, A. L., et al. (2011). Quantitative encoding of the effect of a partial agonist on individual opioid receptors by multisite phosphorylation and threshold detection. *Science Signaling, 4*(185), ra52. http://dx.doi.org/10.1126/scisignal.2001748.

Leri, F., Zhou, Y., Goddard, B., Cummins, E., & Kreek, M. J. (2006). Effects of high-dose methadone maintenance on cocaine place conditioning, cocaine self-administration, and mu-opioid receptor mRNA expression in the rat brain. *Neuropsychopharmacology, 31*(7), 1462–1474. http://dx.doi.org/10.1038/sj.npp.1300927.

Leri, F., Zhou, Y., Goddard, B., Levy, A., Jacklin, D., & Kreek, M. J. (2009). Steady-state methadone blocks cocaine seeking and cocaine-induced gene expression alterations in the rat brain. *European Neuropsychopharmacology, 19*(4), 238–249. http://dx.doi.org/10.1016/j.euroneuro.2008.09.004.

Ling, W., & Wesson, D. R. (2003). Clinical efficacy of buprenorphine: Comparisons to methadone and placebo. *Drug and Alcohol Dependence, 70*(2 Suppl.), S49–S57.

Lutfy, K., Eitan, S., Bryant, C. D., Yang, Y. C., Saliminejad, N., Walwyn, W., et al. (2003). Buprenorphine-induced antinociception is mediated by mu-opioid receptors and compromised by concomitant activation of opioid receptor-like receptors. *Journal of Neuroscience, 23*(32), 10331–10337.

Maisonneuve, I. M., Ho, A., & Kreek, M. J. (1995). Chronic administration of a cocaine "binge" alters basal extracellular levels in male rats: An in vivo microdialysis study. *Journal of Pharmacology and Experimental Therapeutics, 272*(2), 652–657.

Martin, J. A., Campbell, A., Killip, T., Kotz, M., Krantz, M. J., Kreek, M. J., et al. (2011). QT interval screening in methadone maintenance treatment: Report of a SAMHSA expert panel. *Journal of Addictive Diseases, 30*(4), 283–306. http://dx.doi.org/10.1080/10550887.2011.610710.

Mathews, J. L., Peng, X. M., Xiong, W. A., Zhang, A., Negus, S. S., Neumeyer, J. L., et al. (2005). Characterization of a novel bivalent morphinan possessing kappa agonist and mu agonist/antagonist properties. *Journal of Pharmacology and Experimental Therapeutics, 315*(2), 821–827. http://dx.doi.org/10.1124/jpet.105.084343.

McCance-Katz, E. F., Sullivan, L. E., & Nallani, S. (2010). Drug interactions of clinical importance among the opioids, methadone and buprenorphine, and other frequently prescribed medications: A review. *American Journal on Addictions, 19*(1), 4–16. http://dx.doi.org/10.1111/j.1521-0391.2009.00005.x.

McCann, D. J. (2008). Potential of buprenorphine/naltrexone in treating polydrug addiction and co-occurring psychiatric disorders. *Clinical Pharmacology and Therapeutics, 83*(4), 627–630. http://dx.doi.org/10.1038/sj.clpt.6100503.

Mello, N. K., Kamien, J. B., Lukas, S. E., Drieze, J., & Mendelson, J. H. (1993). The effects of nalbuphine and butorphanol treatment on cocaine and food self-administration by rhesus monkeys. *Neuropsychopharmacology, 8*(1), 45–55. http://dx.doi.org/10.1038/npp.1993.6.

Mello, N. K., Lukas, S. E., Mendelson, J. H., & Drieze, J. (1993). Naltrexone-buprenorphine interactions: Effects on cocaine self-administration. *Neuropsychopharmacology, 9*(3), 211–224. http://dx.doi.org/10.1038/npp.1993.57.

Mello, N. K., & Negus, S. S. (1998). Effects of kappa opioid agonists on cocaine- and food-maintained responding by rhesus monkeys. *Journal of Pharmacology and Experimental Therapeutics, 286*(2), 812–824.

Mello, N. K., & Negus, S. S. (2000). Interactions between kappa opioid agonists and cocaine. Preclinical studies. *Annals of New York Academy of Sciences, 909,* 104–132.

Mendelson, J. H., & Mello, N. K. (1996). Management of cocaine abuse and dependence. *New England Journal of Medicine, 334*(15), 965–972. http://dx.doi.org/10.1056/nejm199604113341507.

Montoya, I. D., Gorelick, D. A., Preston, K. L., Schroeder, J. R., Umbricht, A., Cheskin, L. J., et al. (2004). Randomized trial of buprenorphine for treatment of concurrent opiate and cocaine dependence. *Clinical Pharmacology and Therapeutics, 75*(1), 34–48. http://dx.doi.org/10.1016/j.clpt.2003.09.004.

Mooney, L. J., Nielsen, S., Saxon, A., Hillhouse, M., Thomas, C., Hasson, A., et al. (2013). Cocaine use reduction with buprenorphine (CURB): Rationale, design, and methodology. *Contemporary Clinical Trials, 34*(2), 196–204. http://dx.doi.org/10.1016/j.cct.2012.11.002.

Murnane, K. S., Winschel, J., Schmidt, K. T., Stewart, L. M., Rose, S. J., Cheng, K., et al. (2013). Serotonin 2A receptors differentially contribute to abuse-related effects of cocaine and cocaine-induced nigrostriatal and mesolimbic dopamine overflow in non-human primates. *Journal of Neuroscience, 33*(33), 13367–13374. http://dx.doi.org/10.1523/jneurosci.1437-13.2013.

Negus, S. S., Bidlack, J. M., Mello, N. K., Furness, M. S., Rice, K. C., & Brandt, M. R. (2002). Delta opioid antagonist effects of buprenorphine in rhesus monkeys. *Behavioural Pharmacology, 13*(7), 557–570.

Negus, S. S., & Mello, N. K. (2002). Effects of mu-opioid agonists on cocaine- and food-maintained responding and cocaine discrimination in rhesus monkeys: Role of mu-agonist efficacy. *Journal of Pharmacology and Experimental Therapeutics, 300*(3), 1111–1121.

Negus, S. S., Mello, N. K., Lamas, X., & Mendelson, J. H. (1996). Acute and chronic effects of flupenthixol on the discriminative stimulus and reinforcing effects of cocaine in rhesus monkeys. *Journal of Pharmacology and Experimental Therapeutics, 278*(2), 879–890.

Negus, S. S., Mello, N. K., Portoghese, P. S., & Lin, C. E. (1997). Effects of kappa opioids on cocaine self-administration by rhesus monkeys. *Journal of Pharmacology and Experimental Therapeutics, 282*(1), 44–55.

Neumeyer, J. L., Bidlack, J. M., Zong, R. S., Bakthavachalam, V., Gao, P., Cohen, D. J., et al. (2000). Synthesis and opioid receptor affinity of morphinan and benzomorphan derivatives: Mixed kappa agonists and mu agonists/antagonists as potential pharmacotherapeutics for cocaine dependence. *Journal of Medicinal Chemistry, 43*(1), 114–122. http://dx.doi.org/10.1021/jm9903343.

Neumeyer, J. L., Zhang, B., Zhang, T. Z., Sromek, A. W., Knapp, B. I., Cohen, D. J., et al. (2012). Synthesis, binding affinity, and functional in vitro activity of 3-benzylaminomorphinan and 3-benzylaminomorphine ligands at opioid receptors. *Journal of Medicinal Chemistry, 55*(8), 3878–3890. http://dx.doi.org/10.1021/jm3001086.

Nutt, D. J. (2010). Antagonist–agonist combinations as therapies for heroin addiction: Back to the future? *Journal of Psychopharmacology, 24*(2), 141–145. http://dx.doi.org/10.1177/0269881109356129.

Patkar, K. A., Murray, T. F., & Aldrich, J. V. (2009). The effects of C-terminal modifications on the opioid activity of [N-benzylTyr(1)]dynorphin A-(1–11) analogues. *Journal of Medicinal Chemistry, 52*(21), 6814–6821. http://dx.doi.org/10.1021/jm900715m.

Patkar, K. A., Wu, J., Ganno, M. L., Singh, H. D., Ross, N. C., Rasakham, K., et al. (2013). Physical presence of nor-binaltorphimine in mouse brain over 21 days after a single administration corresponds to its long-lasting antagonistic effect on kappa-opioid receptors. *Journal of Pharmacology and Experimental Therapeutics, 346*(3), 545–554. http://dx.doi.org/10.1124/jpet.113.206086.

Patkar, K. A., Yan, X., Murray, T. F., & Aldrich, J. V. (2005). [Nalpha-benzylTyr1, cyclo (D-Asp5, Dap8)]-dynorphin A-(1–11)NH$_2$ cyclized in the "address" domain is a novel kappa-opioid receptor antagonist. *Journal of Medicinal Chemistry, 48*(14), 4500–4503. http://dx.doi.org/10.1021/jm050105i.

Peles, E., Kreek, M. J., Kellogg, S., & Adelson, M. (2006). High methadone dose significantly reduces cocaine use in methadone maintenance treatment (MMT) patients. *Journal of Addictive Diseases, 25*(1), 43–50. http://dx.doi.org/10.1300/J069v25n01_07.

Pettinati, H. M., Kampman, K. M., Lynch, K. G., Suh, J. J., Dackis, C. A., Oslin, D. W., et al. (2008). Gender differences with high-dose naltrexone in patients with co-occurring cocaine and alcohol dependence. *Journal of Substance Abuse Treatment, 34*(4), 378–390. http://dx.doi.org/10.1016/j.jsat.2007.05.011.

Pettit, H. O., Ettenberg, A., Bloom, F. E., & Koob, G. F. (1984). Destruction of dopamine in the nucleus accumbens selectively attenuates cocaine but not heroin self-administration in rats. *Psychopharmacology, 84*(2), 167–173.

Picetti, R., Schlussman, S. D., Zhou, Y., Ray, B., Ducat, E., Yuferov, V., et al. (2013). Addictions and stress: Clues for cocaine pharmacotherapies. *Current Pharmaceutical Design, 19*, 7065–7080, PMID: 23574443.

Pickworth, W. B., Lee, E. M., Abreu, M. E., Umbricht, A., & Preston, K. L. (2004). A laboratory study of hydromorphone and cyclazocine on smoking behavior in residential polydrug users. *Pharmacology Biochemistry and Behavior, 77*(4), 711–715. http://dx.doi.org/10.1016/j.pbb.2004.01.022.

Preston, K. L., Umbricht, A., Schroeder, J. R., Abreu, M. E., Epstein, D. H., & Pickworth, W. B. (2004). Cyclazocine: Comparison to hydromorphone and interaction with cocaine. *Behavioural Pharmacology, 15*(2), 91–102. http://dx.doi.org/10.1097/01.fbp.0000125793.85076.47.

Provencher, B. A., Sromek, A., Li, W., Russell, S., Chartoff, E., Knapp, B. I., et al. (2013). Synthesis and pharmacological evaluation of mixed mu/kappa aminothiazolomorphinans. *Journal of Medicinal Chemistry, 56*, 8872–8878.

Redila, V. A., & Chavkin, C. (2008). Stress-induced reinstatement of cocaine seeking is mediated by the kappa opioid system. *Psychopharmacology (Berlin), 200*(1), 59–70. http://dx.doi.org/10.1007/s00213-008-1122-y.

Ritz, M. C., Lamb, R. J., Goldberg, S. R., & Kuhar, M. J. (1987). Cocaine receptors on dopamine transporters are related to self-administration of cocaine. *Science, 237*(4819), 1219–1223.

Ross, N. C., Kulkarni, S. S., McLaughlin, J. P., & Aldrich, J. V. (2010). Synthesis of CJ-15,208, a novel kappa-opioid receptor antagonist. *Tetrahedron Letters, 51*(38), 5020–5023. http://dx.doi.org/10.1016/j.tetlet.2010.07.086.

Ross, N. C., Reilley, K. J., Murray, T. F., Aldrich, J. V., & McLaughlin, J. P. (2012). Novel opioid cyclic tetrapeptides: Trp isomers of CJ-15,208 exhibit distinct opioid receptor agonism and short-acting kappa opioid receptor antagonism. *British Journal of Pharmacology, 165*(4b), 1097–1108. http://dx.doi.org/10.1111/j.1476-5381.2011.01544.x.

Rothman, R. B., Gorelick, D. A., Heishman, S. J., Eichmiller, P. R., Hill, B. H., Norbeck, J., et al. (2000). An open-label study of a functional opioid kappa antagonist in the treatment of opioid dependence. *Journal of Substance Abuse Treatment, 18*(3), 277–281.

Ruedi-Bettschen, D., Rowlett, J. K., Spealman, R. D., & Platt, D. M. (2010). Attenuation of cocaine-induced reinstatement of drug seeking in squirrel monkeys: Kappa opioid and serotonergic mechanisms. *Psychopharmacology, 210*(2), 169–177. http://dx.doi.org/10.1007/s00213-009-1705-2.

Saito, T., Hirai, H., Kim, Y. J., Kojima, Y., Matsunaga, Y., Nishida, H., et al. (2002). CJ-15,208, a novel kappa opioid receptor antagonist from a fungus, Ctenomyces serratus ATCC15502. *The Journal of Antibiotics (Tokyo), 55*(10), 847–854.

Schattauer, S. S., Miyatake, M., Shankar, H., Zietz, C., Levin, J. R., Liu-Chen, L. Y., et al. (2012). Ligand directed signaling differences between rodent and human kappa-opioid receptors. *Journal of Biological Chemistry, 287*(50), 41595–41607. http://dx.doi.org/10.1074/jbc.M112.381368.

Schindler, A. G., Messinger, D. I., Smith, J. S., Shankar, H., Gustin, R. M., Schattauer, S. S., et al. (2012). Stress produces aversion and potentiates cocaine reward by releasing endogenous dynorphins in the ventral striatum to locally stimulate serotonin reuptake. *Journal of Neuroscience, 32*(49), 17582–17596. http://dx.doi.org/10.1523/jneurosci.3220-12.2012.

Selley, D. E., Sim, L. J., Xiao, R., Liu, Q., & Childers, S. R. (1997). mu-Opioid receptor-stimulated guanosine-5′-O-(gamma-thio)-triphosphate binding in rat thalamus and cultured cell lines: Signal transduction mechanisms underlying agonist efficacy. *Molecular Pharmacology, 51*(1), 87–96.

Shippenberg, T. S., Zapata, A., & Chefer, V. I. (2007). Dynorphin and the pathophysiology of drug addiction. *Pharmacology & Therapeutics, 116*(2), 306–321. http://dx.doi.org/10.1016/j.pharmthera.2007.06.011.

Sim, L. J., Selley, D. E., & Childers, S. R. (1995). In vitro autoradiography of receptor-activated G proteins in rat brain by agonist-stimulated guanylyl 5′-[gamma-[^{35}S]thio]-triphosphate binding. *Proceedings of the National Academy of Sciences of the United States of America, 92*(16), 7242–7246.

Simonin, F., Befort, K., Gaveriaux-Ruff, C., Matthes, H., Nappey, V., Lannes, B., et al. (1994). The human delta-opioid receptor: Genomic organization, cDNA cloning, functional expression, and distribution in human brain. *Molecular Pharmacology, 46*(6), 1015–1021.

Smith, M. A., Cole, K. T., Iordanou, J. C., Kerns, D. C., Newsom, P. C., Peitz, G. W., et al. (2013). The mu/kappa agonist nalbuphine attenuates sensitization to the behavioral effects of cocaine. *Pharmacology Biochemistry and Behavior, 104*, 40–46. http://dx.doi.org/10.1016/j.pbb.2012.12.026.

Smith, M. A., Gordon, K. A., Craig, C. K., Bryant, P. A., Ferguson, M. E., French, A. M., et al. (2003). Interactions between opioids and cocaine on locomotor activity in rats: Influence of an opioid's relative efficacy at the mu receptor. *Psychopharmacology, 167*(3), 265–273. http://dx.doi.org/10.1007/s00213-003-1388-z.

Sofuoglu, M., Singha, A., Kosten, T. R., McCance-Katz, F. E., Petrakis, I., & Oliveto, A. (2003). Effects of naltrexone and isradipine, alone or in combination, on cocaine responses in humans. *Pharmacology Biochemistry and Behavior, 75*(4), 801–808.

Sorge, R. E., & Stewart, J. (2006). The effects of chronic buprenorphine on intake of heroin and cocaine in rats and its effects on nucleus accumbens dopamine levels during self-administration. *Psychopharmacology, 188*(1), 28–41. http://dx.doi.org/10.1007/s00213-006-0485-1.

Soyka, M., & Rosner, S. (2008). Opioid antagonists for pharmacological treatment of alcohol dependence—A critical review. *Current Drug Abuse Reviews, 1*(3), 280–291.

Spagnolo, B., Calo, G., Polgar, W. E., Jiang, F., Olsen, C. M., Berzetei-Gurske, I., et al. (2008). Activities of mixed NOP and mu-opioid receptor ligands. *British Journal of Pharmacology, 153*(3), 609–619. http://dx.doi.org/10.1038/sj.bjp.0707598.

Spanagel, R., Herz, A., & Shippenberg, T. S. (1990). The effects of opioid peptides on dopamine release in the nucleus accumbens: An in vivo microdialysis study. *Journal of Neurochemistry, 55*(5), 1734–1740.

Spangler, R., Unterwald, E. M., & Kreek, M. J. (1993). 'Binge' cocaine administration induces a sustained increase of prodynorphin mRNA in rat caudate-putamen. *Brain Research. Molecular Brain Research, 19*(4), 323–327.

Stevenson, G. W., Wentland, M. P., Bidlack, J. M., Mello, N. K., & Negus, S. S. (2004). Effects of the mixed-action kappa/mu opioid agonist 8-carboxamidocyclazocine on cocaine- and food-maintained responding in rhesus monkeys. *European Journal of Pharmacology*, *506*(2), 133–141. http://dx.doi.org/10.1016/j.ejphar.2004.10.051.

Sullivan, M. A., Bisaga, A., Mariani, J. J., Glass, A., Levin, F. R., Comer, S. D., et al. (2013). Naltrexone treatment for opioid dependence: Does its effectiveness depend on testing the blockade? *Drug and Alcohol Dependence*, *133*, 80–85. http://dx.doi.org/10.1016/j.drugalcdep.2013.05.030.

Toll, L., Khroyan, T. V., Polgar, W. E., Husbands, S. M., & Zaveri, N. T. (2013). Pharmacology of mixed NOP/Mu ligands. In *Research and Development of Opioid-Related Ligands:1131*. (pp. 369–391). American Chemical Society.

Traynor, J. R., & Nahorski, S. R. (1995). Modulation by mu-opioid agonists of guanosine-5'-O-(3-[^{35}S]thio)triphosphate binding to membranes from human neuroblastoma SH-SY5Y cells. *Molecular Pharmacology*, *47*(4), 848–854.

Violin, J. D., & Lefkowitz, R. J. (2007). Beta-arrestin-biased ligands at seven-transmembrane receptors. *Trends in Pharmacological Sciences*, *28*(8), 416–422. http://dx.doi.org/10.1016/j.tips.2007.06.006.

Walsh, S. L., Geter-Douglas, B., Strain, E. C., & Bigelow, G. E. (2001). Enadoline and butorphanol: Evaluation of kappa-agonists on cocaine pharmacodynamics and cocaine self-administration in humans. *Journal of Pharmacology and Experimental Therapeutics*, *299*(1), 147–158.

Wang, J. B., Johnson, P. S., Persico, A. M., Hawkins, A. L., Griffin, C. A., & Uhl, G. R. (1994). Human mu opiate receptor. cDNA and genomic clones, pharmacologic characterization and chromosomal assignment. *FEBS Letters*, *338*(2), 217–222.

Wang, Y. J., Tao, Y. M., Li, F. Y., Wang, Y. H., Xu, X. J., Chen, J., et al. (2009). Pharmacological characterization of ATPM [(−)-3-aminothiazolo[5,4-b]-N-cyclopropylmethylmorphinan hydrochloride], a novel mixed kappa-agonist and mu-agonist/-antagonist that attenuates morphine antinociceptive tolerance and heroin self-administration behavior. *Journal of Pharmacology and Experimental Therapeutics*, *329*(1), 306–313. http://dx.doi.org/10.1124/jpet.108.142802.

Wee, S., & Koob, G. F. (2010). The role of the dynorphin-kappa opioid system in the reinforcing effects of drugs of abuse. *Psychopharmacology*, *210*(2), 121–135. http://dx.doi.org/10.1007/s00213-010-1825-8.

Wee, S., Orio, L., Ghirmai, S., Cashman, J. R., & Koob, G. F. (2009). Inhibition of kappa opioid receptors attenuated increased cocaine intake in rats with extended access to cocaine. *Psychopharmacology (Berlin)*, *205*(4), 565–575. http://dx.doi.org/10.1007/s00213-009-1563-y.

Wee, S., Vendruscolo, L. F., Misra, K. K., Schlosburg, J. E., & Koob, G. F. (2012). A combination of buprenorphine and naltrexone blocks compulsive cocaine intake in rodents without producing dependence. *Science Translational Medicine*, *4*(146), 146ra110. http://dx.doi.org/10.1126/scitranslmed.3003948.

Wentland, M. P., Lou, R. L., Dehnhardt, C. M., Duan, W. H., Cohen, D. J., & Bidlack, J. M. (2001). 3-Carboxamido analogues of morphine and naltrexone: Synthesis and opioid receptor binding properties. *Bioorganic & Medicinal Chemistry Letters*, *11*(13), 1717–1721. http://dx.doi.org/10.1016/s0960-894x(01)00278-5.

Wentland, M. P., Lou, R., Lu, Q., Bu, Y., Denhardt, C., Jin, J., et al. (2009). Syntheses of novel high affinity ligands for opioid receptors. *Bioorganic & Medicinal Chemistry Letters*, *19*(8), 2289–2294. http://dx.doi.org/10.1016/j.bmcl.2009.02.078.

Wentland, M. P., Lou, R., Lu, Q., Bu, Y., VanAlstine, M. A., Cohen, D. J., et al. (2009). Syntheses and opioid receptor binding properties of carboxamido-substituted opioids. *Bioorganic & Medicinal Chemistry Letters*, *19*(1), 203–208. http://dx.doi.org/10.1016/j.bmcl.2008.10.134.

Wentland, M. P., Lou, R. L., Ye, Y. C., Cohen, D. J., Richardson, G. P., & Bidlack, J. M. (2001). 8-Carboxamidocyclazocine analogues: Redefining the structure-activity relationships of 2,6-methano-3-benzazocines. *Bioorganic & Medicinal Chemistry Letters*, *11*(5), 623–626. http://dx.doi.org/10.1016/s0960-894x(01)00014-2.

Wentland, M. P., Lu, Q., Lou, R. L., Bu, Y. G., Knapp, B. I., & Bidlack, J. M. (2005). Synthesis and opioid receptor binding properties of a highly potent 4-hydroxy analogue of naltrexone. *Bioorganic & Medicinal Chemistry Letters*, *15*(8), 2107–2110. http://dx.doi.org/10.1016/j.bmcl.2005.02.032.

Wentland, M. P., VanAlstine, M., Kucejko, R., Lou, R. L., Cohen, D. J., Parkhill, A. L., et al. (2006). Redefining the structure-activity relationships of 2,6-methano-3-benzazocines. 4. Opioid receptor binding properties of 8- N-(4′-phenyl)-phenethyl)carboxamido analogues of cyclazocine and ethylketocyclazocine. *Journal of Medicinal Chemistry*, *49*(18), 5635–5639. http://dx.doi.org/10.1021/jm060278n.

Zhang, Y., Schlussman, S. D., Rabkin, J., Butelman, E. R., Ho, A., & Kreek, M. J. (2013). Chronic escalating cocaine exposure, abstinence/withdrawal, and chronic re-exposure: Effects on striatal dopamine and opioid systems in C57BL/6J mice. *Neuropharmacology*, *67*, 259–266. http://dx.doi.org/10.1016/j.neuropharm.2012.10.015.

Zhang, A., Xiong, W. N., Bidlack, J. M., Hilbert, J. E., Knapp, B. I., Wentland, M. P., et al. (2004). 10-Ketomorphinan and 3-substituted-3-desoxymorphinan analogues as mixed kappa and mu opioid ligands: Synthesis and biological evaluation of their binding affinity at opioid receptors. *Journal of Medicinal Chemistry*, *47*(1), 165–174. http://dx.doi.org/10.1021/jm0304156.

Zhang, A., Xiong, W. N., Hilbert, J. E., DeVita, E. K., Bidlack, J. M., & Neumeyer, J. L. (2004). 2-Aminothiazole-derived opioids. Bioisosteric replacement of phenols. *Journal of Medicinal Chemistry*, *47*(8), 1886–1888. http://dx.doi.org/10.1021/jm049978n.

Zhang, T. Z., Yan, Z. H., Sromek, A., Knapp, B. I., Scrimale, T., Bidlack, J. M., et al. (2011). Aminothiazolomorphinans with mixed kappa and mu opioid activity. *Journal of Medicinal Chemistry*, *54*(6), 1903–1913. http://dx.doi.org/10.1021/jm101542c.

Zhu, J., Chen, C., Xue, J. C., Kunapuli, S., DeRiel, J. K., & Liu-Chen, L. Y. (1995). Cloning of a human kappa opioid receptor from the brain. *Life Sciences*, *56*(9), 1201–1207.

CHAPTER ELEVEN

The Combination of Metyrapone and Oxazepam for the Treatment of Cocaine and Other Drug Addictions

Nicholas E. Goeders[1], Glenn F. Guerin, Christopher D. Schmoutz
Department of Pharmacology, Toxicology & Neuroscience, LSU Health Sciences Center, Shreveport, Louisiana, USA
[1]Corresponding author: e-mail address: ngoede@lsuhsc.edu

Contents

Advances in Pharmacology, Volume 69
ISSN 1054-3589
http://dx.doi.org/10.1016/B978-0-12-420118-7.00011-1

Abstract

Although scientists have been investigating the neurobiology of psychomotor stimulant reward for many decades, there is still no FDA-approved treatment for cocaine
or methamphetamine abuse. Research in our laboratory has focused on the relationship
between stress, the subsequent activation of the hypothalamic–pituitary–adrenal (HPA)
axis, and psychomotor stimulant reinforcement for almost 30 years. This research has led
to the development of a combination of low doses of the cortisol synthesis inhibitor,
metyrapone, and the benzodiazepine, oxazepam, as a potential pharmacological treatment for cocaine and other substance use disorders. In fact, we have conducted a pilot
clinical trial that demonstrated that this combination can reduce cocaine craving and
cocaine use. Our initial hypothesis underlying this effect was that the combination of
metyrapone and oxazepam reduced cocaine seeking and taking by decreasing activity
within the HPA axis. Even so, doses of the metyrapone and oxazepam combination
that consistently reduced cocaine taking and seeking did not reliably alter plasma
corticosterone (or cortisol in the pilot clinical trial). Furthermore, subsequent research
has demonstrated that this drug combination is effective in adrenalectomized rats,
suggesting that these effects must be mediated above the level of the adrenal gland.
Our evolving hypothesis is that the combination of metyrapone and oxazepam produces its effects by increasing the levels of neuroactive steroids, most notably
tetrahydrodeoxycorticosterone, in the medial prefrontal cortex and amygdala. Additional research will be necessary to confirm this hypothesis and may lead to the development of improved and specific pharmacotherapies for the treatment of psychomotor
stimulant use.

ABBREVIATIONS

11β-HSD 11β-hydroxysteroid dehydrogenase
20α-HSD 20α-hydroxysteroid dehydrogenase
6-OHDA 6-hydroxydopamine
ACTH adrenocorticotropic hormone
ALLO allopregnanolone
CRF corticotropin-releasing factor

FR fixed ratio
GABA γ-aminobutyric acid
HPA hypothalamic–pituitary–adrenal
POMC proopiomelanocortin
PTZ pentylenetetrazole
PVN paraventricular nucleus
THDOC tetrahydrodeoxycorticosterone
TSPO translocator protein of 18 kDa
VTA ventral tegmental area

1. INTRODUCTION

Research conducted in our laboratory has demonstrated that the combination of the 11β-hydroxylase inhibitor, metyrapone, and the benzodiazepine, oxazepam, delivered at doses that have no measurable effect when delivered as individual agents, can affect addiction-related behaviors for a variety of drugs. Our hypothesis was that by combining drugs that affect the physiological/brain responses to stress through divergent mechanisms, the drugs might be able to be delivered at significantly reduced doses, thereby minimizing their potential toxic and unwanted side effects while still reducing drug intake.

In December of 2004, Embera NeuroTherapeutics Inc. (Embera), a venture capital-based biotechnology company designed to fund clinical trials investigating the effects of stress-related medications, the combination of metyrapone and oxazepam in particular, on cocaine craving and use in humans, was founded. Embera was incorporated on 15 August 2005. Over the next 3 years, a business plan was put together, a scientific team and scientific advisory board were recruited, and $1.7 M was raised to conduct the first proof-of-principle clinical trial. This was a placebo-controlled, double-blind study conducted by Dr. Anita Kablinger at the Psychopharmacology Research Unit at the LSU Health Sciences Center in Shreveport, investigating the effects of two low-dose combinations of metyrapone and oxazepam (Kablinger et al., 2012). The first subject was enrolled into this study on 14 January 2008, and the final subject completed the study on 14 November 2008. Forty-five subjects were enrolled into the 6-week study: 15 in the placebo group, 15 in an ultralow-dose combination group, and 15 in a low-dose combination group. Approximately 50% of the enrolled subjects completed the study in each of the three arms. No serious adverse events attributable to study medication were observed, and any reported adverse events were relatively minor. Pretreatment with the low-dose combination of metyrapone and oxazepam resulted in statistically significant reductions in cocaine craving measured using the 10-item version of the cocaine-craving questionnaire (CCQ-Brief) (Paliwal, Hyman, & Sinha, 2008), in positive urine screens for cocaine, and in the excretion of the cocaine metabolite benzoylecgonine. Notably, the excretion of benzoylecgonine was significantly reduced in the low-dose group compared to placebo ($p = 0.0011$) during the final 2 weeks of the study. Although this study will obviously have to be replicated in larger clinical trials, these highly translational data demonstrated that the low-dose metyrapone–oxazepam combination was safe and effective in reducing cocaine craving and cocaine taking in humans. This chapter will review the scientific research that led to the development of EMB-001, the combination of low doses of metyrapone and oxazepam, for the treatment of drug and other addictions.

2. STRESS AND ADDICTION

2.1. Historical aspects

Even though our lab has been investigating the relationship between stress and drug craving and relapse—the basis for the highly translational clinical trial described earlier—for over 25 years, this is not a novel concept; this phenomenon has been known to the lay public for many years. An excellent example can be found in the 1980 movie *Airplane!* (Paramount Pictures, Hollywood, CA). Air traffic controller Steve McCroskey (played by Lloyd Bridges) is responsible for the safe landing of a pilotless passenger airliner in this comedy feature. As more mishaps befall the stricken aircraft, McCroskey is heard to say, "Looks like I picked the wrong week to quit drinking." This was subsequently followed by smoking, amphetamines, and sniffing glue, which was an undeniable reference to the stress of the situation increasing McCroskey's desire to use these substances. In general, addictive drugs (including alcohol, cigarettes, and psychomotor stimulants) tend to alter activity within the primary mediator of stress in the body, the hypothalamic–pituitary–adrenal (HPA) axis (Kreek et al., 1984; Lovallo, 2006). Thus, it should come as no surprise that scientists and clinicians alike have reported a connection between substance abuse and stress. Recovering addicts often claim that their drug use was controllable until they were faced with what they perceived as a stressful life situation. Obviously, drug addiction is a much more complex physical and psychological phenomenon than a simple cause and effect based on HPA axis activation, and increasing evidence suggests that an addict's belief that his or her drug of choice provides relief from stress or control over life's stressors has a biological basis, mediated in the central nervous system via "brain stress systems."

Stress is perceived differently by different individuals, and individual responses to stressors are just as varied. However, people generally tend to focus on the negative ramifications associated with exposure to stress. For example, some individuals might complain about stress on the job, stress from dealing with family or friends, or stress related to a traumatic event, and in each case, they would likely describe the unpleasant impact the stressor produced, which could include problems sleeping, increased anxiety, ulcers, heart disease, depression, or other more serious psychiatric disorders. However, despite popular belief, "stress" does not have to be exclusively associated with negative events. The modern definition of stress and its implication for disease were developed by the pioneering neuroendocrinologist Hans Selye, who defined stress as the nonspecific response of the body to any demand placed upon it to adapt, whether that demand produces pleasure or pain (Selye, 1975). Therefore, positive events can be just as "stressful" to the body as negative events. Accordingly, stress can result from the loss of a loved one or from a marriage or birth of a child, a job promotion or the loss of a job, moving into a new house or losing one's home, or any number of events that impact upon an individual's daily life.

2.2. Physiology of stress

Stressors produce an activation of two functionally related biological systems, the sympathetic nervous system and the HPA axis (Koob, 2008; Stratakis & Chrousos, 1995). The activation of these systems makes it possible for an individual to cope with or adapt to an environmental event through the production of a stress response or the "stress cascade." The stress-induced activation of the sympathetic nervous system, mediated through the neurotransmitter norepinephrine, results in an increase in heart rate, a rise in blood pressure, a shift in blood flow to skeletal muscles, an increase in blood glucose, a dilation of the pupils, and an increase in respiration. This automatic response, also called the "fight or flight" response, makes it possible for the individual to face the stressor or attempt to escape from it and occurs below the level of consciousness. In reality, however, people cannot run away from many of life's stressors but instead must learn to adapt to both external and internal environmental changes. During positive events, an individual may believe that his or her increased heart rate represents feelings of happiness and joy, while an increased heart rate resulting from a negative event may be associated with anger or fear. Many abused substances also produce changes in the activity of the sympathetic nervous system (Koob, 2008; Sinha et al., 2003), and these effects are felt differently by different individuals. One person may relish the increased heart rate produced by cocaine, interpreting it as part of the "rush" and euphoria of cocaine use, while the same autonomic response may cause another individual to experience feelings of panic. Activation of the sympathetic nervous system may be responsible for the acute effects of many drugs; however, activation of the HPA axis facilitates long-term adaptation to life's stressors.

The HPA axis consists of a complex, well-regulated interaction between the brain, the anterior pituitary gland, and the adrenal cortex (Goeders, 2002a, 2002b, 2004; Koob, 2008; Koob et al., 2014). The initial step in the activation of the HPA axis is the neuronal-regulated secretion of the peptide corticotropin-releasing factor (CRF). Although CRF is distributed in a number of brain regions, it is those CRF-containing neurons localized in the medial parvocellular subdivision of the paraventricular nucleus (PVN) of the hypothalamus projecting to the external zone of the median eminence that initiate HPA axis activity (Koob, 2008). These neurons release the peptide into the adenohypophyseal portal circulation in a circadian manner or in response to neuronal stimulation. The interaction of CRF with CRF_1 receptors located on anterior pituitary corticotrophs results in the synthesis of proopiomelanocortin (POMC), a large precursor protein that is proteolytically cleaved to produce several smaller biologically active peptides, including β-endorphin and adrenocorticotropic hormone (ACTH). Vasopressin is also released from the parvocellular neurons of the PVN and, when combined with CRF, produces synergistic effects on ACTH release. POMC-derived ACTH diffuses through the general circulation until it reaches the adrenal gland in the abdomen. There, it stimulates the biosynthesis of adrenocorticosteroids, most notably the glucocorticoids, cortisol (in humans), and corticosterone (in rats), and results in their secretion from the adrenal cortex (Lovallo, 2006). Two types of adrenocorticosteroid receptors have been identified, both of which bind corticosterone (Joels & de Kloet, 1994). The type I mineralocorticoid receptor has a higher affinity for corticosterone and is usually fully occupied at basal concentrations of the hormone. This receptor also displays a high affinity for the mineralocorticoid, aldosterone. In contrast, the type II glucocorticoid receptor has a lower affinity for corticosterone and is more likely to be occupied when plasma corticosterone is elevated (e.g., during the stress response). The HPA axis is finely tuned through feedback inhibition coupled to the plasma concentration of circulating cortisol at the level of the anterior pituitary and the PVN (Koob, 2008).

However, glucocorticoid receptors are also localized in brain regions above the hypothalamus, including the hippocampus, the limbic system (e.g., amygdala and bed nucleus of the stria terminalis), and the prefrontal cortex (Lovallo, 2006; McEwen, Weiss, & Schwartz, 1968; Sanchez, Young, Plotsky, & Insel, 2000), suggesting that these higher brain centers are involved in the psychological stress response. It is relevant to note that these same higher brain centers have also been implicated in drug reward (Koob, 2008) and that both stress and addictive drugs produce a similar excitation of dopamine in these brain regions (Saal, Dong, Bonci, & Malenka, 2003).

2.3. Cocaine, anxiety, and the HPA axis

Behaviorally, cocaine use in humans has been reported to produce profound subjective feelings of well-being and a decrease in anxiety (Gawin & Ellinwood, 1988, 1989). In fact, a subpopulation of chronic cocaine users may actually be self-medicating to regulate "painful feelings" and psychiatric symptoms via their drug use (Gawin, 1986; Khantzian, 1985; Kleber & Gawin, 1984), especially since increased rates of affective disorders and anxiety are observed in these individuals (Brady & Lydiard, 1992; Kilbey, Breslau, & Andreski, 1992; Rounsaville et al., 1991). However, cocaine use itself has actually been reported to precipitate episodes of panic attack in some individuals (Anthony, Tien, & Petronis, 1989; Aronson & Craig, 1986; Washton & Tatarsky, 1984). Since panic disorder only became apparent following chronic cocaine use in many of these cases, the drug may have functioned as a precipitating and a causative factor in neurobiologically vulnerable individuals (Aronson & Craig, 1986). As a sympathomimetic drug, cocaine is also able to increase stress-related monoamines such as epinephrine and norepinephrine, which may enhance the subjective feelings of panic (Wilkins, 1992). Furthermore, some of the major symptoms observed during withdrawal from chronic cocaine intoxication can often include severe anxiety and restlessness, agitation, and depression (Gawin & Ellinwood, 1989).

Cocaine-induced anxiogenic effects have also been observed in non-human animals using a variety of behavioral paradigms. For example, cocaine has been reported to augment the aversion for a white illuminated area in the mouse black and white test box model (Costall, Kelly, Naylor, & Onaivi, 1989), to further reduce punished behavior in rats responding under a conflict schedule (Fontana & Commissaris, 1989), to increase defensive withdrawal in rats (Yang, Gorman, Dunn, & Goeders, 1992), and to decrease the number of entries into and time spent in the open arms of an elevated plus maze in mice (Yang et al., 1992) and rats (Rogerio & Takahashi, 1992). Interestingly, even contextual cues previously paired with cocaine delivery can elicit anxiety-like responses in drug-free rats tested in the elevated plus maze (DeVries & Pert, 1998). Withdrawal following repeated cocaine injections has also been reported to induce anxiogenic responses in the elevated plus maze (Sarnyai et al., 1995), and withdrawal from chronic self-administration enhances startle-induced ultrasonic distress vocalizations (Barros & Miczek, 1996; Mutschler & Miczek, 1998a, 1998b). Cocaine withdrawal-induced anxiogenic responses have also been demonstrated in drug discrimination studies. Pentylenetetrazole (PTZ) is a convulsant drug with discriminative stimulus properties that are related to the production of an anxiogenic response (Shearman & Lal, 1980). Cocaine withdrawal produces PTZ-appropriate responding in rats trained to discriminate PTZ from saline (Wood & Lal, 1987). However, acute cocaine injections also generalize to PTZ in rats trained to discriminate the drug from saline (Shearman & Lal, 1981), suggesting that cocaine itself can be anxiogenic. In fact, it has been demonstrated that the drug can act as a reinforcer while simultaneously producing aversive anxiogenic-like effects in rats trained to self-administer cocaine by traversing a straight-arm runway to a goal box (Ettenberg & Geist, 1991). We have also investigated the purported anxiogenic effects of cocaine using the drug discrimination model. In these experiments, rats were trained to discriminate cocaine from saline using a two-lever, food-reinforced responding design. When rats were injected with saline and then exposed to 15 min of restraint stress (Mantsch & Goeders, 1998), significant cocaine-appropriate responding was observed, indicating that a component of cocaine's subjective effects may be associated with stress or anxiety. CRF has been reported to be involved in a variety of neuropsychiatric disorders including depression and anxiety (Nemeroff, 1988; Pitts et al., 1995), suggesting that the anxiety associated with cocaine use and withdrawal may depend, in part, on the effects of the drug on the release of this endogenous stress-related peptide and the resulting activation of the HPA axis.

Scientists have been aware of the existence of a complex relationship between HPA axis activation and the endocrine and neurobehavioral effects of cocaine for several years now (Goeders, 1997). Acute, noncontingent cocaine administration increases plasma levels of ACTH, β-endorphin, and corticosterone in rats (Forman & Estilow, 1988; Levy et al., 1991;

Moldow & Fischman, 1987; Saphier, Welch, Farrar, & Goeders, 1993) and in nonhuman primates (Saphier et al., 1993). These cocaine-induced increases in ACTH and corticosterone are blocked in rats by pretreatment with the CRF receptor antagonist α-helical CRF9-41 (Sarnyai, Biro, Penke, & Telegdy, 1992), by the immunoneutralization of CRF with an anti-CRF antibody (Rivier & Vale, 1987; Sarnyai et al., 1992), or by bilateral electrolytic lesions of the PVN (Rivier & Lee, 1994), indicating that these increases are mediated by the cocaine-induced release of CRF from parvocellular neurons in the PVN. In fact, cocaine can even stimulate the release of CRF from rat hypothalamic organ culture systems *in vitro* (Calogero, Gallucci, Kling, Chrousos, & Gold, 1989). Acute cocaine administration has also been reported to decrease CRF-like immunoreactivity in the hypothalamus, hippocampus, and frontal cortex, while increasing it in the amygdala (Sarnyai et al., 1993), indicating that cocaine can also affect CRF activity in areas located outside the hypothalamus. Similarly, chronic exposure to cocaine decreases CRF receptor binding in brain regions primarily associated with the mesocorticolimbic dopaminergic system (Goeders, Bienvenu, & De Souza, 1990). In clinical studies, the intranasal administration of cocaine has been reported to increase cortisol secretion in male volunteers without a history of drug abuse (Heesch et al., 1995). In chronic cocaine users, the acute, intravenous administration of cocaine has also been reported to increase the secretion of cortisol (Baumann et al., 1995) and ACTH (Mendelson, Mello, Teoh, Ellingboe, & Cochin, 1989; Mendelson, Teoh, Mello, Ellingboe, & Rhoades, 1992). Interestingly, chronic cocaine use may actually attenuate the ability to release cortisol in response to other stressful stimuli (Heesch et al., 1995; Vescovi, Coiro, Volpi, Giannini, & Passeri, 1992). Plasma cortisol, β-endorphin, and ACTH are elevated in cocaine addicts on the day of admission into treatment centers (Vescovi, Coiro, Volpi, & Passeri, 1992), and cocaine-dependent individuals often display abnormal patterns of HPA axis activity (Mendelson, Sholar, Mello, Teoh, & Sholar, 1998). Cocaine appears to produce these HPA axis-related effects by increasing the peak amplitude of secretory pulses of these hormones without altering pulse frequency, which indicates that these increases are likely driven by hypothalamic CRF (Mendelson et al., 1989; Sarnyai, Mello, Mendelson, Eros-Sarnyai, & Mercer, 1996; Teoh et al., 1994). However, as reviewed in the succeeding text, our laboratory and others have also collected data that suggest that many of these effects are mediated through sites outside of the hypothalamus. The prefrontal cortex, or more specifically the medial prefrontal cortex, may function as an interface between the HPA axis and the central nervous system to regulate the interaction between conditioned reward and the stress response.

Thus, cocaine has been reported to stimulate HPA axis activity in a manner analogous to various stressors, which indicates that this system has the potential to influence many of the neurochemical and behavioral effects of the drug. Therefore, we initially selected the combination of oxazepam and metyrapone for the treatment of cocaine addiction since these drugs reduce stress-related anxiety and the HPA axis response to stress. In the following sections of this chapter, we will review the research leading up to the selection of these drugs and the subsequent changes that we have made in our original hypotheses.

3. COCAINE AND BENZODIAZEPINES

3.1. Benzodiazepine receptors

The finding that cocaine and stressors produce similar discriminative stimulus effects (Mantsch & Goeders, 1998) suggests that these two stimuli activate one or more common pharmacological effector systems, which may provide useful information regarding how stressors interact with cocaine-seeking behavior. Benzodiazepines are among the most widely prescribed drugs for the pharmacological management of anxiety (Farnsworth, 1990; Hirschfeld, 1990). Perhaps not coincidentally, some of the major symptoms associated with cocaine withdrawal often include severe anxiety, restlessness, and agitation (Farnsworth, 1990; Gawin & Ellinwood, 1989; Tarr & Macklin, 1987), suggesting that benzodiazepines may be useful for alleviating these negative symptoms during the early stages of withdrawal. These drugs are also useful in the emergency room for the treatment of some of the medical complications associated with cocaine overdose. For example, overdose-related seizures and myocardial ischemia can be treated with intravenous diazepam (Gay, 1981, 1982; Lange & Hillis, 2001; Tarr & Macklin, 1987). Interestingly, the number of benzodiazepine receptors in platelets from chronic cocaine users has been reported to be augmented when compared to those obtained from alcoholics or normal controls (Chesley et al., 1990). In addition, peripheral benzodiazepine receptors (recently renamed translocator protein of 18kDa (TSPO)) labeled with [^{3}H]PK11195 were decreased in neutrophil membranes from the blood of male inpatients following 3 weeks of cocaine abstinence (Javaid et al., 1994). These data indicate that cocaine may affect benzodiazepine receptors or related proteins such as TSPO in humans during various stages of drug use and prompted our further exploration of these interactions in preclinical models.

In our initial study on cocaine and benzodiazepine receptors, chronic, daily noncontingent injections of cocaine (20 or 40 mg/kg, IP) for 15 days resulted in differential effects on central benzodiazepine receptor binding in various regions of the rat brain (Goeders, Bell, Guidroz, & McNulty, 1990). In general, cocaine decreased binding in terminal fields for the mesocorticolimbic dopaminergic system while increasing binding in terminal fields for the nigrostriatal system. Statistically significant decreases in binding in the medial prefrontal cortex and increases in the ventral tegmental area (VTA) were still observed for up to 2 weeks following the final injection of cocaine, suggesting that benzodiazepine receptors in these brain regions may be especially sensitive to the effects of the drug. These cocaine-induced changes in binding appeared to be mediated, at least in part, through the effects of the drug on dopaminergic neuronal activity since intraventricular injections of the neurotoxin 6-hydroxydopamine (6-OHDA) attenuated or reversed these effects (Goeders, Bell, et al., 1990). We have reported similar effects on CRF receptors measured autoradiographically in the rat brain following a similar cocaine dosing regimen (Goeders, Bienvenu, et al., 1990), and these effects were also attenuated in 6-OHDA-lesioned rats, further suggesting a role for CRF and the HPA axis in the behavioral effects of cocaine. Continuous exposure to cocaine also alters benzodiazepine receptor binding in various structures of the rat brain (Lipton, Olsen, & Ellison, 1995; Zeigler, Lipton, Toga, & Ellison, 1991). Unfortunately, these early experiments did not address the potential involvement of benzodiazepine receptors in cocaine reinforcement since the noncontingent administration of a drug is not, by definition, reinforcing. A reinforcer is an event that increases the probability of the behavior that resulted in its presentation (Ferster, 2002). In fact, different behavioral and neurobiological effects are seen when comparing contingent to noncontingent administration (Dworkin, Mirkis, & Smith, 1995; Fumagalli et al., 2013; Palamarchouk, Smagin, & Goeders, 2009; Stefanski et al., 2007; Suto, Ecke, You, & Wise, 2010; Twining, Bolan, & Grigson, 2009). The following experiment was therefore designed to investigate the effects of self-administered cocaine on benzodiazepine receptor binding in rats.

Benzodiazepine receptors were visualized using [^{3}H] flumazenil under standard autoradiographic conditions in animals that self-administered cocaine and in littermates that received simultaneous, yoked infusions of cocaine or saline (Goeders, 1991). The general pharmacological effects of response-independent cocaine administration were estimated by comparing receptor binding changes in the brains of the yoked-cocaine animals with those from the yoked-saline littermates. Differences in binding between the self-administration and yoked-saline littermates likely represented a combination of the general pharmacological and the reinforcing actions of cocaine. Benzodiazepine receptor binding was increased in the frontal cortex and decreased in the substantia nigra and VTA in both the self-administration and the yoked-cocaine groups when compared to their yoked-saline littermates. Comparisons between the yoked-cocaine and yoked-saline animals also revealed significant reductions in binding in the hippocampus. However, changes in receptor binding that were more specifically related to cocaine reinforcement were determined by comparing binding in the self-administration group with that from animals that had received yoked, noncontingent infusions of the drug. Benzodiazepine receptor binding was significantly increased in the medial prefrontal cortex and nucleus accumbens and decreased in the caudate nucleus and globus pallidus of the self-administration rats compared to yoked-cocaine animals. Binding was also decreased significantly more in the VTA of the self-administration rats compared to yoked-cocaine controls. Interestingly, the medial prefrontal cortex is thought to be involved in many of the behavioral effects of cocaine including the development of sensitization (Goeders, Irby, Shuster, & Guerin, 1997; Schenk & Snow, 1994; Sorg, Chen, & Kalivas, 1993) and the initiation of reinforcement (Goeders & Smith, 1983). These data demonstrate that benzodiazepine receptor binding was significantly altered in reinforcement-relevant brain regions associated with ascending dopaminergic systems (e.g., nucleus accumbens and medial prefrontal cortex), suggesting that these effects may indeed be related to cocaine reinforcement. As reviewed earlier, we demonstrated an effect of cocaine on benzodiazepine and CRF receptor binding, especially in reward-relevant regions of the mesocorticolimbic dopamine system, suggesting an interaction between stress and cocaine.

3.2. Benzodiazepines and cocaine reinforcement

In our earliest work in this area, we reported that pretreatment with the benzodiazepine receptor agonist, chlordiazepoxide, significantly decreased intravenous cocaine self-administration in rats (Goeders, McNulty, Mirkis, & McAllister, 1989). This effect was attenuated when the unit dose of cocaine was increased, suggesting that chlordiazepoxide decreased the efficacy of cocaine as a reinforcer. In pilot experiments, diazepam also attenuated intravenous cocaine self-administration maintained under a progressive-ratio schedule of reinforcement in rats (Dworkin, D'Costa, Goeders, & Hoffman, 1989). However, since these decreases in drug intake may have resulted from a nonspecific disruption of the ability of the rats to respond, an additional study was conducted. Alprazolam was tested in adult male Wistar rats responding under a multiple schedule of intravenous cocaine presentation and food reinforcement, with cocaine available during 1 h of the session and food presentations available during the other (Goeders, McNulty, & Guerin, 1993). Food reinforcement was used to generate a control performance to evaluate whether or not the effects of alprazolam were specific for cocaine-maintained responding. Initially, responding maintained by both food and cocaine was reduced following exposure to alprazolam. However, tolerance quickly developed to the sedative effects of alprazolam on food-maintained responding during subsequent testing. On the other hand, no tolerance was observed in the ability of alprazolam to reduce cocaine self-administration. The results of these experiments demonstrate that upon repeated administration, alprazolam could decrease cocaine self-administration without affecting food-maintained responding. This outcome suggests that these effects may result from specific actions on cocaine reinforcement rather than nonspecific effects on the ability of the rats to respond. These studies have been supported by other findings demonstrating that benzodiazepines can attenuate the behavioral effects of cocaine in rats, nonhuman primates, and human subjects (Barrett, Negus, Mello, & Caine, 2005; Negus, Mello, & Fivel, 2000; Rush, Stoops, Wagner, Hays, & Glaser, 2004).

4. STRESS AND COCAINE REINFORCEMENT

At the same time that we were investigating the effects of cocaine on benzodiazepine receptors and the effects of benzodiazepines on the behavioral effects of cocaine, we also began investigating the effects of stress and stress-related drugs on intravenous cocaine self-administration in rats. Our initial studies investigated the role for stress in the acquisition of cocaine self-administration in rats. Other researchers had shown that the acquisition of amphetamine and cocaine self-administration was enhanced in rats exposed to social isolation (Schenk, Lacelle, Gorman, & Amit, 1987) or tail pinch (Piazza, Deminiere, le Moal, & Simon, 1990), in rats witnessing other rats being subjected to electric footshock (Ramsey & Van Ree, 1993), and in rats born of female rats exposed to restraint during pregnancy (Deminiere et al., 1992). Housing with female rats also increases psychomotor stimulant self-administration by male rats (Lemaire, Deminiere, & Mormede, 1994), as do other forms of "social stress" including female rats exposed to an attack by a lactating female rat (Haney, Maccari, Le Moal, Simon, & Piazza, 1995) or male rats exposed to an attack by an aggressive male (Haney et al., 1995), exposed to the threat of attack following several defeats (Tidey & Miczek, 1997), or exposed to only the threat of attack (Miczek & Mutschler, 1996). In addition, research has demonstrated that social hierarchy-related stressors also increase cocaine intake in rhesus monkeys (reviewed in Nader, Czoty, Nader, & Morgan, 2012). These reports are in agreement with the clinical data reviewed in the preceding text, which indicated that stress increases the vulnerability for drug addiction in humans.

4.1. Effects of uncontrollable stress

We first investigated the effects of exposure to response-contingent (controllable stress) and noncontingent (uncontrollable stress) electric footshock on the acquisition of intravenous cocaine self-administration in rats (Goeders & Guerin, 1994). In these experiments, one rat from a group of three randomly received an electric footshock through an electrified floor grid when it pressed a response lever that also resulted in the presentation of food (response-contingent shock). Although this resulted in a conflict between obtaining food reinforcement and avoiding footshock, these animals were in some control over the timing and frequency of the stressor. Shock presentation for the second rat in each triad was yoked to the first rat, so that the second rat received a footshock regardless of its own lever responding behavior (noncontingent shock). Therefore, these rats had no control over the timing or frequency of the delivery of the stressor. The third rat in each triad responded under the same schedule of food reinforcement as the other two rats but was never shocked. When responding under this food reinforcement/electric footshock schedule stabilized for all three rats, tail blood was collected for the determination of plasma corticosterone and testing for the acquisition of cocaine self-administration commenced. These rats were initially tested with an extremely low dose of cocaine (i.e., 0.031 mg/kg/infusion) for 1 week, and this concentration was subsequently doubled weekly through 0.5 mg/kg/infusion, a dose that is readily self-administered by rats. Doses were tested in an ascending order in all of our acquisition experiments since exposure to higher doses of psychomotor stimulants can sensitize rats to lower doses (Schenk & Partridge, 1997), resulting in the acquisition of self-administration at doses of these drugs that would not otherwise maintain responding. In this experiment, animals without control over electric footshock presentation (noncontingent shock) were more sensitive to cocaine. Exposure to noncontingent footshock shifted the ascending limb of the cocaine dose–response curve upward and to the left, indicating that these rats were more sensitive to the reinforcing effects of low doses of cocaine (i.e., 0.125 mg/kg/infusion or lower) than rats exposed to response-contingent or no shock. In general, rats from these other two groups did not self-administer cocaine until higher concentrations were tested (i.e., 0.25 or 0.5 mg/kg/infusion). In addition, when the rats from these other treatment groups did self-administer the drug, rates of self-administration were generally lower than observed in rats exposed to noncontingent shock. Interestingly, increased sensitivity to cocaine was positively correlated with stress-induced increases in plasma corticosterone, and self-administration did not occur unless plasma corticosterone was increased above a critical level or threshold (Goeders & Guerin, 1996b). Electric footshock did not affect responding maintained by higher doses of cocaine that fell on the descending limb of the dose–response curve, possibly because the cocaine infusions alone were sufficient to increase plasma corticosterone above this critical reward threshold. This phenomenon appears to be relatively specific for the acquisition phase of cocaine self-administration since in our laboratory, neither exposure to footshock (Goeders & Guerin, 1996b) nor exogenous injections of corticosterone (Goeders and Guerin, 1999) affect ongoing self-administration during the maintenance phase. Thus, it appears that once this "reward threshold" is crossed, further stress-induced increases in plasma corticosterone are without additional influence on drug intake.

4.2. Effects of exogenous corticosterone

Since stress-induced increases in plasma corticosterone were positively associated with the ability of noncontingent electric footshock to shift the ascending limb of the acquisition dose–response curve upward and to the left, the following experiment was designed to determine the effects of exogenous injections of corticosterone on the acquisition of cocaine self-administration (Mantsch, Saphier, & Goeders, 1998). As reviewed earlier, corticosterone (cortisol in humans) is the last hormone in the cascade of HPA axis activation, so we hypothesized that the stress-induced increase in corticosterone secretion above a critical threshold may have mediated the increased sensitivity to cocaine we observed in rats exposed to non-contingent electric footshock. In this experiment, adult male Wistar rats were treated daily, 15 min prior to each self-administration session, with corticosterone (2.0 mg/kg, IP, suspended in saline) or saline. These injections began 2 weeks prior to the start of self-administration testing to mimic the stress experiment described earlier as closely as possible since exposure to electric footshock also began approximately 2 weeks before self-administration testing began (Goeders & Guerin, 1996b). Similar to what we observed with electric footshock, daily pretreatment with corticosterone also produced a leftward shift in the ascending limb of the dose–response curve for the acquisition of self-administration, indicating that corticosterone-treated rats were more sensitive to the reinforcing effects of low doses of cocaine. All of the corticosterone-treated rats acquired self-administration at the 0.0625-mg/kg/infusion dose or lower, whereas none of the saline-treated rats acquired this behavior until the 0.125-mg/kg/infusion dose or higher.

4.3. Effects of adrenalectomy

The results from the experiments described earlier suggested that increasing plasma corticosterone, either through exposure to stress or via exogenous injections of the hormone, can influence the acquisition of intravenous cocaine self-administration in rats. The following experiments were therefore designed to further examine the role for the HPA axis in cocaine reinforcement by investigating the effects of adrenalectomy on the acquisition of cocaine self-administration in rats (Goeders & Guerin, 1996a). Plasma corticosterone was significantly reduced in adrenalectomized rats compared to sham-operated controls, but there were no differences between these rats with respect to responding under a food reinforcement schedule, indicating that adrenalectomized rats could still learn to make the response necessary for the delivery of a food reinforcer. However, while a typical inverted "U"-shaped dose–response curve for cocaine self-administration was generated by the sham rats, adrenalectomized rats did not learn to self-administer cocaine at any dose tested. These data support the results and conclusions obtained in the experiments described earlier and suggest that corticosterone may be necessary for the acquisition of cocaine self-administration to occur in rats.

In summary, we have shown that exposure to uncontrollable electric footshock facilitates the acquisition of cocaine self-administration. We initially hypothesized that these effects were most likely mediated through the activation of the HPA axis since this increased sensitivity was positively correlated with stress-induced elevations in plasma corticosterone. In fact, similar effects were also seen in rats injected chronically with corticosterone. Electric footshock or exogenous injections of corticosterone each selectively shifted the ascending limb for the acquisition of cocaine self-administration upward and to the left, which indicated that animals receiving such treatments were more sensitive to low doses of the drug. Neither stress nor corticosterone pretreatment affected the descending limb of the acquisition dose–response curve, suggesting that low cocaine doses are especially sensitive to the influence of the HPA axis. Reductions in plasma corticosterone, either pharmacologically or surgically induced, prevent the acquisition of cocaine self-administration over a wide range of doses, further suggesting that the HPA axis is critical to this process.

4.4. Effects of stress-related drugs
4.4.1 Ketoconazole and metyrapone
In addition to benzodiazepines, we also investigated the effects of corticosterone synthesis inhibitors on cocaine reinforcement since our data had suggested a role for stress and the HPA axis in the acquisition of cocaine self-administration in rats. As reviewed earlier, corticosterone is the end product in the activation of the HPA axis (Lovallo, 2006). Ketoconazole is an oral antimycotic agent with a broad spectrum of activity and low toxicity (Sonino, 1987) that is approved by the FDA for the treatment of a number of superficial and systemic fungal infections. This drug also inhibits the 11β-hydroxylation and 18-hydroxylation steps in the synthesis of adrenocorticosteroids (Engelhardt, Dorr, Jaspers, & Knorr, 1985) and may also function as a glucocorticoid receptor antagonist (Loose, Stover, & Feldman, 1983), which makes it a potentially useful drug with which to study the effects of corticosterone in cocaine reinforcement. Furthermore, several clinical trials suggested that 11β-hydroxylase inhibitors such as ketoconazole and metyrapone are also effective in the treatment of hypercortisolemic depression that is resistant to standard antidepressant therapy (Ghadirian et al., 1995; Murphy, Ghadirian, & Dhar, 1998; Thakore & Dinan, 1995; Wolkowitz et al., 1993). This is especially germane since depression and anxiety are often manifested during cocaine withdrawal in humans (Gawin & Ellinwood, 1989) and recent users of cocaine are more likely to experience panic attacks than the general population (Kelley et al., 2012). The following experiment was therefore designed to investigate the effects of ketoconazole on intravenous cocaine self-administration

in rats (Goeders, Peltier, & Guerin, 1998). In these experiments, adult male Wistar rats were allowed alternating 15 min periods of access to food reinforcement and cocaine self-administration during daily 2 h sessions. Pretreatment with ketoconazole reduced low-dose (i.e., 0.125–0.25 mg/kg/ infusion) cocaine self-administration without affecting food-reinforced responding. In fact, pretreatment with ketoconazole resulted in rates and patterns of self-administration at these doses of cocaine that were indistinguishable from those observed during cocaine extinction, when responding only resulted in infusions of saline. However, these effects were attenuated when the highest dose of cocaine tested was self-administered (i.e., 0.5 mg/kg/infusion). Although basal levels were not altered, ketoconazole also reduced plasma corticosterone in rats trained with the lower doses of cocaine but did not significantly affect the hormone when the highest dose was self-administered. These data suggest that ketoconazole may have reduced drug intake, at least in part, through its effects on corticosterone. These data also imply that the use of more effective and/or efficient corticosterone synthesis inhibitors might potentially decrease plasma corticosterone and reduce the self-administration of higher doses of cocaine without producing nonspecific effects. This proved to be true for metyrapone.

Metyrapone blocks the 11β-hydroxylation reaction in the production of corticosterone, thereby resulting in decreases in plasma concentrations of the hormone (Haleem, Kennett, & Curzon, 1988; Haynes, 1990). Pretreatment with metyrapone resulted in significant dose-related decreases in both plasma corticosterone and ongoing cocaine self-administration, suggesting that corticosterone is involved in the maintenance and the acquisition of cocaine self-administration (Goeders & Guerin, 1996a).

4.4.2 Benzodiazepines

The ability of benzodiazepines to decrease cocaine self-administration may have also been related to the effects of these drugs on corticosterone and other "stress" hormones and peptides. These drugs can decrease plasma corticosterone (Keim & Sigg, 1977), cortisol, and ACTH (Meador-Woodruff & Greden, 1988; Torpy et al., 1993), or they can attenuate cocaine-induced increases in plasma corticosterone (Yang et al., 1992) to decrease cocaine reinforcement.

4.5. CRF

As reviewed earlier, ketoconazole (as well as metyrapone) reduces cocaine self-administration in rats (Goeders & Guerin, 1996a; Goeders et al., 1998).

However, we sometimes observed that a rat's initial behavioral response to ketoconazole was somewhat different than subsequent exposures to the drug (Goeders & Guerin, 1997). Therefore, the following experiment was designed to investigate the effects of acute, repeated, and chronic ketoconazole administration on HPA axis activity and CRF content in hypothalamic and extrahypothalamic brain sites in rats (Smagin & Goeders, 2004). Ketoconazole (25 mg/kg, IP) was administered acutely, repeatedly (i.e., two injections separated by 7 days), and chronically for 7 or 14 days. All treatments significantly increased the concentrations of ACTH in blood without affecting corticosterone or testosterone. There was a significant increase (~269%) in CRF content in the median eminence after the acute administration of ketoconazole that just failed to reach statistical significance following repeated or chronic administration. The chronic administration of ketoconazole for 7 days resulted in a significant increase in CRF content in the amygdala (~200%) and the PVN of the hypothalamus (~214%). Interestingly, chronic 14-day administration of ketoconazole also significantly increased CRF content in the nucleus accumbens and medial prefrontal cortex, brain regions where cocaine specifically affected benzodiazepine and CRF receptor binding (Goeders, 1991; Goeders, Bell, et al., 1990; Goeders, Bienvenu, et al., 1990). These data suggest that single, repeated, and chronic ketoconazole administration affects the HPA axis and hypothalamic and extrahypothalamic CRF content in the brain, with a clearly distinct pattern of activation. Since the medial prefrontal cortex and CRF have been implicated in the neurobiology of cocaine addiction (Goeders, 1997; Goeders & Smith, 1983; Guzman, Moscarello, & Ettenberg, 2009), CRF-induced alterations in dopaminergic neurotransmission may play an important role in this peptide's effects on cocaine responsiveness. Interestingly, metyrapone has also been shown to increase CRF messenger RNA levels in the PVN in rhesus monkeys, indicating an increase in neuroendocrine CRF secretion (Van Vugt, Piercy, Farley, Reid, & Rivest, 1997). Taken together, these data suggest that corticosterone synthesis inhibitors, as well as CRF receptor antagonists and benzodiazepines, may affect cocaine reward, at least in part, through interactions with dopamine and CRF within the medial prefrontal cortex (Goeders, 2004).

4.5.1 CRF receptor antagonists
Since both our behavioral and neurobiological experiments indicated a potential role for CRF in cocaine reinforcement, the following experiments were designed to investigate the role for CRF receptor antagonists on

cocaine self-administration in rats (Goeders & Guerin, 2000). We chose to use the small molecule, nonpeptide, CRF_1 receptor antagonist CP-154,526 in these experiments since CP-154,526 enters the brain following systemic administration (McCarthy, Heinrichs, & Grigoriadis, 1999; Schulz et al., 1996), which makes it a potentially more useful tool for investigating the effects of CRF in cocaine reinforcement. Adult male Wistar rats were trained to respond under the multiple, alternating schedule of food rein-forcement and cocaine self-administration described previously (Goeders & Guerin, 2008). Prior to testing, these rats were also exposed to multiple cocaine extinction probes (i.e., saline substitutions) until repro-ducible decreases in responding during extinction were observed (Peltier, Guerin, Dorairaj, & Goeders, 2001). Pretreatment with CP-154,526 did not affect food-maintained responding. However, cocaine self-administration was significantly attenuated and, in some cases, completely eliminated, fol-lowing pretreatment with CP-154,526. Drug intake was decreased across all doses of cocaine tested, with the dose–response curve for cocaine self-administration effectively shifted downward and flattened, suggesting that CP-154,526 decreased cocaine reinforcement. Interestingly, pretreatment with this compound did not produce reliable, reproducible effects on plasma corticosterone (Goeders & Guerin, 2000; Gurkovskaya & Goeders, 2001). Also of note, responding on the cocaine lever following CP-154,526 pre-treatment was significantly suppressed even during the first 15 min of the session, a time when rats typically sample the cocaine lever during extinction (Goeders et al., 1998), suggesting that CRF may be involved in the condi-tioned effects of cocaine as well (DeVries & Pert, 1998; Gurkovskaya & Goeders, 2001). These data underscore a potential role for CRF in cocaine reinforcement and further suggested a role for the HPA axis in cocaine addiction and withdrawal.

In summary, ongoing cocaine self-administration can be attenuated by drugs that reduce corticosterone secretion (i.e., benzodiazepines, ketocona-zole, and metyrapone), but the magnitude of this effect depends in part on the unit dose of cocaine. With lower doses of cocaine, the inhibition of corticosterone synthesis and/or secretion reduces concentrations of the hor-mone below a critical threshold for reward and cocaine self-administration is significantly attenuated. If the dose of cocaine is sufficiently increased, cocaine-induced increases in corticosterone can still reach this threshold even though synthesis is suppressed, and drug taking is not significantly affected. Once this threshold has been crossed, however, further increases in corticosterone do not appear to affect ongoing self-administration.

Finally, cocaine self-administration can also be decreased by drugs that block CRF receptors (e.g., by pretreatment with CP-154,526). In this case, however, increasing the cocaine dose does not overcome the attenuation of self-administration and the dose–response curve is effectively shifted downward and flattened, which further underscores an important role for CRF in the maintenance phase of cocaine self-administration. Unfortunately, at the time this chapter was written, there were no CRF receptor antagonists available for use in humans and the translational potential of CRF receptor antagonists against cocaine-related behaviors in monkeys has been questioned, at least with respect to antalarmin (Lee, Tiefenbacher, Platt, & Spealman, 2003; Mello, Negus, Rice, & Mendelson, 2006). However, since effects on CRF were produced indirectly, at least by ketoconazole, the use of cortisol synthesis inhibitors may provide an alternate approach to alter the activity of CRF.

5. STRESS AND RELAPSE

We have also investigated the effects of various stress-related drugs on the reinstatement of cocaine seeking, an animal model of relapse (de Wit & Stewart, 1983; Erb, Shaham, & Stewart, 1996; Meil & See, 1996). Understanding the factors that contribute to the precipitation of relapse is integral to the development of more effective and efficient strategies for the treatment of addiction. Using this reinstatement model, rats are trained to self-administer a given drug. Once stable self-administration is observed, the rats are subjected to repeated extinction whereby responding is no longer reinforced by the delivery of the drug. Once extinction has been successful, the rats are exposed to various stimuli in an attempt to reinstate drug-seeking behavior. In humans and nonhumans, the acute reexposure to the self-administered drug itself is a potent event for provoking relapse to drug seeking (Shaham, Shalev, Lu, De Wit, & Stewart, 2003; Stewart, 2000). Exposure to stress (Shiffman, Read, & Jarvik, 1985), or simply the presentation of stress-related imagery (Sinha, Catapano, & O'Malley, 1999), is another stimulus demonstrated to be important for relapse in humans. Exposure to external cues or triggers previously associated with drug use can also induce craving and relapse in recovering addicts (Kilgus & Pumariega, 1994; Robbins, Ehrman, Childress, & O'Brien, 1992; Sinha & Li, 2007). We have investigated the ability of a cue previously paired with cocaine self-administration (Meil & See, 1996; See, 2005) to reinstate extinguished cocaine-seeking behavior (Goeders & Clampitt, 2002). In this experiment, responding during reinstatement testing resulted in the contingent presentation of a tone and house light cue that had been paired with cocaine delivery during self-administration training, which reliably reinstated extinguished cocaine-seeking behavior. Conditioned increases in plasma corticosterone were evident during cocaine extinction and during reinstatement (Goeders & Clampitt, 2002). However, while plasma corticosterone returned to basal levels by the end of the session during extinction, it remained elevated through the end of the 2-h session during reinstatement, indicating the involvement of a stress-like physiological response in cue-induced cocaine seeking. In humans, exposure to drug-related cues also increases plasma cortisol and ACTH and activates the sympathetic nervous system (Hyman, Fox, Hong, Doebrick, & Sinha, 2007; Sinha, Garcia, Paliwal, Kreek, & Rounsaville, 2006; Sinha et al., 2003), suggesting an important involvement of the stress response during drug cue-induced cocaine craving. A better understanding of how these cues contribute to the precipitation of relapse may lead to the development of more effective and efficient strategies for the treatment of addiction.

5.1. Stress-related drugs

5.1.1 Ketoconazole

We investigated the effects of ketoconazole on the cocaine-induced (Mantsch & Goeders, 1999b) and the stress-induced reinstatement of extinguished cocaine-seeking behavior (Mantsch & Goeders, 1999a). Adult male Wistar rats were trained to self-administer cocaine during daily 2-h sessions. After 15 sessions of stable self-administration, this behavior was extinguished over the course of 10 consecutive sessions. The ability of cocaine (5–20 mg/kg, IP) to reinstate cocaine seeking was then evaluated. Interestingly, ketoconazole did not affect cocaine-induced reinstatement (Mantsch & Goeders, 1999b). In another experiment, the rats were trained as above and then placed into extinction. In this case, intermittent footshock (15 min) was delivered immediately prior to the reinstatement test session, which was otherwise identical to the extinction conditions. Electric footshock significantly increased responding on the cocaine lever compared to that observed during the previous extinction sessions, and this reinstatement was blocked in animals pretreated with ketoconazole prior to exposure to the stressor. Although plasma corticosterone was still slightly elevated above basal levels, ketoconazole pretreatment significantly decreased the rise in plasma corticosterone produced by electric footshock.

We also tested the effects of ketoconazole on the cue-induced reinstatement of extinguished cocaine seeking (Goeders & Clampitt, 2002). Rats were trained to self-administer cocaine (0.25 mg/kg/infusion; FR4) during daily 2 h sessions. During self-administration training, a lever light was illuminated above the drug lever to indicate the availability of cocaine. After the fixed-ratio (FR) requirement was met, the drug lever light was turned off and cocaine was delivered over 5.6 s accompanied by the presentation of a tone/house light combination (i.e., conditioned cue). After drug delivery, the tone/house light compound stimulus continued during a 20-s time-out period. Once stable rates of cocaine self-administration were observed (i.e., less than 10% variation for 3 consecutive days), drug responding was extinguished. During extinction, the drug lever light and response lever were present, but responses were not reinforced with either cocaine delivery or the compound conditioned stimulus. After drug lever responding was extinguished to 20% of baseline self-administration, rats were tested for reinstatement. During reinstatement testing, rats were either pretreated with ketoconazole or vehicle. Lever pressing during reinstatement resulted in the presentation of the tone/house light combination without cocaine delivery. Pretreatment with ketoconazole reversed the conditioned cue-induced reinstatement of extinguished cocaine-seeking behavior and also blocked the conditioned increases in plasma corticosterone observed during reinstatement (Goeders & Clampitt, 2002), suggesting an important role for corticosterone in the ability of a stressor (electric footshock) or conditioned cues to reinstate cocaine-seeking behavior in rats.

5.1.2 CRF receptor antagonists

Other labs have reported that CRF_1 receptor antagonists decrease the stress- (Erb, 2010; Shaham, Erb, Leung, Buczek, & Stewart, 1998) and cocaine- (Erb, Shaham, & Stewart, 1998) induced reinstatement of extinguished cocaine-seeking behavior in rats. We have shown that pretreatment with the CRF_1 receptor antagonist CP-154,526 also reduces the ability of conditioned cues to reinstate extinguished cocaine (Goeders & Clampitt, 2002) and methamphetamine (Moffett & Goeders, 2007) seeking behaviors. We also conducted another series of related experiments (Gurkovskaya & Goeders, 2001) based on the observation that animals will continue to respond for days during extinction when presented with cues that had been previously paired with cocaine, which is another model of cue-induced cocaine seeking (Weiss et al., 2000). Rats were trained to self-administer cocaine, and when responding stabilized, saline was substituted for cocaine and the animals were tested for extinction for the first time. Other rats were allowed to self-administer cocaine for an additional 30 days, and extinction was tested once again. CP-154,526-treated animals responded significantly less than vehicle-treated animals during extinction on the first day of testing and also after 30 days of self-administration training. Interestingly, CP-154,526 did not suppress plasma corticosterone, suggesting that the effects of this compound were acting, in part, independently of the HPA axis and were likely mediated at sites located outside of the hypothalamus. Nevertheless, these data do underscore an important role for CRF in the ability of environmental cues to stimulate cocaine-seeking behavior in rats.

5.1.3 Benzodiazepines

In other experiments (Goeders, Clampitt, Keller, Sharma, & Guerin, 2009), we investigated the effects of oxazepam or alprazolam on the cue-induced reinstatement of extinguished cocaine seeking. Control rats responded at higher rates during reinstatement testing when compared to the last day of extinction. In contrast, the behavior of rats pretreated with alprazolam did not differ from the last day of extinction training. These data suggest that benzodiazepine therapy may be useful in combating craving induced by conditioned cues associated with cocaine use.

6. RATIONALE FOR TESTING DRUG COMBINATIONS

Thus far, we have shown that benzodiazepine receptor agonists, CRF receptor antagonists, and corticosterone synthesis inhibitors reduce cocaine self-administration. As noted earlier, at the time of this writing, there were no CRF receptor antagonists available for use in humans. Therefore, we decided to focus our efforts on benzodiazepines, corticosterone synthesis inhibitors, and drugs affecting γ-aminobutyric acid (GABA) receptors. Of concern however was the fact that both benzodiazepines and corticosterone synthesis inhibitors have potential side effects that could limit their usefulness in the treatment of cocaine addiction. For example, benzodiazepines are not usually recommended as the treatment of choice for cocaine dependence since these drugs have the potential for abuse (Chouinard, 2004; Lilja, Larsson, Skinhoj, & Hamilton, 2001; O'Brien, 2005), worrying some that the use of these drugs might result in a secondary dependence (Wesson & Smith, 1985). Corticosterone synthesis inhibitors have the potential to produce adrenal insufficiency, among other things, which could also limit the utility of this class of drugs. However, the incidence of side effects produced by these two classes of drugs may be mitigated by reducing the dose, which is the basis for the design of the following experiments. Our hypothesis was that by combining drugs that affect HPA axis activity through divergent mechanisms and delivering these drugs at concentrations that have no effect when administered alone, we would minimize their potential toxic and unwanted side effects while still reducing cocaine intake. Rats were tested with various combinations of these drugs while responding under a multiple, alternating schedule of cocaine and food self-administration (Goeders & Guerin, 2008). The rats were tested with various doses of these drugs until the minimally effective dose that reduced cocaine self-administration without affecting food-maintained responding during the same session was identified for each compound. This was selected as the "effective" dose of the drug. The dose was then reduced until we observed no effects on cocaine self-administration or food-maintained responding, and this was the "ineffective" dose selected for subsequent drug combination experiments. We evaluated combinations of drugs from three different classes: (1) corticosterone synthesis inhibitors, (2) CRF receptor antagonists, and (3) benzodiazepines and other drugs affecting GABAergic neurotransmission. We have previously found that drugs from each of these three classes reduce cocaine self-administration, and each has a unique action on physiological responses to stressors. Therefore, there was every reason to believe that these drugs might produce an additive effect when administered in combination.

6.1. Drug combinations tested

We tested combinations of the various drugs against three doses of self-administered cocaine (i.e., 0.125, 0.25 [our standard dose], and 0.5 mg/kg/infusion). We tested the $GABA_A$ receptor agonist muscimol (1–4 mg/kg, IP), the benzodiazepines and $GABA_A$ receptor agonists oxazepam (5–40 mg/kg, IP) and alprazolam (1–4 mg/kg, IP), the corticosterone synthesis inhibitors metyrapone (50–150 mg/kg, IP) and ketoconazole (25–150 mg/kg, IP), and the CRF receptor antagonist CP-154,526 (20–80 mg/kg, IP). The various combinations that we tested included CP-154,526 and oxazepam, ketoconazole and oxazepam, metyrapone and oxazepam, alprazolam and ketoconazole, CP-154,526 and ketoconazole, CP-154,526 and muscimol, muscimol and metyrapone, and metyrapone and oxazepam. Each of these combinations was effective to some degree in reducing cocaine self-administration without affecting food-maintained responding.

6.1.1 Why metyrapone and oxazepam were selected

We ultimately decided to focus our research on the metyrapone and oxazepam combination for several reasons. First, muscimol was only effective within a very narrow dose range, and we also observed significant variability among the rats in their responses to muscimol. Since the benzodiazepines oxazepam and alprazolam were also effective in reducing cocaine self-administration, did so more reliably than muscimol, and are widely used clinically (Baldessarini, 1996), we determined that benzodiazepines would be more useful than muscimol as a GABA$_A$ receptor agonist (Kostowski, 1995; Luddens & Korpi, 1995; Oreland, 1988) in a combination product. Although CP-154,526 was effective in reducing cocaine self-administration alone and in combination with GABA$_A$ receptor agonists and corticosterone synthesis inhibitors, there are no CRF receptor antagonists currently approved for human use, thus limiting the possible utility of this class of drugs in a combination formulation. However, our data with CP-154,526 do indicate a significant involvement of CRF in cocaine taking and cocaine seeking, suggesting that future combinations might contain a CRF receptor antagonist if one is identified as safe and effective in humans. Metyrapone and ketoconazole were each effective in reducing cocaine self-administration both alone and in combination with GABA$_A$ receptor agonists and CRF receptor antagonists. Ketoconazole, in addition to its previously stated effects, is also a cytochrome P450 inhibitor (Venkatakrishnan et al., 2009) that has significant side effects including hepatotoxicity (Van Cauteren et al., 1989, 1990) and significant drug interactions with a variety of drugs including benzodiazepines (Venkatakrishnan et al., 2009). These side effects limit the usefulness of ketoconazole in a combination formulation. Metyrapone does not produce the side effects observed with ketoconazole (Haleem et al., 1988; Haynes, 1990), does not interfere with the metabolism of benzodiazepines, and has been used clinically for a relatively long period of time, suggesting that metyrapone is superior to ketoconazole for use in a combination product. Alprazolam and oxazepam were each effective in reducing cocaine self-administration alone and in combination with corticosterone synthesis inhibitors and CRF receptor antagonists. However, alprazolam also has a relatively significant potential for abuse. Oxazepam has been reported to be much less preferred by methadone-maintained opiate addicts when compared to other benzodiazepines such as alprazolam or diazepam (Griffiths & Johnson, 2005; Iguchi, Handelsman, Bickel, & Griffiths, 1993), suggesting that oxazepam is less rewarding than alprazolam. The overall design of these experiments was to test these drugs on intravenous cocaine self-administration and cocaine-seeking behavior in combination at doses that produced no measurable effects when they were tested separately. If such combinations reduced cocaine self-administration and cocaine seeking, this would suggest that they were producing an additive effect on cocaine reward. Accordingly, novel pharmacotherapies could be designed using such combinations of these drugs that would reduce cocaine craving and cocaine use with a significantly reduced risk of side effects.

6.2. Effects of metyrapone and oxazepam on cocaine self-administration

Adult male Wistar rats were trained to self-administer cocaine and food under a multiple alternating schedule of reinforcement (Goeders & Guerin, 2008). Three doses of cocaine (0.125, 0.25, or 0.5 mg/kg/infusion) were tested. Rats were also periodically trained with saline substitution (cocaine extinction) and food extinction during the same session. We have studied extinction behavior in detail (Peltier et al., 2001) and have found that erroneous conclusions can sometimes be drawn from drug pretreatment data if extinction has not been sufficiently trained. Once consistent and reproducible behavior during self-administration and extinction was obtained, the animals received vehicle (5% Emulphor in 0.9% saline) pretreatment 30 min before the start of the behavioral session to establish baseline behaviors. Then, the "effective" and "ineffective" doses of metyrapone and oxazepam were individually determined for each rat. The "effective" dose of each drug was the dose that reduced cocaine-maintained responding by at least 50% without affecting responding on the food-associated lever. The "ineffective" dose was that dose that reduced cocaine-maintained responding by less than 10%. These doses were individually determined to ensure that each drug combination consisted of an ineffective dose of each drug for each rat. The effective and ineffective doses were determined for one drug (either metyrapone or oxazepam) before the doses for the second drug were identified, and the drug that was tested first was randomly divided among the rats. The rats only received pretreatments with oxazepam or metyrapone when the baselines for cocaine and food self-administration were stable, and at least two sessions elapsed between each pretreatment. The rats were initially pretreated with either vehicle or a dose of metyrapone or oxazepam that had been shown in previous and pilot studies to be an effective dose in most rats (i.e., 10 mg/kg oxazepam or 50 mg/kg metyrapone). If cocaine self-administration was not reduced by at least

50% without affecting food-maintained responding, the dose was increased (e.g., to 20 mg/kg oxazepam or 100 mg/kg metyrapone) for the next pretreatment. The dose continued to be increased in this way until the effective dose of each drug was identified for each rat. The dose of each drug was then incrementally reduced in the same manner until cocaine intake was altered by less than 10%. When the "effective" and "ineffective" doses for each drug were identified, combination pharmacotherapy testing began. During this phase of the experiment, rats were pretreated with a combination of the individually determined "ineffective" doses of metyrapone and oxazepam. Stable baselines of responding were required between tests. Once combination testing during cocaine self-administration at the 0.25-mg/kg/infusion dose was completed, the dose of cocaine was increased to 0.5 mg/kg/infusion or decreased to 0.125 mg/kg/infusion, and self-administration was allowed to stabilize at the new cocaine dose. Vehicle and extinction probes were conducted at each dose. Once self-administration and extinction met the criteria described earlier, the rats were tested with the same individually determined dose combinations of metyrapone and oxazepam that were tested when 0.25 mg/kg/infusion was the cocaine dose self-administered. Following these tests, the third dose of cocaine was made available for self-administration and the same combinations of metyrapone and oxazepam were tested as described earlier. The decision to initially increase or decrease the cocaine dose was randomly determined for each rat. Responding on the cocaine lever was significantly reduced during cocaine extinction and following pretreatment with the high doses of metyrapone and oxazepam compared to pretreatment with vehicle. In contrast, the effects of pretreatment with the ineffective doses of metyrapone and oxazepam were no different from pretreatment with vehicle. However, pretreatment with a combination of the ineffective doses of metyrapone and oxazepam significantly reduced cocaine self-administration compared to pretreatment with vehicle and was not significantly different from responding observed during extinction. The number of infusions delivered during each of the four 15 min self-administration bins per session following pretreatment with the combination of oxazepam and metyrapone was also significantly decreased compared to vehicle pretreatment. In addition, there were no differences in the number of infusions among the four bins for each treatment condition, indicating that the combination reduced cocaine seeking throughout the behavioral sessions. The combination of oxazepam and metyrapone had no significant effect on food-maintained responding. Similar effects on self-administration were observed when the cocaine unit dose was either increased or decreased. We also measured plasma corticosterone following pretreatment with the combination of metyrapone and oxazepam, and surprisingly we saw no significant effects of these combinations on corticosterone, suggesting that the effects of combinations of metyrapone and oxazepam may be mediated via sites other than the adrenal gland. Finally, we investigated the pharmacokinetics of pretreatment with the combination of metyrapone and oxazepam on cocaine self-administration (Goeders & Guerin, 2008). We measured cocaine and its metabolites ecgonine methyl ester and benzoylecgonine, metyrapone and its metabolite metyrapol, and oxazepam using GC/MS, but the only effects that we saw were minor and unrelated to the effects of the combination on cocaine self-administration.

6.3. Effects of metyrapone and oxazepam on cocaine and methamphetamine cue reactivity

We also investigated the effects of the combination of metyrapone and oxazepam on cue reactivity, a variation of the reinstatement protocol that does not include extinguishing lever pressing (Buffalari, Feltenstein, & See, 2013). We investigated both cocaine and methamphetamine cue reactivity in these experiments (Keller, Cornett, Guerin, & Goeders, 2013). Adult male Wistar rats were trained to self-administer cocaine (0.25 mg/kg/infusion) or methamphetamine (0.06 mg/kg/infusion) under a FR4 schedule of reinforcement. Each completion of the response requirement resulted in an intravenous infusion of drug and the concurrent presentation of a house light and a tone compound stimulus. Once stable drug self-administration was observed for a minimum of 10 days, the rats were placed into abstinence whereby they remained in their home cages for 14 days, and then cue-reactivity testing commenced. The rats were placed into the experimental chambers, both levers were extended and the active stimulus light was illuminated as during self-administration training. During cue-reactivity testing, responding on the active lever resulted in a 5.6-s presentation of the conditioned reinforcer (i.e., the house light and tone compound stimulus previously paired with cocaine or methamphetamine delivery), but no drug was delivered. In the acute experiment, rats were tested with a combination of metyrapone (25–50 mg/kg, IP) and oxazepam (5–10 mg/kg, IP) or vehicle (5% Emulphor in 0.9% saline) 30 min before the start of the behavioral session. In the chronic study, rats were pretreated with vehicle or the same combination of metyrapone and oxazepam (50 mg/kg metyrapone and 10 mg/kg oxazepam, IP) daily for 14 days while in their home cages during abstinence. On the cue-reactivity test day, the rats were treated with the combination 30 min before the start of the test session. The acute combination of metyrapone and oxazepam resulted in dose-related decreases in both methamphetamine and cocaine cue reactivity. Importantly, this reduction in drug seeking was maintained following 2 weeks of chronic administration, suggesting that tolerance does not rapidly develop to the effects of the combination of metyrapone and oxazepam on drug seeking in rats.

6.4. Effects of metyrapone and oxazepam on nicotine self-administration

In one final example, we also tested the combination of metyrapone and oxazepam on nicotine self-administration in rats. Rats were trained to self-administer nicotine (0.03 mg/kg/infusion, IV). When stable baselines of nicotine self-administration were obtained, the rats were pretreated with vehicle and various dose combinations of metyrapone and oxazepam 30 min before the start of the behavioral session. Pretreatment with the combination of metyrapone and oxazepam resulted in dose-related decreases in nicotine self-administration (Goeders et al., 2012), with an efficacy comparable to varenicline, a partial agonist selective for the alpha4beta2 acetylcholine-receptor subtype (Hays & Ebbert, 2008; Hays, Ebbert, & Sood, 2008; Jorenby et al., 2006; Potts & Garwood, 2007; Zierler-Brown & Kyle, 2007) that has become the first-line pharmacotherapy for nicotine dependence.

6.5. Effects of metyrapone and oxazepam in the elevated plus maze

The hypothesis guiding the design of the experiments testing the combination of metyrapone and oxazepam is that drugs or combinations of drugs that affect the body's responses to stressors will alter drug-taking and drug-seeking behaviors. We have demonstrated that the combination of oxazepam and metyrapone is effective in reducing cocaine taking and seeking both in rats (Goeders & Guerin, 2008) and in humans in our pilot clinical trial (Kablinger et al., 2012), but it was important to demonstrate that the combination was effective in reducing stress or anxiety-like behaviors if our hypothesis was accurate. Therefore, we tested this drug combination in male Wistar rats using the elevated plus maze (Pellow, Chopin, File, & Briley, 1985; Pellow & File, 1986). The elevated plus-maze apparatus consists of a wooden structure including two open arms and two enclosed arms (Goeders & Goeders, 2004). Both open and enclosed arms, measuring

50×10 cm, were arranged opposite the arm of same type forming a "plus" shape. A 40-cm high perimeter wall surrounded the two enclosed arms. The arms were connected by a central square measuring 10×10 cm. The plus maze was mounted on a wooden base that elevated the apparatus 50 cm above the floor. The maze was situated in a room lit by a dim, red light. Each drug combination (5–10 mg/kg oxazepam and 25–50 mg/kg metyrapone, IP) was tested acutely and chronically. For the acute experiment, rats were treated with one of the dose combinations or vehicle 30 min before being placed in the center of the maze. In the chronic experiment, rats received daily injections of one of the dose combinations or vehicle (5% Emulphor in 0.9% saline) in their individual home cages. On the 15th day, the rats were treated with the same dose combination or vehicle 30 min before being placed in the center of the elevated plus maze. The chronic administration of all dose combinations was effective in increasing the time spent in the open arms of the plus maze, indicating an anxiolytic effect. Most combinations were also effective acutely, except for the highest dose tested, which was likely the result of a decrease in locomotor activity, and tolerance rapidly developed to this motor effect with chronic administration. The results of this experiment demonstrate that the combination of metyrapone and oxazepam, even at relatively low doses, is effective in reducing anxiety-like behaviors in the elevated plus maze.

7. OUR HYPOTHESIS CHANGES

Over the past 25–30 years, research in our laboratory has been driven by the hypothesis that reducing activity within the HPA axis will decrease drug taking and drug seeking, and we have generated a variety of data supporting this hypothesis (reported above). However, we have recently collected compelling data that have forced us to rethink this hypothesis. Thus, while stress is certainly involved in the etiology of drug addiction and relapse, the biology of this phenomenon is more likely to involve extra-adrenal mechanisms.

7.1. Metyrapone and oxazepam attenuate cocaine self-administration in adrenalectomized rats

One unexpected finding that we made was that the combination of metyrapone and oxazepam was still effective in reducing cocaine self-administration in adrenalectomized rats. In these experiments, adult male Wistar rats were trained to self-administer cocaine (0.25 mg/kg/infusion) under a FR4 schedule of reinforcement. Once responding stabilized under this schedule, the rats received a bilateral adrenalectomy or sham surgery. Following recovery from surgery, the rats were allowed to self-administer cocaine for another 3 weeks. In contrast to what we have observed during the acquisition of cocaine self-administration (Goeders & Guerin, 1996a), where adrenalectomy prevented the acquisition of cocaine self-administration, adrenalectomy had little or no effect on cocaine self-administration once this behavior was established. Self-administration was maintained at a lower rate following adrenalectomy but was remarkably stable. These data suggest that while adrenal-derived corticosterone is critically important for the acquisition of cocaine self-administration, it is not necessary for the maintenance of this behavior. Perhaps the cocaine-induced release of corticosterone produces effects within the central nervous system that are important for cocaine reward, and once these effects are produced, adrenal-derived corticosterone is no longer necessary for continued cocaine self-administration. In addition, we conducted an experiment to assess the efficacy of the combination of metyrapone and oxazepam in a separate group of adrenalectomized rats. Contrary to our initial hypotheses, the combination treatment was still effective in reducing cocaine self-administration when the adrenalectomized rats were tested with various doses. In fact, the reduction in cocaine self-administration following administration of the combination was augmented in adrenalectomized rats compared to presurgery behaviors. This observation suggests that removal of the adrenal gland enhanced the effects of metyrapone and oxazepam. The mechanisms mediating these unexpected findings are unclear at this time, but these results are likely mediated, at least in part, through effects on 11β-hydroxylase. It has been shown that CYP11B1 expression is increased in the hippocampus and hypothalamus following adrenalectomy (Ye et al., 2008). Increased ACTH, also a resultant effect of reduced corticosterone mediated through negative feedback mechanisms, also increases CYP11B1 mRNA in the hypothalamus and cerebral cortex (Ye et al., 2008). Thus, the augmentation of the effects of metyrapone, oxazepam, and their combination on cocaine self-administration in adrenalectomized rats may be related to the resultant increase in 11β-hydroxylase in the brain. Interestingly, adrenalectomy has also been shown to increase benzodiazepine receptors in discrete regions of the rat brain (De Souza, Goeders, & Kuhar, 1986; Goeders, De Souza, & Kuhar, 1986; Miller, Greenblatt, Barnhill, Thompson, & Shaderh, 1988). Such increases in the number of benzodiazepine receptors may also modulate the increased effects of oxazepam on cocaine self-administration in adrenalectomized rats.

7.2. Brain-derived corticosterone

How does the concept of brain-derived corticosterone enter the picture? It is well known that metyrapone inhibits the activity of 11β-hydroxylase (Haleem et al., 1988; Haynes, 1990), which is encoded by the CYP11B1 gene, resulting in a decrease in plasma corticosterone (in rats) or cortisol (in humans). Benzodiazepines have also been demonstrated to inhibit 11β-hydroxylase under certain conditions (Thomson, Fraser, & Kenyon, 1995). However, while the adrenal gland is the primary target for metyrapone's actions (Temple & Liddle, 1970), increasing evidence suggests that CYP11B1 is found in other tissues (Baulieu & Robel, 1990; Stromstedt & Waterman, 1995), including the brain (MacKenzie, Clark, Fraser, et al., 2000). In fact, data from several sources demonstrate that the brain is a major site of extra-adrenal corticosteroid production (Gomez-Sanchez et al., 1996; MacKenzie, Clark, Fraser, et al., 2000; Ye et al., 2008) since corticosterone can be synthesized *de novo* from cholesterol in the brain (Gomez-Sanchez et al., 1996, 1997; MacKenzie, Clark, Fraser, et al., 2000; MacKenzie, Clark, Ingram, et al., 2000). The highest levels of CYP11B1 are found in the cortex and brain stem, although all regions in the brain express this gene (Ye et al., 2008). These data argue for a biological role for 11β-hydroxylase activity within the brain. Thus, the effects of the combination of metyrapone and oxazepam on cocaine self-administration may be mediated via effects on 11β-hydroxylase in specific brain regions, especially in adrenalectomized rats.

P45011β is the rate-limiting step of corticosterone synthesis and converts deoxycorticosterone into corticosterone. This enzyme is present in the adrenal glands (main site of corticosterone biosynthesis) and the brain, demonstrating that corticosterone can be synthesized in the periphery and CNS (Gomez-Sanchez et al., 1996; MacKenzie, Clark, Fraser, et al., 2000; Ye et al., 2008). The decrease in corticosterone synthesis is readily apparent at higher doses of metyrapone but may not be responsible for its behavioral actions against cocaine-related behavior (Goeders & Guerin, 2008). Furthermore, in addition to the inhibition of 11β-hydroxylase activity (Haleem et al., 1988; Haynes, 1990), metyrapone also decreases corticosterone levels via an inhibition of the reductase activity of 11β-hydroxysteroid dehydrogenase (11β-HSD1; Raven, Checkley, & Taylor, 1995; Sampath-Kumar, Yu, Khalil, & Yang, 1997). 11β-HSD is a tissue-specific regulator of local corticosterone concentrations, which interconverts inactive 11-dehydrocorticosterone and active corticosterone (Monder, Lakshmi, & Miroff, 1991). It is present in many target tissues of glucocorticoids including brain, liver, and adipose tissue. The 11β-HSD enzyme has two isoforms that catalyze the activation (reduction via 11β-HSD1) or inactivation (oxidation via 11β-HSD2) of cortisol and corticosterone (Edwards, Benediktsson, Lindsay, & Seckl, 1996). Inhibiting 11β-HSD1 activity prevents any inert 11-keto steroids from being reactivated to active steroids in these tissues, thereby decreasing glucocorticoid-induced effects (Holmes, Yau, Kotelevtsev, Mullins, & Seckl, 2003). Metyrapone has been shown to be a selective inhibitor of the 11β-HSD1 isoform and can modulate local tissue levels of corticosterone via this mechanism (Raven et al., 1995; Sampath-Kumar et al., 1997). This mechanism may also contribute to metyrapone's increased potency in adrenalectomized animals.

7.3. Neuroactive steroids

Although P45011-β inhibition is thought of as the straightforward mode of action for metyrapone, the consequences of this activity are complex. The inhibition of 11β-hydroxylase activity by metyrapone can also increase the upstream precursors of corticosterone such as progesterone and deoxycorticosterone. In this way, metyrapone has been shown to shift steroidogenesis toward the formation of $GABA_A$-active inhibitory neurosteroids such as tetrahydrodeoxycorticosterone (THDOC) and allopregnanolone (ALLO; Jain, Khan, Krishna, & Subhedar, 1994; Raven, O'Dwyer, Taylor, & Checkley, 1996; Rupprecht et al., 1998). Neurosteroids are defined as those steroids that are both synthesized in the nervous system, de novo either from cholesterol or from steroid hormone precursors, and that accumulate in the nervous system independently of peripheral steroid gland secretion rates (Baulieu & Robel, 1990; Robel & Baulieu, 1995). All steroid derivatives are produced from the cholesterol backbone (Robel & Baulieu, 1995), and in contrast to classical endocrine-derived steroids, neuroactive steroids influence membrane-bound receptors and have little to no direct genomic action (Wehling, 1997). This allows the neurosteroids to exert rapid effects, mainly through ligand-gated ion channels, on a number of neurotransmitter receptors including $GABA_A$ receptors (Barbaccia, Serra, Purdy, & Biggio, 2001; Paul & Purdy, 1992; Purdy, Moore, Morrow, & Paul, 1992), where they bind with a high affinity and positively modulate the action of GABA at these receptors, thereby producing anticonvulsant, antidepressant, and anxiolytic effects (Belelli & Lambert, 2005; Lambert, Belelli, Peden, Vardy, & Peters, 2003). As their name implies, neuroactive steroids are derivatives of the steroid biosynthetic pathway, as a branch product of progesterone or deoxycorticosterone (Robel & Baulieu,

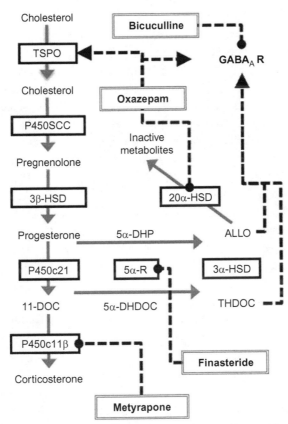

Figure 11.1 Neurosteroid biosynthesis pathway and interactions with relevant drugs. GABA-active neurosteroids are derived from progesterone and deoxycorticosterone (11-DOC) by sequential reactions with α-reductase (5α-R) and 3α-hydroxysteroid dehydrogenase (3α-HSD). Metyrapone inhibits β-hydroxylase (P450c11β) to decrease corticosterone production and increase neurosteroid synthesis. Oxazepam activates the translocator protein of 18kDa (TSPO) and GABA$_A$ receptors and inhibits 20α-hydroxysteroid dehydrogenase to increase neurosteroids and neuronal inhibition. Bicuculline and finasteride prevent metyrapone-induced neurosteroids from affecting GABA$_A$ receptors. Enzymes are styled as boxed capital letters. Important experimental ligands are styled as boxed lowercase letters. Dotted lines indicate the interactions with relevant targets with arrows representing activation and circles representing inhibition.

1995). Figure 11.1 outlines the neurosteroid biosynthesis pathway in a simplified manner and identifies the interactions of related ligands with the pathway. In the brain, progesterone is converted to 5α-dihydroprogesterone by 5α-reductase, which is then converted to the GABA-active ALLO by 3α-hydroxysteroid dehydrogenase in the cytoplasm (Barbaccia et al., 2001). Deoxycorticosterone can also be converted into THDOC by the sequential actions of 5α-reductase and 3α-hydroxysteroid dehydrogenase (Barbaccia et al., 2001). These structural changes convey activity at $GABA_A$ receptors while decreasing activity at nuclear receptors (Agis-Balboa et al., 2006). When 11β-hydroxylase activity is blocked by metyrapone or other substances, the conversion of cholesterol is shifted from corticosterone production to the synthesis of neurosteroids such as ALLO and THDOC (Hirani, Sharma, Jain, Ugale, & Chopde, 2005; Ugale, Mittal, Hirani, & Chopde, 2004; Ugale et al., 2007). Via this indirect mechanism, metyrapone can influence $GABA_A$-mediated phenomena such as alcohol withdrawal, anticonvulsant effects, and anxiety-like behavior (Dhir & Rogawski, 2012; Hirani et al., 2005; Kaminski & Rogawski, 2011; Ugale et al., 2004, 2007). This may have implications for the treatment of drug addiction since neurosteroids such as dehydroepiandrosterone (Doron et al., 2006; Maayan et al., 2006) and ALLO (Anker & Carroll, 2010a, 2010b; Anker, Holtz, Zlebnik, & Carroll, 2009; Anker, Zlebnik, & Carroll, 2010) have been reported to decrease cocaine seeking and cocaine taking in rats. Data from our lab (detailed in the succeeding text) show that finasteride, which inhibits the final step of neurosteroid biosynthesis (Steiner, 1993; Sudduth & Koronkowski, 1993), and bicuculline, a $GABA_A$ receptor antagonist (Chebib & Johnston, 1999), can partially block metyrapone-induced decreases in cocaine self-administration.

In the first experiment, we investigated the effects of bicuculline (Johnston, 1992; Sanger, 1985) on the effects of metyrapone and oxazepam on cocaine self-administration. In this experiment, adult male Wistar rats were trained to self-administer cocaine. When responding stabilized, rats were pretreated with a high dose of metyrapone (or oxazepam) and allowed to self-administer cocaine. Pretreatment with either drug virtually eliminated cocaine-taking behavior. Pretreatment with bicuculline (5 mg/kg, IP) 15 min before the injection of oxazepam or metyrapone reversed the effects of both drugs. Since oxazepam is known to bind to the benzodiazepine binding site on the $GABA_A$ receptor (Bergman, 1986; Martin, 1987; Soderpalm, 1987), it was not surprising that bicuculline attenuated the effects of this benzodiazepine receptor agonist. However, bicuculline also partially reversed the effects of metyrapone, suggesting that the actions of metyrapone were also mediated, at least in part, through $GABA_A$ receptors, and that these effects might be mediated through neuroactive steroids since these compounds also bind to the $GABA_A$ receptor (Baulieu, 1991, 1997; Lambert, Belelli, Hill-Venning, Callachan, & Peters, 1996; Lambert et al., 2003). In the second experiment, we investigated the effects of finasteride, a 5α-reductase inhibitor (Darbra & Pallares, 2010; Gorin,

Crabbe, Tanchuck, Long, & Finn, 2005; Mukai, Higashi, Nagura, & Shimada, 2008). Since 5α-reductase is the rate-limiting step in the synthesis of neurosteroids, an inhibition of the activity of this enzyme will reduce the brain concentrations of these compounds (Mukai et al., 2008). In this experiment, adult male Wistar rats were trained to self-administer cocaine. When responding stabilized, rats were pretreated with metyrapone with or without pretreatment with finasteride (50 mg/kg, IP; two injections 24 h apart). Finasteride partially reversed the effects of metyrapone, again suggesting that metyrapone reduces cocaine taking, at least in part, through the action of neuroactive steroids.

And as noted earlier, the combination of oxazepam and metyrapone has significant anxiolytic actions in the elevated plus-maze model, possibly through direct or indirect actions at the GABA$_A$ receptor. The involvement of neurosteroids in metyrapone's actions may also have implications for cocaine-dependent subjects who also have a mood disorder. Drug-dependent subjects who also experience a significant psychiatric event (e.g., panic attack and major depressive episode) are over twice as likely to have used cocaine in the past year (Kelley et al., 2012). Clinical researchers suggest that treatment of both cocaine dependence and mood disorders concurrently would result in the best outcome for the dually diagnosed individual (Extein & Gold, 1993; Rounsaville, 2004). Numerous studies have demonstrated that neurosteroids possess potent anxiolytic and antidepressant actions in both rodents and humans (Czlonkowska et al., 2003; Dubrovsky, 2005; Longone et al., 2008; Pinna & Rasmusson, 2012; Spivak et al., 2000; Zorumski, Paul, Izumi, Covey, & Mennerick, 2013). Using ALLO or THDOC to treat both cocaine dependence and codiagnosed mood disorders may provide extra efficacy to reduce relapse and psychiatric symptoms.

7.4. Oxazepam and the translocator protein

The involvement of neurosteroids and GABA$_A$ receptors in metyrapone's actions has also prompted us to explore the importance of neurosteroidogenesis in the actions of oxazepam, a weak benzodiazepine. Oxazepam increases inhibitory conductance and decreases neuronal excitability by binding to the GABA$_A$ receptor at the benzodiazepine-positive allosteric modulatory site (Lelas, Rowlett, & Spealman, 2001; Maksay, Tegyey, & Simonyi, 1991). By increasing the affinity of GABA for the receptor, benzodiazepines increase the frequency of channel opening and facilitate the influx of chloride ions resulting in a hyperpolarization of the membrane and decreased action potential propagation. This classical mechanism of action applies to nearly all benzodiazepines, including oxazepam.

In addition to binding to the $GABA_A$ receptor, oxazepam may also increase $GABA_A$-active inhibitory neurosteroids by several mechanisms to facilitate inhibitory neurotransmission. Many benzodiazepines bind to both the $GABA_A$ receptor and the translocator protein of 18kDa (TSPO, formerly called the peripheral benzodiazepine receptor; Groh & Muller, 1985; Papadopoulos et al., 2006; Spero, 1985; Wang, Taniguchi, & Spector, 1984). TSPO is responsible for catalyzing the first steps of steroidogenesis by translocating cholesterol from the cytoplasm into the mitochondrial matrix. This allows side-chain cleavage by P450scc to convert cholesterol to pregnenolone, the first enzymatic conversion in the steroid biosynthesis cascade (Mukhin, Papadopoulos, Costa, & Krueger, 1989; Papadopoulos, Berkovich, & Krueger, 1991; Romeo et al., 1993). The structural requirements for benzodiazepines that bind the TSPO strongly suggest that oxazepam may fall into this class (Wang et al., 1984). Supporting this, in vitro homogenate binding assays performed in our laboratory with diazepam, alprazolam, and oxazepam confirm the dual affinity of oxazepam for the $GABA_A$ receptor and TSPO. In this assay, oxazepam and diazepam bound with similar affinity to both $GABA_A$ receptors and TSPO, while alprazolam exhibited negligible TSPO binding and strong $GABA_A$ binding. New evidence demonstrates that selective TSPO agonists have anxiolytic properties without the common side effects of benzodiazepines such as dependence, tolerance, and withdrawal (Nothdurfter et al., 2012; Rupprecht et al., 2010, 2009). It has been recently demonstrated that the anxiolytic effects of oxazepam in the elevated plus maze can be attenuated by PK11195 (a TSPO antagonist) (Trapani, Palazzo, de Candia, Lasorsa, & Trapani, 2013) and flumazenil (a $GABA_A$ receptor antagonist) (Amrein, Leishman, Bentzinger, & Roncari, 1987; File & Pellow, 1986), signifying that the behavioral effects of oxazepam may be due to these two distinct mechanisms: direct binding to the $GABA_A$ receptor and indirect $GABA_A$-mediated inhibition via TSPO-induced increases in $GABA_A$-active neurosteroids. These behavioral actions were confirmed with midazolam, a benzodiazepine with known affinity for TSPO (Dhir & Rogawski, 2012; Joo et al., 2009; Tokuda, O'Dell, Izumi, & Zorumski, 2010). The binding properties of oxazepam may also explain the differences between it and alprazolam (a benzodiazepine with negligible TSPO binding) in behavioral and neuroendocrine assays.

Griffiths and colleagues have systematically studied the abuse liabilities of multiple benzodiazepine drugs. Their findings indicate that oxazepam is one of the least desirable benzodiazepines for drug-dependent individuals (Griffiths, McLeod, Bigelow, Liebson, & Roache, 1984; Griffiths & Weerts, 1997; Iguchi et al., 1993). In contrast, alprazolam is consistently related as one of the most-abused benzodiazepines (Griffiths & Wolf, 1990; Sellers et al., 1993; Wolf & Griffiths, 1991). This difference between oxazepam and alprazolam is one of the major reasons we have focused on oxazepam in treating dependent subjects. Griffiths attributes the difference in abuse liability between these two drugs to the longer time of onset of oxazepam's euphoric effects. However, it is possible that these differences are also due to GABA$_A$ versus TSPO binding (Mumford, Evans, Fleishaker, & Griffiths, 1995).

In addition to activating TSPO and increasing neurosteroidogenesis, benzodiazepines also inhibit the enzyme responsible for the inactivation of GABA$_A$-active neurosteroids. Much like the role of 11β-HSD in regulating glucocorticoid activation, 20α-hydroxysteroid dehydrogenase (20α-HSD) converts active ALLO into inert 5alpha-pregnan-3alpha, 20alpha-diol (Brozic, Smuc, Gobec, & Rizner, 2006; Higaki et al., 2003). Several benzodiazepines can inhibit this activity to increase active neurosteroids and prolong neuronal inhibition. Although other benzodiazepines such as medazepam and diazepam are more potent, oxazepam has been demonstrated to inhibit 20α-HSD (Usami et al., 2002). These data suggest that along with increasing neurosteroid biosynthesis by TSPO activation, oxazepam prolongs neurosteroid actions by inhibiting the degradation of these compounds.

8. MEDIAL PREFRONTAL CORTEX AND COCAINE

8.1. Clinical data

Data that we have collected over the years have suggested a role for the medial prefrontal cortex in cocaine reinforcement (Goeders & Smith, 1983, 1993) and in the effects of cocaine on benzodiazepine and CRF receptor binding (Goeders, 1991; Goeders, Bell, et al., 1990; Goeders, Bienvenu, et al., 1990). In humans, exposure to cocaine-related cues induces craving and results in changes in blood flow and metabolic activity in the orbitofrontal cortex and the dorsolateral and anterior cingulate cortices (Childress et al., 1999; London, Ernst, Grant, Bonson, & Weinstein, 2000), which loosely correspond to the prefrontal cortex in rats (Ongur & Price, 2000). Increases in glucose metabolism using 18F-fluorodeoxyglucose were observed in the dorsolateral cortex and medial orbitofrontal cortex after the presentation of cues associated with cocaine when compared to neutral cues (Grant et al., 1996). In another study, increases in glucose metabolism were found in the right superior frontal gyrus in the dorsolateral prefrontal cortex and the left lateral orbitofrontal cortex (Bonson et al., 2002). In contrast, glucose metabolism in the left medial prefrontal cortex and the ventromedial frontal pole decreased after the presentation of cocaine-associated cues. Wang and colleagues demonstrated that an interview with the subjects about cocaine use produced increases in metabolism in the orbitofrontal gyrus, but not in the frontal cortex or cingulate gyrus (Wang et al., 1999). Both the anterior cingulate cortex and the dorsolateral prefrontal cortex were activated after the subjects watched a cocaine-related video as measured by blood oxygenation using functional magnetic resonance imaging, fMRI (Maas et al., 1998).

In a more extensive study, the activation of the left dorsolateral cortex and the left anterior cingulate cortex and the left posterior cingulate cortex was also identified using fMRI (Garavan et al., 2000). Finally, cerebral blood flow, measured using 15O-labeled water, increased in the anterior cingulate cortex (Childress et al., 1999; Kilts et al., 2001), but not in the orbitofrontal cortex, in research subjects after internally generated craving (Kilts et al., 2001) or following the presentation of a cocaine-related video (Childress et al., 1999). Taken together, these data highlight the importance of the frontal cortex in cocaine craving in humans, and taken with the preclinical data reviewed earlier, these data further suggest that the prefrontal cortex may mediate the induction of craving resulting from the cue-induced activation of a stress-like physiological response.

8.2. Medial prefrontal cortex corticosterone and cocaine reinforcement

In line with these data, we have conducted a series of experiments designed to measure differences in the neurochemical and neuroendocrine responses to cocaine during response-contingent and response-independent cocaine administration in rats. Male rats were implanted with chronic jugular catheters and microdialysis guide cannulae aimed at the medial prefrontal cortex and were subsequently divided into triads: one rat was selected as the self-administration rat, while the other two rats were designated as the yoked-cocaine and yoked-saline rats, respectively. Self-administration rats were trained to self-administer cocaine, and each infusion was accompanied by an identical simultaneous cocaine infusion to the yoked-cocaine rat and saline to the yoked-saline rat. Once stable self-administration was observed, corticosterone was measured in selected brain regions using *in vivo* microdialysis. Baseline corticosterone in the medial prefrontal cortex was low and stable in all groups prior to the start of the self-administration session and remained stable throughout the entire experiment in the yoked-saline rats, suggesting that the procedure itself was not unduly stressful. Medial prefrontal cortex corticosterone was significantly elevated in the microdialysates from the self-administration rats during cocaine self-administration (269% increases), while corticosterone was increased 553% above baseline in the medial prefrontal cortex of the yoked-cocaine rats (Palamarchouk et al., 2009). Medial prefrontal cortex corticosterone was significantly higher in the yoked-cocaine rats compared to the self-administration rats. We conducted similar experiments in the amygdala and the nucleus accumbens, but we did not detect similar changes in corticosterone in these brain regions. These data suggest that small increases in corticosterone in the medial prefrontal cortex may mediate cocaine reward (e.g., in the self-administration rats), while larger increases are linked to noncontingent infusions and may be indicative of the stress-reducing effects of drug administration contingency, further highlighting the role for this brain region in addiction and suggesting that the medial prefrontal cortex may also serve as an interface between the central nervous system and the HPA axis.

8.3. Medial prefrontal cortex corticosterone and cocaine cue reactivity

We also have preliminary data that indicate that exposure to cocaine-associated cues also alters corticosterone in the medial prefrontal cortex, which is in accord with the human imaging studies reviewed earlier (Childress et al., 1999; Kilts et al., 2001; Maas et al., 1998). Adult male Wistar rats were implanted with chronic jugular catheters and microdialysis guide cannulae aimed at the medial prefrontal cortex. Following recovery from surgery, the rats were randomly divided into two groups: self-administration and yoked-saline. Each completion of the response requirement resulted in an intravenous infusion of cocaine to the self-administration rat, a simultaneous infusion of saline to the yoked-saline rat, and the concurrent presentation of a house light and a tone compound stimulus to both groups of rats. A 20-s time-out period followed each infusion. Lever presses by the yoked-saline rats were counted but produced no programmed consequences at any time. Once responding stabilized under a FR4 schedule of reinforcement, the rats were placed into extinction whereby responding on the "cocaine" lever by the self-administration rats produced no programmed consequences. Extinction training continued until responding decreased to less than 20% of baseline self-administration, at which time the microdialysis procedure was initiated during reinstatement testing. The rats were placed into the experimental chambers, connected to the microdialysis probes, and several 20 min baseline samples were collected. During reinstatement, both levers were extended into the chambers, and the active stimulus light was illuminated as during self-administration training. Responding on the active lever by the self-administration rat resulted in a 5.6-s presentation of the cocaine-associated cues (i.e., a house light and tone compound stimulus that had been paired with the cocaine infusions) to both groups of rats. Baseline corticosterone concentrations in the medial prefrontal cortex were low and stable in both groups prior to the start of the self-administration session. Exposure to the conditioned cues during reinstatement testing resulted in an increase in corticosterone in the medial prefrontal cortex, especially when compared to the yoked–saline rats. These control rats were exposed to the same compound stimulus, but this stimulus had only been paired with saline, never with cocaine. Although these data are preliminary, they do suggest that exposure to cocaine-associated cues increases corticosterone levels in the medial prefrontal cortex. What do these cocaine-induced alterations in brain corticosterone mean, and how do they relate to the effects of the combination of metyrapone and oxazepam? Our evolving hypothesis is that neurosteroids must be involved.

9. NEUROSTEROIDS AND THE COMBINATION OF METYRAPONE AND OXAZEPAM

The involvement of neurosteroids in the actions of both metyrapone and oxazepam provides a plausible mechanism for their additive interaction and efficacy against cocaine-related behaviors. Metyrapone-induced neurosteroids and oxazepam bind to distinct sites on the $GABA_A$ receptor, resulting in positive cooperativity and enhanced chloride influx. Ultimately through increased GABAergic conductance, both drugs may decrease the excitability of brain regions such as the prefrontal cortex or amygdala and decrease the propensity to resume cocaine-seeking behaviors. We have collected exciting new data that supports our new hypothesis.

9.1. Metyrapone and oxazepam and medial prefrontal cortex corticosterone

We have demonstrated that corticosterone in the medial prefrontal cortex is significantly elevated in the microdialysates collected from rats self-administering cocaine, suggesting that cocaine specifically influences corticosterone in this brain region (Palamarchouk et al., 2009). The following experiment was designed to determine the effects of pretreatment with metyrapone and oxazepam on cocaine-induced increases in medial prefrontal cortex corticosterone. Rats were implanted with microdialysis cannulae aimed at the medial prefrontal cortex. Following recovery from surgery, rats were placed into the microdialysis chamber and allowed to acclimate overnight. Dialysate samples were collected over a 5-h period. Baseline samples were collected for 2 h before the rats were injected with vehicle (IP). This was followed by an injection of cocaine (10 mg/kg, IP) 30 min later. Samples were collected for an hour, and subsequently, these same rats were injected with vehicle or the combination of metyrapone (50 mg/kg, IP) and oxazepam (10 mg/kg, IP) followed by another injection of cocaine. Samples were again collected via microdialysis for an hour following the second cocaine injection. Cocaine reliably increased corticosterone in the medial prefrontal cortex, and this increase was blocked by pretreatment with the combination of metyrapone and oxazepam (Fig. 11.2). These data suggest that this drug combination can act centrally to influence brain concentrations of corticosterone that have been increased by cocaine.

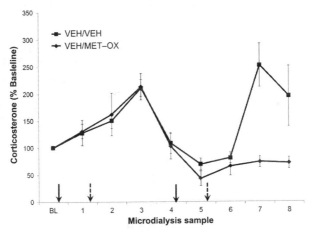

Figure 11.2 The combination of metyrapone and oxazepam (MET–OX) reduces cocaine-induced corticosterone in the medial prefrontal cortex. Rats were implanted with microdialysis probes, and corticosterone was analyzed in the medial prefrontal cortex following cocaine injections and MET–OX pretreatment. The first solid arrow indicates an injection of vehicle, while the second represents either an injection of MET–OX or vehicle. Both dashed arrows represent IP injections of cocaine. Pretreatment with the MET–OX combination decreased corticosterone in this brain region following cocaine injection. $N = 3$–5/group.

9.2. Metyrapone and oxazepam and neurosteroids

When metyrapone blocks the 11β-hydroxylase reaction to inhibit the synthesis of corticosterone, the cholesterol metabolic pathway shifts to produce ALLO and THDOC, which are $GABA_A$-active neurosteroids that produce behavioral effects similar to benzodiazepines. We have shown that ALLO reduces cocaine cue reactivity following forced abstinence but does not affect cocaine self-administration when administered peripherally. The current experiment was designed to measure ALLO and THDOC in the medial prefrontal cortex and amygdala following treatment with the combination of metyrapone and oxazepam in rats self-administering cocaine to determine if the drug combination alters neurosteroid levels in brain areas that are major components of the cocaine reward circuit. Pairs of adult male rats were implanted with chronic indwelling jugular catheters. One of the pair (self-administration) was trained to respond on a FR4 schedule of cocaine reinforcement (0.25 mg/kg/infusion), while the second rat (yoked-saline) only received simultaneous yoked infusions of saline during daily 2 h sessions. Each pair was randomly assigned to one of two groups. One group received vehicle, while the other group received the combination of metyrapone (50 mg/kg, IP) and oxazepam (10 mg/kg, IP). All injections were given 30 min prior to the start of the session. After responding stabilized and a baseline established for each self-administration rat, the pairs were tested three times each, allowing stable responding to return between each test. Thirty minutes after the start of the third test, the rats were sacrificed and the brains rapidly dissected on ice, quick frozen on dry ice, and stored at −80 °C. Neurosteroids were extracted from the brain homogenate and derivatized with hydroxyl amine and their levels measured using an Orbitrap Velos mass spectrometer equipped with a Waters' Acquity UPLC. The combination of metyrapone and oxazepam completely blocked cocaine self-administration during the first 30 min of the behavioral test. The treatment also decreased plasma corticosterone, while corticosterone in the control group increased. ALLO was not different across the four groups in either the medial prefrontal cortex or the amygdala, except for slightly higher values in the cocaine self-administration rats that received metyrapone and oxazepam (Fig. 11.3). THDOC was dramatically higher in the groups receiving metyrapone and oxazepam in both the medial prefrontal cortex and amygdala when compared to vehicle. The animals that self-administered cocaine also had higher levels than those receiving yoked-saline infusions. As expected, the low-dose combination of metyrapone and oxazepam blocked

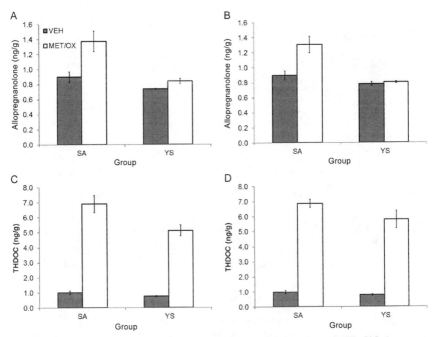

Figure 11.3 The combination of metyrapone and oxazepam (MET–OX) increases GABA-active neurosteroids in the amygdala and medial prefrontal cortex. MET–OX pretreatment significantly increased ALLO (panels A and B) and THDOC (panels C and D) in both the medial prefrontal cortex (panels A and C) and amygdala (panels B and D). This effect was more pronounced in animals self-administering cocaine (SA group) compared to yoked-saline rats (YS group). $N = 3$/group.

cocaine self-administration and partially blocked corticosterone production, which led to increased levels of THDOC, but not ALLO, in two brain areas that are critical parts of both the cocaine reward circuit and the HPA axis stress system. These data are in agreement with the experiment earlier. If metyrapone and oxazepam block the cocaine-induced increase in corticosterone in the medial prefrontal cortex, this would suggest that the metabolism of cholesterol must have been shifted from the production of corticosterone to the synthesis of neuroactive steroids. The increase in THDOC reported here suggests that the combination of metyrapone and oxazepam is doing just as we predicted. Taken together, these data are contributing to our understanding of the mechanisms underlying the effects of the combination of metyrapone and oxazepam on cocaine reinforcement.

10. CONCLUSION

There is a clear relationship between the body's response to stressors and drug addiction. Recovering addicts often claim that their drug use was controllable until they were faced with what they perceived as a stressful life situation. The combination of metyrapone and oxazepam was developed to address this relationship. Our initial hypothesis was that by blocking the ability of conditioned cues or triggers in the environment to activate the HPA axis response to stress, we would reduce the ability of those triggers to promote craving that leads to relapse. We demonstrated that the combination of metyrapone and oxazepam is effective in reducing cocaine and nicotine self-administration in rats, cocaine and methamphetamine cue reactivity in rats, and cocaine craving and cocaine taking in humans. Thus, this drug combination may be effective for treating dependence on a variety of drugs. However, upon further examination, we discovered that a reduction in HPA axis activity is not necessary for the combination of metyrapone and oxazepam to be effective in reducing cocaine reinforcement in rats, suggesting that other mechanisms must be involved. Cocaine also increases corticosterone locally in the brain, and this effect may be independent of the HPA axis. Preliminary data suggest that the peripheral administration of metyrapone and oxazepam attenuates the cocaine-induced increase in corticosterone in the medial prefrontal cortex of the rat brain. Other experiments have shown that the drug combination can also increase levels of neuroactive steroids, especially THDOC, in the medial prefrontal cortex, the same brain region where we saw reductions in brain-derived corticosterone. These data suggest that the combination of metyrapone and oxazepam may reduce cocaine seeking by increasing neuroactive steroid levels in important addiction-related brain areas. Additional research investigating THDOC and other neurosteroids in drug reward and dependence may lead to the development of more effective and novel pharmacotherapies for the treatment of substance abuse.

CONFLICT OF INTEREST

Nicholas Goeders is a founder of Embera NeuroTherapeutics, Inc. He and Glenn Guerin are coinventors on one of the patent applications related to the development of metyrapone and oxazepam for the treatment of addiction, and they receive royalty payments through the license with the LSU Health Sciences Center in Shreveport. Dr. Goeders is also the coinventor on the other Embera patent applications and holds equity interest in the company. Dr. Christopher Schmoutz has no conflicts of interest to declare.

REFERENCES

Agis-Balboa, R. C., Pinna, G., Zhubi, A., Maloku, E., Veldic, M., Costa, E., et al. (2006). Characterization of brain neurons that express enzymes mediating neurosteroid biosynthesis. *Proceedings of the National Academy of Sciences of the United States of America, 103*(39), 14602–14607.

Amrein, R., Leishman, B., Bentzinger, C., & Roncari, G. (1987). Flumazenil in benzodiazepine antagonism. Actions and clinical use in intoxications and anaesthesiology. *Medical Toxicology and Adverse Drug Experience, 2*(6), 411–429.

Anker, J. J., & Carroll, M. E. (2010a). Reinstatement of cocaine seeking induced by drugs, cues, and stress in adolescent and adult rats. *Psychopharmacology, 208*(2), 211–222.

Anker, J. J., & Carroll, M. E. (2010b). Sex differences in the effects of allopregnanolone on yohimbine-induced reinstatement of cocaine seeking in rats. *Drug and Alcohol Dependence, 107*(2–3), 264–267.

Anker, J. J., Holtz, N. A., Zlebnik, N., & Carroll, M. E. (2009). Effects of allopregnanolone on the reinstatement of cocaine-seeking behavior in male and female rats. *Psychopharmacology, 203*(1), 63–72.

Anker, J. J., Zlebnik, N. E., & Carroll, M. E. (2010). Differential effects of allopregnanolone on the escalation of cocaine self-administration and sucrose intake in female rats. *Psychopharmacology, 212*(3), 419–429.

Anthony, J. C., Tien, A. Y., & Petronis, K. R. (1989). Epidemiologic evidence on cocaine use and panic attacks. *American Journal of Epidemiology, 129*(3), 543–549.

Aronson, T. A., & Craig, T. J. (1986). Cocaine precipitation of panic disorder. *The American Journal of Psychiatry, 143*(5), 643–645.

Baldessarini, R. J. (1996). Drugs and the treatment of psychiatric disorders: Psychosis and anxiety. In J. G. Hardman, L. E. Limbird, P. B. Molinoff, R. W. Ruddon, & A. G. Gilman (Eds.), *Goodman & Gilman's the pharmacological basis of therapeutics* (9th ed., pp. 399–430). New York, NY: McGraw-Hill.

Barbaccia, M. L., Serra, M., Purdy, R. H., & Biggio, G. (2001). Stress and neuroactive steroids. *International Review of Neurobiology, 46*, 243–272.

Barrett, A. C., Negus, S. S., Mello, N. K., & Caine, S. B. (2005). Effect of GABA agonists and GABA-A receptor modulators on cocaine- and food-maintained responding and cocaine discrimination in rats. *The Journal of Pharmacology and Experimental Therapeutics, 315*(2), 858–871.

Barros, H. M., & Miczek, K. A. (1996). Withdrawal from oral cocaine in rate: Ultrasonic vocalizations and tactile startle. *Psychopharmacology, 125*(4), 379–384.

Baulieu, E. E. (1991). Neurosteroids: A new function in the brain. *Biology of the Cell, 71*(1–2), 3–10.

Baulieu, E. E. (1997). Neurosteroids: Of the nervous system, by the nervous system, for the nervous system. *Recent Progress in Hormone Research, 52*, 1–32.

Baulieu, E. E., & Robel, P. (1990). Neurosteroids: A new brain function? *The Journal of Steroid Biochemistry and Molecular Biology, 37*(3), 395–403.

Baumann, M. H., Gendron, T. M., Becketts, K. M., Henningfield, J. E., Gorelick, D. A., & Rothman, R. B. (1995). Effects of intravenous cocaine on plasma cortisol and prolactin in human cocaine abusers. *Biological Psychiatry, 38*(11), 751–755.

Belelli, D., & Lambert, J. J. (2005). Neurosteroids: Endogenous regulators of the GABA(A) receptor. *Nature Reviews. Neuroscience, 6*(7), 565–575.

Bergman, S. A. (1986). The benzodiazepine receptor. *Anesthesia Progress, 33*(5), 213–219.

Bonson, K. R., Grant, S. J., Contoreggi, C. S., Links, J. M., Metcalfe, J., Weyl, H. L., et al. (2002). Neural systems and cue-induced cocaine craving. *Neuropsychopharmacology*, *26*(3), 376–386.

Brady, K. T., & Lydiard, R. B. (1992). Bipolar affective disorder and substance abuse. *Journal of Clinical Psychopharmacology*, *12*(1 Suppl.), 17S–22S.

Brozic, P., Smuc, T., Gobec, S., & Rizner, T. L. (2006). Phytoestrogens as inhibitors of the human progesterone metabolizing enzyme AKR1C1. *Molecular and Cellular Endocrinology*, *259*(1–2), 30–42.

Buffalari, D. M., Feltenstein, M. W., & See, R. E. (2013). The effects of varied extinction procedures on contingent cue-induced reinstatement in Sprague-Dawley rats. *Psychopharmacology*, *230*(2), 319–327.

Calogero, A. E., Gallucci, W. T., Kling, M. A., Chrousos, G. P., & Gold, P. W. (1989). Cocaine stimulates rat hypothalamic corticotropin-releasing hormone secretion in vitro. *Brain Research*, *505*(1), 7–11.

Chebib, M., & Johnston, G. A. (1999). The 'ABC' of GABA receptors: A brief review. *Clinical and Experimental Pharmacology & Physiology*, *26*(11), 937–940.

Chesley, S. F., Schatzki, A. D., DeUrrutia, J., Greenblatt, D. J., Shader, R. I., & Miller, L. G. (1990). Cocaine augments peripheral benzodiazepine binding in humans. *The Journal of Clinical Psychiatry*, *51*(10), 404–406.

Childress, A. R., Mozley, P. D., McElgin, W., Fitzgerald, J., Reivich, M., & O'Brien, C. P. (1999). Limbic activation during cue-induced cocaine craving. *The American Journal of Psychiatry*, *156*(1), 11–18.

Chouinard, G. (2004). Issues in the clinical use of benzodiazepines: Potency, withdrawal, and rebound. *The Journal of Clinical Psychiatry*, *65*(Suppl. 5), 7–12.

Costall, B., Kelly, M. E., Naylor, R. J., & Onaivi, E. S. (1989). The actions of nicotine and cocaine in a mouse model of anxiety. *Pharmacology, Biochemistry, and Behavior*, *33*(1), 197–203.

Czlonkowska, A. I., Zienowicz, M., Bidzinski, A., Maciejak, P., Lehner, M., Taracha, E., et al. (2003). The role of neurosteroids in the anxiolytic, antidepressive- and anticonvulsive effects of selective serotonin reuptake inhibitors. *Medical Science Monitor*, *9*(11), RA270–RA275.

Darbra, S., & Pallares, M. (2010). Alterations in neonatal neurosteroids affect exploration during adolescence and prepulse inhibition in adulthood. *Psychoneuroendocrinology*, *35*(4), 525–535.

Deminiere, J. M., Piazza, P. V., Guegan, G., Abrous, N., Maccari, S., Le Moal, M., et al. (1992). Increased locomotor response to novelty and propensity to intravenous amphetamine self-administration in adult offspring of stressed mothers. *Brain Research*, *586*(1), 135–139.

De Souza, E. B., Goeders, N. E., & Kuhar, M. J. (1986). Benzodiazepine receptors in rat brain are altered by adrenalectomy. *Brain Research*, *381*(1), 176–181.

DeVries, A. C., & Pert, A. (1998). Conditioned increases in anxiogenic-like behavior following exposure to contextual stimuli associated with cocaine are mediated by corticotropin-releasing factor. *Psychopharmacology*, *137*(4), 333–340.

de Wit, H., & Stewart, J. (1983). Drug reinstatement of heroin-reinforced responding in the rat. *Psychopharmacology*, *79*(1), 29–31.

Dhir, A., & Rogawski, M. A. (2012). Role of neurosteroids in the anticonvulsant activity of midazolam. *British Journal of Pharmacology*, *165*(8), 2684–2691.

Doron, R., Fridman, L., Gispan-Herman, I., Maayan, R., Weizman, A., & Yadid, G. (2006). DHEA, a neurosteroid, decreases cocaine self-administration and reinstatement of cocaine-seeking behavior in rats. *Neuropsychopharmacology*, *31*(10), 2231–2236.

Dubrovsky, B. O. (2005). Steroids, neuroactive steroids and neurosteroids in psychopathology. *Progress in Neuro-Psychopharmacology & Biological Psychiatry*, *29*(2), 169–192.

Dworkin, S. I., D'Costa, A., Goeders, N. E., & Hoffman, E. (1989). A progressive-ratio schedule for cocaine administration: Effects of cocaine dose and diazepam. *Neuroscience Abstracts, 15*, 802.

Dworkin, S. I., Mirkis, S., & Smith, J. E. (1995). Response-dependent versus response-independent presentation of cocaine: Differences in the lethal effects of the drug. *Psychopharmacology, 117*(3), 262–266.

Edwards, C. R., Benediktsson, R., Lindsay, R. S., & Seckl, J. R. (1996). 11 beta-Hydroxysteroid dehydrogenases: Key enzymes in determining tissue-specific glucocorticoid effects. *Steroids, 61*(4), 263–269.

Engelhardt, D., Dorr, G., Jaspers, C., & Knorr, D. (1985). Ketoconazole blocks cortisol secretion in man by inhibition of adrenal 11 beta-hydroxylase. *Klinische Wochenschrift, 63*(13), 607–612.

Erb, S. (2010). Evaluation of the relationship between anxiety during withdrawal and stress-induced reinstatement of cocaine seeking. *Progress in Neuro-Psychopharmacology & Biological Psychiatry, 34*(5), 798–807.

Erb, S., Shaham, Y., & Stewart, J. (1996). Stress reinstates cocaine-seeking behavior after prolonged extinction and a drug-free period. *Psychopharmacology, 128*(4), 408–412.

Erb, S., Shaham, Y., & Stewart, J. (1998). The role of corticotropin-releasing factor and corticosterone in stress- and cocaine-induced relapse to cocaine seeking in rats. *The Journal of Neuroscience, 18*(14), 5529–5536.

Ettenberg, A., & Geist, T. D. (1991). Animal model for investigating the anxiogenic effects of self-administered cocaine. *Psychopharmacology, 103*(4), 455–461.

Extein, I. L., & Gold, M. S. (1993). Hypothesized neurochemical models for psychiatric syndromes in alcohol and drug dependence. *Journal of Addictive Diseases, 12*(3), 29–43.

Farnsworth, M. G. (1990). Benzodiazepine abuse and dependence: Misconceptions and facts. *The Journal of Family Practice, 31*(4), 393–400.

Ferster, C. B. (2002). Schedules of reinforcement with Skinner. 1970. *Journal of the Experimental Analysis of Behavior, 77*(3), 303–311.

File, S. E., & Pellow, S. (1986). Intrinsic actions of the benzodiazepine receptor antagonist Ro 15-1788. *Psychopharmacology, 88*(1), 1–11.

Fontana, D. J., & Commissaris, R. L. (1989). Effects of cocaine on conflict behavior in the rat. *Life Sciences, 45*(9), 819–827.

Forman, L. J., & Estilow, S. (1988). Cocaine influences beta-endorphin levels and release. *Life Sciences, 43*(4), 309–315.

Fumagalli, F., Moro, F., Caffino, L., Orru, A., Cassina, C., Giannotti, G., et al. (2013). Region-specific effects on BDNF expression after contingent or non-contingent cocaine i.v. self-administration in rats. *The International Journal of Neuropsychopharmacology, 16*(4), 913–918.

Garavan, H., Pankiewicz, J., Bloom, A., Cho, J. K., Sperry, L., Ross, T. J., et al. (2000). Cue-induced cocaine craving: Neuroanatomical specificity for drug users and drug stimuli. *The American Journal of Psychiatry, 157*(11), 1789–1798.

Gawin, F. H. (1986). New uses of antidepressants in cocaine abuse. *Psychosomatics, 27*(11 Suppl.), 24–29.

Gawin, F. H., & Ellinwood, E. H., Jr. (1988). Cocaine and other stimulants. Actions, abuse, and treatment. *The New England Journal of Medicine, 318*(18), 1173–1182.

Gawin, F. H., & Ellinwood, E. H., Jr. (1989). Cocaine dependence. *Annual Review of Medicine, 40*, 149–161.

Gay, G. R. (1981). You've come a long way, baby! Coke time for the new American lady of the eighties. *Journal of Psychoactive Drugs, 13*(4), 297–318.

Gay, G. R. (1982). Clinical management of acute and chronic cocaine poisoning. *Annals of Emergency Medicine, 11*(10), 562–572.

Ghadirian, A. M., Engelsmann, F., Dhar, V., Filipini, D., Keller, R., Chouinard, G., et al. (1995). The psychotropic effects of inhibitors of steroid biosynthesis in depressed patients refractory to treatment. *Biological Psychiatry, 37*(6), 369–375.

Goeders, N. E. (1991). Cocaine differentially affects benzodiazepine receptors in discrete regions of the rat brain: Persistence and potential mechanisms mediating these effects. *The Journal of Pharmacology and Experimental Therapeutics, 259*(2), 574–581.

Goeders, N. E. (1997). A neuroendocrine role in cocaine reinforcement. *Psychoneuroendocrinology, 22*(4), 237–259.

Goeders, N. E. (2002a). The HPA axis and cocaine reinforcement. *Psychoneuroendocrinology, 27*(1–2), 13–33.

Goeders, N. E. (2002b). Stress and cocaine addiction. *The Journal of Pharmacology and Experimental Therapeutics, 301*(3), 785–789.

Goeders, N. E. (2004). Stress, motivation, and drug addiction. *Current Directions in Psychological Science, 13*(1), 33–35.

Goeders, N., Bell, V., Guidroz, A., & McNulty, M. (1990). Dopaminergic involvement in the cocaine-induced up-regulation of benzodiazepine receptors in the rat caudate nucleus. *Brain Research, 515*(1–2), 1–8.

Goeders, N. E., Bienvenu, O. J., & De Souza, E. B. (1990). Chronic cocaine administration alters corticotropin-releasing factor receptors in the rat brain. *Brain Research, 531*(1–2), 322–328.

Goeders, N. E., & Clampitt, D. M. (2002). Potential role for the hypothalamo-pituitary-adrenal axis in the conditioned reinforcer-induced reinstatement of extinguished cocaine seeking in rats. *Psychopharmacology, 161*(3), 222–232.

Goeders, N. E., Clampitt, D. M., Keller, C., Sharma, M., & Guerin, G. F. (2009). Alprazolam and oxazepam block the cue-induced reinstatement of extinguished cocaine seeking in rats. *Psychopharmacology, 201*(4), 581–588.

Goeders, N. E., Cohen, A., Fox, B. S., Azar, M. R., George, O., & Koob, G. F. (2012). Effects of the combination of metyrapone and oxazepam on intravenous nicotine self-administration in rats. *Psychopharmacology, 223*(1), 17–25.

Goeders, N. E., De Souza, E. B., & Kuhar, M. J. (1986). Benzodiazepine receptor GABA ratios: Regional differences in rat brain and modulation by adrenalectomy. *European Journal of Pharmacology, 129*(3), 363–366.

Goeders, J. E., & Goeders, N. E. (2004). Effects of oxazepam on methamphetamine-induced conditioned place preference. *Pharmacology, Biochemistry, and Behavior, 78*(1), 185–188.

Goeders, N. E., & Guerin, G. F. (1994). Non-contingent electric footshock facilitates the acquisition of intravenous cocaine self-administration in rats. *Psychopharmacology, 114*(1), 63–70.

Goeders, N. E., & Guerin, G. F. (1996a). Effects of surgical and pharmacological adrenalectomy on the initiation and maintenance of intravenous cocaine self-administration in rats. *Brain Research, 722*(1–2), 145–152.

Goeders, N. E., & Guerin, G. F. (1996b). Role of corticosterone in intravenous cocaine self-administration in rats. *Neuroendocrinology, 64*(5), 337–348.

Goeders, N. E., & Guerin, G. F. (1997). Effects of ketoconazole on intravenous cocaine self-administration in rats. In L. S. Harris (Ed.), *NIDA Research Monograph 174, Problems of Drug Dependence, 1996* (p. 180). NIH publication number 97–4236.

Goeders, N. E., & Guerin, G. F. (1999). Pretreatment with corticosterone or dexamethasone fails to affect ongoing cocaine self-administration in rats. *Neuroscience Abstracts, 25*, 1872.

Goeders, N. E., & Guerin, G. F. (2000). Effects of the CRH receptor antagonist CP-154,526 on intravenous cocaine self-administration in rats. *Neuropsychopharmacology, 23*(5), 577–586.

Goeders, N. E., & Guerin, G. F. (2008). Effects of the combination of metyrapone and oxazepam on cocaine and food self-administration in rats. *Pharmacology, Biochemistry, and Behavior, 91*(1), 181–189.

Goeders, N. E., Irby, B. D., Shuster, C. C., & Guerin, G. F. (1997). Tolerance and sensitization to the behavioral effects of cocaine in rats: Relationship to benzodiazepine receptors. *Pharmacology, Biochemistry, and Behavior, 57*(1–2), 43–56.

Goeders, N. E., McNulty, M. A., & Guerin, G. F. (1993). Effects of alprazolam on intravenous cocaine self-administration in rats. *Pharmacology, Biochemistry, and Behavior, 44*(2), 471–474.

Goeders, N. E., McNulty, M. A., Mirkis, S., & McAllister, K. H. (1989). Chlordiazepoxide alters intravenous cocaine self-administration in rats. *Pharmacology, Biochemistry, and Behavior, 33*(4), 859–866.

Goeders, N. E., Peltier, R. L., & Guerin, G. F. (1998). Ketoconazole reduces low dose cocaine self-administration in rats. *Drug and Alcohol Dependence, 53*(1), 67–77.

Goeders, N. E., & Smith, J. E. (1983). Cortical dopaminergic involvement in cocaine reinforcement. *Science, 221*(4612), 773–775.

Goeders, N. E., & Smith, J. E. (1993). Intracranial cocaine self-administration into the medial prefrontal cortex increases dopamine turnover in the nucleus accumbens. *The Journal of Pharmacology and Experimental Therapeutics, 265*(2), 592–600.

Gomez-Sanchez, C. E., Zhou, M. Y., Cozza, E. N., Morita, H., Eddleman, F. C., & Gomez-Sanchez, E. P. (1996). Corticosteroid synthesis in the central nervous system. *Endocrine Research, 22*(4), 463–470.

Gomez-Sanchez, C. E., Zhou, M. Y., Cozza, E. N., Morita, H., Foecking, M. F., & Gomez-Sanchez, E. P. (1997). Aldosterone biosynthesis in the rat brain. *Endocrinology, 138*(8), 3369–3373.

Gorin, R. E., Crabbe, J. C., Tanchuck, M. A., Long, S. L., & Finn, D. A. (2005). Effects of finasteride on chronic and acute ethanol withdrawal severity in the WSP and WSR selected lines. *Alcoholism, Clinical and Experimental Research, 29*(6), 939–948.

Grant, S., London, E. D., Newlin, D. B., Villemagne, V. L., Liu, X., Contoreggi, C., et al. (1996). Activation of memory circuits during cue-elicited cocaine craving. *Proceedings of the National Academy of Sciences of the United States of America, 93*(21), 12040–12045.

Griffiths, R. R., & Johnson, M. W. (2005). Relative abuse liability of hypnotic drugs: A conceptual framework and algorithm for differentiating among compounds. *The Journal of Clinical Psychiatry, 66*(Suppl. 9), 31–41.

Griffiths, R. R., McLeod, D. R., Bigelow, G. E., Liebson, I. A., & Roache, J. D. (1984). Relative abuse liability of diazepam and oxazepam: Behavioral and subjective dose effects. *Psychopharmacology, 84*(2), 147–154.

Griffiths, R. R., & Weerts, E. M. (1997). Benzodiazepine self-administration in humans and laboratory animals—Implications for problems of long-term use and abuse. *Psychopharmacology, 134*(1), 1–37.

Griffiths, R. R., & Wolf, B. (1990). Relative abuse liability of different benzodiazepines in drug abusers. *Journal of Clinical Psychopharmacology, 10*(4), 237–243.

Groh, B., & Muller, W. E. (1985). A comparison of the relative in vitro and in vivo binding affinities of various benzodiazepines and related compounds for the benzodiazepine receptor and for the peripheral benzodiazepine binding site. *Research Communications in Chemical Pathology and Pharmacology, 49*(3), 463–466.

Gurkovskaya, O., & Goeders, N. E. (2001). Effects of CP-154,526 on responding during extinction from cocaine self-administration in rats. *European Journal of Pharmacology, 432*(1), 53–56.

Guzman, D., Moscarello, J. M., & Ettenberg, A. (2009). The effects of medial prefrontal cortex infusions of cocaine in a runway model of drug self-administration: Evidence of reinforcing but not anxiogenic actions. *European Journal of Pharmacology, 605*(1–3), 117–122.

Haleem, D. J., Kennett, G., & Curzon, G. (1988). Adaptation of female rats to stress: Shift to male pattern by inhibition of corticosterone synthesis. *Brain Research, 458*(2), 339–347.

Haney, M., Maccari, S., Le Moal, M., Simon, H., & Piazza, P. V. (1995). Social stress increases the acquisition of cocaine self-administration in male and female rats. *Brain Research, 698*(1–2), 46–52.

Haynes, R. C., Jr. (1990). Adrenocorticotropic hormone; adrenocortical steroids and their synthetic analogs; inhibitors of the synthesis and actions of adrenocortical hormones. In A. G. Gilman, T. W. Rall, A. S. Nies, & P. Taylor (Eds.), *The pharmacological basis of therapeutics* (pp. 1431–1462). New York, NY: Pergamon Press.

Hays, J. T., & Ebbert, J. O. (2008). Varenicline for tobacco dependence. *The New England Journal of Medicine, 359*(19), 2018–2024.

Hays, J. T., Ebbert, J. O., & Sood, A. (2008). Efficacy and safety of varenicline for smoking cessation. *The American Journal of Medicine, 121*(4 Suppl. 1), S32–S42.

Heesch, C. M., Negus, B. H., Keffer, J. H., Snyder, R. W., 2nd., Risser, R. C., & Eichhorn, E. J. (1995). Effects of cocaine on cortisol secretion in humans. *The American Journal of the Medical Sciences, 310*(2), 61–64.

Higaki, Y., Usami, N., Shintani, S., Ishikura, S., El-Kabbani, O., & Hara, A. (2003). Selective and potent inhibitors of human 20alpha-hydroxysteroid dehydrogenase (AKR1C1) that metabolizes neurosteroids derived from progesterone. *Chemico-Biological Interactions, 143–144*, 503–513.

Hirani, K., Sharma, A. N., Jain, N. S., Ugale, R. R., & Chopde, C. T. (2005). Evaluation of GABAergic neuroactive steroid 3alpha-hydroxy-5alpha-pregnane-20-one as a neurobiological substrate for the anti-anxiety effect of ethanol in rats. *Psychopharmacology, 180*(2), 267–278.

Hirschfeld, R. M. (1990). Future directions in the treatment of anxiety. *Journal of Psychiatric Research, 24*(Suppl. 2), 163–167.

Holmes, M. C., Yau, J. L., Kotelevtsev, Y., Mullins, J. J., & Seckl, J. R. (2003). 11 Beta-hydroxysteroid dehydrogenases in the brain: Two enzymes two roles. *Annals of the New York Academy of Sciences, 1007*, 357–366.

Hyman, S. M., Fox, H., Hong, K. I., Doebrick, C., & Sinha, R. (2007). Stress and drug-cue-induced craving in opioid-dependent individuals in naltrexone treatment. *Experimental and Clinical Psychopharmacology, 15*(2), 134–143.

Iguchi, M. Y., Handelsman, L., Bickel, W. K., & Griffiths, R. R. (1993). Benzodiazepine and sedative use/abuse by methadone maintenance clients. *Drug and Alcohol Dependence, 32*(3), 257–266.

Jain, M. R., Khan, F. A., Krishna, N. S., & Subhedar, N. (1994). Intracranial metyrapone stimulates CRF-ACTH axis in the teleost, Clarias batrachus: Possible role of neurosteroids. *Neuroreport, 5*(16), 2093–2096.

Javaid, J. I., Notorangelo, M. P., Pandey, S. C., Reddy, P. L., Pandey, G. N., & Davis, J. M. (1994). Peripheral benzodiazepine receptors are decreased during cocaine withdrawal in humans. *Biological Psychiatry, 36*(1), 44–50.

Joels, M., & de Kloet, E. R. (1994). Mineralocorticoid and glucocorticoid receptors in the brain. Implications for ion permeability and transmitter systems. *Progress in Neurobiology, 43*(1), 1–36.

Johnston, G. A. (1992). GABAA agonists as targets for drug development. *Clinical and Experimental Pharmacology & Physiology, 19*(1), 73–78.

Joo, H. K., Oh, S. C., Cho, E. J., Park, K. S., Lee, J. Y., Lee, E. J., et al. (2009). Midazolam inhibits tumor necrosis factor-alpha-induced endothelial activation: Involvement of the peripheral benzodiazepine receptor. *Anesthesiology, 110*(1), 106–112.

Jorenby, D. E., Hays, J. T., Rigotti, N. A., Azoulay, S., Watsky, E. J., Williams, K. E., et al. (2006). Efficacy of varenicline, an alpha4beta2 nicotinic acetylcholine receptor partial agonist, vs placebo or sustained-release bupropion for smoking cessation: A randomized controlled trial. *JAMA, 296*(1), 56–63.

Kablinger, A. S., Lindner, M. A., Casso, S., Hefti, F., DeMuth, G., Fox, B. S., et al. (2012). Effects of the combination of metyrapone and oxazepam on cocaine craving and cocaine taking: A double-blind, randomized, placebo-controlled pilot study. *Journal of Psychopharmacology, 26*(7), 973–981.

Kaminski, R. M., & Rogawski, M. A. (2011). 11beta-Hydroxylase inhibitors protect against seizures in mice by increasing endogenous neurosteroid synthesis. *Neuropharmacology, 61*(1–2), 133–137.

Keim, K. L., & Sigg, E. B. (1977). Plasma corticosterone and brain catecholamines in stress: Effect of psychotropic drugs. *Pharmacology, Biochemistry, and Behavior, 6*(1), 79–85.

Keller, C. M., Cornett, E. M., Guerin, G. F., & Goeders, N. E. (2013). Combinations of oxazepam and metyrapone attenuate cocaine and methamphetamine cue reactivity. *Drug and Alcohol Dependence, 133*(2), 405–412.

Kelley, A. M., Athy, J. R., Cho, T. H., Erickson, B., King, M., & Cruz, P. (2012). Risk propensity and health risk behaviors in U.S. army soldiers with and without psychological disturbances across the deployment cycle. *Journal of Psychiatric Research, 46*(5), 582–589.

Khantzian, E. J. (1985). The self-medication hypothesis of addictive disorders: Focus on heroin and cocaine dependence. *The American Journal of Psychiatry, 142*(11), 1259–1264.

Kilbey, M. M., Breslau, N., & Andreski, P. (1992). Cocaine use and dependence in young adults: Associated psychiatric disorders and personality traits. *Drug and Alcohol Dependence, 29*(3), 283–290.

Kilgus, M. D., & Pumariega, A. J. (1994). Experimental manipulation of cocaine craving by videotaped environmental cues. *Southern Medical Journal, 87*(11), 1138–1140.

Kilts, C. D., Schweitzer, J. B., Quinn, C. K., Gross, R. E., Faber, T. L., Muhammad, F., et al. (2001). Neural activity related to drug craving in cocaine addiction. *Archives of General Psychiatry, 58*(4), 334–341.

Kleber, H. D., & Gawin, F. H. (1984). Cocaine abuse: A review of current and experimental treatments. *NIDA Research Monograph, 50*, 111–129.

Koob, G. F. (2008). A role for brain stress systems in addiction. *Neuron, 59*(1), 11–34.

Koob, G. F., Buck, C. L., Cohen, A., Edwards, S., Park, P. E., Schlosburg, J. E., et al. (2014). Addiction as a stress surfeit disorder. *Neuropharmacology, 76*(Part B), 370–382.

Kostowski, W. (1995). Recent advances in the GABA-A-benzodiazepine receptor pharmacology. *Polish Journal of Pharmacology, 47*(3), 237–246.

Kreek, M. J., Ragunath, J., Plevy, S., Hamer, D., Schneider, B., & Hartman, N. (1984). ACTH, cortisol and beta-endorphin response to metyrapone testing during chronic methadone maintenance treatment in humans. *Neuropeptides, 5*(1–3), 277–278.

Lambert, J. J., Belelli, D., Hill-Venning, C., Callachan, H., & Peters, J. A. (1996). Neurosteroid modulation of native and recombinant GABAA receptors. *Cellular and Molecular Neurobiology, 16*(2), 155–174.

Lambert, J. J., Belelli, D., Peden, D. R., Vardy, A. W., & Peters, J. A. (2003). Neurosteroid modulation of GABAA receptors. *Progress in Neurobiology, 71*(1), 67–80.

Lange, R. A., & Hillis, L. D. (2001). Cardiovascular complications of cocaine use. *The New England Journal of Medicine, 345*(5), 351–358.

Lee, B., Tiefenbacher, S., Platt, D. M., & Spealman, R. D. (2003). Role of the hypothalamic-pituitary-adrenal axis in reinstatement of cocaine-seeking behavior in squirrel monkeys. *Psychopharmacology, 168*(1–2), 177–183.

Lelas, S., Rowlett, J. K., & Spealman, R. D. (2001). Triazolam discrimination in squirrel monkeys distinguishes high-efficacy agonists from other benzodiazepines and nonbenzodiazepine drugs. *Psychopharmacology, 154*(1), 96–104.

Lemaire, V., Deminiere, J. M., & Mormede, P. (1994). Chronic social stress conditions differentially modify vulnerability to amphetamine self-administration. *Brain Research,* *649*(1–2), 348–352.

Levy, A. D., Li, Q. A., Kerr, J. E., Rittenhouse, P. A., Milonas, G., Cabrera, T. M., et al. (1991). Cocaine-induced elevation of plasma adrenocorticotropin hormone and corticosterone is mediated by serotonergic neurons. *The Journal of Pharmacology and Experimental Therapeutics,* *259*(2), 495–500.

Lilja, J., Larsson, S., Skinhoj, K. T., & Hamilton, D. (2001). Evaluation of programs for the treatment of benzodiazepine dependency. *Substance Use & Misuse,* *36*(9–10), 1213–1231.

Lipton, J. W., Olsen, R. W., & Ellison, G. D. (1995). Length of continuous cocaine exposure determines the persistence of muscarinic and benzodiazepine receptor alterations. *Brain Research,* *676*(2), 378–385.

London, E. D., Ernst, M., Grant, S., Bonson, K., & Weinstein, A. (2000). Orbitofrontal cortex and human drug abuse: Functional imaging. *Cerebral Cortex,* *10*(3), 334–342.

Longone, P., Rupprecht, R., Manieri, G. A., Bernardi, G., Romeo, E., & Pasini, A. (2008). The complex roles of neurosteroids in depression and anxiety disorders. *Neurochemistry International,* *52*(4–5), 596–601.

Loose, D. S., Stover, E. P., & Feldman, D. (1983). Ketoconazole binds to glucocorticoid receptors and exhibits glucocorticoid antagonist activity in cultured cells. *The Journal of Clinical Investigation,* *72*(1), 404–408.

Lovallo, W. R. (2006). The hypothalamic-pituitary-adrenocortical axis in addiction. *International Journal of Psychophysiology,* *59*(3), 193–194.

Luddens, H., & Korpi, E. R. (1995). Biological function of GABAA/benzodiazepine receptor heterogeneity. *Journal of Psychiatric Research,* *29*(2), 77–94.

Maas, L. C., Lukas, S. E., Kaufman, M. J., Weiss, R. D., Daniels, S. L., Rogers, V. W., et al. (1998). Functional magnetic resonance imaging of human brain activation during cue-induced cocaine craving. *The American Journal of Psychiatry,* *155*(1), 124–126.

Maayan, R., Lotan, S., Doron, R., Shabat-Simon, M., Gispan-Herman, I., Weizman, A., et al. (2006). Dehydroepiandrosterone (DHEA) attenuates cocaine-seeking behavior in the self-administration model in rats. *European Neuropsychopharmacology,* *16*(5), 329–339.

MacKenzie, S. M., Clark, C. J., Fraser, R., Gomez-Sanchez, C. E., Connell, J. M., & Davies, E. (2000). Expression of 11beta-hydroxylase and aldosterone synthase genes in the rat brain. *Journal of Molecular Endocrinology,* *24*(3), 321–328.

MacKenzie, S. M., Clark, C. J., Ingram, M. C., Lai, M., Seckl, J., Gomez-Sanchez, C. E., et al. (2000). Corticosteroid production by fetal rat hippocampal neurons. *Endocrine Research,* *26*(4), 531–535.

Maksay, G., Tegyey, Z., & Simonyi, M. (1991). Central benzodiazepine receptors: In vitro efficacies and potencies of 3-substituted 1,4-benzodiazepine stereoisomers. *Molecular Pharmacology,* *39*(6), 725–732.

Mantsch, J. R., & Goeders, N. E. (1998). Generalization of a restraint-induced discriminative stimulus to cocaine in rats. *Psychopharmacology,* *135*(4), 423–426.

Mantsch, J. R., & Goeders, N. E. (1999a). Ketoconazole blocks the stress-induced reinstatement of cocaine-seeking behavior in rats: Relationship to the discriminative stimulus effects of cocaine. *Psychopharmacology,* *142*(4), 399–407.

Mantsch, J. R., & Goeders, N. E. (1999b). Ketoconazole does not block cocaine discrimination or the cocaine-induced reinstatement of cocaine-seeking behavior. *Pharmacology, Biochemistry, and Behavior,* *64*(1), 65–73.

Mantsch, J. R., Saphier, D., & Goeders, N. E. (1998). Corticosterone facilitates the acquisition of cocaine self-administration in rats: Opposite effects of the type II glucocorticoid receptor agonist dexamethasone. *The Journal of Pharmacology and Experimental Therapeutics,* *287*(1), 72–80.

Martin, I. L. (1987). The benzodiazepines and their receptors: 25 years of progress. *Neuropharmacology*, 26(7B), 957–970.

McCarthy, J. R., Heinrichs, S. C., & Grigoriadis, D. E. (1999). Recent advances with the CRF1 receptor: Design of small molecule inhibitors, receptor subtypes and clinical indications. *Current Pharmaceutical Design*, 5(5), 289–315.

McEwen, B. S., Weiss, J. M., & Schwartz, L. S. (1968). Selective retention of corticosterone by limbic structures in rat brain. *Nature*, 220(5170), 911–912.

Meador-Woodruff, J. H., & Greden, J. F. (1988). Effects of psychotropic medications on hypothalamic-pituitary-adrenal regulation. *Endocrinology and Metabolism Clinics of North America*, 17(1), 225–234.

Meil, W. M., & See, R. E. (1996). Conditioned cued recovery of responding following prolonged withdrawal from self-administered cocaine in rats: An animal model of relapse. *Behavioural Pharmacology*, 7(8), 754–763.

Mello, N. K., Negus, S. S., Rice, K. C., & Mendelson, J. H. (2006). Effects of the CRF1 antagonist antalarmin on cocaine self-administration and discrimination in rhesus monkeys. *Pharmacology, Biochemistry, and Behavior*, 85(4), 744–751.

Mendelson, J. H., Mello, N. K., Teoh, S. K., Ellingboe, J., & Cochin, J. (1989). Cocaine effects on pulsatile secretion of anterior pituitary, gonadal, and adrenal hormones. *The Journal of Clinical Endocrinology and Metabolism*, 69(6), 1256–1260.

Mendelson, J. H., Sholar, M., Mello, N. K., Teoh, S. K., & Sholar, J. W. (1998). Cocaine tolerance: Behavioral, cardiovascular, and neuroendocrine function in men. *Neuropsychopharmacology*, 18(4), 263–271.

Mendelson, J. H., Teoh, S. K., Mello, N. K., Ellingboe, J., & Rhoades, E. (1992). Acute effects of cocaine on plasma adrenocorticotropic hormone, luteinizing hormone and prolactin levels in cocaine-dependent men. *The Journal of Pharmacology and Experimental Therapeutics*, 263(2), 505–509.

Miczek, K. A., & Mutschler, N. H. (1996). Activational effects of social stress on IV cocaine self-administration in rats. *Psychopharmacology*, 128(3), 256–264.

Miller, L. G., Greenblatt, D. J., Barnhill, J. G., Thompson, M. L., & Shaderh, R. I. (1988). Modulation of benzodiazepine receptor binding in mouse brain by adrenalectomy and steroid replacement. *Brain Research*, 446(2), 314–320.

Moffett, M. C., & Goeders, N. E. (2007). CP-154,526, a CRF type-1 receptor antagonist, attenuates the cue-and methamphetamine-induced reinstatement of extinguished methamphetamine-seeking behavior in rats. *Psychopharmacology*, 190(2), 171–180.

Moldow, R. L., & Fischman, A. J. (1987). Cocaine induced secretion of ACTH, beta-endorphin, and corticosterone. *Peptides*, 8(5), 819–822.

Monder, C., Lakshmi, V., & Miroff, Y. (1991). Kinetic studies on rat liver 11 beta-hydroxysteroid dehydrogenase. *Biochimica et Biophysica Acta*, 1115(1), 23–29.

Mukai, Y., Higashi, T., Nagura, Y., & Shimada, K. (2008). Studies on neurosteroids XXV. Influence of a 5alpha-reductase inhibitor, finasteride, on rat brain neurosteroid levels and metabolism. *Biological & Pharmaceutical Bulletin*, 31(9), 1646–1650.

Mukhin, A. G., Papadopoulos, V., Costa, E., & Krueger, K. E. (1989). Mitochondrial benzodiazepine receptors regulate steroid biosynthesis. *Proceedings of the National Academy of Sciences of the United States of America*, 86(24), 9813–9816.

Mumford, G. R., Evans, S. M., Fleishaker, J. C., & Griffiths, R. R. (1995). Alprazolam absorption kinetics affects abuse liability. *Clinical Pharmacology and Therapeutics*, 57(3), 356–365.

Murphy, B. E., Ghadirian, A. M., & Dhar, V. (1998). Neuroendocrine responses to inhibitors of steroid biosynthesis in patients with major depression resistant to antidepressant therapy. *Canadian Journal of Psychiatry*, 43(3), 279–286.

Mutschler, N. H., & Miczek, K. A. (1998a). Withdrawal from a self-administered or non-contingent cocaine binge: Differences in ultrasonic distress vocalizations in rats. *Psychopharmacology, 136*(4), 402–408.

Mutschler, N. H., & Miczek, K. A. (1998b). Withdrawal from i.v. cocaine "binges" in rats: Ultrasonic distress calls and startle. *Psychopharmacology, 135*(2), 161–168.

Nader, M. A., Czoty, P. W., Nader, S. H., & Morgan, D. (2012). Nonhuman primate models of social behavior and cocaine abuse. *Psychopharmacology, 224*(1), 57–67. http://dx.doi.org/10.1007/s00213-012-2843-5.

Negus, S. S., Mello, N. K., & Fivel, P. A. (2000). Effects of GABA agonists and GABA-A receptor modulators on cocaine discrimination in rhesus monkeys. *Psychopharmacology, 152*(4), 398–407.

Nemeroff, C. B. (1988). The role of corticotropin-releasing factor in the pathogenesis of major depression. *Pharmacopsychiatry, 21*(2), 76–82. http://dx.doi.org/10.1055/s-2007-1014652.

Nothdurfter, C., Rammes, G., Baghai, T. C., Schule, C., Schumacher, M., Papadopoulos, V., et al. (2012). Translocator protein (18 kDa) as a target for novel anxiolytics with a favourable side-effect profile. *Journal of Neuroendocrinology, 24*(1), 82–92.

O'Brien, C. P. (2005). Benzodiazepine use, abuse, and dependence. *The Journal of Clinical Psychiatry, 66*(Suppl. 2), 28–33.

Ongur, D., & Price, J. L. (2000). The organization of networks within the orbital and medial prefrontal cortex of rats, monkeys and humans. *Cerebral Cortex, 10*(3), 206–219.

Oreland, L. (1988). The benzodiazepines: A pharmacological overview. *Acta Anaesthesiologica Scandinavica. Supplementum, 88*, 13–16.

Palamarchouk, V., Smagin, G., & Goeders, N. E. (2009). Self-administered and passive cocaine infusions produce different effects on corticosterone concentrations in the medial prefrontal cortex (MPC) of rats. *Pharmacology, Biochemistry, and Behavior, 94*(1), 163–168.

Paliwal, P., Hyman, S. M., & Sinha, R. (2008). Craving predicts time to cocaine relapse: Further validation of the Now and Brief versions of the cocaine craving questionnaire. *Drug and Alcohol Dependence, 93*(3), 252–259.

Papadopoulos, V., Baraldi, M., Guilarte, T. R., Knudsen, T. B., Lacapere, J. J., Lindemann, P., et al. (2006). Translocator protein (18 kDa): New nomenclature for the peripheral-type benzodiazepine receptor based on its structure and molecular function. *Trends in Pharmacological Sciences, 27*(8), 402–409.

Papadopoulos, V., Berkovich, A., & Krueger, K. E. (1991). The role of diazepam binding inhibitor and its processing products at mitochondrial benzodiazepine receptors: Regulation of steroid biosynthesis. *Neuropharmacology, 30*(12B), 1417–1423.

Paul, S. M., & Purdy, R. H. (1992). Neuroactive steroids. *The FASEB Journal, 6*(6), 2311–2322.

Pellow, S., Chopin, P., File, S. E., & Briley, M. (1985). Validation of open: Closed arm entries in an elevated plus-maze as a measure of anxiety in the rat. *Journal of Neuroscience Methods, 14*(3), 149–167.

Pellow, S., & File, S. E. (1986). Anxiolytic and anxiogenic drug effects on exploratory activity in an elevated plus-maze: A novel test of anxiety in the rat. *Pharmacology, Biochemistry, and Behavior, 24*(3), 525–529.

Peltier, R. L., Guerin, G. F., Dorairaj, N., & Goeders, N. E. (2001). Effects of saline substitution on responding and plasma corticosterone in rats trained to self-administer different doses of cocaine. *The Journal of Pharmacology and Experimental Therapeutics, 299*(1), 114–120.

Piazza, P. V., Deminiere, J. M., le Moal, M., & Simon, H. (1990). Stress- and pharmacologically-induced behavioral sensitization increases vulnerability to acquisition of amphetamine self-administration. *Brain Research, 514*(1), 22–26.

Pinna, G., & Rasmusson, A. M. (2012). Up-regulation of neurosteroid biosynthesis as a pharmacological strategy to improve behavioural deficits in a putative mouse model of post-traumatic stress disorder. *Journal of Neuroendocrinology, 24*(1), 102–116.

Pitts, A. F., Samuelson, S. D., Meller, W. H., Bissette, G., Nemeroff, C. B., & Kathol, R. G. (1995). Cerebrospinal fluid corticotropin-releasing hormone, vasopressin, and oxytocin concentrations in treated patients with major depression and controls. *Biological Psychiatry, 38*(5), 330–335.

Potts, L. A., & Garwood, C. L. (2007). Varenicline: The newest agent for smoking cessation. *American Journal of Health-System Pharmacy, 64*(13), 1381–1384.

Purdy, R. H., Moore, P. H., Jr., Morrow, A. L., & Paul, S. M. (1992). Neurosteroids and GABAA receptor function. *Advances in Biochemical Psychopharmacology, 47*, 87–92.

Ramsey, N. F., & Van Ree, J. M. (1993). Emotional but not physical stress enhances intravenous cocaine self-administration in drug-naive rats. *Brain Research, 608*(2), 216–222.

Raven, P. W., Checkley, S. A., & Taylor, N. F. (1995). Extra-adrenal effects of metyrapone include inhibition of the 11-oxoreductase activity of 11 beta-hydroxysteroid dehydrogenase: A model for 11-HSD I deficiency. *Clinical Endocrinology, 43*(5), 637–644.

Raven, P. W., O'Dwyer, A. M., Taylor, N. F., & Checkley, S. A. (1996). The relationship between the effects of metyrapone treatment on depressed mood and urinary steroid profiles. *Psychoneuroendocrinology, 21*(3), 277–286.

Rivier, C., & Lee, S. (1994). Stimulatory effect of cocaine on ACTH secretion: Role of the hypothalamus. *Molecular and Cellular Neurosciences, 5*(2), 189–195.

Rivier, C., & Vale, W. (1987). Cocaine stimulates adrenocorticotropin (ACTH) secretion through a corticotropin-releasing factor (CRF)-mediated mechanism. *Brain Research, 422*(2), 403–406.

Robbins, S. J., Ehrman, R. N., Childress, A. R., & O'Brien, C. P. (1992). Using cue reactivity to screen medications for cocaine abuse: A test of amantadine hydrochloride. *Addictive Behaviors, 17*(5), 491–499.

Robel, P., & Baulieu, E. E. (1995). Neurosteroids: Biosynthesis and function. *Critical Reviews in Neurobiology, 9*(4), 383–394.

Rogerio, R., & Takahashi, R. N. (1992). Anxiogenic properties of cocaine in the rat evaluated with the elevated plus-maze. *Pharmacology, Biochemistry, and Behavior, 43*(2), 631–633.

Romeo, E., Cavallaro, S., Korneyev, A., Kozikowski, A. P., Ma, D., Polo, A., et al. (1993). Stimulation of brain steroidogenesis by 2-aryl-indole-3-acetamide derivatives acting at the mitochondrial diazepam-binding inhibitor receptor complex. *The Journal of Pharmacology and Experimental Therapeutics, 267*(1), 462–471.

Rounsaville, B. J. (2004). Treatment of cocaine dependence and depression. *Biological Psychiatry, 56*(10), 803–809.

Rounsaville, B. J., Anton, S. F., Carroll, K., Budde, D., Prusoff, B. A., & Gawin, F. (1991). Psychiatric diagnoses of treatment-seeking cocaine abusers. *Archives of General Psychiatry, 48*(1), 43–51.

Rupprecht, R., Papadopoulos, V., Rammes, G., Baghai, T. C., Fan, J., Akula, N., et al. (2010). Translocator protein (18 kDa) (TSPO) as a therapeutic target for neurological and psychiatric disorders. *Nature Reviews. Drug Discovery, 9*(12), 971–988.

Rupprecht, R., Rammes, G., Eser, D., Baghai, T. C., Schule, C., Nothdurfter, C., et al. (2009). Translocator protein (18 kD) as target for anxiolytics without benzodiazepine-like side effects. *Science, 325*(5939), 490–493.

Rupprecht, R., Strohle, A., Hermann, B., di Michele, F., Spalletta, G., Pasini, A., et al. (1998). Neuroactive steroid concentrations following metyrapone administration in depressed patients and healthy volunteers. *Biological Psychiatry, 44*(9), 912–914.

Rush, C. R., Stoops, W. W., Wagner, F. P., Hays, L. R., & Glaser, P. E. (2004). Alprazolam attenuates the behavioral effects of d-amphetamine in humans. *Journal of Clinical Psychopharmacology, 24*(4), 410–420.

Saal, D., Dong, Y., Bonci, A., & Malenka, R. C. (2003). Drugs of abuse and stress trigger a common synaptic adaptation in dopamine neurons. *Neuron, 37*(4), 577–582.

Sampath-Kumar, R., Yu, M., Khalil, M. W., & Yang, K. (1997). Metyrapone is a competitive inhibitor of 11beta-hydroxysteroid dehydrogenase type 1 reductase. *The Journal of Steroid Biochemistry and Molecular Biology, 62*(2–3), 195–199.

Sanchez, M. M., Young, L. J., Plotsky, P. M., & Insel, T. R. (2000). Distribution of corticosteroid receptors in the rhesus brain: Relative absence of glucocorticoid receptors in the hippocampal formation. *The Journal of Neuroscience, 20*(12), 4657–4668.

Sanger, D. J. (1985). GABA and the behavioral effects of anxiolytic drugs. *Life Sciences, 36*(16), 1503–1513.

Saphier, D., Welch, J. E., Farrar, G. E., & Goeders, N. E. (1993). Effects of intracerebroventricular and intrahypothalamic cocaine administration on adrenocortical secretion. *Neuroendocrinology, 57*(1), 54–62.

Sarnyai, Z., Biro, E., Gardi, J., Vecsernyes, M., Julesz, J., & Telegdy, G. (1993). Alterations of corticotropin-releasing factor-like immunoreactivity in different brain regions after acute cocaine administration in rats. *Brain Research, 616*(1–2), 315–319.

Sarnyai, Z., Biro, E., Gardi, J., Vecsernyes, M., Julesz, J., & Telegdy, G. (1995). Brain corticotropin-releasing factor mediates 'anxiety-like' behavior induced by cocaine withdrawal in rats. *Brain Research, 675*(1–2), 89–97.

Sarnyai, Z., Biro, E., Penke, B., & Telegdy, G. (1992). The cocaine-induced elevation of plasma corticosterone is mediated by endogenous corticotropin-releasing factor (CRF) in rats. *Brain Research, 589*(1), 154–156.

Sarnyai, Z., Mello, N. K., Mendelson, J. H., Eros-Sarnyai, M., & Mercer, G. (1996). Effects of cocaine on pulsatile activity of hypothalamic-pituitary-adrenal axis in male rhesus monkeys: Neuroendocrine and behavioral correlates. *The Journal of Pharmacology and Experimental Therapeutics, 277*(1), 225–234.

Schenk, S., Lacelle, G., Gorman, K., & Amit, Z. (1987). Cocaine self-administration in rats influenced by environmental conditions: Implications for the etiology of drug abuse. *Neuroscience Letters, 81*(1–2), 227–231.

Schenk, S., & Partridge, B. (1997). Sensitization and tolerance in psychostimulant self-administration. *Pharmacology, Biochemistry, and Behavior, 57*(3), 543–550.

Schenk, S., & Snow, S. (1994). Sensitization to cocaine's motor activating properties produced by electrical kindling of the medial prefrontal cortex but not of the hippocampus. *Brain Research, 659*(1–2), 17–22.

Schulz, D. W., Mansbach, R. S., Sprouse, J., Braselton, J. P., Collins, J., Corman, M., et al. (1996). CP-154,526: A potent and selective nonpeptide antagonist of corticotropin releasing factor receptors. *Proceedings of the National Academy of Sciences of the United States of America, 93*(19), 10477–10482.

See, R. E. (2005). Neural substrates of cocaine-cue associations that trigger relapse. *European Journal of Pharmacology, 526*(1–3), 140–146.

Sellers, E. M., Ciraulo, D. A., DuPont, R. L., Griffiths, R. R., Kosten, T. R., Romach, M. K., et al. (1993). Alprazolam and benzodiazepine dependence. *The Journal of Clinical Psychiatry, 54*(Suppl.), 64–75, Discussion 67–76.

Selye, H. (1975). Stress and distress. *Comprehensive Therapy, 1*(8), 9–13.

Shaham, Y., Erb, S., Leung, S., Buczek, Y., & Stewart, J. (1998). CP-154,526, a selective, non-peptide antagonist of the corticotropin-releasing factor1 receptor attenuates stress-induced relapse to drug seeking in cocaine- and heroin-trained rats. *Psychopharmacology, 137*(2), 184–190.

Shaham, Y., Shalev, U., Lu, L., De Wit, H., & Stewart, J. (2003). The reinstatement model of drug relapse: History, methodology and major findings. *Psychopharmacology, 168*(1–2), 3–20.

Shearman, G. T., & Lal, H. (1980). Generalization and antagonism studies with convulsant, GABAergic and anticonvulsant drugs in rats trained to discriminate pentylenetetrazol from saline. *Neuropharmacology, 19*(5), 473–479.

Shearman, G. T., & Lal, H. (1981). Discriminative stimulus properties of cocaine related to an anxiogenic action. *Progress in Neuro-Psychopharmacology, 5*(1), 57–63.

Shiffman, S., Read, L., & Jarvik, M. E. (1985). Smoking relapse situations: A preliminary typology. *The International Journal of the Addictions, 20*(2), 311–318.

Sinha, R., Catapano, D., & O'Malley, S. (1999). Stress-induced craving and stress response in cocaine dependent individuals. *Psychopharmacology, 142*(4), 343–351.

Sinha, R., Garcia, M., Paliwal, P., Kreek, M. J., & Rounsaville, B. J. (2006). Stress-induced cocaine craving and hypothalamic-pituitary-adrenal responses are predictive of cocaine relapse outcomes. *Archives of General Psychiatry, 63*(3), 324–331.

Sinha, R., & Li, C. S. (2007). Imaging stress- and cue-induced drug and alcohol craving: Association with relapse and clinical implications. *Drug and Alcohol Review, 26*(1), 25–31.

Sinha, R., Talih, M., Malison, R., Cooney, N., Anderson, G. M., & Kreek, M. J. (2003). Hypothalamic-pituitary-adrenal axis and sympatho-adreno-medullary responses during stress-induced and drug cue-induced cocaine craving states. *Psychopharmacology, 170*(1), 62–72.

Smagin, G. N., & Goeders, N. E. (2004). Effects of acute and chronic ketoconazole administration on hypothalamo–pituitary–adrenal axis activity and brain corticotropin-releasing hormone. *Psychoneuroendocrinology, 29*(10), 1223–1228.

Soderpalm, B. (1987). Pharmacology of the benzodiazepines; with special emphasis on alprazolam. *Acta Psychiatrica Scandinavica. Supplementum, 335*, 39–46.

Sonino, N. (1987). The use of ketoconazole as an inhibitor of steroid production. *The New England Journal of Medicine, 317*(13), 812–818.

Sorg, B. A., Chen, S. Y., & Kalivas, P. W. (1993). Time course of tyrosine hydroxylase expression after behavioral sensitization to cocaine. *The Journal of Pharmacology and Experimental Therapeutics, 266*(1), 424–430.

Spero, L. (1985). Modulation of specific [3H]phenytoin binding by benzodiazepines. *Neurochemical Research, 10*(6), 755–765.

Spivak, B., Maayan, R., Kotler, M., Mester, R., Gil-Ad, I., Shtaif, B., et al. (2000). Elevated circulatory level of GABA(A)—Antagonistic neurosteroids in patients with combat-related post-traumatic stress disorder. *Psychological Medicine, 30*(5), 1227–1231.

Stefanski, R., Ziolkowska, B., Kusmider, M., Mierzejewski, P., Wyszogrodzka, E., Kolomanska, P., et al. (2007). Active versus passive cocaine administration: Differences in the neuroadaptive changes in the brain dopaminergic system. *Brain Research, 1157*, 1–10.

Steiner, J. F. (1993). Finasteride: A 5 alpha-reductase inhibitor. *Clinical Pharmacy, 12*(1), 15–23.

Stewart, J. (2000). Pathways to relapse: The neurobiology of drug- and stress-induced relapse to drug-taking. *Journal of Psychiatry & Neuroscience, 25*(2), 125–136.

Stratakis, C. A., & Chrousos, G. P. (1995). Neuroendocrinology and pathophysiology of the stress system. *Annals of the New York Academy of Sciences, 771*, 1–18.

Stromstedt, M., & Waterman, M. R. (1995). Messenger RNAs encoding steroidogenic enzymes are expressed in rodent brain. *Brain Research. Molecular Brain Research, 34*(1), 75–88.

Sudduth, S. L., & Koronkowski, M. J. (1993). Finasteride: The first 5 alpha-reductase inhibitor. *Pharmacotherapy, 13*(4), 309–325Discussion 309–325.

Suto, N., Ecke, L. E., You, Z. B., & Wise, R. A. (2010). Extracellular fluctuations of dopamine and glutamate in the nucleus accumbens core and shell associated with lever-pressing during cocaine self-administration, extinction, and yoked cocaine administration. *Psychopharmacology*, *211*(3), 267–275.

Tarr, J. E., & Macklin, M. (1987). Cocaine. *Pediatric Clinics of North America*, *34*(2), 319–331.

Temple, T. E., & Liddle, G. W. (1970). Inhibitors of adrenal steroid biosynthesis. *Annual Review of Pharmacology*, *10*, 199–218.

Teoh, S. K., Sarnyai, Z., Mendelson, J. H., Mello, N. K., Springer, S. A., Sholar, J. W., et al. (1994). Cocaine effects on pulsatile secretion of ACTH in men. *The Journal of Pharmacology and Experimental Therapeutics*, *270*(3), 1134–1138.

Thakore, J. H., & Dinan, T. G. (1995). Cortisol synthesis inhibition: A new treatment strategy for the clinical and endocrine manifestations of depression. *Biological Psychiatry*, *37*(6), 364–368.

Thomson, I., Fraser, R., & Kenyon, C. J. (1995). Regulation of adrenocortical steroidogenesis by benzodiazepines. *The Journal of Steroid Biochemistry and Molecular Biology*, *53*(1–6), 75–79.

Tidey, J. W., & Miczek, K. A. (1997). Acquisition of cocaine self-administration after social stress: Role of accumbens dopamine. *Psychopharmacology*, *130*(3), 203–212.

Tokuda, K., O'Dell, K. A., Izumi, Y., & Zorumski, C. F. (2010). Midazolam inhibits hippocampal long-term potentiation and learning through dual central and peripheral benzodiazepine receptor activation and neurosteroidogenesis. *The Journal of Neuroscience*, *30*(50), 16788–16795.

Torpy, D. J., Grice, J. E., Hockings, G. I., Walters, M. M., Crosbie, G. V., & Jackson, R. V. (1993). Alprazolam blocks the naloxone-stimulated hypothalamo-pituitary-adrenal axis in man. *The Journal of Clinical Endocrinology and Metabolism*, *76*(2), 388–391.

Trapani, A., Palazzo, C., de Candia, M., Lasorsa, F. M., & Trapani, G. (2013). Targeting of the translocator protein 18 kDa (TSPO): A valuable approach for nuclear and optical imaging of activated microglia. *Bioconjugate Chemistry*, *24*, 1415–1428.

Twining, R. C., Bolan, M., & Grigson, P. S. (2009). Yoked delivery of cocaine is aversive and protects against the motivation for drug in rats. *Behavioral Neuroscience*, *123*(4), 913–925.

Ugale, R. R., Mittal, N., Hirani, K., & Chopde, C. T. (2004). Essentiality of central GABAergic neuroactive steroid allopregnanolone for anticonvulsant action of fluoxetine against pentylenetetrazole-induced seizures in mice. *Brain Research*, *1023*(1), 102–111.

Ugale, R. R., Sharma, A. N., Kokare, D. M., Hirani, K., Subhedar, N. K., & Chopde, C. T. (2007). Neurosteroid allopregnanolone mediates anxiolytic effect of etifoxine in rats. *Brain Research*, *1184*, 193–201.

Usami, N., Yamamoto, T., Shintani, S., Ishikura, S., Higaki, Y., Katagiri, Y., et al. (2002). Substrate specificity of human 3(20)alpha-hydroxysteroid dehydrogenase for neurosteroids and its inhibition by benzodiazepines. *Biological & Pharmaceutical Bulletin*, *25*(4), 441–445.

Van Cauteren, H., Lampo, A., Vandenberghe, J., Vanparys, P., Coussement, W., De Coster, R., et al. (1989). Toxicological profile and safety evaluation of antifungal azole derivatives. *Mycoses*, *32*(Suppl. 1), 60–66.

Van Cauteren, H., Lampo, A., Vandenberghe, J., Vanparys, P., Coussement, W., De Coster, R., et al. (1990). Safety aspects of oral antifungal agents. *British Journal of Clinical Practice. Supplement*, *71*, 47–49.

Van Vugt, D. A., Piercy, J., Farley, A. E., Reid, R. L., & Rivest, S. (1997). Luteinizing hormone secretion and corticotropin-releasing factor gene expression in the paraventricular nucleus of rhesus monkeys following cortisol synthesis inhibition. *Endocrinology*, *138*(6), 2249–2258.

Venkatakrishnan, K., Rader, M., Ramanathan, R. K., Ramalingam, S., Chen, E., Riordan, W., et al. (2009). Effect of the CYP3A inhibitor ketoconazole on the pharmacokinetics and pharmacodynamics of bortezomib in patients with advanced solid tumors: A prospective, multicenter, open-label, randomized, two-way crossover drug-drug interaction study. *Clinical Therapeutics, 31*(Pt. 2), 2444–2458.

Vescovi, P. P., Coiro, V., Volpi, R., Giannini, A., & Passeri, M. (1992). Hyperthermia in sauna is unable to increase the plasma levels of ACTH/cortisol, beta-endorphin and prolactin in cocaine addicts. *Journal of Endocrinological Investigation, 15*(9), 671–675.

Vescovi, P. P., Coiro, V., Volpi, R., & Passeri, M. (1992). Diurnal variations in plasma ACTH, cortisol and beta-endorphin levels in cocaine addicts. *Hormone Research, 37*(6), 221–224.

Wang, J. K., Taniguchi, T., & Spector, S. (1984). Structural requirements for the binding of benzodiazepines to their peripheral-type sites. *Molecular Pharmacology, 25*(3), 349–351.

Wang, G. J., Volkow, N. D., Fowler, J. S., Cervany, P., Hitzemann, R. J., Pappas, N. R., et al. (1999). Regional brain metabolic activation during craving elicited by recall of previous drug experiences. *Life Sciences, 64*(9), 775–784.

Washton, A. M., & Tatarsky, A. (1984). Adverse effects of cocaine abuse. *NIDA Research Monograph, 49*, 247–254.

Wehling, M. (1997). Specific, nongenomic actions of steroid hormones. *Annual Review of Physiology, 59*, 365–393.

Weiss, F., Maldonado-Vlaar, C. S., Parsons, L. H., Kerr, T. M., Smith, D. L., & Ben-Shahar, O. (2000). Control of cocaine-seeking behavior by drug-associated stimuli in rats: Effects on recovery of extinguished operant-responding and extracellular dopamine levels in amygdala and nucleus accumbens. *Proceedings of the National Academy of Sciences of the United States of America, 97*(8), 4321–4326.

Wesson, D. R., & Smith, D. E. (1985). Cocaine: Treatment perspectives. *NIDA Research Monograph, 61*, 193–203.

Wilkins, J. N. (1992). Brain, lung, and cardiovascular interactions with cocaine and cocaine-induced catecholamine effects. *Journal of Addictive Diseases, 11*(4), 9–19.

Wolf, B., & Griffiths, R. R. (1991). Physical dependence on benzodiazepines: Differences within the class. *Drug and Alcohol Dependence, 29*(2), 153–156.

Wolkowitz, O. M., Reus, V. I., Manfredi, F., Ingbar, J., Brizendine, L., & Weingartner, H. (1993). Ketoconazole administration in hypercortisolemic depression. *The American Journal of Psychiatry, 150*(5), 810–812.

Wood, D. M., & Lal, H. (1987). Anxiogenic properties of cocaine withdrawal. *Life Sciences, 41*(11), 1431–1436.

Yang, X. M., Gorman, A. L., Dunn, A. J., & Goeders, N. E. (1992). Anxiogenic effects of acute and chronic cocaine administration: Neurochemical and behavioral studies. *Pharmacology, Biochemistry, and Behavior, 41*(3), 643–650.

Ye, P., Kenyon, C. J., Mackenzie, S. M., Nichol, K., Seckl, J. R., Fraser, R., et al. (2008). Effects of ACTH, dexamethasone, and adrenalectomy on 11beta-hydroxylase (CYP11B1) and aldosterone synthase (CYP11B2) gene expression in the rat central nervous system. *The Journal of Endocrinology, 196*(2), 305–311.

Zeigler, S., Lipton, J., Toga, A., & Ellison, G. (1991). Continuous cocaine administration produces persisting changes in brain neurochemistry and behavior. *Brain Research, 552*(1), 27–35.

Zierler-Brown, S. L., & Kyle, J. A. (2007). Oral varenicline for smoking cessation. *The Annals of Pharmacotherapy, 41*(1), 95–99.

Zorumski, C. F., Paul, S. M., Izumi, Y., Covey, D. F., & Mennerick, S. (2013). Neurosteroids, stress and depression: Potential therapeutic opportunities. *Neuroscience and Biobehavioral Reviews, 37*(1), 109–122.

CHAPTER TWELVE

Salvinorin A Analogs and Other Kappa-Opioid Receptor Compounds as Treatments for Cocaine Abuse

Bronwyn M. Kivell[*], **Amy W.M. Ewald**[*], **Thomas E. Prisinzano**[†,1]

[*]School of Biological Sciences, Centre for Biodiscovery, Victoria University of Wellington, Wellington, New Zealand
[†]Department of Medicinal Chemistry, University of Kansas, Lawrence, Kansas, USA
[1]Corresponding author: e-mail address: prisinza@ku.edu

Contents

Abstract

Acute activation of kappa-opioid receptors produces anti-addictive effects by regulating dopamine levels in the brain. Unfortunately, classic kappa-opioid agonists have undesired side effects such as sedation, aversion, and depression, which restrict their clinical use. Salvinorin A (Sal A), a novel kappa-opioid receptor agonist extracted from the plant *Salvia divinorum*, has been identified as a potential therapy for drug abuse and addiction. Here, we review the preclinical effects of Sal A in comparison with traditional kappa-opioid agonists and several new analogs. Sal A retains the anti-addictive properties of traditional kappa-opioid receptor agonists with several improvements including reduced side effects. However, the rapid metabolism of Sal A makes it undesirable

Advances in Pharmacology, Volume 69
ISSN 1054-3589
http://dx.doi.org/10.1016/B978-0-12-420118-7.00012-3

481

for clinical development. In an effort to improve the pharmacokinetics and tolerability of this compound, kappa-opioid receptor agonists based on the structure of Sal A have been synthesized. While work in this field is still in progress, several analogs with improved pharmacokinetic profiles have been shown to have anti-addictive effects. While in its infancy, it is clear that these compounds hold promise for the future development of anti-addictive therapeutics.

ABBREVIATIONS

5-HT serotonin
CB$_1$ cannabinoid receptor type 1
CPP conditioned place preference
CREB cAMP response element-binding protein
DA dopamine
DAT dopamine transporter
DMSO dimethyl sulfoxide
dStr dorsal striatum
ED$_{50}$ effective dose for 50% of maximal response
ERK1/2 extracellular signal-regulated kinases
FST forced swim test
GTP-γS [^{35}S]guanosine 5′-O-[gamma-thio]triphosphate
i.p. intraperitoneal
KOPr kappa-opioid receptor
MAPK mitogen-activated protein kinase
NA noradrenaline
NAcb nucleus accumbens
nor-BNI norbinaltorphimine
Sal A Salvinorin A
s.c. subcutaneous
SN substantia nigra
U50,488 2-(3,4-dichlorophenyl)-N-methyl-N-[(2R)-2-pyrrolidin-1-ylcyclohexyl] acetamide
U69,593 N-methyl-2-phenyl-N-[(5R,7S,8S)-7-pyrrolidin-1-yl-1-oxaspiro[4.5]decan-8-yl]acetamide
VTA ventral tegmental area

1. INTRODUCTION

Salvinorin A (Sal A) is the active compound isolated from *Salvia divinorum*, a member of the Lamiaceae (mint) family (Ortega, Blount, & Manchand, 1982) classified in 1962 by Epling and Jativa (Epling & Jativa-M, 1962). Traditionally, *S. divinorum* has been used as a medicine of the Mazatec Indians of Oaxaca, Mexico. It has hallucinogenic effects in humans

(Siebert, 1994) and is reported to be the most potent naturally occurring hallucinogen. Unlike other known hallucinogens, it does not bind or activate serotonergic pathways (5-HT$_{2A}$) and is a potent and selective kappa-opioid receptor (KOPr) agonist (Roth et al., 2002). In humans, Sal A does not produce the same effects in resting electroencephalogram when compared to other hallucinogens such as mescaline or ketamine suggesting that it has different psychomimetic actions (Ranganathan et al., 2012). Another unique property of Sal A is that it was the first identified KOPr agonist with a nonnitrogenous structure.

Sal A was found to be a full agonist at the KOPr (Roth et al., 2002) and has similar efficacy to 2-(3,4-dichlorophenyl)-N-methyl-N-[(2R)-2-pyrrolidin-1-ylcyclohexyl]acetamide (U50,488), N-methyl-2-phenyl-N-[(5R,7S,8S)-7-pyrrolidin-1-yl-1-oxaspiro[4.5]decan-8-yl]acetamide (U69,593), and the endogenous KOPr peptide dynorphin A in [^{35}S] guanosine 5'-O-[gamma-thio]triphosphate (GTP-γS) assays (Chavkin et al., 2004; Prevatt-Smith et al., 2011).

The novel properties of Sal A have led many researchers to reevaluate the KOPr system for potential therapies known to be modulated by kappa-mediated pathways including anti-addictive effects, often in comparison with the endogenous KOPr ligands and traditional arylacetamide KOPr agonists (Morani, Kivell, Prisinzano, & Schenk, 2009; Shippenberg, Zapata, & Chefer, 2007; Wang, Sun, Tao, Chi, & Liu, 2010) (see Wee & Koob, 2010, for recent review). Sal A reduces the adverse actions of morphine such as tolerance, reward, learning, and memory (reviewed in Wang et al., 2010) and can be used to treat pain (for review, see McCurdy, Sufka, Smith, Warnick, & Nieto, 2006), particularly when KOPr agonists are peripherally restricted (reviewed in Kivell & Prisinzano, 2010). Sal A has also been investigated as a nonaddictive analgesic (Groer et al., 2007; McCurdy et al., 2006) and neuroprotective agent (Su, Riley, Kiessling, Armstead, & Liu, 2011; Wang, Ma, Riley, Armstead, & Liu, 2012). While Sal A has been found to have many actions similar to traditional kappa-opioid agonists, there are many differences in its actions. Sal A has been shown to induce analgesia (McCurdy et al., 2006) and has both aversive (behavioral conditional place aversion models) (Zhang, Butelman, Schlussman, Ho, & Kreek, 2005) and rewarding effects (Braida et al., 2008) as well as prodepressive (Carlezon et al., 2006; Morani, Schenk, Prisinzano, & Kivell, 2012) and antidepressive effects (Braida et al., 2007; Hanes, 2001). While many of these contradicting effects can be explained by the use of different doses and acute versus chronic administration, a clearer understanding of these effects and their underlying mechanisms is needed. Recent developments in the understanding of "functional selectivity" or "biased agonism" whereby multiple agonists acting on the same receptor are able to have different effects have led to greater interest into the effects of KOPr agonists and potential signaling pathways relating to various behavioral effects. There is renewed hope that KOPr agonists possessing desirable anti-addictive effects without unwanted side effects may be identified.

To this end, many of the studies conducted to determine the biological and cellular effects of Sal A have been done in comparison to classic KOPr agonists such as U50,488 or U69,593, enadoline, or dynorphin A. These compounds have all been investigated for their ability to modulate addiction-related behaviors and are briefly outlined here followed by the comparisons with the effects of Sal A.

2. KAPPA-OPIOID RECEPTORS AND THE ENDOGENOUS OPIOID SYSTEM

KOPr is a pertussis toxin-sensitive G-protein-coupled receptor that exerts its effects in the brain and intestines (Avidorreiss et al., 1995). There are three known pharmacological variants of KOPr—KOPr1, KOPr2, and KOPr3—but the only subtype that has been cloned to date is KOPr1 (Heyliger, Jackson, Rice, & Rothman, 1999; Horan et al., 1993; Yasuda et al., 1993). KOPr is enriched in brain circuitry involved in the control of motivation and mood and is found in various neocortical areas, including the olfactory blub, amygdala, basal ganglia, external globus pallidus, hippocampus, thalamus, hypothalamus, ventral tegmental area (VTA), and locus coeruleus (Simonin et al., 1995).

Dynorphin is a posttranslational product of the PDYN gene. Prodynorphin is cleaved into several types of dynorphin by proprotein convertase 2 including dynorphin A, dynorphin B, and big dynorphin (Marinova et al., 2005). Dynorphins are widely distributed throughout the central nervous system (Watson, Khachaturian, Coy, Taylor, & Akil, 1982) with high levels found in the substantia nigra (SN), hypothalamus, caudate nucleus, globus pallidus, and putamen (Gramsch, Hollt, Pasi, Mehraein, & Herz, 1982). Lower amounts of dynorphin can also be found in the amygdala, hippocampus, periaqueductal gray, colliculi, pons, medulla, and area postrema (Gramsch et al., 1982). Dynorphin A (1–17), the most active form of dynorphin, preferentially activates KOPr although it does have some affinity for mu-opioid receptor and delta-opioid receptor (Chavkin, James, & Goldstein, 1982; Merg et al., 2006).

The activation of the endogenous KOPr system leads to several negative behavioral effects including stress and aversion (Wee & Koob, 2010), depression (Knoll & Carlezon, 2010), anxiety (Van't Veer & Carlezon, 2013), hypothermia (Spencer, Hruby, & Burks, 1988), increased submissive behavior (Shippenberg et al., 2007), sedation (Dykstra, Gmerek, Winger, & Woods, 1987), and modulation of drug-seeking behaviors (Bruchas, Land, & Chavkin, 2010; Butelman, Yuferov, & Kreek, 2012; Liu-Chen, 2004; reviewed in Wee & Koob, 2010). It is generally accepted that stimulation of the KOPr/dynorphin system antagonizes the hedonic or rewarding effects of drugs of abuse (Nestler, 2001; Shippenberg et al., 2007). It has also been suggested that these effects are via punishment or aversive-like effects, which directly oppose the actions of the mu-opioid system. Accordingly, the KOPr system is upregulated by acute and chronic exposure to drugs of abuse such as cocaine and morphine (Tjon et al., 1997; Unterwald, Rubenfeld, & Kreek, 1994; Wang et al., 1999).

Stimulation of the dopaminergic system with cocaine has also been shown to increase dynorphin levels (Daunais, Roberts, & McGinty, 1993; Spangler, Unterwald, & Kreek, 1993). Further support for the role of KOPr in depressive-like behaviors and anhedonia following KOPr activation is that these behavioral effects are blocked by prior administration of KOPr antagonists (Chartoff et al., 2012; Shirayama et al., 2004; Zhang, Shi, Woods, Watson, & Ko, 2007). The dysphoric and aversive effects of KOPr activation have been shown to require intact mesoaccumbal dopamine (DA) neurotransmission, and studies also indicate that decreased DA neurotransmission underlies these dysphoric effects (Dichiara & Imperato, 1988; Shippenberg, Balskubik, & Herz, 1993; Wee & Koob, 2010). KOPr activation also decreases serotonin (5-HT) release in freely moving rats (Tao & Auerbach, 2002, 2005) and mediates stress-induced anxiety-like behaviors in mice (Bruchas, Land, Lemos, & Chavkin, 2009). Recently, a review of positron-emission tomography studies highlighted the importance of the KOPr/dynorphin system in the regulation of DA transmission contributing to the hypodopaminergic state observed in cocaine addiction (Trifilieff & Martinez, 2013).

3. KAPPA-OPIOID REGULATION OF DOPAMINE SYSTEMS

KOPrs are located in tyrosine hydroxylase-positive neurons that are found in locations directly opposed to dopamine transporters (DATs) (Svingos, Chavkin, Colago, & Pickel, 2001). DAT is a Na^+/Cl^- symporter protein from the SLC6 gene family that is expressed in neurons located in the VTA, SN, dorsal striatum (dStr), and nucleus accumbens (NAcb), areas crucial to the brain reward pathway (Boja & Kuhar, 1989; Scheffel, Pogun, Stathis, Boja, & Kuhar, 1991). Dopaminergic neurons that innervate the NAcb were found to contain DAT protein on their axons, dendrites, and cell bodies (Nirenberg et al., 1997). DAT functions as a major regulator of DA levels in the synapse and acts by reuptaking DA into presynaptic terminals, where it is either recycled for further use or degraded by monoamine oxidases or catechol-O-methyltransferase (Guo et al., 2007). Administration of synthetic KOPr agonists has been shown to regulate extracellular DA concentrations by both decreasing DA release and increasing DAT activity in the NAcb core and shell (Thompson et al., 2000).

The cell-surface expression of DAT is regulated by DA, with acute exposure leading to increased DAT expression and chronic exposure leading to a decrease in DAT cell-surface expression (Chi & Reith, 2003; Furman et al., 2009; Gulley, Doolen, & Zahniser, 2002; Saunders et al., 2000). Thompson et al. (2000) found that the administration of KOPr agonists increased DAT activity, effectively reducing the concentration of extracellular DA. It has been suggested that this is one of the possible mechanisms by which KOPr agonists exert their effects. These KOPr effects on DA uptake and release functionally oppose the actions of cocaine and other drugs of abuse that reduce DA uptake (Collins, D'Addario, & Izenwasser, 2001; Thompson et al., 2000). Activation of mesoaccumbal DA neurotransmission and a decrease in dopamine D_1 receptor activation have been shown to underlie the aversive effects of KOPr agonists (Shippenberg et al., 1993; Shippenberg, Bals-Kubik, Huber, & Herz, 1991; Shippenberg & Herz, 1987, 1988). Differential regulation of DA levels by multiple signaling pathways and mechanism, such as DA release and reuptake in various brain regions, is another possible mechanism by which Sal A and novel KOPr agonists may regulate addiction, stress, depression, sedation, and aversion.

4. EFFECTS OF DRUGS OF ABUSE ON THE KAPPA-OPIOID SYSTEM

Both acute and chronic administrations of drugs of abuse upregulate the kappa-opioid system. Spangler et al. (1997) found that preprodynorphin mRNA in the caudate putamen of rats was increased after acute administration of cocaine. This was shortly followed by preproenkephalin mRNA and KOPr mRNA after the second day of "binge" cocaine (Spangler et al.,

1997). Initial cocaine exposure in rhesus monkeys self-administering cocaine also activated the PDYN mRNA expression in the caudate putamen (Fagergren et al., 2003).

Chronic cocaine administration upregulates KOPr expression in the NAcb shell, caudate putamen, claustrum, and endopiriform nucleus (Collins et al., 2002). This increase is also accompanied by an elevation in preprodynorphin mRNA levels (Collins et al., 2001, 2002; Tzaferis & McGinty, 2001). The kappa-opioid system remains upregulated for several days following cocaine use, which has been linked to dysphoric effects during withdrawal (Hurd & Herkenham, 1993; Kreek, 1996; Sivam, 1989; Smiley, Johnson, Bush, Gibb, & Hanson, 1990). Repeated cocaine also alters mesoaccumbal, mesocortical (Gehrke, Chefer, & Shippenberg, 2008), and nigrostriatal DA neurotransmissions and results in decreased basal DA neurotransmission during cocaine withdrawal in mice (Zhang et al., 2013).

5. EFFECTS OF KAPPA-OPIOID RECEPTOR AGONISTS ON DRUG ADDICTION

KOPr agonists have little abuse potential and are not self-administered (Tang & Collins, 1985). The ability of KOPr agonists to have profound effects on motivational reward and emotional states has led to studies manipulating this system with the aim of identifying the way KOPr agonists exert anti-addictive effects. In the same manner, the ability of KOPr antagonists to modulate depressive and anxiety-related behaviors, particularly relating to stress-induced relapse, is also studied.

There are three major stages of the addiction cycle: the initial binging stage, followed by withdrawal (and the negative effects associated with withdrawal), and finally the preoccupation or anticipation stage that leads to further drug taking (Koob & Le Moal, 2008). These hypotheses of the drug addiction cycle incorporate reinforcement of the drugs of abuse and neuroadaptations in the reward and stress systems within the brain (Koob, 2008). KOPr agonists are hypothesized to play a role in combating addiction at the binge or intoxication phase by attenuating the rewarding effects of drugs of abuse. The mesolimbic DA system, containing DA projections from the VTA to the NAcb, is modulated by KOPr agonists including endogenous dynorphin, which functions to decrease the rewarding effects of drugs of abuse (for recent reviews, see Butelman et al., 2012; Picetti et al., 2013; Shippenberg, 2009; Wee & Koob, 2010). On the other hand, KOPr antagonists are of potential therapeutic use later in the addiction cycle as they have been shown to modulate stress pathways in addiction. KOPr antagonists hold therapeutic promise for their ability to reduce stress-induced relapse (Chavkin, 2011; Picetti et al., 2013). The *in vivo* effects of KOPr antagonists are variable with long-lasting increases in alcohol self-administration seen in rats exposed to a single injection of norbinaltorphimine (nor-BNI). These results also suggest that the effects of KOPr agonists are due to direct modulation of the reward circuitry, rather than by increasing the aversive effects of KOPr agonists (Mitchell, Liang, & Fields, 2005). Other studies show that nor-BNI decreases ethanol self-administration in ethanol-dependent rats (Walker, Zorrilla, & Koob, 2010). nor-BNI alone did not alter cocaine self-administration in rhesus monkeys but did prevent KOPr agonist-induced decreases in cocaine self-administration in rhesus monkeys (Glick, Maisonneuve, Raucci, & Archer, 1995) and rats (Negus, Mello, Portoghese, & Lin, 1997) and in an extended cocaine access model in rats attenuated cocaine intake (Wee, Orio, Ghirmai, Cashman, & Koob, 2009). Studies suggested that the KOPr antagonist JDTic attenuates alcohol self-administration in the rat (Schank et al., 2012). Recently, attenuation of stress-induced drug-seeking behavior by KOPr antagonists has been shown to hold promise for potential therapeutics (Beardsley, Pollard, Howard, & Carroll, 2010; Butelman et al., 2012) (for recent review of preclinical and clinical effects of KOPr antagonists, see Carroll & Carlezon, 2013). Here, we will focus on KOPr agonists and their potential role in the development of pharmacotherapies to reduce the rewarding effects of drugs of abuse, particularly cocaine.

The activation of the kappa-opioid system opposes the actions of the mu-opioid system. It is generally accepted, based on the large body of evidence in animal models, that stimulation of the kappa-system antagonizes the rewarding effects of drugs of abuse (Mello & Negus, 2000; Shippenberg, Chefer, Zapata, & Heidbreder, 2001) by modulating DA levels in the central nervous system (Dichiara & Imperato, 1988; Jackisch, Hotz, & Hertting, 1993; Margolis, Hjelmstad, Bonci, & Fields, 2003; Spanagel, Herz, & Shippenberg, 1992; Suzuki, Kishimoto, Ozaki, & Narita, 2001; Werling, Frattali, Portoghese, Takemori, & Cox, 1988). It has also been suggested that these effects are via punishment or aversive-like effects. In particular, KOPr activation modulates DA uptake in the NAcb via DAT in the rat (Thompson et al., 2000) and directly inhibits DA neurons in the midbrain in whole-cell patch-clamp recordings in rat brain slices (Margolis et al., 2003). Repeated treatment with the traditional KOPr agonist U69,593 also alters dopamine D_2 receptor mRNA levels (Perreault et al., 2007) and function in the rat (Acri, Thompson, & Shippenberg, 2001). Recently, Mori et al. (2013) showed that in discriminative stimulus tests in the rat, the dopamine D_2 receptor agonist sulpiride generalized to the effects of U50,488 (3 mg/kg), an effect that was not seen with the dopamine D_1 antagonist SCH23390. This suggests that postsynaptic dopamine D_2 receptors are critical for the induction of the discriminative stimulus effects induced by U50,488. This was also suggested to be due to the suppression of the Akt pathway (Mori et al., 2013). Given the recently identified physical and functional interaction between dopamine D_2 receptors and DAT (Bolan et al., 2007) and regulation of DAT by KOPr agonists, there is further need for investigations into the role KOPr agonists have on these proteins regulating DA levels.

Chronic cocaine exposure results in adaptations in the kappa-opioid system (Butelman et al., 2012; Gehrke et al., 2008), while KOPr-activating drugs prevent alterations in brain function that occur as a consequence of repeated drug use (Chefer et al., 2005; Chefer, Moron, Hope, Rea, & Shippenberg, 2000; El Daly, Chefer, Sandill, & Shippenberg, 2000). These studies reinforce the function of the kappa-opioid system as a part of a negative feedback loop that buffers the increases in DA levels in response to cocaine and functions to maintain a steady state (Chefer et al., 2005; Spanagel et al., 1992). These studies strongly support the potential of KOPr agonists as anti-addictive pharmacotherapies. Unfortunately, classic selective and potent KOPr agonists such as U50,488 and U69,593 produce undesired side effects such as aversion, depression, dysphoria, emesis, and sedation (Prisinzano, Tidgewell, & Harding, 2005; Shippenberg et al., 2007; Todtenkopf, Marcus, Portoghese, & Carlezon, 2004; Wee & Koob, 2010). Clinically, activation of the kappa-opioid system has been associated with adverse effects such as confusion, hallucinations, and visual distortions (Johnson, MacLean, Reissig, Prisinzano, & Griffiths, 2011; Pfeiffer, Brantl, Herz, & Emrich, 1986; Walsh, Geter-Douglas, Strain, & Bigelow, 2001). These side effects have restricted the use of classic KOPr agonists as anti-addictive agents (Walsh, Strain, Abreu, & Bigelow, 2001). Several strategies are being employed to develop KOPr-based pharmacotherapies with varying binding and selectivity for kappa- and other-opioid receptors.

Previous studies have shown that dynorphin A (1) blocks cocaine-induced increases in striatal dopamine levels, (2) blocks cocaine-induced place preference, and (3) attenuates cocaine-induced locomotor activity (Zhang, Butelman, Schlussman, Ho, & Kreek, 2004). However, the therapeutic potential of KOPr agonist-selective peptides is relatively unexplored compared to small molecules. This is likely to continue given the difficulties in overcoming pharmacokinetic problems and rapid metabolism.

The structurally unique properties of Sal A have identified this novel KOPr-activating compound as a lead for the development of new anti-addictive pharmacotherapies. There are studies that show differences between Sal A and traditional KOPr agonists in terms of structural binding, activation, and behavioral and cellular effects. In the following sections, we will discuss both the behavioral and cellular effects of Sal A and its analogs.

6. ANIMAL STUDIES WITH SAL A

Sal A has been shown to decrease the effects of cocaine in preclinical models. Studies have shown that Sal A modulates cocaine-seeking behavior and attenuates behavioral sensitization by modulating DA levels within the reward pathways. Recently, Sal A (0.3 mg/kg) was shown to attenuate cocaine prime-induced reinstatement, similar to U69,593 (0.3 mg/kg), U50,488 (30 mg/kg), and spiradoline (1 mg/kg) (Morani et al., 2009). Sal A also attenuated the expression of cocaine-induced behavioral sensitization in rats (Morani et al., 2012) comparable to U69,593 (Heidbreder, Babovicvuksanovic, Shoaib, & Shippenberg, 1995). The decrease in cocaine self-administration with traditional KOPr agonist U69,593 was accompanied by a decrease in food intake in rhesus monkeys (Mello & Negus, 1998; Negus et al., 1997), and decreases in self-administration were only apparent when rats were trained with a cue (Schenk, Partridge, & Shippenberg, 1999). These data suggest that traditional KOPr agonists may decrease the general responding of lab animals rather than specifically targeting the rewarding effects of cocaine. In contrast to these effects, Sal A did not attenuate responses for a natural reward in rats (10% sucrose solution) at the dose (0.3 mg/kg) (intraperitoneal, i.p.) that attenuated cocaine prime-induced reinstatement (Morani et al., 2009). Morani et al. (2012) also showed that 0.3 mg/kg of Sal A had no effect on spontaneous locomotion, cocaine-induced stereotypy, cocaine-induced hyperactivity, or conditioned taste aversion, suggesting that the Sal A dose sufficient to produce attenuation of drug-seeking behavior in rats does not cause sedation or aversion. However, decreased swimming and increased immobility times were observed in the forced swim test (FST) indicating that prodepressive effects are still seen at this dose. Together, these data distinguish, in part, the behavioral effects of Sal A from traditional KOPr agonists.

Studies to compare the effects of Sal A with traditional KOPr agonists in their ability to modulate mesocortical limbic DA signaling have also been conducted recently. Gehrke et al. (2008) utilized quantitative microdialysis techniques to show that acute, locally administered (200 nM), but not repeated, systemic Sal A (5 days 3.2 mg/kg) decreased DA levels in the dStr in a KOPr-dependent manner in the mouse. This is similar to traditional KOPr agonists, which were shown to decrease DA release in rat striatal synaptosomes (Ronken, Mulder, & Schoffelmeer, 1993) and in mice following intra-NAcb perfusion of U69,593 (Chefer et al., 2005). DA levels in the NAcb have an important role in modulating the rewarding effects of drugs of abuse, food, and sex (Nestler & Carlezon, 2006; Wise, 1998), and decreased levels of DA within the NAcb have been previously shown to lead to anhedonia in the rat (Weiss, Markou, Lorang, & Koob, 1992).

Regulation of DA levels in the NAcb may be the mechanism underlying the behavioral effects of Sal A. Further evidence to support this is a recent study by Ebner, Roitman, Potter, Rachlin, and Chartoff (2010) who showed that Sal A (2 mg/kg) decreased phasic DA release in the rat NAcb 5–135 min postinjection without increasing DA reuptake, with max effects seen at 15 min. A lower dose of Sal A (0.25 mg/kg) did not alter DA release in the NAcb (Ebner et al., 2010), which is in contrast to the study in mice by Gehrke et al. (2008). However, species differences and the route of Sal A administration (local vs. systemic administration) are the likely explanations for the difference seen in these studies. The timing of these effects on decreased DA release in the NAcb is consistent with the rapid pharmacokinetic effects of Sal A (Butelman, Prisinzano, Deng, Rus, & Kreek, 2009; Ranganathan et al., 2012; Schmidt et al., 2005; Teksin et al., 2009).

Acute U69,593 administration increases DA uptake in the NAcb in addition to decreasing DA release (Thompson et al., 2000), an effect that is not seen with Sal A in the dStr (Gehrke et al., 2008) or NAcb (Ebner et al., 2010). Further studies are needed to confirm whether acute Sal A modulates DA uptake in the NAcb following local administration. However, results to date indicate significant differences in DA uptake between Sal A and traditional KOPr agonists U50,488 and U69,593.

Sal A (100 nM) also inhibited 5-HT and DA release and induced noradrenaline (NA) overflow in mouse striatal and prefrontal cortex synaptosomes, effects that were not observed in the presence of pertussis toxin or nor-BNI. This is in contrast to U69,593, which had no effect on NA levels. These effects were not mediated by mu-opioid receptors, but the delta-opioid receptor antagonist naltrindole did have an effect (Grilli et al., 2009). Again, this is another example highlighting different effects of Sal A compared to traditional KOPr agonists.

When a compound fully substitutes for another in the discriminative stimulus test, it suggests that these compounds are similar in their actions (Peet & Baker, 2011). Sal A has been found to reliably and fully substitute for U69,593 and U50,488 in drug-discriminating studies in rodents following Sal A (1 mg/kg) (i.p.) (Baker et al., 2009) and also in primates (0.001–0.032 mg/kg) (subcutaneous, s.c.) (Butelman, Harris, & Kreek, 2004; Butelman, Rus, Prisinzano, & Kreek, 2010). Butelman et al. (2004) showed a reversal of the discriminative stimulus effects of Sal A (0.001–0.032 mg/kg) (s.c.) by the KOPr antagonist quadazocine but not another KOPr antagonist 5'-guanidinonaltrindole. This may be due to a different binding site for Sal A compared to traditional KOPr agonists or differences in selectivity, onset of action, or pharmacokinetic properties. These effects were also not blocked by the 5-HT$_2$ antagonist ketanserin (0.1 mg/kg) (Butelman et al., 2010). The onset of the Sal A effects started at 5–15 min and dissipated by 120 min. In addition to these studies, Sal A was shown to have effects on the neuroendocrine system by increasing prolactin levels in rhesus monkeys (Butelman et al., 2007). Discriminative stimulus effects of Sal A were not substituted for by serotonergic hallucinogens, ketamine, or cannabinoids (Butelman et al., 2007; Killinger, Peet, & Baker, 2010; Walentiny et al., 2010). These effects combined further support the KOPr selectivity of Sal A *in vivo* and also highlight the differences between Sal A and traditional KOPr agonists.

The behavioral effects of Sal A differ according to the duration of exposure (acute vs. chronic) or the administered dose (low vs. high). Sal A does not modulate cocaine-induced locomotion in mice (Gehrke et al., 2008) or rats (Morani et al., 2009) in contrast to U69,593, which shows attenuation of cocaine-induced locomotor activity (Collins et al., 2001; Heidbreder, Schenk, Partridge, & Shippenberg, 1998). However, acute Sal A at 2 mg/kg has also been shown to attenuate cocaine-induced locomotor activity in the rat, while repeated Sal A potentiated cocaine-induced locomotor activity (Chartoff, Potter, Damez-Werno, Cohen, & Carlezon, 2008). Repeated Sal A administration at a high dose (3.2 mg/kg) showed a different effect to U69,593, with increased cocaine-evoked DA levels in the dStr without decreasing cocaine-induced hyperactivity in the rat (Gehrke et al., 2008). A high acute dose of Sal A (2 mg/kg) lowered the breakpoint in progressive-ratio responding to sucrose, suggesting a decrease in the reinforcing effects of sucrose. This effect was seen between 20 and 40 min postinjection. A lower dose of Sal A (0.25 mg/kg) had no effect on progressive-ratio responding. These data showing that low-dose Sal A does not alter the rewarding properties of sucrose (Ebner et al., 2010) support results from previous studies that showed no differences in sucrose responding based on a fixed ratio schedule following 0.3 or 1 mg/kg Sal A over a 60 min time period (Morani et al., 2009). Previous studies comparing progressive and fixed ratio self-administration schedules suggest that the two paradigms typically produce similar effects in reinforcement (Winger & Woods, 1985). Another study in mice showed that Sal A (1.0 and 3.2 mg/kg (i.p.)) caused conditioned place aversion and decreased locomotor activity. There was no change in DA levels in the NAcb, but there were significantly decreased DA levels in the caudate putamen (Zhang et al., 2005).

Given these data, it is likely that high doses of Sal A (2 mg/kg) have predominantly aversive effects including the ability to decrease DA release, reward, and motivation. It also attenuates the effects of cocaine hyperactivity when administered acutely but potentiates the same effects when chronically administered. On the other hand, low doses of Sal A (<0.25 mg/kg) (i.p.) consistently display less aversive effects (Morani et al., 2009, 2012) and are within the range with known anticocaine effects. Given this, Sal A possesses desirable anti-addictive effects with fewer side effects compared to traditional KOPr agonists. Although the pharmacokinetic properties of Sal A are not desirable as an anticocaine pharmacotherapy (discussed in the succeeding text), its novel structure may aid in the development of new compounds with better pharmacokinetics and side effect profiles.

7. EFFECTS OF SAL A ON DEPRESSION

Sal A has been shown to have both pro- (Morani et al., 2012) and antidepressive effects *in vivo* (Braida et al., 2007, 2008, 2009; Harden, Smith, Niehoff, McCurdy, & Taylor, 2012). In contrast, the effects traditional KOPr agonists such as U69,593 tend to be consistently prodepressive and aversive (Van't Veer & Carlezon, 2013). Known KOPr-mediated effects on depression and stress-related behaviors, particularly in the ability of KOPr agonists to potentiate stress-induced relapse, have been a major limiting factor in the development of KOPr agonist-based anti-addictive pharmacotherapies. In this regard, the effects of Sal A are somewhat different to traditional KOPrs. Major differences in these effects are reviewed in the succeeding text.

8. ANTIDEPRESSIVE EFFECTS OF SAL A

In zebra fish, swimming behavior and conditioned place preference (CPP) tests have shown that low doses of Sal A have antidepressive effects (Braida et al., 2007). It is generally accepted that the effects of Sal A on depression are not due to the effects of reduced locomotion or a reduced ability to perform tasks, particularly at the lower Sal A doses (<0.5 mg/kg) where no changes in locomotor activity are reported in rats (Carlezon et al., 2006; Chartoff et al., 2008; Morani et al., 2009). The antidepressant-like effects of Sal A have also been reported with low doses of Sal A (10 μg/kg) in rats and mice (0.001 and 10 μg/kg). At these doses, Sal A decreased immobility and increased swimming times in the FST in a KOPr-dependent and cannabinoid receptor type 1 (CB_1)-dependent manner as the effects were blocked by respective antagonists. Low-dose Sal A (0.1–40 μg/kg) also showed cocaine CPP and intracerebroventricular self-administration, suggestive of rewarding effects (Braida et al., 2009). The low doses of Sal A used in this study can potentially account for the variation in effects seen, with low-dose Sal A being considered antidepressive (Braida et al., 2007, 2008, 2009) or neutral and higher doses being considered prodepressive (Carlezon et al., 2006; Morani et al., 2012; Potter, Damez-Werno, Carlezon, Cohen, & Chartoff, 2011). DA levels in the NAcb shell were also increased with the administration of low-dose Sal A (40 μg/kg), indicative of reward. Sal A (0.1–160 μg/kg) has also been shown to have anxiolytic effects 20 min postinjection (i.p.) in rats. These effects were shown to be nor-BNI-reversible at the lowest 0.1 μg/kg dose, indicating selective KOPr-mediated effects. However, effects were also reversed by the CB_1 antagonist AM251 indicating a role of CB_1 in these effects (Braida et al., 2009). However, a more recent study has suggested that this reversal is explained by the actions of AM251 at the KOPr not CB_1 receptors (Walentiny et al., 2010). Recently, additional studies have also suggested a biphasic effect of Sal A on reward (Potter et al., 2011). Utilizing an intracranial self-stimulation (ICSS) model to measure reward sensitivity, Potter et al. (2011) showed that repeated high-dose Sal A (2 mg/kg/day) resulted in increased baseline thresholds indicating that Sal A decreased the reward-potentiating effects of a cocaine challenge. However, when the same doses used in rats and mice by Braida et al. (2009) were used in this study, no effects on ICSS baseline thresholds were seen in rats (Potter et al., 2011). A recent study by Harden et al. (2012) assessed the effects of Sal A on chronic mild stress in rats. In this study, Sal A (1 mg/kg) reversed anhedonia. The authors chose this model as it is believed to be a superior model to the FST model of depression because it does not apply the stressor at the same time as performing the test. In this same study, Sal A had no effect on sucrose intake in the absence of chronic mild stress suggesting that Sal A does not alter the hedonic effects of sucrose. This study supports the study conducted by Morani et al. (2009) where Sal A (0.3 and 1 mg/kg) also did not alter sucrose responding.

9. PRODEPRESSIVE EFFECTS OF SAL A

Activation of KOPrs by both traditional KOPr agonists and Sal A has been shown to produce prodepressive effects in laboratory animals. In the FST, Carlezon et al. (2006) showed that Sal A decreased swimming and increased immobility times following systemic administration at doses of 0.25–2 mg/kg (i.p.). Sal A also dose-dependently elevated ICSS thresholds, with significant increases seen at doses ranging from 0.5 to 2 mg/kg (i.p.) in the rat. Elevated ICSS thresholds have been shown to be representative of depressive effects in humans (Carlezon et al., 2006). No attenuation of locomotor activity was observed within these doses, consistent with other findings for Sal A, and in contrast to traditional agonists such as U69,593, which show sedative effects at similar doses. Decreased DA levels were also seen in the NAcb, at the dose where Sal A shows prodepressive effects in the FST and ICSS models. No changes in 5-HT concentrations were observed, suggesting a specific KOPr-mediated effect. This correlation suggests that decreased DA levels within the NAcb may contribute to these depressive effects.

It is clear from these studies that there are no consistent effects for Sal A in its ability to modulate both pro- and antidepressive behaviors. However, it is clear that the properties of Sal A differ from that of traditional KOPr agonists. Further studies are needed to evaluate these differences at both the behavioral and cellular levels to determine the mechanisms underlying these actions. Based on the studies listed earlier, there is evidence to suggest that Sal A has the potential to yield compounds that have anti-addictive properties without inducing depression.

10. SIGNALING PATHWAYS REGULATED BY SAL A

Some recent studies have investigated the ability of Sal A to regulate known KOPr signaling pathways and compared these with traditional KOPr agonists. The transcription factor cAMP response element-binding protein (CREB) is known to regulate dynorphin levels (Carlezon et al., 1998). Phosphorylated CREB levels in the rat have been shown to increase in the NAcb in response to stress (Pliakas et al., 2001), an effect that is behaviorally correlated to an increase in immobility in the FST, a preclinical measure of depression (Porsolt, 1979). The stress-related effects of corticotrophin-releasing factor have recently been shown to be mediated by KOPrs (Land et al., 2009). Elevations in CREB have also been shown to reduce the rewarding effects of cocaine (a measure of anhedonia). Endogenously, in the NAcb, elevated CREB-mediated dynorphin levels lead to decreased DA and prodepressive behaviors. In the presence of cocaine, the endogenous KOPr system decreases DA levels in the NAcb, opposing the actions of cocaine (and other stimulants). This is also the same mechanism hypothesized to be responsible for prodepressive effects and other undesirable effects associated with drug withdrawal. Dynorphin-mediated activation of CREB is postulated to be the cause of relapse, where drug-taking activities are resumed in order to decrease the adverse effects of withdrawal. For a recent review on the role of CREB and dynorphin, see Muschamp and Carlezon (2013). The role of Sal A in modulating CREB levels remains to be determined. One study has shown that acute Sal A (2 mg/kg) does not change CREB protein levels in the NAcb or caudate putamen but repeated Sal A increases CREB activation in the NAcb of the rat (Potter et al., 2011).

CREB is activated by extracellular signal-regulated kinases (ERK1/2), and both KOPr and DAT proteins have been shown to signal via ERK1/2 pathways (Potter et al., 2011; Rothman, Dersch, Carroll, & Ananthan, 2002; Yoshizawa et al., 2011). Activation of ERK1/2 leads to an increase in DAT function and cell-surface expression (Bolan et al., 2007; Moron et al., 2003), and ERK1/2 inhibitors (but not P38 mitogen-activated protein kinase (MAPK) inhibitors) cause a concentration- and time-dependent decrease in DA uptake, an effect shown to be due to decreased DAT cell-surface expression (Moron et al., 2003). ERK1/2 activation is known to have both β-arrestin-dependent and β-arrestin-independent phases (McLennan et al., 2008). The early ERK1/2 activation phase (5–15 min) is via activation of Gβγ-subunits that are phosphoinositide-3-kinase-, Ca^{2+}-, and protein kinase-ç-dependent (Belcheva et al., 2005), whereas the late ERK1/2 activation phase (2 h) requires recruitment of β-arrestin (McLennan et al., 2008). Both acute and repeated Sal A increased ERK1/2 phosphorylation in the NAcb. Acute Sal A increased ERK1/2 phosphorylation rapidly at 15 min, while repeated Sal A induced a delayed increase in ERK1/2 phosphorylation (Potter et al., 2011).

P38-α MAPK activation by KOPr agonists in the dorsal raphe has been shown to be required for KOPr-mediated dysphoria (Land et al., 2009) and behavioral stress effects in the mouse (Bruchas et al., 2011). This is also believed to require β-arrestin recruitment (Bruchas et al., 2007). In theory, should this hold true, then KOPr agonists that do not activate P38-α MAPK or β-arrestin may be devoid of dysphoric effects (Muschamp, Van't Veer, & Carlezon, 2011). Previous studies have shown that MOM Sal B fails to recruit β-arrestin (Beguin et al., 2012), but Morani et al. (manuscript submitted for review) still report prodepressive effects in the rat with MOM Sal B (0.3 mg/kg) (i.p.) in the FST with the same dose that displayed anti-addictive effects. The differences seen between assays may be due in part to the pharmacokinetic properties of MOM Sal B. However, there is little information on the signaling pathways activated by Sal A and even less is known about the signaling pathways of novel Sal A analogs. The correlation between cellular, behavioral, and pharmacokinetic effects is likely to lead to a better understanding of the complex signaling mechanisms responsible for both the desired anti-addictive effects and unwanted side effects.

11. PHARMACOKINETICS OF SAL A

Sal A is well known to have a short half-life and rapid onset of action (Butelman et al., 2009; Hooker et al., 2008; Ranganathan et al., 2012; Teksin et al., 2009). Behavioral studies in humans consistently report very short-lasting psychoactive effects with the onset of seconds to minutes (MacLean, Johnson, Reissig, Prisinzano, & Griffiths, 2013). Sal A concentration in plasma peaks at 10 min and returns to baseline within 30 min (Ranganathan et al., 2012). In primates, Sal A had peak effects on facial relaxation and ptosis at between 5 and 15 min following s.c. injection and 1–2 min following intravenous administration of Sal A (0.001–0.032 mg/kg) (Butelman et al., 2010). Teksin et al. (2009) showed that following a 10 mg/kg dose of Sal A, the T_{max} was 10–15 min in both plasma and brain with a half-life of 36 min in the brain. This study also showed that Sal A increased the activity of permeability glycoprotein ATPase activity suggesting that it is a substrate for this protein (Teksin et al., 2009). These studies correlate well with behavioral data in animals showing that Sal A pretreatment of longer than 20 min often failed to have behavioral effects. Characterization of new Sal A analogs with longer-acting effects has the potential to lead to new more effective KOPr-activating compounds with improved pharmacokinetics to Sal A.

12. SAL A ANALOGS

One of the most important factors to consider in the development of Sal A analogs is an improved pharmacokinetic profile. With this in mind, several groups have utilized the neoclerodane diterpene structure of Sal A to develop novel compounds with varying opioid-binding properties (Lovell et al., 2012; Munro, Rizzacasa, Roth, Toth, & Yan, 2005; Prevatt-Smith et al., 2011; Prisinzano, 2009; Prisinzano & Rothman, 2008; Tidgewell et al., 2004; Valdes, Chang, Visger, & Koreeda, 2001; Vortherms & Roth, 2006) (reviewed in Grundmann, Phipps, Zadezensky, and Butterweck (2007)).

Ethoxymethyl ether salvinorin B (EOM Sal B) and methoxymethyl ether salvinorin B (MOM Sal B) are two potent and selective analogs with C-2 substitutions (Fig. 12.1). Both MOM Sal B and EOM Sal B have been shown to have a longer half-life *in vivo* compared to Sal A (Baker et al., 2009; Wang et al., 2008). Hooker, Patel, Kothari, and Schiffer (2009) compared EOM Sal B to the parent compound Sal A and showed that EOM Sal B had increased metabolic stability and decreased plasma protein affinity, which are likely mechanisms for its increased duration of effects (Hooker et al., 2009).

In vitro studies indicate that MOM Sal B is five- and sevenfold more potent at KOPr in GTP-γS assays than U50,488 and Sal A, respectively (Wang et al., 2008). EOM Sal B and MOM Sal B have increased binding to KOPr compared to Sal A (Munro et al., 2008), and MOM Sal B has been shown to be longer-acting *in vivo* than Sal A in hotplate and hypothermic assays in the rat (Wang, 2008). In a study by Hooker (2009), EOM Sal B gave threefold higher levels in the brain 65 min following i.p. injection, indicating slower metabolism. A recent study by Peet and Baker (2011) compared MOM Sal B and EOM Sal B for their ability to produce discriminative stimulus effects in rats trained to discriminate Sal A. The discrimination assays are a method to investigate similarities between known drugs of abuse and novel compounds with respect to their interoceptive stimulus properties. Male Sprague–Dawley rats were trained to discriminate Sal A (2 mg/kg) from vehicle (75% DMSO, 25% water) prior to stimulus generalization testing with EOM Sal B and MOM Sal B. Time course tests showed that both EOM Sal B and MOM Sal B had greater potency and substituted fully for U50,488 and Sal A (Peet & Baker, 2011). It is also worth

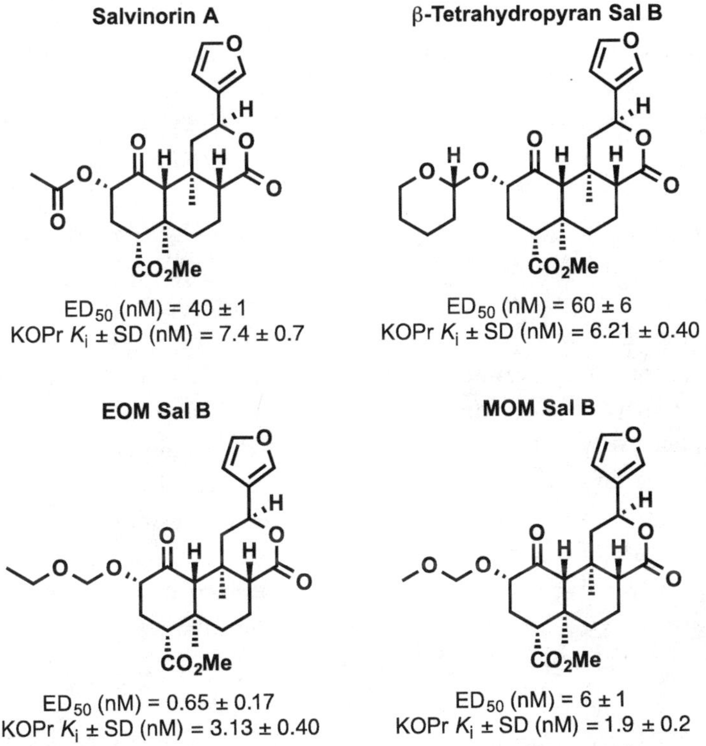

Figure 12.1 Kappa-opioid receptor agonists. Opioid receptor binding ([^{3}H] U69,593) in CHO cells expressing human KOP receptors ($K_i \pm$ SD nM). ED$_{50}$ = effective dose for 50% of maximal response in [^{35}S] GTP-γS binding. *Data for EOM Sal B, MOM Sal B, and β-tetrahydropyran Sal B taken from Prevatt-Smith et al. (2011) and data for Sal A taken from Lozama et al. (2011).*

noting that, although EOM Sal B (ED$_{50}$ 0.65 nM) is 10 times more potent (ED$_{50}$ in GTP-γS assays) than MOM Sal B (ED$_{50}$ 6 nM) *in vitro* (Munro et al., 2008), the study by Peet and Baker (2011) did not show this magnitude of effect *in vivo*. Therefore, further characterization of effects *in vivo* is necessary to identify the bioavailability and pharmacokinetic effects of these Sal A analogs. To our knowledge, this is the first study showing that the synthetic derivatives of Sal A produce similar discriminative stimulus effects. Differences between Sal A, EOM Sal B, and MOM Sal B were also noted, in that, unlike Sal A, they also partially substituted for ketamine and lysergic acid diethylamide (LSD). It remains to be determined if these compounds have other differences *in vivo* including anti–addictive effects and effects on mood, locomotion, and aversion.

In an attempt to address these important issues (Morani et al., 2013), we tested the effects of MOM Sal B on cocaine-seeking behavior using the cocaine prime-induced reinstatement paradigm in rats. We also investigated the side effects of MOM Sal B such as modulation of motor function (spontaneous locomotion and cocaine-induced hyperactivity), reward reinforcement (sucrose reinforcement), aversion (conditioned taste aversion), and depression (FST). These results were consistent with the effects previously reported for Sal A (Morani et al., 2009, 2012). This study showed that MOM Sal B (0.3 mg/kg) attenuated cocaine primed-induced reinstatement in a similar way to Sal A (0.3 mg/kg), with no change in activity in either cocaine-induced hyperactivity or spontaneous open-field activity tests. However, MOM Sal B, unlike Sal A, attenuated sucrose reinforcement indicating that its anti-addictive effects may be nonspecific, by altering natural reward pathways. Increased immobility and decreased swimming times in the FST were also observed. This indicates that MOM Sal B has an improved side effect profile compared to traditional KOPr agonists; however, prodepressive effects and effects on natural reward remain. MOM Sal B has a much higher potency in GTP-γS assays at KOPr receptors ($ED_{50} = 6 \pm 1$) compared to Sal A ($ED_{50} = 40$ nM ± 10), and this may be responsible for the increased side effects seen in this study.

Recently, a novel Sal A analog lacking a hydrolysable ester at C-2, a modification that is likely to yield longer-acting compound, was synthesized (Wang et al., 2008). β-Tetrahydropyran Sal B (Fig. 12.1) was also shown to have anti-addictive effects using the preclinical self-administration model of cocaine prime-induced relapse (Prevatt-Smith et al., 2011). β-Tetrahydropyran Sal B attenuated cocaine prime-induced drug-seeking behavior at a dose of 1 mg/kg in a similar way to Sal A (0.3 mg/kg). The increased dose required to see these effects may be explained by differences in absorption, distribution, metabolism, and excretion as β-tetrahydropyran Sal B has similar potency in GTP-γS assays ($ED_{50} = 60$ nM ± 6) to Sal A ($ED_{50} = 40$ nM ± 10).

These findings form the proof of principal that Sal A analogs have anti-addictive effects. It remains to be determined if these compounds also have improved side effect profiles. It is clear from these behavioral results that highly potent selective KOPr agonists such as MOM Sal B, while having reduced side effects compared to traditional KOPrs, still exhibit undesirable prodepressive effects, which are likely to limit their therapeutic utility. However, valuable information gained will aid the development of further compounds and develop a selection criterion for additional compounds to test preclinically.

Partial agonists or functional agonists that are able to activate signaling pathways differentially may hold the key to the discovery of analogs with anti-addictive effects without unwanted side effects. No derivatives of Sal A have been identified as KOPr partial agonists or antagonists to date. It is possible, by studying the signaling activity of Sal A and novel analogs, particularly with their abilities to recruit β-arrestin and induce phosphorylation of kinases including ERK(1/2) and P38, that compounds with the desired effects may be identified. In order to do this, further studies on KOPr signaling pathways is needed.

13. CONCLUSION

Recent studies have investigated the preclinical effects of Sal A on behaviors such as reward, aversion, and depression. However, many of these studies show conflicting results. It has become clear that the choice of behavioral model, dose of Sal A administered, and duration of Sal A administration is responsible for the majority of the differences seen. While high doses of Sal A cause side effects typical of traditional KOPr agonists, lower doses of Sal A do not present these effects. It is therefore exciting to note that the anti-addictive/antireward effects of Sal A are present at levels below the threshold of many known side effects such as sedation, aversion, and attenuation of natural reward. Although Sal A has been found to display prodepressive effects, the reduced side effect profile of Sal A compared to classic KOPr agonists makes Sal A a compound of high therapeutic promise in treating drug abuse.

The potential of Sal A as a pharmacotherapy can be further determined by characterization of the cellular signaling pathways responsible for each of these behavioral effects seen and whether it is, in fact, possible to separate these undesirable side effects from the anti-addictive effects. It has been hypothesized that partial KOPr agonists or "functional agonists" that are able to activate signaling pathways differentially may hold the key to the development of anti-addictive compounds without the side effects. Recently, p38 activation, β-arrestin recruitment, and late activation of ERK have been identified as potential candidates responsible for undesirable side effects. Sal A analogs have recently been synthesized in an effort to improve the behavioral effects and pharmacokinetic properties of Sal A. None of these derivatives have been identified as KOPr partial agonists or antagonists to date. However, as there is currently limited information on the behavioral effects and cellular signaling pathways of these compounds, the potential of these analogs as an anti-addictive therapy remains to be seen. Further studies in this field are warranted as Sal A and its analogs hold definite promise as treatments for drug abuse.

CONFLICT OF INTEREST

The authors have no conflicts of interest to declare.

REFERENCES

Acri, J. B., Thompson, A. C., & Shippenberg, T. (2001). Modulation of pre- and postsynaptic dopamine D2 receptor function by the selective kappa-opioid receptor agonist U69593. Synapse, 39(4), 343–350.

Avidorreiss, T., Zippel, R., Levy, R., Saya, D., Ezra, V., Barg, J., et al. (1995). Kappa-opioid receptor-transfected cell-lines—Modulation of adenylyl-cyclase activity following acute and chronic opioid treatments. FEBS Letters, 361(1), 70–74.

Baker, L. E., Panos, J. J., Killinger, B. A., Peet, M. M., Bell, L. M., Haliw, L. A., et al. (2009). Comparison of the discriminative stimulus effects of salvinorin A and its derivatives to U69,593 and U50,488 in rats. Psychopharmacology, 203(2), 203–211.

Beardsley, P. M., Pollard, G. T., Howard, J. L., & Carroll, F. I. (2010). Effectiveness of analogs of the kappa opioid receptor antagonist (3R)-7-hydroxy-N-((1S)-1-{[(3R,4R)-4-(3-hydroxyphenyl)-3,4-dimethyl-1-piperidinyl]methyl}-2-methylpropyl)-1,2,3,4-tetrahydro-3-isoquinolinecarboxamide (JDTic) to reduce U50,488-induced diuresis and stress-induced cocaine reinstatement in rats. Psychopharmacology, 210(2), 189–198.

Beguin, C., Potuzak, J., Xu, W., Liu-Chen, L.-Y., Streicher, J. M., Groer, C. E., et al. (2012). Differential signaling properties at the kappa opioid receptor of 12-epi-salvinorin A and its analogues. Bioorganic & Medicinal Chemistry Letters, 22(2), 1023–1026.

Belcheva, M. M., Clark, A. L., Haas, P. D., Serna, J. S., Hahn, J. W., Kiss, A., et al. (2005). mu and kappa opioid receptors activate ERK/MAPK via different protein kinase c isoforms and secondary messengers in astrocytes. Journal of Biological Chemistry, 280(30), 27662–27669.

Boja, J. W., & Kuhar, M. J. (1989). [³H]Cocaine binding and inhibition of [³H]dopamine uptake is similar in both the rat striatum and nucleus accumbens. European Journal of Pharmacology, 173, 215–217.

Bolan, E. A., Kivell, B., Jaligam, V., Oz, M., Jayanthi, L. D., Han, Y., et al. (2007). D-2 receptors regulate dopamine transporter function via an extracellular signal-regulated kinases 1 and 2-dependent and phosphoinositide 3 kinase-independent mechanism. Molecular Pharmacology, 71(5), 1222–1232.

Braida, D., Capurro, V., Zani, A., Rubino, T., Vigano, D., Parolaro, D., et al. (2009). Potential anxiolytic- and antidepressant-like effects of salvinorin A, the main active ingredient of Salvia Divinorum, in rodents. British Journal of Pharmacology, 157(5), 844–853.

Braida, D., Limonta, V., Capurro, V., Fadda, P., Rubino, T., Mascia, P., et al. (2008). Involvement of kappa-opioid and endocannabinoid system on salvinorin A-induced reward. Biological Psychiatry, 63(3), 286–292.

Braida, D., Limonta, V., Pegorini, S., Zani, A., Guerini-Rocco, C., Gori, E., et al. (2007). Hallucinatory and rewarding effect of salvinorin A in zebrafish: Kappa-opioid and CB1-cannabinoid receptor involvement. Psychopharmacology, 190(4), 441–448.

Bruchas, M. R., Land, B. B., Aita, M., Xu, M., Barot, S. K., Li, S., et al. (2007). Stress-induced p38 mitogen-activated protein kinase activation mediates kappa-opioid-dependent dysphoria. *Journal of Neuroscience, 27*(43), 11614–11623.

Bruchas, M., Land, B., & Chavkin, C. (2010). The dynorphin/kappa opioid system as a modulator of stress-induced and pro-addictive behaviors. *Brain Research, 1314*, 44–55.

Bruchas, M. R., Land, B. B., Lemos, J. C., & Chavkin, C. (2009). CRF1-R activation of the dynorphin/kappa opioid system in the mouse basolateral amygdala mediates anxiety-like behavior. *PLoS ONE, 4*(12), e8528.

Bruchas, M. R., Schindler, A. G., Shankar, H., Messinger, D. I., Miyatake, M., Land, B. B., et al. (2011). Selective p38 alpha MAPK deletion in serotonergic neurons produces stress resilience in models of depression and addiction. *Neuron, 71*(3), 498–511.

Butelman, E. R., Harris, T. J., & Kreek, M. J. (2004). The plant-derived hallucinogen, salvinorin A, produces kappa-opioid agonist-like discriminative effects in rhesus monkeys. *Psychopharmacology, 172*(2), 220–224.

Butelman, E. R., Mandau, M., Tidgewell, K., Prisinzano, T. E., Yuferov, V., & Kreek, M. J. (2007). Effects of salvinorin A, a kappa-opioid hallucinogen, on a neuroendocrine biomarker assay in nonhuman primates with high kappa-receptor homology to humans. *Journal of Pharmacology and Experimental Therapeutics, 320*(1), 300–306.

Butelman, E. R., Prisinzano, T. E., Deng, H., Rus, S., & Kreek, M. J. (2009). Unconditioned behavioral effects of the powerful kappa-opioid hallucinogen salvinorin A in nonhuman primates: Fast onset and entry into cerebrospinal fluid. *Journal of Pharmacology and Experimental Therapeutics, 328*(2), 588–597.

Butelman, E. R., Rus, S., Prisinzano, T. E., & Kreek, M. J. (2010). The discriminative effects of the kappa-opioid hallucinogen salvinorin A in nonhuman primates: Dissociation from classic hallucinogen effects. *Psychopharmacology, 210*(2), 253–262.

Butelman, E. R., Yuferov, V., & Kreek, M. J. (2012). Kappa-opioid receptor/dynorphin system: Genetic and pharmacotherapeutic implications for addiction. *Trends in Neurosciences, 35*(10), 587–596.

Carlezon, W. A., Beguin, C., DiNieri, J. A., Baumann, M. H., Richards, M. R., Todtenkopf, M. S., et al. (2006). Depressive-like effects of the kappa-opioid receptor agonist salvinorin A on behavior and neurochemistry in rats. *Journal of Pharmacology and Experimental Therapeutics, 316*(1), 440–447.

Carlezon, W. A., Jr., Thome, J., Olson, V. G., Lane-Ladd, S. B., Brodkin, E. S., Hiroi, N., et al. (1998). Regulation of cocaine reward by CREB. *Science, 282*(5397), 2272–2275.

Carroll, F. I., & Carlezon, W. A. Jr. (2013). Development of kappa-opioid receptor antagonists. *Journal of Medicinal Chemistry, 56*(6), 2178–2195. http://www.ncbi.nlm.nih.gov/pubmed/23360448.

Chartoff, E. H., Potter, D., Damez-Werno, D., Cohen, B. M., & Carlezon, W. A. (2008). Exposure to the selective kappa-opioid receptor agonist salvinorin A modulates the behavioral and molecular effects of cocaine in rats. *Neuropsychopharmacology, 33*(11), 2676–2687.

Chartoff, E., Sawyer, A., Rachlin, A., Potter, D., Pliakas, A., & Carlezon, W. A. (2012). Blockade of kappa opioid receptors attenuates the development of depressive-like behaviors induced by cocaine withdrawal in rats. *Neuropharmacology, 62*(1), 167–176.

Chavkin, C. (2011). The therapeutic potential of kappa-opioids for treatment of pain and addiction. *Neuropsychopharmacology, 36*(1), 369–370.

Chavkin, C., James, I. F., & Goldstein, A. (1982). Dynorphin is a specific endogenous ligand of the kappa-opioid receptor. *Science, 215*(4531), 413–415.

Chavkin, C., Sud, S., Jin, W. Z., Stewart, J., Zjawiony, J. K., Siebert, D. J., et al. (2004). Salvinorin A, an active component of the hallucinogenic sage Salvia divinorum is a highly efficacious kappa-opioid receptor agonist: Structural and functional considerations. *Journal of Pharmacology and Experimental Therapeutics, 308*(3), 1197–1203.

Chefer, V. I., Czyzyk, T., Bolan, E. A., Moron, J., Pintar, J. E., & Shippenberg, T. S. (2005). Endogenous kappa-opioid receptor systems regulate mesoaccumbal dopamine dynamics and vulnerability to cocaine. *Journal of Neuroscience, 25*(20), 5029–5037.

Chefer, V. I., Moron, J. A., Hope, B., Rea, W., & Shippenberg, T. S. (2000). Kappa-opioid receptor activation prevents alterations in mesocortical dopamine neurotransmission that occur during abstinence from cocaine. *Neuroscience, 101*(3), 619–627.

Chi, L., & Reith, M. E. (2003). Substrate-induced trafficking of the dopamine transporter in heterologously expressing cells and in rat striatal synaptosomal preparations. *The Journal of Pharmacology and Experimental Therapeutics, 307*(2), 729–736.

Collins, S. L., D'Addario, C., & Izenwasser, S. (2001). Effects of kappa-opioid receptor agonists on long-term cocaine use and dopamine neurotransmission. *European Journal of Pharmacology, 426*(1–2), 25–34.

Collins, S. L., Kunko, P. M., Ladenheim, B., Cadet, J. L., Carroll, F. I., & Izenwasser, S. (2002). Chronic cocaine increases kappa-opioid receptor density: Lack of effect by selective dopamine uptake inhibitors. *Synapse, 45*(3), 153–158.

Daunais, J. B., Roberts, D. C. S., & McGinty, J. F. (1993). Cocaine self-administration increases preprodynorphin, but not c-fos, messenger-RNA in rat striatum. *Neuroreport, 4*(5), 543–546.

Dichiara, G., & Imperato, A. (1988). Opposite effects of mu-opiate and kappa-opiate agonists on dopamine release in the nucleus accumbens and in the dorsal caudate of freely moving rats. *Journal of Pharmacology and Experimental Therapeutics, 244*(3), 1067–1080.

Dykstra, L., Gmerek, D. E., Winger, G., & Woods, J. H. (1987). Kappa opioids in rhesus monkeys. I. Diuresis, sedation, analgesia and discriminative stimulus effects. *Journal of Pharmacology and Experimental Therapeutics, 242*(2), 413–420.

Ebner, S. R., Roitman, M. F., Potter, D. N., Rachlin, A. B., & Chartoff, E. H. (2010). Depressive-like effects of the kappa opioid receptor agonist salvinorin A are associated with decreased phasic dopamine release in the nucleus accumbens. *Psychopharmacology, 210*(2), 241–252.

El Daly, E., Chefer, V., Sandill, S., & Shippenberg, T. S. (2000). Modulation of the neurotoxic effects of methamphetamine by the selective kappa-opioid receptor agonist U69593. *Journal of Neurochemistry, 74*(4), 1553–1562.

Epling, C., & Jativa-M, C. D. (1962). A new species of Salvia S. divinorum sp. nov. (Labiatae) from Mexico. *Botanical Museum Leaflets, Harvard University, 20*(3), 75–76.

Fagergren, P., Smith, H. R., Daunais, J. B., Nader, M. A., Porrino, L. J., & Hurd, Y. L. (2003). Temporal upregulation of prodynorphin mRNA in the primate striatum after cocaine self-administration. *European Journal of Neuroscience, 17*(10), 2212–2218.

Furman, C. A., Chen, R., Guptaroy, B., Zhang, M., Holz, R. W., & Gnegy, M. (2009). Dopamine and amphetamine rapidly increase dopamine transporter trafficking to the surface: Live-cell imaging using total internal reflection fluorescence microscopy. *Journal of Neuroscience, 29*(10), 3328–3336.

Gehrke, B. J., Chefer, V. I., & Shippenberg, T. S. (2008). Effects of acute and repeated administration of salvinorin A on dopamine function in the rat dorsal striatum. *Psychopharmacology, 197*(3), 509–517.

Glick, S. D., Maisonneuve, I. M., Raucci, J., & Archer, S. (1995). Kappa opioid inhibition of morphine and cocaine self-administration in rats. *Brain Research, 681*, 147–152.

Gramsch, C., Hollt, V., Pasi, A., Mehraein, P., & Herz, A. (1982). Immunoreactive dynorphin in human-brain and pituitary. *Brain Research, 233*(1), 65–74.

Grilli, M., Neri, E., Zappettini, S., Massa, F., Bisio, A., Romussi, G., et al. (2009). Salvinorin A exerts opposite presynaptic controls on neurotransmitter exocytosis from mouse brain nerve terminals. *Neuropharmacology, 57*(5–6), 523–530.

Groer, C. E., Tidgewell, K., Moyer, R. A., Harding, W. W., Rothman, R. B., Prisinzano, T. E., et al. (2007). An opioid agonist that does not induce mu-opioid receptor—Arrestin interactions or receptor internalization. *Molecular Pharmacology, 71*(2), 549–557.

Grundmann, O., Phipps, S. M., Zadezensky, I., & Butterweck, V. (2007). Salvia divinorum and salvinorin A: An update on pharmacology and analytical methodology. *Planta Medica, 73*(10), 1039–1046.

Gulley, J. M., Doolen, S., & Zahniser, N. R. (2002). Brief, repeated exposure to substrates down-regulates dopamine transporter function in Xenopus oocytes in vitro and rat dorsal striatum in vivo. *Journal of Neurochemistry, 83*(2), 400–411.

Guo, S., Zhou, D. F., Sun, H. Q., Wu, G. Y., Haile, C. N., Kosten, T. A., et al. (2007). Association of functional catechol O-methyl transferase (COMT) Val108Met polymorphism with smoking severity and age of smoking initiation in Chinese male smokers. *Psychopharmacology, 190*(4), 449–456.

Hanes, K. R. (2001). Antidepressant effects of the herb salvia divinorum: A case report. *Journal of Clinical Psychopharmacology, 21*(6), 634–635.

Harden, M. T., Smith, S. E., Niehoff, J. A., McCurdy, C. R., & Taylor, G. T. (2012). Antidepressive effects of the kappa-opioid receptor agonist salvinorin A in a rat model of anhedonia. *Behavioural Pharmacology, 23*(7), 710–715.

Heidbreder, C. A., Babovicvuksanovic, D., Shoaib, M., & Shippenberg, T. S. (1995). Development of behavioral sensitization to cocaine—Influence of kappa-opioid receptor agonists. *Journal of Pharmacology and Experimental Therapeutics, 275*(1), 150–163.

Heidbreder, C. A., Schenk, S., Partridge, B., & Shippenberg, T. S. (1998). Increased responsiveness of mesolimbic and mesostriatal dopamine neurons to cocaine following repeated administration of a selective kappa-opioid receptor agonist. *Synapse, 30*(3), 255–262.

Heyliger, S. O., Jackson, C., Rice, K. C., & Rothman, R. B. (1999). Opioid peptide receptor studies. 10. Nor-BNI differentially inhibits kappa receptor agonist-induced G-protein activation in the guinea pig caudate: Further evidence of kappa receptor heterogeneity. *Synapse, 34*(4), 256–265.

Hooker, J. M., Patel, V., Kothari, S., & Schiffer, W. K. (2009). Metabolic changes in the rodent brain after acute administration of salvinorin A. *Molecular Imaging and Biology, 11*(3), 137–143.

Hooker, J. M., Xu, Y., Schiffer, W., Shea, C., Carter, P., & Fowler, J. S. (2008). Pharmacokinetics of the potent hallucinogen, salvinorin A in primates parallels the rapid onset and short duration of effects in humans. *NeuroImage, 41*(3), 1044–1050.

Horan, P. J., Decosta, B. R., Rice, K., Haaseth, R. C., Hruby, V. J., & Porreca, F. (1993). Differential antagonism of bremazocine-induced and U69,593-induced antinociception by quadazocine—Further functional evidence of opioid kappa-receptor multiplicity in the mouse. *Journal of Pharmacology and Experimental Therapeutics, 266*(2), 926–933.

Hurd, Y. L., & Herkenham, M. (1993). Molecular alterations in the neostriatum of human cocaine addicts. *Synapse, 13*(4), 357–369.

Jackisch, R., Hotz, H., & Hertting, G. (1993). No evidence for presynaptic opioid receptors on cholinergic, but presence of kappa-receptors on dopaminergic-neurons in the rabbit caudate-nucleus—Involvement of endogenous opioids. *Naunyn-Schmiedebergs Archives of Pharmacology, 348*(3), 234–241.

Johnson, M. W., MacLean, K. A., Reissig, C. J., Prisinzano, T. E., & Griffiths, R. R. (2011). Human psychopharmacology and dose-effects of salvinorin A, a kappa opioid agonist hallucinogen present in the plant Salvia divinorum. *Drug and Alcohol Dependence, 115*(1–2), 150–155.

Killinger, B. A., Peet, M. M., & Baker, L. E. (2010). Salvinorin A fails to substitute for the discriminative stimulus effects of LSD or ketamine in Sprague–Dawley rats. *Pharmacology, Biochemistry, and Behavior, 96*(3), 260–265.

Kivell, B., & Prisinzano, T. E. (2010). Kappa opioids and the modulation of pain. *Psychopharmacology, 210*(2), 109–119.

Knoll, A. T., & Carlezon, W. A., Jr. (2010). Dynorphin, stress, and depression. *Brain Research*, *1314*, 56–73.

Koob, G. F. (2008). A role for brain stress systems in addiction. *Neuron*, *59*(1), 11–34.

Koob, G. F., & Le Moal, M. (2008). Addiction and the brain antireward system. *Annual Review of Psychology*, *59*, 29–53.

Kreek, M. J. (1996). Cocaine, dopamine and the endogenous opioid system. *Journal of Addictive Diseases*, *15*(4), 73–96.

Land, B. B., Bruchas, M. R., Schattauer, S., Giardino, W. J., Aita, M., Messinger, D., et al. (2009). Activation of the kappa opioid receptor in the dorsal raphe nucleus mediates the aversive effects of stress and reinstates drug seeking. *Proceedings of the National Academy of Sciences of the United States of America*, *106*(45), 19168–19173.

Liu-Chen, L. Y. (2004). Agonist-induced regulation and trafficking of kappa opioid receptors. *Life Sciences*, *75*(5), 511–536.

Lovell, K. M., Vasiljevik, T., Araya, J. J., Lozama, A., Prevatt-Smith, K. M., Day, V. W., et al. (2012). Semisynthetic neoclerodanes as kappa opioid receptor probes. *Bioorganic & Medicinal Chemistry*, *20*(9), 3100–3110.

Lozama, A., Cunningham, C. W., Caspers, M. J., Douglas, J. T., Dersch, C. M., Rothman, R. B., et al. (2011). Opioid receptor probes derived from cycloaddition of the hallucinogen natural product salvinorin A. *Journal of Natural Products*, *74*(4), 718–726.

MacLean, K. A., Johnson, M. W., Reissig, C. J., Prisinzano, T. E., & Griffiths, R. R. (2013). Dose-related effects of salvinorin A in humans: Dissociative, hallucinogenic, and memory effects. *Psychopharmacology*, *226*(2), 381–392.

Margolis, E. B., Hjelmstad, G. O., Bonci, A., & Fields, H. L. (2003). Kappa-opioid agonists directly inhibit midbrain dopaminergic neurons. *Journal of Neuroscience*, *23*(31), 9981–9986.

Marinova, Z., Vukojevic, V., Surcheva, S., Yakovleva, T., Cebers, G., Pasikova, N., et al. (2005). Translocation of dynorphin neuropeptides across the plasma membrane—A putative mechanism of signal transmission. *Journal of Biological Chemistry*, *280*(28), 26360–26370.

McCurdy, C. R., Sufka, K. J., Smith, G. H., Warnick, J. E., & Nieto, M. J. (2006). Antinociceptive profile of salvinorin A, a structurally unique kappa opioid receptor agonist. *Pharmacology, Biochemistry, and Behavior*, *83*(1), 109–113.

McLennan, G. P., Kiss, A., Miyatake, M., Belcheva, M. M., Chambers, K. T., Pozek, J. J., et al. (2008). Kappa opioids promote the proliferation of astrocytes via G beta gamma and beta-arrestin 2-dependent MAPK-mediated pathways. *Journal of Neurochemistry*, *107*(6), 1753–1765.

Mello, N. K., & Negus, S. S. (1998). Effects of kappa opioid agonists on cocaine- and food-maintained responding by rhesus monkeys. *Journal of Pharmacology and Experimental Therapeutics*, *286*(2), 812–824.

Mello, N. K., & Negus, S. S. (2000). Interactions between kappa opioid agonists and cocaine. Preclinical studies. *Annals of the New York Academy of Sciences*, *909*, 104–132.

Merg, F., Filliol, D., Usynin, I., Bazov, I., Bark, N., Hurd, Y. L., et al. (2006). Big dynorphin as a putative endogenous ligand for the kappa-opioid receptor. *Journal of Neurochemistry*, *97*(1), 292–301.

Mitchell, J. M., Liang, M. T., & Fields, H. I. (2005). A single injection of the kappa opioid antagonist norbinaltorphimine increases ethanol consumption in rats. *Psychopharmacology*, *182*, 384–392.

Morani, A. S., Kivell, B., Prisinzano, T. E., & Schenk, S. (2009). Effect of kappa-opioid receptor agonists U69593, U50488H, spiradoline and salvinorin A on cocaine-induced drug-seeking in rats. *Pharmacology, Biochemistry, and Behavior*, *94*(2), 244–249.

Morani, A. S., Schenk, S., Prisinzano, T. E., & Kivell, B. M. (2012). A single injection of a novel kappa opioid receptor agonist salvinorin A attenuates the expression of cocaine-induced behavioral sensitization in rats. *Behavioural Pharmacology*, *23*(2), 162–170.

Morani, A. S., Ewald, A., Prevatt-Smith, K. M., Prisinzano, T. E., & Kivell, B. M. (2013). The 2-methoxy methyl analogue of salvinorin A attenuates cocaine-induced drug seeking and sucrose reinforcements in rats. *European Journal of Pharmacology*, *720*(1–3), 69–76.

Mori, T., Yoshizawa, K., Ueno, T., Nishiwaki, M., Shimizu, N., Shibasaki, M., et al. (2013). Involvement of dopamine D2 receptor signal transduction in the discriminative stimulus effects of the kappa-opioid receptor agonist U-50,488H in rats. *Behavioural Pharmacology*, *24*(4), 275–281.

Moron, J. A., Zakharova, I., Ferrer, J. V., Merrill, G. A., Hope, B., Lafer, E. M., et al. (2003). Mitogen-activated protein kinase regulates dopamine transporter surface expression and dopamine transport capacity. *Journal of Neuroscience*, *23*(24), 8480–8488.

Munro, T. A., Duncan, K. K., Xu, W., Wang, Y., Liu-Chen, L.-Y., Carlezon, W. A., Jr., et al. (2008). Standard protecting groups create potent and selective kappa opioids: Salvinorin B alkoxymethyl ethers. *Bioorganic & Medicinal Chemistry*, *16*(3), 1279–1286.

Munro, T. A., Rizzacasa, M. A., Roth, B. L., Toth, B. A., & Yan, F. (2005). Studies toward the pharmacophore of salvinorin A, a potent kappa opioid receptor agonist. *Journal of Medicinal Chemistry*, *48*(2), 345–348.

Muschamp, J. W., & Carlezon, W. A., Jr. (2013). Roles of nucleus accumbens CREB and dynorphin in dysregulation of motivation. *Cold Spring Harbor Perspectives in Medicine*, *3*(2), a012005.

Muschamp, J. W., Van't Veer, A., & Carlezon, W. A., Jr. (2011). Tracking down the molecular substrates of stress: New roles for p38alpha MAPK and kappa-opioid receptors. *Neuron*, *71*(3), 383–385.

Negus, S. S., Mello, N. K., Portoghese, P. S., & Lin, C. E. (1997). Effects of kappa opioids on cocaine self-administration by rhesus monkeys. *Journal of Pharmacology and Experimental Therapeutics*, *282*(1), 44–55.

Nestler, E. J. (2001). Molecular basis of long-term plasticity underlying addiction. *Nature Reviews. Neuroscience*, *2*(2), 119–128.

Nestler, E. J., & Carlezon, W. A. (2006). The mesolimbic dopamine reward circuit in depression. *Biological Psychiatry*, *59*(12), 1151–1159.

Nirenberg, M. J., Chan, J., Pohorille, A., Vaughan, R. A., Uhl, G. R., Kuhar, M. J., et al. (1997). The dopamine transporter: Comparative ultrastructure of dopaminergic axons in limbic and motor compartments of the nucleus accumbens. *The Journal of Neuroscience*, *17*, 6899–6907.

Ortega, A., Blount, J. F., & Manchand, P. S. (1982). Salvinorin, a new trans-neoclerodane diterpene from Salvia divinorum (Labiatae). *Journal of the Chemical Society, Perkin Transactions 1*, 2505–2508.

Peet, M. M., & Baker, L. E. (2011). Salvinorin B derivatives, EOM-Sal B and MOM-Sal B, produce stimulus generalization in male Sprague–Dawley rats trained to discriminate salvinorin A. *Behavioural Pharmacology*, *22*(5–6), 450–457.

Perreault, M. L., Graham, D., Scattolon, S., Wang, Y., Szechtman, H., & Foster, J. A. (2007). Cotreatment with the kappa opioid agonist U69593 enhances locomotor sensitization to the D2/D3 dopamine agonist quinpirole and alters dopamine D2 receptor and prodynorphin mRNA expression in rats. *Psychopharmacology*, *194*(4), 485–496.

Pfeiffer, A., Brantl, V., Herz, A., & Emrich, H. M. (1986). Psychotomimesis mediated by kappa-opiate receptors. *Science*, *233*(4765), 774–776.

Picetti, R., Schlussman, S. D., Zhou, Y., Ray, B., Ducat, E., Yuferov, V., et al. (2013). Addictions and stress: clues for cocaine pharmacotherapies. *Current Pharmaceutical Design*, *19*(40), 7065–7080.

Pliakas, A. M., Carlson, R. R., Neve, R. L., Konradi, C., Nestler, E. J., & Carlezon, W. A., Jr. (2001). Altered responsiveness to cocaine and increased immobility in the forced swim test associated with elevated cAMP response element-binding protein expression in nucleus accumbens. *The Journal of Neuroscience*, *21*(18), 7397–7403.

Porsolt, R. D. (1979). Animal-model of depression. *Biomedicine*, *30*(3), 139–140.

Potter, D. N., Damez-Werno, D., Carlezon, W. A., Cohen, B. M., & Chartoff, E. H. (2011). Repeated exposure to the kappa-opioid receptor agonist salvinorin A modulates extracellular signal-regulated kinase and reward sensitivity. *Biological Psychiatry*, *70*(8), 744–753.

Prevatt-Smith, K. M., Lovell, K. M., Simpson, D. S., Day, V. W., Douglas, J. T., Bosch, P., et al. (2011). Potential drug abuse therapeutics derived from the hallucinogenic natural product salvinorin A. *Medicinal Chemistry Communications*, *2*(12), 1217–1222.

Prisinzano, T. E. (2009). Natural products as tools for neuroscience: Discovery and development of novel agents to treat drug abuse. *Journal of Natural Products*, *72*(3), 581–587.

Prisinzano, T. E., & Rothman, R. B. (2008). Salvinorin A analogs as probes in opioid pharmacology. *Chemical Reviews*, *108*(5), 1732–1743.

Prisinzano, T. E., Tidgewell, K., & Harding, W. W. (2005). Kappa opioids as potential treatments for stimulant dependence. *AAPS Journal*, *7*(3), E592–E599.

Ranganathan, M., Schnakenberg, A., Skosnik, P. D., Cohen, B. M., Pittman, B., Sewell, R. A., et al. (2012). Dose-related behavioral, subjective, endocrine, and psychophysiological effects of the kappa opioid agonist salvinorin A in humans. *Biological Psychiatry*, *72*(10), 871–879.

Ronken, E., Mulder, A. H., & Schoffelmeer, A. N. (1993). Interacting presynaptic kappa-opioid and GABAA receptors modulate dopamine release from rat striatal synaptosomes. *Journal of Neurochemistry*, *61*(5), 1634–1639.

Roth, B. L., Baner, K., Westkaemper, R., Siebert, D., Rice, K. C., Steinberg, S., et al. (2002). Salvinorin A: A potent naturally occurring nonnitrogenous kappa opioid selective agonist. *Proceedings of the National Academy of Sciences of the United States of America*, *99*(18), 11934–11939.

Rothman, R. B., Dersch, C. M., Carroll, F. I., & Ananthan, S. (2002). Studies of the biogenic amine transporters. VIII: Identification of a novel partial inhibitor of dopamine uptake and dopamine transporter binding. *Synapse*, *43*(4), 268–274.

Saunders, C., Ferrer, J. V., Shi, L., Chen, J., Merrill, G., Lamb, M. E., et al. (2000). Amphetamine-induced loss of human dopamine transporter activity: An internalization-dependent and cocaine-sensitive mechanism. *Proceedings of the National Academy of Sciences of the United States of America*, *97*(12), 6850–6855.

Schank, J. R., Goldstein, A. L., Rowe, K. E., King, C. E., Marusich, J. A., Wiley, J. L., et al. (2012). The kappa opioid receptor antagonist JDTic attenuates alcohol seeking and withdrawal anxiety. *Addiction Biology*, *17*, 634–647.

Scheffel, U., Pogun, S., Stathis, M., Boja, J. W., & Kuhar, M. J. (1991). *In vivo* labeling of cocaine binding sites on dopamine transporters with [³H]WIN 35,428. *The Journal of Pharmacology and Experimental Therapeutics*, *257*, 954–958.

Schenk, S., Partridge, B., & Shippenberg, T. S. (1999). U69593, a kappa-opioid agonist, decreases cocaine self-administration and decreases cocaine-produced drug-seeking. *Psychopharmacology*, *144*(4), 339–346.

Schmidt, M. D., Schmidt, M. S., Butelman, E. R., Harding, W. W., Tidgewell, K., Murry, D. J., et al. (2005). Pharmacokinetics of the plant-derived kappa-opioid hallucinogen salvinorin A in nonhuman primates. *Synapse*, *58*(3), 208–210.

Shippenberg, T. S. (2009). The dynorphin/kappa opioid receptor system: A new target for the treatment of addiction and affective disorders? *Neuropsychopharmacology*, *34*(1), 247.

Shippenberg, T. S., Balskubik, R., & Herz, A. (1993). Examination of the neurochemical substrates mediating the motivational effects of opioids—Role of the mesolimbic dopamine system and D-1 vs D-2 dopamine-receptors. *Journal of Pharmacology and Experimental Therapeutics*, *265*(1), 53–59.

Shippenberg, T. S., Bals-Kubik, R., Huber, A., & Herz, A. (1991). Neuroanatomical substrates mediating the aversive effects of D-1 dopamine receptor antagonists. *Psychopharmacology*, *103*(2), 209–214.

Shippenberg, T. S., Chefer, V. I., Zapata, A., & Heidbreder, C. A. (2001). Modulation of the behavioral and neurochemical effects of psychostimulants by kappa-opioid receptor systems. *Annals of the New York Academy of Sciences, 937*, 50–73.

Shippenberg, T. S., & Herz, A. (1987). Place preference conditioning reveals the involvement of D1-dopamine receptors in the motivational properties of mu- and kappa-opioid agonists. *Brain Research, 436*(1), 169–172.

Shippenberg, T. S., & Herz, A. (1988). Motivational effects of opioids: Influence of D-1 versus D-2 receptor antagonists. *European Journal of Pharmacology, 151*(2), 233–242.

Shippenberg, T. S., Zapata, A., & Chefer, V. I. (2007). Dynorphin and the pathophysiology of drug addiction. *Pharmacology & Therapeutics, 116*(2), 306–321.

Shirayama, Y., Ishida, H., Iwata, M., Hazama, G. I., Kawahara, R., & Duman, R. S. (2004). Stress increases dynorphin immunoreactivity in limbic brain regions and dynorphin antagonism produces antidepressant-like effects. *Journal of Neurochemistry, 90*(5), 1258–1268.

Siebert, D. J. (1994). Salvia-divinorum and salvinorin-A—New pharmacological findings. *Journal of Ethnopharmacology, 43*(1), 53–56.

Simonin, F., Gaveriaux-Ruff, C., Befort, K., Matthes, H., Lannes, B., Micheletti, G., et al. (1995). Kappa-opioid receptor in humans: cDNA and genomic cloning, chromosomal assignment, functional expression, pharmacology, and expression pattern in the central nervous system. *Proceedings of the National Academy of Sciences, 92*(15), 7006–7010.

Sivam, S. P. (1989). Cocaine selectively increases striatonigral dynorphin levels by a dopaminergic mechanism. *Journal of Pharmacology and Experimental Therapeutics, 250*(3), 818–824.

Smiley, P. L., Johnson, M., Bush, L., Gibb, J. W., & Hanson, G. R. (1990). Effects of cocaine on extrapyramidal and limbic dynorphin systems. *Journal of Pharmacology and Experimental Therapeutics, 253*(3), 938–943.

Spanagel, R., Herz, A., & Shippenberg, T. S. (1992). Opposing tonically active endogenous opioid systems modulate the mesolimbic dopaminergic pathway. *Proceedings of the National Academy of Sciences of the United States of America, 89*(6), 2046–2050.

Spangler, R., Unterwald, E. M., & Kreek, M. J. (1993). 'Binge' cocaine administration induces a sustained increase of prodynorphin mRNA in rat caudate-putamen. *Molecular Brain Research, 19*(4), 323–327.

Spangler, R., Zhou, Y., Maggos, C. E., Schlussman, S. D., Ho, A., & Kreek, M. J. (1997). Prodynorphin, proenkephalin and kappa opioid receptor mRNA responses to acute "binge" cocaine. *Brain Research. Molecular Brain Research, 44*(1), 139–142.

Spencer, R., Hruby, V., & Burks, T. (1988). Body temperature response profiles for selective mu, delta and kappa opioid agonists in restrained and unrestrained rats. *Journal of Pharmacology and Experimental Therapeutics, 246*(1), 92–101.

Su, D., Riley, J., Kiessling, W. J., Armstead, W. M., & Liu, R. (2011). Salvinorin A produces cerebrovasodilation through activation of nitric oxide synthase, κ receptor, and adenosine triphosphate-sensitive potassium channel. *Anesthesiology, 114*(2), 374.

Suzuki, T., Kishimoto, Y., Ozaki, S., & Narita, M. (2001). Mechanism of opioid dependence and interaction between opioid receptors. *European Journal of Pain (London, England), 5*, 63–65.

Svingos, A. L., Chavkin, C., Colago, E. E., & Pickel, V. M. (2001). Major coexpression of kappa-opioid receptors and the dopamine transporter in nucleus accumbens axonal profiles. *Synapse, 42*(3), 185–192.

Tang, A. H., & Collins, R. J. (1985). Behavioral-effects of a novel kappa-opioid analgesic, U-50488, in rats and rhesus-monkeys. *Psychopharmacology, 85*(3), 309–314.

Tao, R., & Auerbach, S. B. (2002). Opioid receptor subtypes differentially modulate serotonin efflux in the rat central nervous system. *Journal of Pharmacology and Experimental Therapeutics, 303*(2), 549–556.

Tao, R., & Auerbach, S. B. (2005). Mu-opioids disinhibit and kappa-opioids inhibit serotonin efflux in the dorsal raphe nucleus. *Brain Research*, *1049*(1), 70–79.

Teksin, Z. S., Lee, I. J., Nemieboka, N. N., Othman, A. A., Upreti, V. V., Hassan, H. E., et al. (2009). Evaluation of the transport, in vitro metabolism and pharmacokinetics of salvinorin A, a potent hallucinogen. *European Journal of Pharmaceutics and Biopharmaceutics*, *72*(2), 471–477.

Thompson, A. C., Zapata, A., Justice, J. B., Vaughan, R. A., Sharpe, L. G., & Shippenberg, T. S. (2000). Kappa-opioid receptor activation modifies dopamine uptake in the nucleus accumbens and opposes the effects of cocaine. *Journal of Neuroscience*, *20*(24), 9333–9340.

Tidgewell, K., Harding, W. W., Schmidt, M., Holden, K. G., Murry, D. J., & Prisinzano, T. E. (2004). A facile method for the preparation of deuterium labeled salvinorin A: Synthesis of [2,2,2-2H3]-salvinorin A. *Bioorganic & Medicinal Chemistry Letters*, *14*(20), 5099–5102.

Tjon, G. H. K., Voorn, P., Vanderschuren, L., DeVries, T. J., Michiels, N., Jonker, A. J., et al. (1997). Delayed occurrence of enhanced striatal preprodynorphin gene expression in behaviorally sensitized rats: Differential long-term effects of intermittent and chronic morphine administration. *Neuroscience*, *76*(1), 167–176.

Todtenkopf, M. S., Marcus, J. F., Portoghese, P. S., & Carlezon, W. A. (2004). Effects of kappa-opioid receptor ligands on intracranial self-stimulation in rats. *Psychopharmacology*, *172*(4), 463–470.

Trifilieff, P., & Martinez, D. (2013). Kappa-opioid receptor signaling in the striatum as a potential modulator of dopamine transmission in cocaine dependence. *Frontiers in Psychiatry*, *4*.

Tzaferis, J. A., & McGinty, J. F. (2001). Kappa opioid receptor stimulation decreases amphetamine-induced behavior and neuropeptide mRNA expression in the striatum. *Molecular Brain Research*, *93*(1), 27–35.

Unterwald, E. M., Rubenfeld, J. M., & Kreek, M. J. (1994). Repeated cocaine administration upregulates K and [mu], but not [delta], opioid receptors. *Neuroreport*, *5*(13), 1613–1616.

Valdes, L. J., 3rd., Chang, H. M., Visger, D. C., & Koreeda, M. (2001). Salvinorin C, a new neoclerodane diterpene from a bioactive fraction of the hallucinogenic Mexican mint Salvia divinorum. *Organic Letters*, *3*(24), 3935–3937.

Van't Veer, A., & Carlezon, W. A., Jr. (2013). Role of kappa-opioid receptors in stress and anxiety-related behavior. *Psychopharmacology*, *1–18*.

Vortherms, T. A., & Roth, B. L. (2006). Salvinorin A: From natural product to human therapeutics. *Molecular Interventions*, *6*(5), 257–265.

Walentiny, D. M., Vann, R. E., Warner, J. A., King, L. S., Seltzman, H. H., Navarro, H. A., et al. (2010). Kappa opioid mediation of cannabinoid effects of the potent hallucinogen, salvinorin A, in rodents. *Psychopharmacology*, *210*(2), 275–284.

Walker, B. M., Zorrilla, E. P., & Koob, G. F. (2010). Systemic kappa-opioid receptor antagonism by nor-binaltorphimine reduces dependence-induced excessive alcohol self-administration in rats. *Addiction Biology*, *16*, 116–119.

Walsh, S. L., Geter-Douglas, B., Strain, E. C., & Bigelow, G. E. (2001). Enadoline and butorphanol: Evaluation of kappa-agonists on cocaine pharmacodynamics and cocaine self-administration in humans. *Journal of Pharmacology and Experimental Therapeutics*, *299*(1), 147–158.

Walsh, S. L., Strain, E. C., Abreu, M. E., & Bigelow, G. E. (2001). Enadoline, a selective kappa opioid agonist: Comparison with butorphanol and hydromorphone in humans. *Psychopharmacology*, *157*(2), 151–162.

Wang, Y., Chen, Y., Xu, W., Lee, D. Y. W., Ma, Z., Rawls, S. M., et al. (2008). 2-Methoxymethyl-salvinorin B is a potent kappa opioid receptor agonist with longer lasting action in vivo than salvinorin A. *Journal of Pharmacology and Experimental Therapeutics*, *324*(3), 1073–1083.

Wang, Z., Ma, N., Riley, J., Armstead, W. M., & Liu, R. (2012). Salvinorin A administration after global cerebral hypoxia/ischemia preserves cerebrovascular autoregulation via kappa opioid receptor in piglets. *PLoS ONE*, 7(7), e41724.

Wang, Y. H., Sun, J. F., Tao, Y. M., Chi, Z. Q., & Liu, J. G. (2010). The role of kappa-opioid receptor activation in mediating antinociception and addiction. *Acta Pharmacologica Sinica*, 31(9), 1065–1070.

Wang, X. M., Zhou, Y., Spangler, R., Ho, A., Han, J. S., & Kreek, M. J. (1999). Acute intermittent morphine increases preprodynorphin and kappa opioid receptor mRNA levels in the rat brain. *Molecular Brain Research*, 66(1–2), 184–187.

Watson, S. J., Khachaturian, H., Coy, D., Taylor, L., & Akil, H. (1982). Dynorphin is located throughout the CNS and is often co-localized with alpha-neo-endorphin. *Life Sciences*, 31(16–1), 1773–1776.

Wee, S., & Koob, G. F. (2010). The role of the dynorphin-kappa opioid system in the reinforcing effects of drugs of abuse. *Psychopharmacology*, 210(2), 121–135.

Wee, S., Orio, L., Ghirmai, S., Cashman, J. R., & Koob, G. F. (2009). Inhibition of kappa opioid receptors attenuated increased cocaine intake in rats with extended access to cocaine. *Psychopharmacology*, 205, 565–575.

Weiss, F., Markou, A., Lorang, M. T., & Koob, G. F. (1992). Basal extracellular dopamine levels in the nucleus accumbens are decreased during cocaine withdrawal after unlimited-access self-administration. *Brain Research*, 593(2), 314–318.

Werling, L. L., Frattali, A., Portoghese, P. S., Takemori, A. E., & Cox, B. M. (1988). Kappa-receptor regulation of dopamine release from striatum and cortex of rats and guinea-pigs. *Journal of Pharmacology and Experimental Therapeutics*, 246(1), 282–286.

Winger, G., & Woods, J. H. (1985). Comparison of fixed-ratio and progressive-ratio schedules of maintenance of stimulant drug-reinforced responding. *Drug and Alcohol Dependence*, 15(1–2), 123–130.

Wise, R. A. (1998). Drug-activation of brain reward pathways. *Drug and Alcohol Dependence*, 51(1–2), 13–22.

Yasuda, K., Raynor, K., Kong, H., Breder, C. D., Takeda, J., Reisine, T., et al. (1993). Cloning and functional comparison of kappa-opioid and delta-opioid receptors from mouse-brain. *Proceedings of the National Academy of Sciences of the United States of America*, 90(14), 6736–6740.

Yoshizawa, K., Narita, M., Saeki, M., Narita, M., Isotani, K., Horiuchi, H., et al. (2011). Activation of extracellular signal-regulated kinase is critical for the discriminative stimulus effects induced by U-50,488H. *Synapse*, 65(10), 1052–1061.

Zhang, Y., Butelman, E. R., Schlussman, S. D., Ho, A., & Kreek, M. J. (2004). Effect of the endogenous kappa opioid agonist dynorphin A(1–17) on cocaine-evoked increases in striatal dopamine levels and cocaine-induced place preference in C57BL/6J mice. *Psychopharmacology*, 172(4), 422–429.

Zhang, Y., Butelman, E. R., Schlussman, S. D., Ho, A., & Kreek, M. J. (2005). Effects of the plant-derived hallucinogen salvinorin A on basal dopamine levels in the caudate putamen and in a conditioned place aversion assay in mice: Agonist actions at kappa opioid receptors. *Psychopharmacology*, 179(3), 551–558.

Zhang, Y., Schlussman, S. D., Rabkin, J., Butelman, E. R., Ho, A., & Kreek, M. J. (2013). Chronic escalating cocaine exposure, abstinence/withdrawal, and chronic re-exposure: Effects on striatal dopamine and opioid systems in C57BL/6J mice. *Neuropharmacology*, 67, 259–266.

Zhang, H., Shi, Y. G., Woods, J. H., Watson, S. J., & Ko, M. C. (2007). Central kappa-opioid receptor-mediated antidepressant-like effects of nor-Binaltorphimine: Behavioral and BDNF mRNA expression studies. *European Journal of Pharmacology*, 570(1–3), 89–96.

CHAPTER THIRTEEN

Nicotinic Receptor Antagonists as Treatments for Nicotine Abuse

Peter A. Crooks[*,1], Michael T. Bardo[†], Linda P. Dwoskin[‡]

[*]Department of Pharmaceutical Sciences, College of Pharmacy, University of Arkansas for Medical Sciences, Little Rock, Arizona, USA
[†]Department of Psychology, College of Pharmacy, University of Kentucky, Lexington, Kentucky, USA
[‡]Department of Pharmaceutical Sciences, College of Pharmacy, University of Kentucky, Lexington, Kentucky, USA
[1]Corresponding author: e-mail address: pacrooks@uams.edu

Contents

Abstract

Despite the proven efficacy of current pharmacotherapies for tobacco dependence, relapse rates continue to be high, indicating that novel medications are needed. Currently, several smoking cessation agents are available, including varenicline (Chantix®), bupropion (Zyban®), and cytisine (Tabex®). Varenicline and cytisine are partial agonists at the $\alpha 4\beta 2^*$ nicotinic acetylcholine receptor (nAChR). Bupropion is an antidepressant but is also an antagonist at $\alpha 3\beta 2^*$ ganglionic nAChRs. The rewarding effects of nicotine are mediated, in part, by nicotine-evoked dopamine (DA) release leading to sensitization, which is associated with repeated nicotine administration and nicotine addiction.

Advances in Pharmacology, Volume 69
ISSN 1054-3589
http://dx.doi.org/10.1016/B978-0-12-420118-7.00013-5

Receptor antagonists that selectivity target central nAChR subtypes mediating nicotine-evoked DA release should have efficacy as tobacco use cessation agents with the therapeutic advantage of a limited side-effect profile. While α-conotoxin MII (α-CtxMII)-insensitive nAChRs (e.g., α4β2*) contribute to nicotine-evoked DA release, these nAChRs are widely distributed in the brain, and inhibition of these receptors may lead to non-selective and untoward effects. In contrast, α-CtxMII-sensitive nAChRs mediating nicotine-evoked DA release offer an advantage as targets for smoking cessation, due to their more restricted localization primarily to dopaminergic neurons. Small drug-like molecules that are selective antagonists at α-CtxMII-sensitive nAChR subtypes that contain α6 and β2 subunits have now been identified. Early research identified a variety of quaternary ammonium analogs that were potent and selective antagonists at nAChRs mediating nicotine-evoked DA release. More recent data have shown that novel, non-quaternary bis-1,2,5,6-tetrahydropyridine analogs potently inhibit ($IC_{50} < 1$ nM) nicotine-evoked DA release *in vitro* by acting as antagonists at α-CtxMII-sensitive nAChR subtypes; these compounds also decrease NIC self-administration in rats.

ABBREVIATIONS

ANN artificial neural network
bNDI S-(−)-N,N'-decane-1,10-diyl-bis-nicotinium diiodide
bPiDDB N,N'-dodecane-1,12-diyl-bis-3-picolinium dibromide
bQDDB N,N'-dodecane-1,12-diyl-bis-quinolinium dibromide
BTMPS bis-(2,2,6,6,-tetramethyl-4-piperidinyl) sebacate
DA dopamine
MEC mecamylamine
MLA methyllycaconitine
MLR multiple linear regression
NAc nucleus accumbens
nAChR nicotinic acetylcholine receptor
NDDNI S-(−)-N-n-dodecylnicotinium iodide
NDNI S-(−)-N-n-decylnicotinium iodide
NE norepinephrine
NONI S-(−)-N-n-octylnicotinium iodide
THP 1,2,5,6-tetrahydropyridine
TMP 2,2,6,6-tetramethyl-4-piperidinol
VMAT2 vesicular monoamine transporter-2
α-CtxMII α-conotoxin MII

1. INTRODUCTION

Cigarette smoking is the most preventable cause of death with regard to global health. Despite the known health consequences of chronic smoking, compulsive tobacco use still persists throughout the world. Despite the proven efficacy of some current pharmacotherapies for tobacco dependence, relapse rates continue to be high (George & O'Malley, 2004; Hajek, McRobbie, & Myers, 2013; Hajek, Stead, et al., 2013; Hurt et al., 2003; Wileyto et al., 2004), indicating a need for alternative and more efficacious pharmacotherapies. Cessation therapies are available utilizing either nicotine replacement therapy (i.e., the nicotine patch and gum) or the use of nicotinic acetylcholine receptor (nAChR) partial agonists (e.g., varenicline).

Tobacco dependence is described as a chronic, relapsing disorder in which compulsive drug use persists despite negative consequences (George & O'Malley, 2004; Le Foll & Goldberg, 2009; Rose, 2008). About 80% of those who attempt to quit smoking relapse within the first month, and only 3% remain abstinent at 6 months (Benowitz, 2009), indicating that new medications are needed to specifically address the problem of relapse (George & O'Malley, 2004; Harmey, Griffin, & Kenny, 2012; Hurt et al., 2003; Irvin, Hendricks, & Brandon, 2003). The rewarding effects of nicotine are mediated, at least in part, by nicotine-evoked dopamine (DA) release leading to sensitization, which is associated with repeated nicotine administration and NIC addiction. Based on findings that the nonselective nAChR antagonist mecamylamine (MEC) has efficacy as a tobacco use cessation agent but is limited by peripherally mediated side effects, antagonist molecules with selectivity for central nAChR subtypes mediating nicotine-evoked DA release should have efficacy as tobacco use cessation agents with the therapeutic advantage of a limited side-effect profile.

2. CURRENT SMOKING CESSATION THERAPIES THAT TARGET nAChRs

2.1. Varenicline and cytisine

Varenicline was developed by Pfizer, Inc. and approved by the FDA as a smoking cessation agent in 2006. Varenicline not only acts as a partial agonist at $\alpha4\beta2^*$ nAChRs but also interacts weakly with $\alpha3\beta2^*$ and $\alpha6\beta2^*$ nAChRs and is a full agonist at $\alpha7$ nAChRs (Mihalak, Carroll, & Luetje, 2006). Varenicline has been shown to substitute for nicotine in drug discrimination studies in rats and blocks nicotine self-administration. In a randomized controlled clinical trial, carried out after 1 year of varenicline therapy, the rate of continuous tobacco use abstinence was 10% for placebo and 23% for varenicline; this compared favorably with the rate for bupropion (15%) (Jorenby et al., 2006). A subsequent meta-analysis of

101 clinical studies investigating varenicline showed it to be more effective than both bupropion and nicotine replacement therapy (~1.5 odds ratio) (Mills, Wu, Spurden, Ebbert, & Wilson, 2009).

A public health advisory notice was issued by the FDA in 2008 indicating that patients on varenicline experience serious neuropsychiatric symptoms, including depressed mood, suicidal ideation, and attempted or completed suicide (FDA public health advisory, 2008). In 2009, the FDA required both varenicline and bupropion to carry black box warnings, due to public reports of side effects, including depression, suicidal thoughts, and suicidal actions (FDA public health advisory, 2009). However, a recent a study of the medical records of 119,546 adults who had used a smoking cessation product between 1st September 2006 and 31st October 2011 (Thomas et al., 2013) found no clear evidence of an increased risk of treated depression or suicidal behavior for patients prescribed with varenicline or bupropion when compared to those taking nicotine replacement therapies. The FDA has also issued a recent safety announcement that the use of varenicline may be associated with a small, increased risk of certain cardiovascular adverse events in patients with cardiovascular disease (FDA drug safety communication, 2011).

Cytisine is a natural product isolated from *Cytisus laborinum* that is marketed in Europe as a smoking cessation agent under the trade name Tabex® (Etter, 2006; Zatonski, Cedzynska, Tutka, & West, 2006). Varenicline is a synthetic analog of cytisine. Cytisine was approved as a smoking cessation drug in 2006 in eastern Europe but is currently unavailable in the United States. Cytisine has a long-standing record of efficacy in the treatment of nicotine addiction in Europe and, similar to varenicline, is a selective partial agonist of human $\alpha4\beta2^*$ nAChRs (Lukas, 2007). In addition to its utility in smoking cessation treatments, cytisine has shown antidepressant activity in male C57BL/6J mice (Mineur, Somenzi, & Picciotto, 2007). A recent meta-analysis of eight clinical studies indicated that cytisine has comparable effectiveness to other smoking cessation agents marketed in the United States (Hajek, McRobbie, et al., 2013; Hajek, Stead, et al., 2013).

2.2. Bupropion

Bupropion was originally marketed as an antidepressant molecule due to its ability to inhibit DA and norepinephrine (NE) transport into the presynaptic nerve terminal. Importantly, bupropion inhibits DA uptake into striatal synaptosomes and NE uptake into hypothalamic synaptosomes; it also dose-dependently increases presynaptic vesicular DA uptake and redistributes vesicular monoamine transporter-2 (VMAT2) protein (Rau et al., 2005). Bupropion has also been shown to act as an antagonist at human $\alpha 3\beta 4$ ganglionic nAChRs via an allosteric inhibitory mechanism (Fryer & Lukas, 1999) and inhibits $\alpha 3\beta 2$, $\alpha 4\beta 2$, and $\alpha 7$ nAChRs expressed in *Xenopus* oocytes (Slemmer, Martin, & Damaj, 2000). These studies indicate that bupropion-induced decreases in smoking likely result from both its nAChR antagonism and its DAT and NET inhibition properties (Dwoskin, Pivavarchyk, et al., 2009; Dwoskin, Smith, et al., 2009). The clinical effectiveness of bupropion as a smoking cessation agent has been evaluated (Wu, Wilson, Dimoulas, & Mills, 2006). After 1 year of treatment, the odds of sustaining smoking cessation are 1.5 times higher in the bupropion group compared to the placebo group. The evidence indicates that bupropion is comparable to nicotine replacement therapy but is less effective than varenicline.

2.3. Mecamylamine

MEC is a nonselective noncompetitive channel blocker of nAChRs and was originally introduced as an antihypertensive drug in 1955 (Bacher, Wu, Shytle, & George, 2009). It has more recently been shown to dose-dependently decrease nicotine self-administration in laboratory animal models and to block cue-induced reinstatement of nicotine-seeking behavior (DeNoble & Mele, 2006; Glick, Visker, & Maisonneuve, 1996). Clinical studies with MEC, which acts at both central and peripheral nAChRs, provide precedence for the use of nAChR antagonists as tobacco use cessation agents. MEC reverses both positive and negative subjective effects of i.v. nicotine in smokers (Lundahl, Henningfield, & Lukas, 2000). In a randomized, double-blind placebo-controlled study, MEC combined with a nicotine transdermal patch improved cessation outcome for up to 1 year compared to nicotine alone (Rose, 2006, 2008; Rose et al., 1994). Also, MEC is beneficial in reducing smoking satisfaction (Rose, 2008); however, MEC's clinical utility is limited by anticholinergic side effects (e.g., constipation and hypotension) due to the lack of nAChR selectivity and inhibition of peripheral nAChRs (Rose, 2009). Thus, the development of *selective* small-molecule antagonists targeting central nAChRs mediating nicotine-evoked DA release constitutes a novel approach to the development of treatments for tobacco dependence and relapse prevention.

3. EMERGING POTENTIAL THERAPEUTICS FOR TREATMENT OF TOBACCO DEPENDENCE

Other partial agonists of nAChRs are currently under development. Dianicline, a drug developed by Sanofi-Aventis, is a selective partial agonist, binding primarily to the $\alpha4\beta2^*$ nAChR subtype, and has a similar pharmacological profile to varenicline (Cohen et al., 2003). In drug discrimination studies, dianicline substituted for nicotine but at doses that decreased the rate of responding (Cohen et al., 2003). In clinical studies, dianicline exhibited a 16% success rate compared to 8% for placebo (Fagerstrom & Balfour, 2006). Clinical development of dianicline has been discontinued after reports of unfavorable results in phase 3 studies (Sanofi Pipeline, 2012).

Sazetidine A is a nicotine analog that also acts as a subtype-selective partial agonist at $\alpha4\beta2^*$ nAChRs. Interestingly, this drug interacts as an agonist at $(\alpha4)_2(\beta2)_3$ subtypes and as an antagonist at $(\alpha4)_3(\beta2)_2$ subtypes (Xiao et al., 2006; Zwart et al., 2008). These studies have also shown that both $\alpha4\beta2^*$ and $\alpha62^*$ nAChRs mediate sazetidine A-evoked DA release, which can be blocked by both MEC and dihydro-β-erythroidine (Zwart et al., 2008). The $\alpha6$-selective antagonist, α-conotoxin MII (α-CtxMII), also inhibits sazetidine A-evoked DA release ($I_{max} = 50\%$). Sazetidine A substitutes completely for nicotine in drug discrimination studies in the rat and appears to act as a partial agonist at nAChRs in hippocampus and as a full agonist at nAChRs in striatum (Dwoskin, Pivavarchyk, et al., 2009; Dwoskin, Smith, et al., 2009; Xiao, Woolverton, Sahibzada, Yasuda, & Kellar, 2007).

UCI-30002 is a novel antagonist that acts as a positive allosteric modulator of $GABA_A$ receptors (Johnstone et al., 2004) and, as such, may also have efficacy as a negative allosteric modulator of $\alpha4\beta2$ nAChRs, since this drug inhibits nicotine-evoked currents in *Xenopus* oocytes expressing neuronal $\alpha4\beta2$, $\alpha7$, and $\alpha3\beta4$ nAChRs (Yoshimura et al., 2007). UCI-30002 has been shown to decrease nicotine self-administration utilizing both a fixed ratio and a progressive ratio schedule (Yoshimura et al., 2007), suggesting an effect on nicotine reward, and does not alter food-maintained responding (Yoshimura et al., 2007). Negative allosteric modulators of nAChRs represent a new area of drug discovery in the search for novel smoking cessation agents.

Recently, AT-1001 *N*-(2-bromophenyl)-9-methyl-9-azabicyclo[3.3.1] nonan-3-amine has been reported as a selective, high-affinity $\alpha3\beta4^*$ nAChR antagonist that potently and dose-dependently blocks nicotine self-administration in rats without altering responding for food (Toll et al., 2012). AT-1001 is the first ligand reported with a K_i below 10 nM at $\alpha 3\beta 4^*$ nAChRs and a 90-fold selectivity over $\alpha 4\beta 2^*$ and $\alpha 7^*$ nAChRs. Interestingly, AT-1001 is a poor inhibitor of NIC-induced DA release, compared to MEC and α-CtxMII, suggesting that its inhibition of nicotine self-administration in rats is not directly due to a decrease in DA release in nucleus accumbens, but may involve an indirect pathway mediated by $\alpha 3\beta 4^*$ nAChR inhibition. Nevertheless, these findings highlight the emergence of the $\alpha 3\beta 4^*$ nAChR as a new potential target for the development of clinically useful smoking cessation agents.

4. SMALL-MOLECULE SURROGATES OF α-CtxMII AS SMOKING CESSATION AGENTS

We began our nAChR antagonist research program because we believed that subtype-selective nAChR antagonists that block reward-relevant mesocorticolimbic and nigrostriatal DA release evoked by nicotine might offer patients who do not respond to existing smoking cessation therapies alternative treatment options. Thus, we set out to discover and develop molecules that were selective antagonists at those nAChR subtypes that mediate nicotine-evoked DA release, that is, nAChR subtypes associated with reward produced by tobacco smoking (Crooks, Ravard, Teng, & Dwoskin, 1995; Dwoskin & Crooks, 2001). At the time we initiated this research program, this was considered to be a new and somewhat controversial approach to therapeutic intervention in tobacco addiction.

The seminal discovery that the neuropeptide α-CtxMII blocks nicotine-stimulated DA release in rat striatal synaptosomes (Kulak, Nguyen, Olivera, & McIntosh, 1997) was a key finding of great relevance to the discovery of nAChR antagonists that block nicotine reward. The specific goal was to identify small, drug-like molecules that act as selective antagonists at α-CtxMII-sensitive nAChR subtypes, which contain $\alpha 6$ and $\beta 2$ subunits (i.e., $\alpha 6\beta 2^*$, $\alpha 6\beta 2\beta 3^*$, $\alpha 6\alpha 4\beta 2\beta 3^*$, and $\alpha 4\alpha 6\beta 2^*$). These α-CtxMII-sensitive nAChRs were selected as targets for drug discovery because they are localized primarily to DA neurons that mediate nicotine-evoked DA release leading to nicotine reward. While α-CtxMII-insensitive nAChRs (e.g., $\alpha 4\beta 2^*$) contribute to nicotine-evoked DA release, these nAChRs have a wide distribution in brain, which may lead to nonselective effects.

In contrast, α-CtxMII-sensitive nAChRs mediating nicotine-evoked DA release offer an advantage as a target for smoking cessation due to their more restricted localization primarily to DA neurons. Currently, there are few selective drug-like compounds that differentiate α-CtxMII-sensitive nAChRs from other central and peripheral nAChR subtypes (e.g., $\alpha4\beta2^*$, $\alpha7^*$, and $\alpha3\beta4^*$ nAChRs).

We considered our approach of developing small-molecule surrogates of α-CtxMII to be innovative for a number of reasons. First, no new chemical entities have been synthesized that are small molecules acting as α-CtxMII surrogates. Second, identification of $\alpha6\beta2^*$ nAChRs as targets for the discovery of novel tobacco dependence medications was a novel approach at the time we commenced our studies (Crooks et al., 1995). Third, the overall general strategy is innovative, since currently, there are no *specific* nAChR antagonists approved for smoking cessation, and we believed that antagonist treatment could be useful in providing an alternative clinical option for highly motivated individuals undergoing cessation. Current pharmacotherapeutic approaches are based primarily on replacement therapies, in which full or partial nAChR agonists (e.g., nicotine and varenicline) interact predominantly with $\alpha4\beta2^*$ nAChRs (Coe et al., 2005; Paterson et al., 2010; Rose, Salley, Behm, Bates, & Westman, 2010). nAChR agonists are generally well tolerated and produce good patient compliance, substituting for the reinforcing effect of tobacco use (Garwood & Potts, 2007; Shahan, Odum, & Bickel, 2000). However, partial agonist or agonist replacement therapy is less than optimal (Schuh, Schuh, & Henningfield, 1996); a potential disadvantage is that continued activation of nAChRs maintains receptor desensitization and nicotine dependence. Fourth, the ability to selectively inhibit central nAChRs offers new tools to provide insights on mechanisms involving $\alpha6\beta2^*$ nAChRs. Fifth, our focus on the development of pharmacotherapies to thwart *relapse* is of great significance with regard to developing effective strategies to combat nicotine addiction. While the various factors involved in relapse in humans are complex, including the co-occurrence of alcohol consumption and factors related to impulsivity and stress (Bourque, Mendrek, Dinh-Williams, & Potvin, 2013; Brunzell, 2012; VanderVeen, Cohen, & Watson, 2012), it is also known that smoking-related cues play a role (Le Foll & Goldberg, 2005; Perkins, 1999). To the extent that cue-induced craving is associated with activation of $\alpha6\beta2^*$ nAChRs, it may be possible to develop an antagonist pharmacotherapy that enhances relapse prevention by blocking the effect of these cues.

nAChRs, members of the Cys-loop family of ligand-gated ion channel receptors, consist of pentameric transmembrane proteins with diverse composition (Anand, Conroy, Schoepfer, Whiting, & Lindstrom, 1991; Millar & Gotti, 2009). Although nAChR subtype predominance does not necessarily reflect functional importance, the $\alpha4\beta2$ subtype, probed by high-affinity [^{3}H]-nicotine binding, is predominant in the CNS (Flores, Rogers, Pabreza, Wolfe, & Kellar, 1992; Whiting & Lindstrom, 1987; Zoli, Lena, Picciotto, & Changeux, 1998). Immunoprecipitation studies indicate that more than two different subunits form functional nAChRs and individual neurons elaborate multiple subtypes (Conroy, Vernallis, & Berg, 1992; Forsayeth & Kobrin, 1997; Turner & Kellar, 2005), increasing the complexity associated with elucidation of specific nAChR subtype function. Mammalian homomeric nAChRs consist of $\alpha7$ or $\alpha9$ subunits (Flores et al., 1992; Gotti, Zoli, & Clementi, 2006; McIntosh et al., 2005; Wada et al., 1989). The exact subunit composition and stoichiometry of native nAChRs remain to be elucidated. Nevertheless, subunit composition has an important impact on pharmacological sensitivity, including antagonist affinity (Cachelin & Rust, 1995; Harvey & Luetje, 1996; Harvey, Maddox, & Luetje, 1996). Nicotine activation of nAChRs increases extracellular DA in nucleus accumbens and striatum, mediating, at least in part, nicotine reward (Corrigall, Franklin, Coen, & Clarke, 1992; Rahman et al., 2008). nAChRs modulate synaptic activity and neurotransmitter release (Collins, Salminen, Marks, Whiteaker, & Grady, 2009; Dani & Bertrand, 2007; McGehee & Role, 1995; Quarta et al., 2007). Rat nigral DA neurons express mRNA for $\alpha3$, $\alpha4$, $\alpha5$, $\alpha6$, $\alpha7$, $\beta2$, $\beta3$, and $\beta4$ (Arroyo-Jimenez et al., 1999; Wada et al., 1989). Studies using $\beta2$ knockout mice have revealed that $\beta2$ is necessary for nicotine-evoked DA release (Grady et al., 2001, 2007; Salminen et al., 2004; Whiteaker et al., 2000). Subtype assignment of native nAChRs mediating nicotine-evoked DA release is based largely on the inhibition of agonist-induced responses by subtype-selective antagonists, defined by their inhibitory activity in cell systems expressing nAChR subunits of known composition. A major role for $\alpha6\beta2^*$ in nicotine-evoked striatal DA release is based on α-CtxMII inhibition of nicotine-evoked [^{3}H]-DA release, as well as knockout and gain-of-function studies (Cartier et al., 1996; Cui et al., 2003; Drenan et al., 2010; Drenan, Grady et al., 2008; Drenan, Nashmi, et al., 2008; Kaiser, Soliakov, Harvey, Luetje, & Wonnacott, 1998); $\alpha6$ and $\beta2$ subunits are highly expressed in DA cell bodies (Cui et al., 2003; Goldner, Dineley, & Patrick, 1997; Le Novère, Zoli, & Changeux, 1996).

Results from comprehensive molecular genetics gene deletion studies implicate the α4α6β2β3* subtype in nicotine-evoked DA release and nicotine reward. These studies suggested that nicotine-evoked DA release is mediated by 6 different subtypes, that is, α6β2β3*, α4α6β2β3*, α6β2*, and α4α6β2* (α-CtxMII-sensitive subtypes) and α4β2* and α4α5β2* (α-CtxMII-insensitive subtypes) (Gotti et al., 2005; Salminen et al., 2004). The α4α6β2β3* subtype had the highest sensitivity to nicotine of any native nAChR and constituted approximately 50% of α6-containing nAChRs on DA terminals of wild-type mice (Salminen et al., 2007). From these studies, it is clear that multiple subtypes can mediate nicotine-evoked DA release. The ability to design small-molecule antagonists that can selectively target these subtypes to inhibit nicotine-evoked DA release represents a primary goal for our laboratory. DA neurons have special chaperones for assembling accessory subunits with α6 for transporting nAChRs to the cell surface; α6 concatamers will increase understanding of the functional properties of α6-containing nAChRs (Kuryatov & Lindstrom, 2011). It is important to note that the subtype composition and relative contribution of nicotine-evoked DA release nAChRs are species-dependent, and relative contributions of different subtypes are species-dependent. In mice, α6-containing nAChRs represent 30% of presynaptic nAChRs that mediate nicotine-evoked DA release, while in nonhuman primates, 70% of nAChRs that mediate nicotine-evoked DA release are α6-containing nAChRs (Kulak et al., 1997; McCallum, Collins, Paylor, & Marks, 2006; Salminen et al., 2004). CNS location is also an important factor; α6β2* nAChRs are the predominant subtype that mediates nicotine-evoked DA release in nucleus accumbens, whereas α6β2* nAChRs only contribute in striatum (Exley, Clements, Hartung, McIntosh, & Cragg, 2008). These studies demonstrate that α6β2* nAChRs are major subtypes that mediate nicotine-evoked DA release and nicotine self-administration leading to dependence (Brunzell, 2012; Brunzell, Boschen, Hendrick, Beardsley, & McIntosh, 2010; Drenan et al., 2010; Gotti et al., 2010; Jackson, McIntosh, Brunzell, Sanjakdar, & Damaj, 2009; Moretti et al., 2010; Pons et al., 2008).

Neurotoxin peptides acting as subtype-selective nAChR antagonists are unlikely to be easily developed into treatments for tobacco use cessation, since they are high-molecular-weight peptides and unlikely to not cross the blood–brain barrier. Our current approach aimed to provide potent small-molecule antagonists that inhibit the same nAChR subtypes as α-CtxMII. Pharmacological tools, which differentiate among specific high-affinity heteromeric nAChR subtypes, are few. This situation represents a major hindrance in increasing our understanding of which specific subtypes contribute to nicotine addiction and in the development of effective pharmacotherapies for tobacco dependence. We hypothesize that drug-like nAChR antagonists inhibiting α6β2* nAChR subtypes will decrease nicotine-evoked DA release and nicotine reward, thus providing a new class of cessation agents that prevent relapse. In support of this hypothesis, our drug discovery effort focused initially on the development of nAChR subtype-selective antagonists based on structural modification of the nicotine molecule (Dwoskin & Bardo, 2009; Dwoskin & Crooks, 2001; Dwoskin, Smith, et al., 2009; Dwoskin et al., 2004).

5. MONOQUATERNARY AMMONIUM SALTS DERIVED FROM *N*-METHYLNICOTINIUM ION AS NICOTINIC RECEPTOR ANTAGONISTS

Based upon early findings that the *N*-methylnicotinium ion inhibited DA uptake into rat striatal slices (Dwoskin, Leibee, Jewell, Fang, & Crooks, 1992), we initially synthesized and evaluated a series of *N-n*-alkylnicotinium analogs and related compounds for their ability to inhibit nicotine-evoked DA release from rat striatal slices and to displace [³H]-nicotine binding from rat striatal membranes (α4β2* nAChRs) (Crooks et al., 1995). We were particularly interested in the nAChR mediating nicotine-evoked DA release, since we believed that it constituted an excellent therapeutic target for the development of clinical candidates for treating nicotine addiction. The exact subunit composition and stoichiometry of this nAChR receptor were not known at the time our studies began and even today have still not been fully elucidated. The receptor was initially termed the α3β2* subtype but was later renamed as a group of α6* or more recently α6β2* subtypes.

The most effective antagonists screened in our nicotine-evoked DA release assay were those quaternary ammonium nicotine analogs that incorporated an *N-n*-alkyl substituent of three carbons or more in length. The introduction of an aromatic or unsaturated residue into the *N*-alkyl substituent also afforded antagonist molecules. The most potent compound was S-(−)-*N-n*-octylnicotinium iodide (NONI, Fig. 13.1), which had full antagonist potency. Importantly, NONI had low affinity for the high-affinity [³H]-nicotine binding site ($K_i = 20$ μM) and appeared to be somewhat more selective as an antagonist at α6β2* nAChRs (IC$_{50}$ = 0.62 μM) (Crooks et al., 2004). Interestingly, some of the *N*-alkylnicotinium analogs had differential properties at α4β2*, α7*, and α6β2* nAChRs. The related

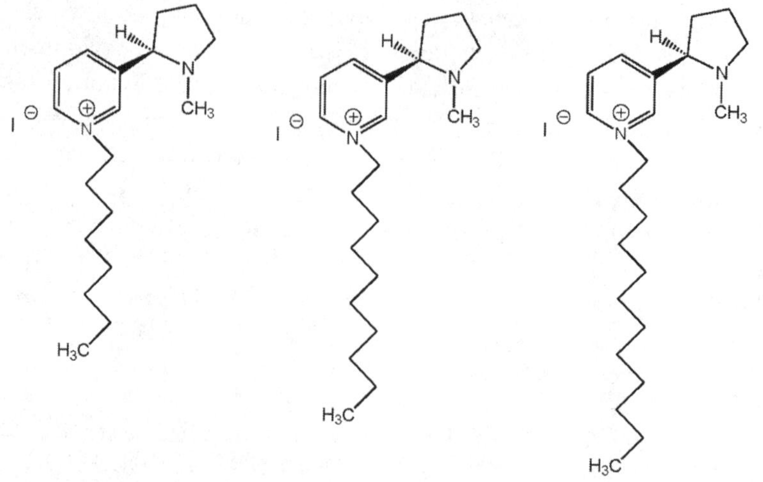

Figure 13.1 Chemical structures of the N-n-alkyl-substituted analogs of S-(−)-nicotine, NONI (S-(−)-N-n-octylnicotinium iodide), NDNI (S-(−)-N-n-decylnicotinium bromide, and NDDNI (S-(−)-N-n-dodecylnicotinium iodide. NONI exhibited an IC$_{50}$ of 0.62 μM at α6-containing nAChRs.

compound S-(−)-N-n-decylnicotinium iodide (NDNI; Fig. 13.1) was not active as an antagonist at α6β2* nAChRs (IC$_{50}$ > 100 μM) but afforded a K_i value of 90 nM in the [^{3}H]-nicotine binding assay. The N-n-dodecyl analog, NDDNI (Fig. 13.1.), was a very potent antagonist at α6β2* nAChRs (IC$_{50}$ = 9 nM) but was nonselective, exhibiting a K_i of 140 nM at α4β2* nAChRs. In the nicotine-evoked ^{86}Rb$^+$ efflux assay, a functional assay for the α4β2* nAChR subtype, NDNI and NONI had IC$_{50}$s of 30 pM and 85 nM, respectively (Dwoskin, Wilkins, Pauly, & Crooks, 1999).

These results were considered key findings, since NONI represented our first lead compound in the search for new tobacco use cessation agents (Dwoskin et al., 2004). These early data also indicated that while NONI was a selective α6β2* nAChR subtype antagonist, NDNI was a potent and selective α4β2* nAChR subtype antagonist and that both compounds might be valuable tools for probing the consequences of activating different subtypes of nicotinic receptor. More importantly, the N-n-alkylnicotinium analogs as a group were found to have good affinity for the blood–brain barrier choline transporter, and [^{3}H]-NONI was shown to act as a substrate for this transporter in brain uptake studies in the rat. NONI exhibited the following saturable blood–brain barrier penetration parameters— $V_{max} = 603 \pm 80$ nmol/min/g, $K_m + 661 \pm 75$ μM, and

$K_d = 7.3 \pm 3.1 \times 10^{-4}$ ml/g—compared to choline, $V_{max} = 3 \pm 0.3$ nmol/min/g, $K_m = 42 \pm 6$ μM, and $K_d = 1.0 \pm 0.06 \times 10^{-4}$ ml/g (Crooks et al., 2004; Lockman et al., 2008), indicating that this molecule, although cationic and polar, is brain-bioavailable. However, the general lack of selectivity of this class of analogs for α6β2* nAChRs prompted us to explore other structural modifications of the nicotine molecule.

5.1. Bis-Quaternary ammonium analogs

During the course of the structure–activity studies on the N-alkylnicotinium analogs, it was observed that significant structural changes could be made to the nicotinium moiety (i.e., the quaternary ammonium "headgroup") with retention of antagonist potency at nAChRs mediating nicotine-evoked DA release. It was found that simple azaheterocycles, such as pyridine and 3-picoline, could be substituted for the S-(−)-nicotine moiety with retention of nAChR inhibitory potency (Dwoskin et al., 2004). The classical bis-quaternary ammonium salts, hexamethonium chloride (N,N'-hexane-1,6-bis-trimethyammonium chloride) and decamethonium chloride (N,N'-decane-1,10-bis-trimethyammonium chloride), which are regarded as simplified analogs of the more conformationally retrained natural product, d-tubocurarine, have been utilized in the past to differentiate between subtypes of different peripheral nicotinic receptors. Thus, decamethonium is a selective inhibitor of neuromuscular nicotinic receptors, while hexamethonium inhibits ganglionic nicotinic receptors (Koelle, 1975). Recent studies (Papke, Wecker, & Stitzel, 2010) have since shown that decamethonium and hexamethonium interact with both peripheral and central nAChRs expressed in Xenopus oocytes. Thus, although decamethonium was shown to be a selective depolarizing blocker of muscle-type nAChRs in these studies, it was also an effective antagonist of mouse neuronal nAChRs and was particularly potent at α7 homomeric receptors. Similarly, hexamethonium exhibited comparable inhibitory potency at both α3-containing nAChRs (ganglionic) and α4β2 nAChRs. These data indicate that the earlier classification of these channel-blocking agents did not take into account the inability of these molecules to cross the blood–brain barrier, which results in functional protection of CNS receptors in whole animal studies.

Based on the earlier studies with the trimethylammonium analogs, a second quaternary ammonium moiety was introduced into the scaffold of the N-alkylnicotinium analogs, in order to determine the effect of bis-cationic analogs on antagonist potency and selectivity and to additionally probe the chemical space around the bis-"headgroups" by replacing the nicotinium headgroup with other azaheterocyclic moieties. Thus, a series of bis-analogs bearing nicotinium, pyridinium, picolinium, quinolinium, and iso-quinolinium headgroups separated by variable-length n-alkane linkers were initially synthesized and evaluated as ligands for $\alpha6\beta2^*$, $\alpha4\beta2^*$, and $\alpha7^*$ nAChRs (Ayers et al., 2002; Crooks et al., 2004). From the observed structure–activity trends, it was clear that the majority of the analogs generally had poor affinity for the $\alpha4\beta2^*$ nAChR, with the exception of the bis-nicotinium analogs. One of these, S-(−)-N,N'-decane-1,10-diyl-bis-nicotinium diiodide (Fig. 13.2), exhibited a K_i value of 330 nM at $\alpha4\beta2^*$ nAChRs and functionally inhibited nicotine-evoked $^{86}Rb^+$ efflux ($IC_{50} = 3.76$ μM) while demonstrating no affinity for $\alpha7^*$ nAChRs. The bis-quinolinium and bis-isoquinolinium analogs all exhibited affinity for $\alpha7^*$ nAChRs, the most potent being N,N'-dodecane-1,12-diyl-bis-quinolinium dibromide (Fig. 13.2), with a K_i value of 1.6 μM, which is comparable to nicotine.

The most interesting series of bis-analogs were the N,N'-n-alkane-diyl-bis-3-picolinium dibromides. These analogs had n-alkane tethers ranging

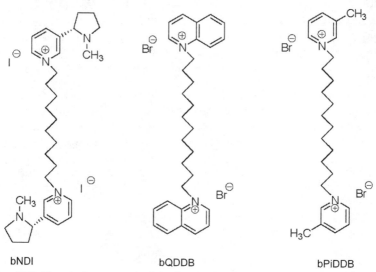

bNDI   bQDDB   bPiDDB

Figure 13.2 Chemical structures of the bis-quaternary ammonium compounds bNDI (S-(−)-N,N-decane-1,10-diyl-bis-nicotinium diiodide), bQDDB (N,N-dodecane-1,12-diyl-bis-quinolinium dibromide), and bPiDDB (N,N-dodecane-1,12-diyl-bis-3-picolinium dibromide). bPiDDB exhibited an IC_{50} of 5 μM at $\alpha6$-containing nAChRs.

from C_6 to C_{12}, and all of the analogs exhibited antagonism of $\alpha6\beta2^*$ nAChRs (Crooks et al., 2004; Dwoskin et al., 2004). The most potent analog was N,N'-dodecane-1,12-diyl-bis-3-picolinium dibromide (bPiDDB; Fig. 13.2), which exhibited a remarkable IC_{50} of 5 nM ($I_{max} = 60\%$) and had little or no affinity for either $\alpha4\beta2^*$ or $\alpha7^*$ nAChRs. We considered bPiDDB to be an important lead candidate for further study, since it had high potency and selectivity at the nAChR mediating nicotine-evoked DA release and, like NONI, was an excellent substrate for the blood–brain barrier choline transporter (i.e., brain-bioavailable). bPiDDB exhibited the following saturable blood–brain barrier penetration parameters—$V_{max} = 4.3 \pm 1.0$ nmol/min/g, $K_m = 5 \pm 2$ μM, and $K_d = 1.1 \pm 0.06 \times 10^{-4}$ ml/g—which are comparable to choline (Lockman et al., 2008). Additionally, we also found that bPiDDB diminished nicotine self-administration in proof-of-concept *in vivo* studies (Fig. 13.3).

In a subsequent study, we synthesized and evaluated an extended series of bis-azaaromatic quaternary ammonium salts (Zheng, Sumithran, Deaciuc, Dwoskin, & Crooks, 2007). This study focused on investigating the possible

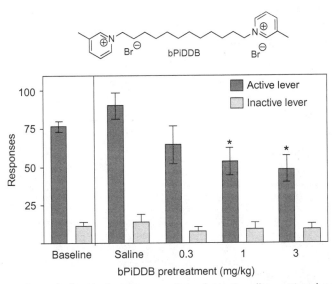

Figure 13.3 General chemical structures of conformationally restricted analogs of bPiDDB that incorporate 1,2-, 1,3-, and 1,4-dialkylphenyl linkers between the two quaternary ammonium headgroups. This structural change generally led to a decrease in the inhibition of nicotine-evoked DA release. (For color version of this figure, the reader is referred to the online version of this chapter.)

binding conformation of these molecules. The design of the model compounds incorporated a phenyl ring into the middle of the N-N' alkane linker moiety, allowing a variety of arrangements of the two smaller methylene linker units around the aromatic "core" unit (i.e., 1,2-, 1,3-, and 1,4-dialkylphenyl linkers) (Fig. 13.4). This approach constrains these molecules into "extended" or "angular" geometries and is a well-known and extensively used strategy in drug design for locking ligands into a desired conformation or geometry, with the goal of increasing activity and selectivity. To increase conformational restriction even further, a triple bond was also introduced into each of the alkane linker units that were attached to the central phenyl ring. The study indicated that the transition from the more conformationally flexible N,N'-alkanyl-diyl-bis-azaheterocyclic analogs, such as bPiDDB, to more conformationally restricted analogs generally resulted in a decrease in inhibition of nicotine-evoked [³H]-DA release and suggested that maintaining flexibility of the alkane linker is important for high inhibitory potency and optimal interaction with nAChRs. The data also suggested that bPiDDB likely binds in an "extended" conformation, rather than an "angular" conformation. It was hypothesized from molecular modeling studies that the greater potency of the more flexible bis-analogs was due to the binding site of the α6-containing nAChR subtype likely being deep inside the channel of the receptor; thus, ligands must be flexible enough to reach this binding site.

In a related study (Zhang, Lockman, et al., 2008; Zhang, Zheng, et al., 2008), a series of novel bis-pyridinium cyclophanes were evaluated as conformationally restricted bis-quaternary ammonium compounds. These analogs were poor antagonists at α6β2* nAChR but were considered worthy of evaluating for their affinity for the blood–brain barrier choline transporter. All the cyclophanes examined exhibited high affinity for the choline

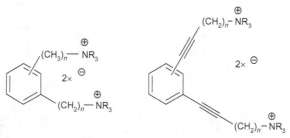

Figure 13.4 Concentration of ¹⁴C-bPiDDB in the plasma and brain after 1 and 3 mg/kg administration of ¹⁴C-bpiDDB in the Sprague–Dawley rat.

transporter when compared to the natural substrate, choline. Of the cyclophanes tested, two analogs N,N'-(1,10-decanediyl)3,3'-(1,9-decadiyn-1,10-diyl)-bis-pyridinium diiodide and N,N'-(1,9-nonanediyl)3,3'-(1,9-decadiyn-1,10-diyl)-bis-pyridinium dibromide exhibited K_i values of 0.8 and 1.4 μM, respectively, and are among the most potent blood–brain barrier choline transporter ligands ever reported. We extended this study to include a series of bis-azaaromatic quaternary ammonium compounds containing both flexible and conformationally restricted polymethylenic linker moieties around a central phenyl core (Zheng et al., 2010). The results from this study suggested that incorporating a linear, conformationally restricted linker into the molecule improves affinity for the choline transporter.

5.1.1 Pharmacokinetic studies with bPiDDB

With bPiDDB as the lead molecule, the pharmacokinetics of [^{14}C-methyl]-bPiDDB was investigated in the rat (Albayati, Dwoskin, & Crooks, 2008). We were interested in determining whether bPiDDB was brain-bioavailable, since we had determined earlier that it was a good substrate for the blood–brain barrier choline transporter (Lockman et al., 2008) and should therefore accumulate in the brain after peripheral administration. Plasma concentrations of [^{14}C-methyl]-bPiDDB after peripheral administration (1, 3, and 5 mg/kg) were determined at 10 time points over 3 h to afford absolute plasma bioavailabilities of 80%, 68%, and 104%, respectively, and C_{max} values of 0.13, 0.33, and 0.43 μg/ml, respectively (Fig. 13.5). T_{max} values were 5.0, 6.7, and 8.8 min, and $t_{1/2}$ values were 76.0, 54.6, and 41.7 min, respectively. No significant metabolic products of bPiDDB could be detected, and moderate protein binding (63–65%) was observed. As anticipated, bPiDDB penetrated the blood–brain barrier, even though it is an extremely polar, dicationic molecule. The blood–brain ratio at 5 min was 0.18, increasing to 0.51 at 60 min, indicating that clearance of bPiDDB from the brain was slower than clearance from plasma. Overall, the results indicated that bPiDDB is distributed rapidly from the site of administration into plasma, affords good plasma concentrations, and reaches brain tissues through facilitated transport via the blood–brain barrier choline transporter to afford therapeutically relevant concentrations in rat brain.

5.1.2 bPiDDB pharmacology

We have shown that repeated nicotine administration in rats robustly increases in vitro bPiDDB inhibitory potency at α6-containing nAChRs by three orders of magnitude compared to similar in vitro assays in naive rats

Concentration of ^{14}C-bPiDDB in plasma and brain homogenates vs time after 1 and 3 mg/kg s.c. administration of ^{14}C-bPiDDB.

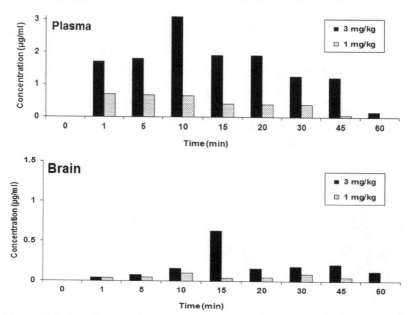

Figure 13.5 Acute bPiDDB (1 and 3 mg/kg) decreases NIC self-administration: bPiDDB (0.3–3 mg/kg, s.c., 15 min pretreatment) decreased the number of nicotine infusions (0.03 mg/kg/infusion) earned (active lever). (For color version of this figure, the reader is referred to the online version of this chapter.)

(Smith et al., 2010) (i.e., $IC_{50} = 5$ pM vs. 6 nM). This finding is relevant to smoking cessation therapy, since tobacco smokers self-administer nicotine repeatedly and animal models incorporating repeated nicotine treatment allow for better mechanistic evaluation of therapeutic candidates following neuroadaptive changes. This study demonstrated that repeated nicotine treatment may differentially regulate the stoichiometry, conformation, and/or composition of $\alpha6\beta2^*$ nAChRs.

We have also shown that bPiDDB inhibits nicotine-evoked norepinephrine release from superfused rat hippocampal slices with an IC_{50} of 430 nM ($I_{max} = 90\%$) and likely acts as an allosteric inhibitor at this nAChR subtype (putative $\alpha3\beta4$) (Smith et al., 2009). Kinetic analysis afforded a Schild regression slope that was different from unity, which is consistent with allosteric inhibition. Thus, bPiDDB has 200-fold more inhibitory potency at $\alpha6\beta2^*$ nAChR subtypes compared to its inhibitory potency at $\alpha3\beta4^*$ nAChRs. This is important because the $\alpha3\beta4^*$ subtype, like the

$\alpha6\beta2^*$ subtype, contributes to nicotine reward (Picciotto & Kenny, 2013; Stoker & Markou, 2013).

In a critical behavioral study, we determined that bPiDDB dose-dependently decreased nicotine self-administration, but not sucrose-maintained responding in the rat (Neugebauer, Zhang, Crooks, Dwoskin, & Bardo, 2006); and in locomotor experiments, bPiDDB attenuated the hyperactivity produced by acute and repeated nicotine dosing in the rat. Thus, bPiDDB continued to be our lead molecule in the search for subtype-selective nAChR antagonists. It should be noted that when administered peripherally, several bis-quaternary ammonium antagonists, including bPiDDB, specifically decreased nicotine self-administration and reinstatement of nicotine seeking in rats, providing proof of concept of this representative class of drug as a new pharmacotherapy for nicotine addiction. Additional behavioral studies in the rat have been carried out on other structurally related N,N'-alkane-diyl-bis-3-picoliniums (Dwoskin et al., 2008; Wooters et al., 2011).

In summary, bPiDDB is a selective, noncompetitive inhibitor of $\alpha6\beta2^*$ nAChRs; bPiDDB inhibits [^{3}H]-nicotine and [^{3}H]-MLA binding ($\alpha4\beta2^*$ and $\alpha7^*$ nAChRs, respectively) only at *high* concentrations ($>10\ \mu M$; Dwoskin et al., 2008) and decreases nicotine self-administration in rats. Furthermore, bPiDDB (1 μM) produced only 15% and 12% inhibition of acetylcholine (1 mM)-induced current at ganglionic-type $\alpha3\beta4$ nAChRs and muscle-type $\alpha1\beta1\epsilon\delta$ nAChRs, respectively, expressed in *Xenopus* oocytes (unpublished data). Subsequent optimization studies (see the succeeding text) were carried out to address the likelihood that this general class of compound would have poor oral bioavailability.

5.2. Tris-Quaternary ammonium salts

A related SAR study to assess the effect of introducing a third picolinium headgroup into the bPiDDB scaffold on inhibition of nicotine-evoked DA release was also carried out. The rationale for this structural modification was to determine if the change from one (mono), to two (bis), to three (tris) cationic headgroups would continue to improve affinity and inhibitory potency for the target nAChR protein. An increase in inhibitory potency in the progression from mono, to bis, to tris would indicate that at least three polar interactions between the cationic groupings in these molecules and the corresponding putative anionic sites on the receptor protein can occur. This approach was based on molecular modeling data that indicated that the binding sites that the bis-analogs interacted with were located in the vestibule area of the nAChR ion channel.

Two series of tris-scaffolds were constructed, that is, the 1,3,5-tri-(pent-1-ynyl-5-azaaromatic quaternary ammonium) benzene series (scaffold A, unsaturated) (Fig. 13.6A) and the 1,3,5-tri-(n-pentanyl-5-azaaromatic quaternary ammonium) benzene series (scaffold B, saturated) (Fig. 13.6B) (Zheng, Zhang, et al., 2007). The tris-azaaromatic quaternary ammonium salts were synthesized utilizing Sonogashira coupling chemistry (Fig. 13.7). A variety of azaaromatic heterocycles were utilized as headgroups. These molecules were then evaluated as antagonists at $\alpha6\beta2^*$ nAChRs and for their affinity for $\alpha4\beta2^*$ and $\alpha7^*$ nAChRs. Three compounds emerged from this study as potent and selective inhibitors of $\alpha6\beta2^*$ nAChRs with IC_{50}s in the range 0.2–4 nM. Two of these were unsaturated picolinium analogs, that is, 1,3,5-tri-{5-[1-(3-picolinium)]-pent-1-ynyl}benzene tribromide (TRIS-1) ($IC_{50} = 0.2$ nM) and 1,3,5-tri-{5-[1-(2-picolinium)]-pent-1-ynyl}benzene tribromide (TRIS-2) ($IC_{50} = 4.0$ nM); the third compound was a saturated 3-picolinium analog: 1,3,5-tri-{5-[1-(3-picolinium)]-pentyl}benzene tribromide (TRIS-3) ($IC_{50} = 2.0$ nM). None of these analogs had any significant affinity for $\alpha4\beta2^*$ and $\alpha7^*$ nAChRs. Thus, these very potent and selective tris-analogs represented additional new leads in our search for potent and selective nAChR antagonists as treatments for nicotine addiction. However, subsequent studies showed that although one of the lead tris-analogs was effective in dose-dependently decreasing nicotine self-administration in the rat, it produced toxicity at the higher concentration range of the dose–response. Additionally, the tris-analogs generally exhibited lower affinity for the blood–brain choline transporter and thus were expected to have poor oral and brain bioavailability.

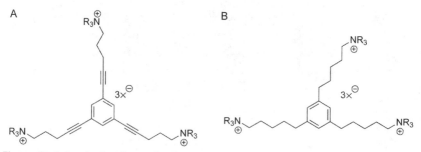

Figure 13.6 Synthetic scheme for the synthesis of tris-3-picolinium analogs.

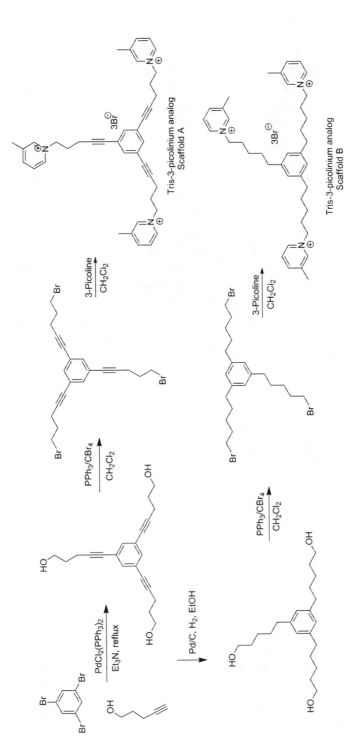

Figure 13.7 Structures of the two tris-quaternary ammonium scaffolds A (1,3,5-tri-{5-[1-(ammonium)-pent-1-ynyl]benzene) and B (1,3,5-tri-{5-[1-(ammonium)-pentyl]benzene); TRIS-1 scaffold A, NR₃ = 3-picolinium; TRIS-2 scaffold A, NR₃ = 2-picolinium; TRIS-3 scaffold B, NR₃ = 3-picolinium.

5.3. Tetrakis-Quaternary ammonium salts

Concomitant with the development of the tris-series of compounds, the incorporation of an additional cationic headgroup into the tris-scaffold was carried out to complete the transition from mono-, to bis-, to tris-, to tetrakis-quaternary ammonium salts. This modification was investigated to determine if further increases in the number of cationic centers in these molecules would enhance antagonist potency and selectivity at $\alpha6\beta2^*$ nAChRs. We generated two series of tetrakis-azaaromatic quaternary ammonium analogs, that is, 1,2,4,5-tetrakis-(pent-1-ynyl-5-azaaromatic quaternary ammonium)benzene salts (scaffold A, unsaturated) (Fig. 13.8A) and 1,2,4,5-tetrakis-(n-pentanyl-5-azaaromatic quaternary ammonium) benzene salts (scaffold B, saturated) (Fig. 13.8B) (Zhang, Lockman, et al., 2008; Zhang, Zheng, et al., 2008), utilizing a similar Sonogashira coupling strategy to that used in the synthesis of the saturated and unsaturated tris-scaffolds (Fig. 13.9). These analogs were evaluated as antagonists at $\alpha6\beta2^*$ nAChRs and as ligands for $\alpha4\beta2^*$ and $\alpha7^*$ nAChRs. Three tetrakis-analogs where identified as potent and selective inhibitors of $\alpha6\beta2^*$ nAChR subtype; these were all members of the saturated tetrakis-series, that is, 1,2,4,5-tetrakis-{5-[1-(3-benzylpyridinium)]-n-pentanyl}benzene tetrabromide (TETRAKIS-1) (IC$_{50}$ = 28 nM), 1,2,4,5-tetrakis-{5-[1-(quinolinium)]-n-pentanyl}benzene tetrabromide (TETRAKIS-2) (IC$_{50}$ = 56 nM), and 1,2,4,5-tetrakis-{5-[1-(3-(3-hydroxypropyl)-pyridinium)]-n-pentanyl}benzene tetrabromide (TETRAKIS-3) (IC$_{50}$ = 3.4 nM). It is noteworthy that 3-picolinium analogs in both tetrakis-series afforded only weak inhibitory activity at $\alpha6\beta2^*$ nAChR subtypes, while a variety of significantly larger and unique quaternary ammonium headgroups were present in the more active analogs.

Unfortunately, the tetrakis-analogs were not substrates for the blood–brain barrier choline transporter and consequently turned out be ineffective

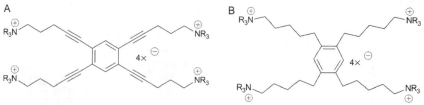

Figure 13.8 Synthetic scheme for the synthesis of tetrakis-3-picolinium and tetrakis-isoquinolinium analogs.

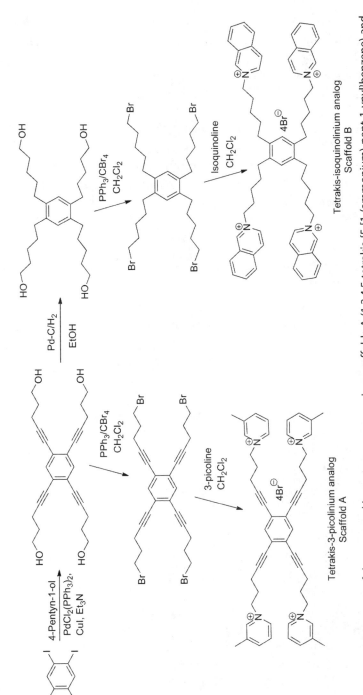

Figure 13.9 Structures of the two tetrakis-quaternary ammonium scaffolds A (1,2,4,5-tetrakis-{5-[1-(ammonium)-pent-1-ynyl]benzene}) and B (1,2,4,5-tetrakis-{5-[1-(ammonium)-pentyl]benzene}); TETRAKIS-1 scaffold A, NR_3 = 3-benzylpyridinium; TETRAKIS-2 scaffold A, NR_3 = quinolinium; TETRAKIS-3 scaffold B, NR_3 = 3-(3-hydroxypropyl)-pyridinium.

in dose-dependently decreasing nicotine self-administration in the rat. Nevertheless, these results and those described earlier for the bis- and tris-analogs suggested that the strategy to identify highly potent nAChR ligands through progressive introduction of cationic moieties around a common phenyl core structure had been successful in affording potent inhibitors of $\alpha6\beta2^*$ nAChRs.

Reviews of our work on the discovery and development of bis-, tris-, and tetrakis-quaternary ammonium salts as potential smoking cessation agents provide a comprehensive account of how new leads from this drug discovery effort were developed in our preclinical pharmacological and behavioral evaluation programs (Dwoskin, Pivavarchyk, et al., 2009; Dwoskin, Smith, et al., 2009).

5.4. QSAR modeling of quaternary ammonium nicotinic receptor antagonists

Since $\alpha6\beta2^*$ nAChRs have not been fully characterized and to gain a better understanding of the relationship between biological activity and antagonist structure, we carried out QSAR modeling studies on the libraries of quaternary ammonium salts as antagonists at $\alpha6\beta2^*$ nAChRs (Zheng et al., 2006). Back-propagation artificial neural networks (ANNs) were trained on a data set of 45 molecules with quantitative IC_{50} values to model structure–activity relationships. The ANN QSAR models produced a reasonable level of correlation between experimental and calculated $\log(1/IC_{50})$ ($r^2 = 0.76$). We have used this predictive model effectively to reduce synthetic and *in vitro* screening activities by eliminating virtual compounds of predicted low activity from the pool of candidate molecules for synthesis. The application of this ANN QSAR model has led to the successful discovery of six new compounds in this study and continues to be utilized as a useful predictive tool for our drug discovery efforts. We were also able to develop a QSAR model to predict maximal inhibition (I_{max}) values for quaternary ammonium antagonists interacting at $\alpha6\beta2^*$ nAChRs (Zheng, McConell, Zhan, Dwoskin, & Crooks, 2009; Zheng, Zheng, et al., 2009). This represented the first reported QSAR study to predict I_{max} values. The study was conducted using multiple linear regression (MLR) analysis and neural network analysis with maximal inhibition values of the antagonists as target values. Both models afforded good correlations (MLR—$r^2 = 0.89$, rmsd $= 9.01$, $q^2 = 0.83$, and loormsd $= 11.1$ and NN—$r^2 = 0.89$, rmsd $= 8.98$, $q^2 = 0.83$, and loormsd $= 11.2$), which provided a basis for rationalizing the selection of virtual compounds for synthesis in the discovery of effective and selective second-generation antagonists of α6β2* nAChRs.

5.5. Bis-, tris-, and tetrakis-tertiary amino analogs

Building on the success of the bis-, tris-, and tetrakis-series of compounds as potent antagonists of α6β2* nAChRs, we initiated a structure–activity study to determine if the azaaromatic headgroups attached to these scaffolds could be replaced with nonaromatic azacyclic tertiary amino headgroups. Our reasoning was based on the properties of the BTMPS molecule [bis-(2,2,6,6,-tetramethyl-4-piperidinyl) sebacate] (Fig. 13.10), a non-competitive, use-dependent antagonist at nAChRs. This molecule incorporates two azacyclic 2,2,6,6-tetramethyl-4-piperidinol (TMP) headgroups separated by a linear sebacate linker and could be considered a structural analog of bPiDDB. One advantage of replacing azaaromatic headgroups with nonaromatic azacyclic headgroups is that this would allow more efficient partitioning of these molecules through cell membranes via passive diffusion, leading to improved oral and brain bioavailability, while still allowing the headgroups to be protonated at physiological pH (since the headgroup moieties would likely have pKas in the range 7–9). Thus, these molecules, like bPiDDB, would be dicationic at physiological pH and may interact with the same receptor binding sites that bPiDDB interacts with. We considered

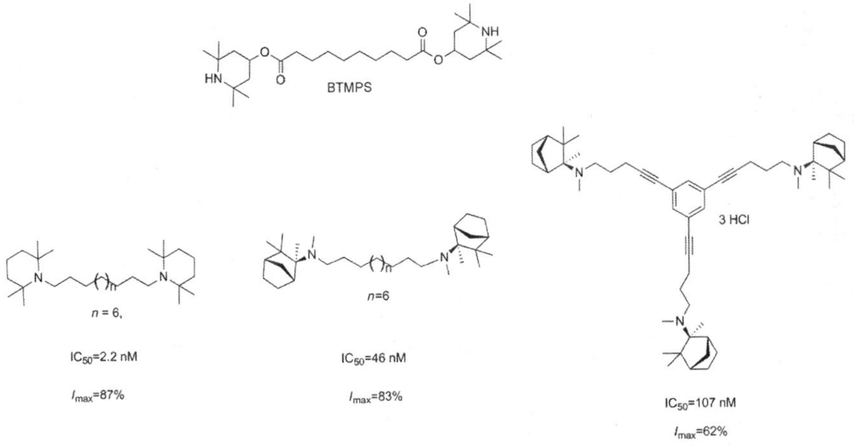

Figure 13.10 Structure of BTMPS and structurally related analogs; IC_{50} and I_{max} values of TMP and mecamylamine analogs in the nicotine-evoked dopamine release assay are also provided.

azacyclic TMP and MEC structures as suitable replacement headgroups for the 3-picolinium headgroups in bPiDDB, since both TMP and MEC have been previously shown to be noncompetitive antagonists at nAChRs. By linking two or three MEC or TMP molecules together via a linear lipophilic bis-methylene linker or a conformationally restricted (unsaturated) tris-scaffold, a series of bis- and tris-tertiary amine analogs were synthesized and evaluated as potent antagonists at $\alpha6$-containing nAChRs (Zhang et al., 2010). Three analogs were identified that exhibited high antagonist potency (Fig. 13.10): the bis-TMP analog, N,N'-dodecane-1,12-diyl-bis-[1-(2,2,6,6-tetramethylpiperidine)] dihydrochloride ($IC_{50} = 2.2$ nM; $I_{max} = 87\%$); the bis-MEC analog, S,S-(+)-N,N'-dodecane-1,12-diyl-bis-1-mecamylamine dichloride ($IC_{50} = 46$ nM; $I_{max} = 90\%$); and the tris-MEC analog, S,S,S-(+)-1,3,5- tri-{5-[1-(mecamylamine)]-pent-1-ynyl}benzene trihydrochloride ($IC_{50} = 107$ nM; $I_{max} = 62\%$). Thus, linking TMP and MEC headgroups to a lipophilic C_{12} n-alkane linker or a conformationally restrained (unsaturated) tris-scaffold with tertiary amino rather than quaternary ammonium headgroups afforded several potent antagonists of $\alpha6\beta2^*$ nAChRs. Such analogs may provide a new strategy for the design of more drug-like molecules that have improved membrane permeation characteristics and high inhibitory potency against $\alpha6\beta2^*$ nAChRs.

The promising results with the bis- and tris-analogs in which azaaromatic quaternary ammonium headgroups had been replaced with nonaromatic azacyclic headgroups prompted us to expand this library of more drug-like molecules. From the synthesis viewpoint, a means to reductively convert our large library of azaaromatic quaternary ammonium bis-, tris-, and tetrakis-analogs into corresponding analogs containing tertiary amino headgroups was sought. This would allow us to generate a large library of more drug-like molecules very efficiently in a single reductive chemical step. We were mindful of the likelihood that exhaustive reduction of the azaaromatic moiety would, in cases where a substituted aromatic heterocyclic headgroup was present (e.g., a 3-picolinium moiety), introduce a chiral center into the resulting azacyclic product, which would cause serious issues with regard to isomer separation in the final product (i.e., multiple diastereomers and their enantiomers). Also, we were aware that the reductive agent to be utilized should be one that would not compromise linkers and/or scaffolds that incorporated double or triple bonds. A suitable reduction methodology utilizing $NaBH_4$ was developed that rapidly and efficiently converted pyridinium and isoquinolinium headgroups into corresponding 1,2,5,6-tetrahydropyridine and 1,2,3,4-tetrahydroisoquinoline headgroups (Zhang et al., 2011). This methodology was selective for azaaromatic moieties and also useful for the reduction of 3-substituted pyridinium headgroups, since the residual double bond in the reduced headgroup prevented the generation of a chiral carbon at C3 of the pyridine ring in the reduced product.

A small library of these more drug-like bis-, tris-, and tetrakis-tertiary amine analogs was generated and evaluated as antagonists of $\alpha6\beta2^*$ nAChRs. Of the analogs tested, several were identified with IC_{50} values in the low nM or sub-nM range. It was observed that the IC_{50} values of these reduced bis-, tris-, and tetrakis-analogs were generally within an order of magnitude of the IC_{50} values of the corresponding parent quaternary ammonium molecule. Also, all the tertiary amino analogs exhibited incomplete inhibition of nicotine-evoked DA release, with I_{max} values ranging from 58% to 76%. The results suggest that the quaternary ammonium lead compounds and their reduced tertiary amine analogs may be interacting at a common site in the channel of the $\alpha6\beta2^*$ nAChR and that the tertiary amine analogs likely interact at these sites in their protonated forms via similar ionic interactions to those involving the quaternary ammonium salts. From a developmental perspective, these tertiary amino analogs that possess better drug-like properties than the parent quaternary ammonium salts are expected to permeate biological membranes more easily, leading to improved oral and brain bioavailability.

A published review (Dwoskin, Pivavarchyk, et al., 2009) provides additional information on the preclinical development of both bPiDDB and reduced bPiDDB (r-bPiDDB or bis-THP3) as nicotinic receptor-based therapeutics and candidates for smoking cessation. Both bPiDDB and bis-THP3 (Fig. 13.11) are effective in decreasing nicotine self-administration in the rat. The ability of bis-THP3 to decrease nicotine self-administration was retained without any loss of effect following seven repeated daily treatments.

More recent studies have now identified several lead molecules that have a common structural scaffold (i.e., two 1,2,5,6-tetrahydropyridino (THP) moieties connected via a C10 or C12 n-alkane linker) that allows for optimization toward drug-likeness and clinical utility (Table 13.1). This scaffold suggests a likely pharmacophore for the antagonist recognition site on α-CtxMII-sensitive nAChRs mediating nicotine-evoked DA release. bis-THP1 (Fig. 13.11) and bis-THP3 (previously known as r-bPiDDB; Dwoskin, Pivavarchyk, et al., 2009; Smith et al., 2010) potently inhibit

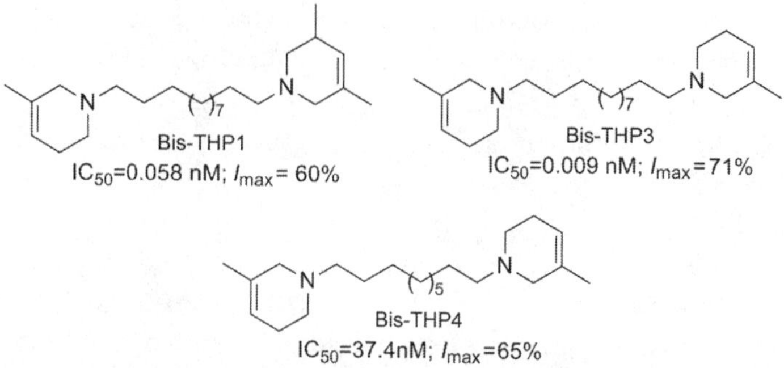

Bis-THP1
$IC_{50}=0.058$ nM; $I_{max}=60\%$

Bis-THP3
$IC_{50}=0.009$ nM; $I_{max}=71\%$

Bis-THP4
$IC_{50}=37.4$nM; $I_{max}=65\%$

Figure 13.11 Structures, IC_{50} and I_{max} values of the three lead analogs, (±)-1-[12-(3-methyl-1,2,5,6-tetrahydropyridin-1-yl)dodecyl]-3,5-dimethyl-1,2,5,6-tetrahydropyridine (bis-THP1), 1,12-bis(3-methyl-1,2,5,6-tetrahydropyridinyl)dodecane (bis-THP3), and 1,10-bis(3-methyl-1,2,5,6-tetrahydropyridinyl)decane (bis-THP4).

Table 13.1 Comparative IC_{50} values, cLog$D$7.4, rotatable bonds, and predicted water solubility (Sw) of a series of nonquaternary ammonium, bis-pyridine analogs

Reduced bis-pyridine analogs	Inhibition of NIC-evoked [³DA] release ($IC_{50} \pm$ SEM, nM)	cLog$D$7.4	Rotatable bonds	Predicted Sw (mg/ml)
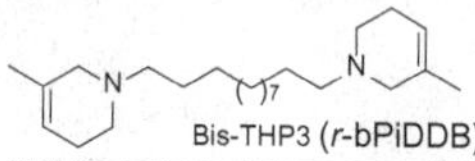 Bis-THP3 (r-bPiDDB)	0.009 ± 0.004	4.6	13	0.02
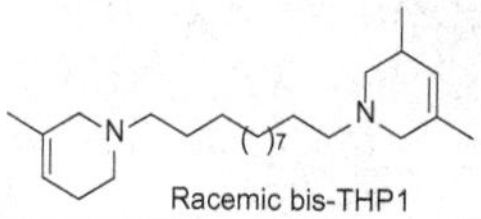 Racemic bis-THP1	0.058 ± 0.020	5.1	13	0.02
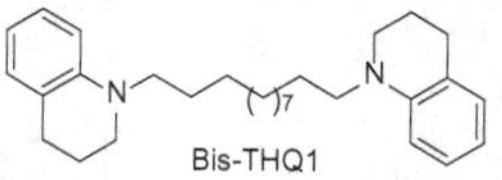 Bis-THQ1	83.5 ± 46.8	9.9	13	<0.01
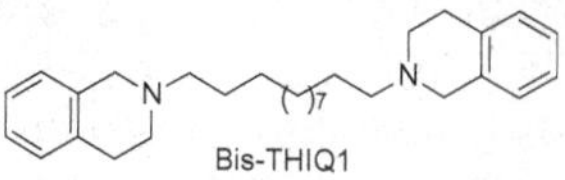 Bis-THIQ1	8.59 ± 3.27	5.9	13	<0.01
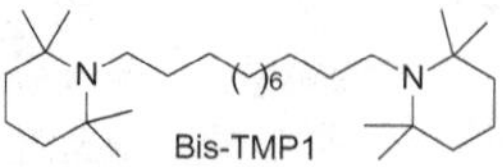 Bis-TMP1	3.51 ± 1.24	7.2	13	0.05

Preliminary results in Dwoskin, Pivavarchyk, et al. (2009), Smith et al. (2010), and Zhang et al. (2010, 2011).

nicotine-evoked DA release ($IC_{50} = 0.009$–0.058 nM; $I_{max} = 60$–74%; Table 13.1 and Fig. 13.11) and inhibit [^{3}H]-nicotine and [^{3}H]-MLA binding only at μM concentrations; note that bis-THP1 is a nonsymmetrical racemic analog and its optical isomers have not yet been evaluated. bis-THP4 (Fig. 13.11), a structurally related analog of bis-THP3 with a C10 linker, exhibits decreased potency ($IC_{50} = 37.4$ nM, $I_{max} = 65\%$) relative to the C12 leads. All the analogs in Table 13.1 are hydrophobic, highly flexible molecules. In terms of drug-likeness, predictive ADMET screening of lead analogs bis-THP1 and bis-THP3 indicates a >75% chance that oral bioavailability will be >30%, with a >20% likelihood that oral bioavailability will be >70%, which is within the acceptable range. However, the Log$D7.4$ is estimated to be in the range 4.6–5.1 for the leads, which is above the ideal range of 1–3 but is still acceptable. Analogs with a Log$D7.4$ of 3–5 are predicted to have good cell membrane permeability, but absorption will be lower, due to lower water solubility, and metabolism will increase owing to increased binding to metabolic enzymes.

The lead bis-THP analogs potently inhibit ($IC_{50} = 9$–58 pM) nicotine-evoked [^{3}H]-DA release at α-CtxMII-sensitive nAChRs (Fig. 13.12, top) (Dwoskin, Pivavarchyk, et al., 2009, unpublished data). Inhibition produced by a maximally effective concentration of bis-THP3 (bPiDDB) was not additive with a maximally effective concentration of α-CtxMII (Fig. 13.12, middle) (Smith et al., 2010), indicating that this lead molecule acts at the same nAChR subtypes as α-CtxMII. Both bis-THP1 and bis-THP3 decreased responding for i.v. nicotine self-administration (Fig. 13.12, bottom) in the rat at doses that had no effect on responding for food and at doses that did not produce any overt signs of toxicity (i.e., lethargy and weight loss) (Dwoskin, Pivavarchyk, et al., 2009, unpublished data). While these behavioral data are encouraging, it is not known if either bis-THP3 or bis-THP1 will block cue-induced reinstatement of nicotine seeking or if these analogs will retain behavioral specificity when given orally. Preliminary results for bis-THP3 reveal a brain–plasma ratio = 2 (60 min post-s.c. dose; 58 μmol/kg).

6. CONCLUSION

Despite the proven efficacy of some current pharmacotherapies for tobacco dependence, relapse rates continue to be high, indicating that novel medications are needed. The rewarding effects of nicotine are mediated, at least in part, by nicotine-evoked DA release leading to sensitization, which is

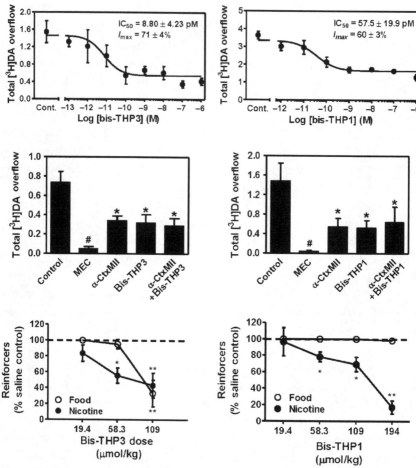

Figure 13.12 *Top*: Concentration-dependent inhibition of NIC-evoked $[^3H]$-DA release by bis-THP3 (bPiDDB) and bis-THP1 in rat striatum *in vitro* (Dwoskin, Pivavarchyk, et al., 2009; Smith et al., 2010). (One-way ANOVAs: bis-THP3, F8, 16 = 33.9, $p < 0.05$; bis-THP1, F7, 27 = 10.7, $p < 0.01$; $n = 9$ and 8, respectively.) *Center*: Inhibition of NIC-evoked $[^3H]$-DA release by maximally effective concentrations of bis-THP3 is not additive with a maximally effective α-CtxMII concentration *in vitro* (one-way ANOVAs:THP3, F4,15 = 82.1, $p < 0.001$ $n = 4$. *$p < 0.05$ compared to control; #$p < 0.05$ compared to α-CtxMII + bis-THP3). *Bottom*: bis-THP3 and bis-THP1 (s.c.) decrease NIC self-administration (i.v.) at doses that do not alter food-maintained responding; $n = 4$–8 per group. *$p < 0.05$, **$p < 0.01$ compared to control.

associated with repeated nicotine administration and nicotine addiction. Based on findings that the nonselective nAChR antagonist MEC has efficacy as a tobacco use cessation agent but is limited by peripherally mediated side effects, we hypothesized that antagonists with selectivity for central nAChR subtypes mediating nicotine-evoked DA release will have efficacy as tobacco use cessation agents with the therapeutic advantage of a limited side-effect profile. While α-CtxMII-insensitive nAChRs (e.g., $\alpha4\beta2^*$) contribute to nicotine-evoked DA release, these nAChRs have a wide distribution in brain, which may lead to nonselective effects. In contrast, α-CtxMII-sensitive nAChRs mediating nicotine-evoked DA release offer an advantage as a target for smoking cessation due to their more restricted localization primarily to DA neurons. Our goal is to identify small drug-like molecules that act as selective antagonists at α-CtxMII-sensitive nAChR subtypes that contain $\alpha6$ and $\beta2$ subunits (i.e., $\alpha6\beta2^*$, $\alpha6\beta2\beta3^*$, $\alpha6\alpha4\beta2\beta3^*$, and $\alpha4\alpha6\beta2^*$). Our earlier research identified quaternary ammonium analogs that act as potent and selective nAChR antagonists. The current focus of our research is to enhance the drug-likeness of these nAChR antagonists, while retaining their high potency and selectivity for $\alpha6\beta2^*$ nAChR subtypes. Our research has shown that novel small molecules can be designed that inhibit ($IC_{50} < 1$ nM) nicotine-evoked DA release *in vitro* by acting as antagonists at α-CtxMII-sensitive nAChR subtypes and by decreasing nicotine self-administration in rats. Thus, our working hypothesis is that novel drug-like bis-THP analogs, which potently and selectively inhibit α-CtxMII-sensitive nAChR subtypes mediating nicotine-evoked DA release, will specifically inhibit nicotine self-administration and/or cue-induced reinstatement of nicotine seeking. Our future research aim is to enhance the drug-likeness of our lead compounds by improving water solubility through introduction of hydrogen-bond acceptor moieties in the linker and by decreasing conformational flexibility toward the goal of identifying orally bioavailable, drug-like preclinical leads for the development as smoking cessation and/or relapse prevention.

CONFLICT OF INTEREST

A potential royalty stream to PAC and LPD may occur consistent with University of Kentucky policy.

ACKNOWLEDGMENTS

This research was supported by NIH grant U19DA017548. The University of Kentucky holds patents on the compounds described in the current work.

REFERENCES

Albayati, Z. A. F., Dwoskin, L. P., & Crooks, P. A. (2008). Pharmacokinetics of the novel nicotinic receptor antagonist N, N'-dodecane-1,12-diyl-bis-3-picolinium dibromide in the rat. *Drug Metabolism and Disposition, 18*, 3870–3873.

Anand, R., Conroy, W. G., Schoepfer, R., Whiting, P., & Lindstrom, J. (1991). Neuronal nicotinic acetylcholine receptors expressed in Xenopus oocytes have a pentameric quaternary structure. Journal of Biological Chemistry, 266, 11192–11198.

Arroyo-Jimenez, M. M., Bourgeois, J. P., Marubio, L. M., Le Sourd, A. M., Ottersen, O. P., Rinvik, E., et al. (1999). Ultrastructural localization of the α4-subunit of the neuronal acetylcholine nicotinic receptor in the rat substantia nigra. Journal of Neuroscience, 19, 6475–6487.

Ayers, J. T., Dwoskin, L. P., Deaciuc, A. G., Grinevich, V. P., Zhu, J., & Crooks, P. A. (2002). bis-Azaaromatic quaternary ammonium analogues: Ligands for α4β2 and α7* subtypes of neuronal nicotinic receptors. Bioorganic and Medicinal Chemistry Letters, 12, 3067–3071.

Bacher, I., Wu, B., Shytle, D. R., & George, T. P. (2009). Mecamylamine—A nicotinic acetylcholine receptor antagonist with potential for the treatment of neuropsychiatric disorders. Expert Opinion on Pharmacotherapy, 10, 2709–2721.

Benowitz, N. L. (2009). Pharmacology of nicotine: Addiction, smoking-induced disease and therapeutics. Annual Review of Pharmacology and Toxicology, 49, 57–71.

Bourque, J., Mendrek, A., Dinh-Williams, S. L., & Potvin, S. (2013). Neural circuitry of impulsivity in a cigarette craving paradigm. Front Psychiatry, 4, 1–9. Article 67.

Brunzell, D. H. (2012). Preclinical evidence that activation of mesolimbic alpha 6 subunit containing nicotinic acetylcholine receptors supports nicotine addiction phenotype. Nicotine & Tobacco Research, 14, 1258–1269.

Brunzell, D. H., Boschen, K. E., Hendrick, E. S., Beardsley, P. M., & McIntosh, J. M. (2010). Alpha-conotoxin MII-sensitive nicotinic acetylcholine receptors in the nucleus accumbens shell regulate progressive ratio responding maintained by nicotine. Neuropsychopharmacology, 35, 665–673.

Cachelin, A. B., & Rust, G. (1995). β-Subunits co-determine the sensitivity of rat neuronal nicotinic receptors to antagonists. Pflugers Archive: European Journal of Physiology, 429, 449.

Cartier, G. E., Yoshikami, D., Gray, W. R., Luo, S., Olivera, B. M., & McIntosh, J. M. (1996). A new α-conotoxin which targets α3β2 nicotinic acetylcholine receptors. Journal of Biological Chemistry, 271, 7522–7528.

Coe, J. W., Brooks, P. R., Vetelino, M. G., Wirtz, M. C., Arnold, E. P., & Huang, J. (2005). Varenicline: An alpha4beta2 nicotinic receptor partial agonist for smoking cessation. Journal of Medicinal Chemistry, 48, 3474–3477.

Cohen, C., Bergis, O. E., Galli, F., Lochead, A. W., Jegham, S., Biton, B., et al. (2003). SSR591813, a novel selective and partial alpha4beta2 nicotinic receptor agonist with potential as an aid to smoking cessation. Journal of Pharmacology and Experimental Therapeutics, 306, 407–420.

Collins, A. C., Salminen, O., Marks, M. J., Whiteaker, P., & Grady, S. R. (2009). The road to discovery of neuronal nicotinic cholinergic receptor subtypes. In Nicotine psychopharmacology. Handbook of experimental pharmacology, Vol. 192, (pp. 85–112). New York, NY: Springer.

Conroy, W. G., Vernallis, A. B., & Berg, D. K. (1992). The α5 gene product assembles with multiple acetylcholine receptor subunits to form distinctive receptor subtypes in brain. Neuron, 9, 679–691.

Corrigall, W. A., Franklin, K. B. J., Coen, K. M., & Clarke, P. B. S. (1992). The mesolimbic dopaminergic system is implicated in the reinforcing properties of nicotine. Psychopharmacology, 107, 285–289.

Crooks, P. A., Ayers, J. T., Rui, X., Sumithran, S. P., Grinevich, V. P., Wilkins, L. W., et al. (2004). Development of subtype-selective nicotinic receptor ligands as receptor antagonists. Bioorganic and Medicinal Chemistry Letters, 14, 1869–1874.

Crooks, P. A., Ravard, A., Teng, L. H., & Dwoskin, L. P. (1995). Inhibition of nicotine-evoked [^{3}H]dopamine release by pyridine N-substituted nicotine analogues: A new class of nicotinic antagonist. *Drug Development Research, 36*, 71–82.

Cui, C., Booker, T. K., Allen, R. S., Grady, S. R., Whiteaker, P., Marks, M. J., et al. (2003). The β3 nicotinic receptor subunit: A component of α-conotoxin MII-binding nicotinic acetylcholine receptors that modulate dopamine release and related behaviors. *Journal of Neuroscience, 23*, 11045–11053.

Dani, J. A., & Bertrand, D. (2007). Nicotinic acetylcholine receptors and nicotinic cholinergic mechanisms of the central nervous system. *Annual Review of Pharmacology and Toxicology, 47*, 699–729.

DeNoble, V. J., & Mele, P. C. (2006). Intravenous nicotine self-administration in rats: Effects of mecamylamine, hexamethonium and naloxone. *Psychopharmacology, 184*, 266–272.

Drenan, R. M., Grady, S. R., Steele, A. D., McKinney, S., Patzlaff, N. E., McIntosh, J. M., et al. (2010). Cholinergic modulation of locomotion and striatal dopamine release is mediated by α6α4* nicotinic acetylcholine receptors. *Journal of Neuroscience, 30*, 9877–9889.

Drenan, R. M., Grady, S. R., Whiteaker, P., McClure-Begley, T., McKinney, S., Miwa, J. M., et al. (2008). In vivo activation of midbrain dopamine neurons via sensitized high affinity α6* nicotinic acetylcholine receptors. *Neuron, 60*, 123–136.

Drenan, R. M., Nashmi, R., Imoukhuede, P., Just, H., McKinney, S., & Lester, H. A. (2008). Subcellular trafficking, pentameric assembly and subunit stoichiometry of neuronal nicotinic acetylcholine receptors containing fluorescently labeled α6 and β3 subunits. *Molecular Pharmacology, 73*, 27–41.

Dwoskin, L. P., & Bardo, M. T. (2009). Targeting nicotinic receptor antagonists as novel pharmacotherapies for tobacco dependence and relapse. *Neuropsychopharmacology, 34*, 244–246.

Dwoskin, L. P., & Crooks, P. A. (2001). Competitive neuronal nicotinic receptor antagonists: A new direction for drug discovery. *Journal of Pharmacology and Experimental Therapeutics, 298*, 395–402.

Dwoskin, L. P., Leibee, L. L., Jewell, A. L., Fang, Z.-X., & Crooks, P. A. (1992). Inhibition of [^{3}H]-dopamine uptake into rat striatal slices by quaternary N-methylated nicotine metabolites. *Life Sciences, 50*, PL233–PL237.

Dwoskin, L. P., Pivavarchyk, M., Joyce, B. M., Neugebauer, N. M., Zheng, G., Zhang, Z., et al. (2009). Targeting reward-relevant nicotinic receptors in the discovery of novel pharmacotherapeutic agents to treat tobacco dependence. In R. A. Bevins & A. R. Caggiula (Eds.), *55th annual Nebraska symposium on motivation: The motivational impact of nicotine and its role in tobacco use* , Vol. 55. (pp. 31–63). New York, NY: Springer.

Dwoskin, L. P., Smith, A. M., Wooters, T. E., Zhang, Z., Crooks, P. A., & Bardo, M. T. (2009). Nicotinic receptor-based therapeutics and candidates for smoking cessation. *Biochemical Pharmacology, 78*, 732–743, NIHMS123315.

Dwoskin, L. P., Sumithran, S. P., Zhu, J., Deaciuc, A. G., Ayers, J. T., & Crooks, P. A. (2004). Subtype-selective nicotinic receptor antagonists: Potential as tobacco use cessation agents. *Bioorganic and Medicinal Chemistry Letters, 14*, 1863–1867.

Dwoskin, L. P., Wilkins, L. H., Pauly, J., & Crooks, P. A. (1999). Development of a novel class of subtype-selective nicotinic receptor antagonist: Pyridine-N-substituted nicotine analogs. In B. Rudy & P. Seeburg (Eds.), *Molecular and functional diversity of ion channels and receptors*, Vol. 868. New York, NY: Wiley Dwoskin (Special Issue).

Dwoskin, L. P., Wooters, T. E., Sumithran, S. P., Siripurapu, K. B., Joyce, B. M., Lockman, P. R., et al. (2008). N, N'-Alkane-diyl-bis-3-picoliniums as nicotinic receptor antagonists: Inhibition of nicotine-induced dopamine release and hyperactivity. *Journal of Pharmacology and Experimental Therapeutics 326*, 563–576.

Etter, J.-F. (2006). Cytisine for smoking cessation: A literature review and a meta-analysis. *Archives of Internal Medicine, 166*, 1553–1559.

Exley, R., Clements, M. A., Hartung, H., McIntosh, M. J., & Cragg, S. J. (2008). α6 Containing nicotinic acetylcholine receptors dominate the nicotine control of dopamine neurotransmission in nucleus accumbens. *Neuropsychopharmacology*, 3, 2158–2166.

Fagerstrom, K., & Balfour, D. J. (2006). Neuropharmacology and potential efficacy of new treatments for tobacco dependence. *Expert Opinion on Investigational Drugs*, 15, 107–116.

FDA Drug Safety Communication (2011). *Chantix (varenicline) may increase the risk of certain cardiovascular adverse events in patients with cardiovascular disease*. http://www.fda.gov/Drugs/DrugSafety/ucm259161.htm.

FDA Public Health Advisory (2008). *Public health advisory on Chantix*. http://www.fda.gov/CDER/Drug/early_comm/varenicline.htm.

FDA Public Health Advisory (2009). *FDA requires new boxed warnings for the smoking cessation drugs Chantix and Zyban*. http://www.fda.gov/Drugs/DrugSafety/PostmarketDrugSafetyInformationforPatientsandProviders/DrugSafetyInformationforHealthcareProfessionals/PublicHealthAdvisories/ucm169988.htm.

Flores, C. M., Rogers, S. W., Pabreza, L. A., Wolfe, B. B., & Kellar, K. J. (1992). A subtype of nicotinic cholinergic receptor in rat brain is composed of alpha4 and beta2 subunits and is up-regulated by chronic nicotine treatment. *Molecular Pharmacology*, 41, 31–37.

Forsayeth, J. R., & Kobrin, E. (1997). Formation of oligomers containing the β3 and β4 subunits of the rat nicotinic receptor. *Journal of Neuroscience*, 17, 1531–1538.

Fryer, J. D., & Lukas, R. J. (1999). Noncompetitive functional inhibition at diverse, human nicotinic acetylcholine receptor subtypes by bupropion, phencyclidine, and ibogaine. *Journal of Pharmacology and Experimental Therapeutics*, 288, 88–92.

Garwood, C. L., & Potts, L. A. (2007). Emerging pharmacotherapies for smoking cessation. *American Journal of Health-System Pharmacy*, 15, 1693–1698.

George, T. P., & O'Malley, S. S. (2004). Current pharmacological treatments for nicotine dependence. *Trends in Pharmacological Sciences*, 25, 42–48.

Glick, S. D., Visker, K. E., & Maisonneuve, J. M. (1996). An oral self-administration model of nicotine preference in rats: Effects of mecamylamine. *Psychopharmacology*, 128, 426–431.

Goldner, F. M., Dineley, K. T., & Patrick, J. W. (1997). Immunohistochemical localization of the nicotinic acetylcholine receptor subunit α6 to dopaminergic neurons in the substantia nigra and ventral tegmental area. *Neuroreport*, 8, 2739–2742.

Gotti, C., Guiducci, S., Tedesco, V., Corbiolo, S., Zanetti, L., Moretti, M., et al. (2010). Nicotinic acetylcholine receptors in the mesolimbic pathway: Primary role of ventral tegmental area α6β2* receptors in mediating systemic nicotine effects on dopamine release, locomotion, and reinforcement. *Journal of Neuroscience*, 30, 5311–5325.

Gotti, C., Moretti, M., Clementi, F., Riganti, F., McIntosh, J. M., Collins, A. C., et al. (2005). Expression of nigrostriatal α6-containing nicotinic acetylcholine receptors is selectively reduced, but not eliminated, by β3 subunit gene deletion. *Molecular Pharmacology*, 67, 2007–2015.

Gotti, C., Zoli, M., & Clementi, F. (2006). Brain nicotinic acetylcholine receptors: Native subtypes and their relevance. *Trends in Pharmacological Sciences*, 27, 482–491.

Grady, S. R., Meinerz, N. M., Cao, J., Reynolds, A. M., Picciotto, M. R., Changeux, J.-P., et al. (2001). Nicotinic agonists stimulate acetylcholine release from mouse interpeduncular nucleus: A function mediated by a different nAChR than dopamine release from striatum. *Journal of Neurochemistry*, 76, 258–268.

Grady, S. R., Salminen, O., Laverty, D. C., Whiteaker, P., McIntosh, J. M., & Collins, A. C. (2007). The subtypes of nicotinic acetylcholine receptors on dopaminergic terminals of mouse striatum. *Biochemical Pharmacology*, 74, 1235–1246.

Hajek, P., McRobbie, H., & Myers, K. (2013). Efficacy of cytisine in helping smokers quit: Systematic review and meta-analysis. *Thorax*. http://dx.doi.org/10.1136/thoraxjnl-2012-203035.

Hajek, P., Stead, L. F., West, R., Jarvis, M., Hartmann-Boyce, J., & Lancaster, T. (2013). Relapse prevention interventions for smoking cessation. *Cochrane Database of Systematic Reviews*, (8). http://dx.doi.org/10.1002/1465188458, Art. No. CD003999.

Harmey, D., Griffin, P. R., & Kenny, P. J. (2012). Development of novel pharmacotherapeutics for tobacco dependence: Progress and future directions. *Nicotine & Tobacco Research*, *14*, 1300–1318.

Harvey, S. C., & Luetje, C. W. (1996). Determinants of competitive antagonist sensitivity on neuronal nicotinic receptor beta subunits. *Journal of Neuroscience*, *16*, 3798–3806.

Harvey, S. C., Maddox, F. N., & Luetje, C. W. (1996). Multiple determinants of dihydro-beta-erythroidine sensitivity on rat neuronal nicotinic receptor alpha subunits. *Journal of Neurochemistry*, *67*, 1953–1959.

Hurt, R. D., Krook, J. E., Croghan, I. T., Loprinzi, C. L., Sloan, J. A., Novotny, P. J., et al. (2003). Nicotine patch therapy based on smoking rate followed by bupropion for prevention of relapse to smoking. *Journal of Clinical Oncology*, *21*, 914–920.

Irvin, J. E., Hendricks, P. S., & Brandon, T. H. (2003). The increasing recalcitrance of smokers in clinical trials II: Pharmacotherapy trials. *Nicotine and Tobacco Research*, *5*, 27–35.

Jackson, K. J., McIntosh, J. M., Brunzell, D. H., Sanjakdar, S. S., & Damaj, M. I. (2009). The role of α6-containing nicotinic acetylcholine receptors in nicotine reward and withdrawal. *Journal of Pharmacology and Experimental Therapeutics*, *331*, 547–554.

Johnstone, T. B., Hogankamp, D. J., Coyne, L., Su, J., Halliwell, R. F., Tran, M. B., et al. (2004). Modifying quinolone antibiotics yields new anxiolytics. *Nature Medicine*, *10*, 31–32.

Jorenby, D. E., Hays, J. T., Rigotti, N. A., Azoulay, S., Watsky, E. J., Williams, K. E., et al. (2006). Efficacy of varenicline, an alpha4beta2 nicotinic acetylcholine receptor partial agonist, vs placebo or sustained-release bupropion for smoking cessation: A randomized controlled trial. *JAMA*, *296*, 56–63.

Kaiser, S. A., Soliakov, L., Harvey, S. C., Luetje, C. W., & Wonnacott, S. (1998). Differential inhibition by α-conotoxin-MII of the nicotinic stimulation of [3H]dopamine release from rat striatal synaptosomes and slices. *Journal of Neurochemistry*, *70*, 1069–1076.

Koelle, G. B. (1975). Neuromuscular blocking agents. In L. S. Goodman & A. Gilman (Eds.), *The pharmacological basis of therapeutic* (pp. 575–588). New York, NY: MacMillan Publishing Co.

Kulak, J. M., Nguyen, T. A., Olivera, B. M., & McIntosh, J. M. (1997). α-Conotoxin MII blocks nicotine-stimulated dopamine release in rat striatal synaptosomes. *Journal of Neuroscience*, *17*, 5263–5270.

Kuryatov, A., & Lindstrom, J. (2011). Expression of functional human $\alpha6\beta2\beta3^*$ acetylcholine receptors in *Xenopus laevis* oocytes achieved through subunit chimeras and concatamers. *Molecular Pharmacology*, *79*, 126–140.

Le Foll, B., & Goldberg, S. R. (2005). Control of the reinforcing effects of nicotine by associated environmental stimuli in animals and humans. *TRENDS in Pharmacological Sciences*, *26*, 287–293.

Le Foll, B., & Goldberg, S. R. (2009). Effects of nicotine in experimental animals and humans: An update on addictive properties. In *Handbook of experimental pharmacology*, Vol. 192, (pp. 335–367). New York, NY: Springer.

Le Novère, N., Zoli, M., & Changeux, J. P. (1996). Neuronal nicotinic receptor alpha6 subunit mRNA is selectively concentrated in catecholaminergic nuclei of the rat brain. *European Journal of Neuroscience*, *8*, 2428–2439.

Lockman, P. R., Geldenhuys, W. J., Manda, V., Thomas, F., Crooks, P. A., Dwoskin, L. P., et al. (2008). Carrier mediated transport at the blood–brain barrier for the quaternary ammonium nicotinic receptor antagonist, N, N-dodecyl-bis-picolinium bromide (bPiDDB). *Journal of Pharmacology and Experimental Therapeutics, 324*, 244–250.

Lukas, R. J. (2007). *Pharmacological effects of nicotine and nicotinic receptor subtype pharmacological profiles*. Boca Raton, FL: CRC Press LLC.

Lundahl, L. H., Henningfield, J. E., & Lukas, S. E. (2000). Mecamylamine blockade of both positive and negative effects of IV nicotine in human volunteers. *Pharmacology, Biochemistry, and Behavior, 66*, 637–643.

McCallum, S. E., Collins, A. C., Paylor, R., & Marks, M. J. (2006). Deletion of the beta2 nicotinic acetylcholine receptor subunit alters development of tolerance to nicotine and eliminates receptor upregulation. *Psychopharmacology, 184*, 314–327.

McGehee, D. S., & Role, L. W. (1995). Physiological diversity of nicotinic acetylcholine receptors expressed by vertebrate neurons. *Annual Review of Physiology, 57*, 521–546.

McIntosh, J. M., Plazas, P. V., Watkins, M., Gomez-Casati, M. E., Olivera, B. M., & Elgoyhen, A. B. (2005). A novel alpha-conotoxin, PeIA, cloned from *Conus pergrandis*, discriminates between rat alpha9alpha10 and alpha7 nicotinic cholinergic receptors. *Journal of Biological Chemistry, 280*, 30107–30112.

Mihalak, K. B., Carroll, F. I., & Luetje, C. W. (2006). Varenicline is a partial agonist at alpha4beta2 and a full agonist at alpha7 neuronal nicotinic receptors. *Molecular Pharmacology, 70*, 801–805.

Millar, N. S., & Gotti, C. (2009). Diversity of vertebrate nicotinic acetylcholine receptors. *Neuropharmacology, 56*, 237–246.

Mills, E. J., Wu, P., Spurden, D., Ebbert, J. O., & Wilson, K. (2009). Efficacy of pharmacotherapies for short-term smoking abstinence: A systematic review and meta-analysis. *Harm Reduction Journal, 6*, 25.

Mineur, Y. S., Somenzi, O., & Picciotto, M. R. (2007). Cytisine, a partial agonist of high-affinity nicotinic acetylcholine receptors, has antidepressant-like properties in male C57BL/6J mice. *Neuropharmacology, 52*, 1256–1262.

Moretti, M., Mugnaini, M., Tessari, M., Zoli, M., Gaimarri, A., Manfredi, I., et al. (2010). A comparative study of the effects of the intravenous self-administration or subcutaneous minipump infusion of nicotine on the expression of brain neuronal nicotinic receptor subtypes. *Molecular Pharmacology, 78*, 287–296.

Neugebauer, N. M., Zhang, Z., Crooks, P. A., Dwoskin, L. P., & Bardo, M. T. (2006). Effect of a novel nicotinic receptor antagonist, N, N′-dodecane-1,12-diyl-bis-3-picolinium dibromide (bPiDDB), on nicotine self-administration and hyperactivity in rats. *Psychopharmacology, 184*, 426–434.

Papke, R. L., Wecker, L., & Stitzel, J. A. (2010). Activation and inhibition of mouse muscle and neuronal nicotinic acetylcholine receptors expressed in *Xenopus* oocytes. *Journal of Pharmacology and Experimental Therapeutics, 333*, 501–518.

Paterson, N. E., Min, W., Hackett, A., Lowe, D., Hanania, T., Caldarone, B., et al. (2010). The high-affinity nAChR partial agonists varenicline and sazetidine-A exhibit reinforcing properties in rats. *Progress in Neuro-Psychopharmacology & Biological Psychiatry, 34*, 1455–1464.

Perkins, K. A. (1999). Nicotine self-administration. *Nicotine and Tobacco Research, 2*, 133–137.

Picciotto, M. R., & Kenny, P. J. (2013). Molecular mechanisms underlying behaviors related to nicotine addiction. *Cold Spring Harbor Perspectives in Medicine, 3*. http://dx.doi.org/10.1101/cshperspect.a012112.

Pons, S., Fattore, L., Cossu, G., Tolu, S., Porcu, E., McIntosh, J. M., et al. (2008). Crucial role of α4 and α6 nicotinic acetylcholine receptor subunits from ventral tegmental area in systemic nicotine self-administration. *Journal of Neuroscience, 28*, 12318–12327.

Quarta, D., Ciruela, F., Patkar, K., Borycz, J., Solinas, M., Lluis, C., et al. (2007). Heteromeric nicotinic acetylcholine-dopamine autoreceptor complexes modulate striatal dopamine release. *Neuropsychopharmacology, 32*, 35–42.

Rahman, S., Zhang, Z., Papke, R. L., Crooks, P. A., Dwoskin, L. P., & Bardo, M. T. (2008). Region-specific effects of the novel nicotinic receptor antagonist N, N'-dodecane-1,12-diyl-bis-3-picolinium bromide (bPiDDB) on the nicotine-induced increase in extracellular dopamine: An in vivo reverse microdialysis study. *British Journal of Pharmacology*, *153*, 792–804.

Rau, K. S., Birdsall, E., Hanson, J. E., Johnson-Davis, K. L., Carroll, F. I., Wilkins, D. G., et al. (2005). Bupropion increases striatal vesicular monoamine transport. *Neuropharmacology*, *49*, 820–830.

Rose, J. E. (2006). Nicotine and non-nicotine factors in cigarette addiction. *Psychopharmacology*, *184*, 274–285.

Rose, J. E. (2008). Disrupting nicotine reinforcement from cigarette to brain. *Annals of the New York Academy of Sciences*, *1141*, 233–256.

Rose, J. E. (2009). New findings on addiction and treatment. In R. A. Bevins & A. R. Caggiula (Eds.), *55th annual Nebraska symposium on motivation: The motivational impact of nicotine and its role in tobacco use*, Vol. 55, (pp. 230–242). New York, NY: Springer.

Rose, J. E., Behm, F. M., Westman, E. C., Levin, E. D., Stein, R. M., & Ripka, G. V. (1994). Mecamylamine combined with nicotine skin patch facilitates smoking cessation beyond nicotine patch treatment alone. *Clinical Pharmacology and Therapeutics*, *56*, 86–99.

Rose, J. E., Salley, A., Behm, F. M., Bates, J. E., & Westman, E. C. (2010). Reinforcing effects of nicotine and non-nicotine components of cigarette smoke. *Psychopharmacology*, *1*, 1–12.

Salminen, O., Drapeau, J. A., McIntosh, J. M., Collins, A. C., Marks, M. J., & Grady, S. R. (2007). Pharmacology of α-conotoxin MII-sensitive subtypes of nicotinic acetylcholine receptors isolated by breeding of null mutant mice. *Molecular Pharmacology*, *71*, 1563–1571.

Salminen, O., Murphy, K. L., McIntosh, J. M., Drago, J., Marks, M. J., Collins, A. C., et al. (2004). Subunit composition and pharmacology of two classes of striatal presynaptic nicotinic acetylcholine receptors mediating dopamine release in mice. *Molecular Pharmacology*, *65*, 1526–1535.

Sanofi Pipeline. (2012). http://en.sanofi-aventis.com/binaries/080212_PDF_Slides_media_tcm28-15767.pdf.

Schuh, L. M., Schuh, K. J., & Henningfield, J. E. (1996). Pharmacologic determinants of tobacco dependence. *American Journal of Therapy*, *3*, 335–341.

Shahan, T. A., Odum, A. L., & Bickel, W. K. (2000). Nicotine gum as a substitute for cigarettes: A behavioral economic analysis. *Behavioral Pharmacology*, *11*, 71–79.

Slemmer, J. E., Martin, B. R., & Damaj, M. I. (2000). Bupropion is a nicotinic antagonist. *Journal of Pharmacology and Experimental Therapeutics*, *295*, 321–327.

Smith, A. M., Dhawan, G. K., Zhang, Z., Siripurapu, K. B., Crooks, P. A., & Dwoskin, L. P. (2009). The novel nicotinic receptor antagonist, N, N'-dodecane-1,12-diyl-bis-3-picolinium dibromide (bPiDDB), inhibits nicotine-evoked [3H]norepinephrine overflow from rat hippocampal slices. *Biochemical Pharmacology*, *78*, 889–897.

Smith, A. M., Pivavarchyk, M., Wooters, T. E., Zhang, Z., McIntosh, J. M., Crooks, P. A., et al. (2010). Repeated nicotine increases bPiDDB potency to inhibit nicotine-evoked DA release from rat striatum. *Biochemical Pharmacology*, *80*, 402–409.

Stoker, A. K., & Markou, A. (2013). Unraveling the neurobiology of nicotine dependence using genetically engineered mice. *Current Opinion in Neurobiology*, *23*, 493–499.

Thomas, K. H., Martin, R. M., Davies, N. M., Metcalfe, C., Windmeijer, F., & Gunnel, D. (2013). Smoking cessation treatment and risk of depression, suicide, and self harm in the Clinical Practice Research Datalink prospective cohort study. *British Journal of Medicine*, *347*, f5704.

Toll, L., Zaveri, N. T., Polgar, W. E., Jiang, F., Khroyan, T. V., Zhou, W., et al. (2012). AT-1001: A high affinity and selective α3β4 nicotinic acetylcholine receptor antagonist blocks nicotine self-administration in rats. *Neuropsychopharmacology*, *37*, 1367–1376.

Turner, J. R., & Kellar, K. J. (2005). Nicotinic cholinergic receptors in the rat cerebellum: Multiple heteromeric subtypes. *Journal of Neuroscience*, *25*, 9258–9265.

VanderVeen, J. W., Cohen, L. M., & Watson, N. L. (2012). Utilizing a multimodal assessment strategy to examine variations of impulsivity among young adults engaged in co-occurring smoking and binge drinking behaviors. *Drug and Alcohol Dependence*, *127*, 150–155.

Wada, E., Wada, K., Boulter, J., Deneris, E., Heinemann, S., Patrick, J., et al. (1989). Distribution of alpha2, alpha3, alpha4, and beta2 neuronal nicotinic receptor subunit mRNAs in the central nervous system: A hybridization histochemical study in the rat. *Journal of Comparative Neurology*, *284*, 314–335.

Whiteaker, P., Marks, M. J., Grady, S. R., Lu, Y., Picciotto, M. R., Changeux, J. P., et al. (2000). Pharmacological and null mutation approaches reveal nicotinic receptor diversity. *European Journal of Pharmacology*, *393*(1–3), 123–135.

Whiting, P., & Lindstrom, J. (1987). Purification and characterization of a nicotinic acetylcholine receptor from rat brain. *Proceedings of the National Academy of Sciences of the United States of America*, *84*, 595–599.

Wileyto, P., Patterson, F., Niaura, R., Epstein, L., Brown, R., Audrain-McGovern, J., et al. (2004). Do small lapses predict relapse to smoking behavior under bupropion treatment? *Nicotine and Tobacco Research*, *6*, 357–366.

Wooters, T. E., Smith, A. M., Pivavarchyk, M., Siripurapu, K. B., McIntosh, J. M., Zhang, Z., et al. (2011). bPiDI: A novel selective α6β2* nicotinic receptor antagonist and preclinical candidate treatment for nicotine abuse. *British Journal of Pharmacology*, *163*, 346–357.

Wu, P., Wilson, K., Dimoulas, P., & Mills, E. J. (2006). Effectiveness of smoking cessation therapies: A systematic review and meta-analysis. *BMC Public Health*, *6*, 300.

Xiao, Y., Fan, H., Musachio, J. L., Wei, Z. L., Chellappan, S. K., Kozikowski, A. P., et al. (2006). Sazetidine-A, a novel ligand that desensitizes alpha4beta2 nicotinic acetylcholine receptors without activating them. *Molecular Pharmacology*, *70*, 1454–1460.

Xiao, Y., Woolverton, W. L., Sahibzada, N., Yasuda, R. P., & Kellar, K. J. (2007). Pharmacological properties of sazetidine-A, a desensitizer of alpha4beta2 nicotinic acetylcholine receptors. *Society for Neuroscience—Abstracts*, *33*, 574.6.

Yoshimura, R. F., Hogenkamp, D. J., Li, W. Y., Tran, M. B., Belluzzi, J. D., Whittemore, E. R., et al. (2007). Negative allosteric modulation of nicotinic acetylcholine receptors blocks nicotine self-administration in rats. *Journal of Pharmacology and Experimental Therapeutics*, *323*, 907–915.

Zatonski, W., Cedzynska, M., Tutka, P., & West, R. (2006). An uncontrolled trial of cytisine (Tabex) for smoking cessation. *Tobacco Control*, *15*, 481–484.

Zhang, Z., Lockman, P. R., Mittapalli, R. K., Allen, D. D., Dwoskin, L. P., & Crooks, P. A. (2008). bis-Pyridinium cyclophanes: Novel ligands with high affinity for the blood–brain barrier choline transporter. *Bioorganic and Medicinal Chemistry Letters*, *18*, 5622–5625.

Zhang, Z., Pivavarchyk, M., Subramanian, K. L., Deaciuc, A. G., Dwoskin, L. P., & Crooks, P. A. (2010). Novel bis-2,2,6,6-tetramethylpiperidine (bis-TMP) and bis-mecamylamine antagonists at neuronal nicotinic receptors mediating nicotine-evoked dopamine release. *Bioorganic and Medicinal Chemistry Letters*, *20*, 1420–1423.

Zhang, Z., Zheng, G., Pivavarchyk, M., Deaciuc, A. G., Dwoskin, L. P., & Crooks, P. A. (2008). tetrakis-Azaaromatic quaternary ammonium: Selective neuronal nicotinic receptor antagonists at subtypes that mediate nicotine-evoked dopamine release. *Bioorganic and Medicinal Chemistry Letters*, *18*, 5753–5757.

Zhang, Z., Zheng, G., Pivavarchyk, M., Deaciuc, A. G., Dwoskin, L. P., & Crooks, P. A. (2011). Novel bis-, tris-, and tetrakis tertiary amino analogs as antagonists at neuronal nicotinic receptors that mediate nicotine-evoked dopamine release. *Bioorganic and Medicinal Chemistry Letters*, *21*, 88–91.

Zheng, F., Bayram, E., Sumithran, S. P., Ayers, J. T., Zhan, C. G., Schmitt, J. D., et al. (2006). QSAR modeling of mono- and bis-quaternary ammonium salts that act as antagonists at neuronal nicotinic acetylcholine receptors mediating dopamine release. *Bioorganic and Medicinal Chemistry*, *14*, 3017–3037.

Zheng, F., McConell, M., Zhan, C.-G., Dwoskin, L. P., & Crooks, P. A. (2009). QSAR study on maximal inhibition (I_{max}) of quaternary ammonium antagonists for S-(-)-nicotine-evoked dopamine release from dopaminergic nerve terminals in rat striatum. *Bioorganic and Medicinal Chemistry*, *17*, 4477–4485.

Zheng, G., Sumithran, S. P., Deaciuc, A. G., Dwoskin, L. P., & Crooks, P. A. (2007). tris-Azaaromatic quaternary ammonium salts: Novel templates as antagonists at nicotinic receptors mediating nicotine-evoked dopamine release. *Bioorganic and Medicinal Chemistry Letters*, *17*, 6701–6706.

Zheng, G., Zhang, Z., Lockman, P. R., Geldenhuys, W. J., Allen, D. D., Dwoskin, L. P., et al. (2010). bis-Azaaromatic quaternary ammonium salts as ligands for the blood–brain barrier choline transporter. *Bioorganic and Medicinal Chemistry Letters*, *20*, 3208–3210.

Zheng, G., Zhang, Z., Pivarvarchyk, M., Deaciuc, A. G., Dwoskin, L. P., & Crooks, P. A. (2007). bis-Azaaromatic quaternary ammonium salts as antagonists at nicotinic receptors mediating nicotine-evoked dopamine release: An investigation of binding conformation. *Bioorganic and Medicinal Chemistry Letters*, *17*, 6734–6738.

Zheng, F., Zheng, G., Deaciuc, A. G., Zhan, C., Dwoskin, L. P., & Crooks, P. A. (2009). Computational neural network analysis of the affinity of N-n-alkylnicotinium salts for the α4β2 nicotinic acetylcholine receptor. *Journal of Enzyme Inhibition and Medicinal Chemistry*, *24*, 157–168.

Zoli, M., Lena, C., Picciotto, M. R., & Changeux, J. P. (1998). Identification of four classes of brain nicotinic receptors using beta2 mutant mice. *Journal of Neuroscience*, *18*, 4461–4472.

Zwart, R., Carbone, A. L., Moroni, M., Bermudez, I., Mogg, A. J., Folly, E. A., et al. (2008). Sazetidine-A is a potent and selective agonist at native and recombinant alpha 4 beta 2 nicotinic acetylcholine receptors. *Molecular Pharmacology*, *73*, 1834–1843.

CHAPTER FOURTEEN

New Directions in Nicotine Vaccine Design and Use

Paul R. Pentel[*,†,‡,1], **Mark G. LeSage**[†,‡,§]
[*]Department of Pharmacology, University of Minnesota, Minneapolis, Minnesota, USA
[†]Department of Medicine, University of Minnesota, Minneapolis, Minnesota, USA
[‡]Minneapolis Medical Research Foundation, Minneapolis, Minnesota, USA
[§]Department of Psychology, University of Minnesota, Minneapolis, Minnesota, USA
[1]Corresponding author: e-mail address: pentel@umn.edu

Contents

Advances in Pharmacology, Volume 69
ISSN 1054-3589
http://dx.doi.org/10.1016/B978-0-12-420118-7.00014-7

553

Abstract

Clinical trials of nicotine vaccines suggest that they can enhance smoking cessation rates but do not reliably produce the consistently high serum antibody concentrations required. A wide array of next-generation strategies are being evaluated to enhance vaccine efficacy or provide antibody through other mechanisms. Protein conjugate vaccines may be improved by modifications of hapten or linker design or by optimizing hapten density. Conjugating hapten to viruslike particles or disrupted virus may allow exploitation of naturally occurring viral features associated with high immunogenicity. Conjugates that utilize different linker positions on nicotine can function as independent immunogens, so that using them in combination generates higher antibody concentrations than can be produced by a single immunogen. Nanoparticle vaccines, consisting of hapten, T cell help peptides, and adjuvants attached to a liposome or synthetic scaffold, are in the early stages of development. Nanoparticle vaccines offer the possibility of obtaining precise and consistent control of vaccine component stoichiometry and spacing and immunogen size and shape. Passive transfer of nicotine-specific monoclonal antibodies offers a greater control of antibody dose, the ability to give very high doses, and an immediate onset of action but is expensive and has a shorter duration of action than vaccines. Viral vector-mediated transfer of genes for antibody production can elicit high levels of antibody expression in animals and may present an alternative to vaccination or passive immunization if the long-term safety of this approach is confirmed. Next-generation immunotherapies are likely to be substantially more effective than first-generation vaccines.

ABBREVIATIONS

3′-AmNic 3-aminonicotine
AAV adeno-associated virus
KLH keyhole limpet hemocyanin
nAChR nicotinic cholinergic receptor
rEPA recombinant *P. aeruginosa* exoprotein A
Th T helper

1. INTRODUCTION

Nicotine vaccines appear quite promising in animals but have been disappointing in initial clinical trials for enhancing smoking cessation rates. There are a number of likely reasons for this lack of translation, most of which should be addressable with improvements in vaccine design or the manner in which vaccines are used. This chapter will focus on understanding the limitations of first-generation nicotine vaccines studied to date and how to overcome them. Readers are referred to other reviews for a more detailed discussion of nicotine vaccine development and the mechanism of action (Bevins, Wilkinson, & Sanderson, 2008; LeSage, Keyler, & Pentel, 2006; Raupach, Hoogsteder, & Onno van Schayck, 2012; Shen, Orson, & Kosten, 2012).

2. STATUS OF FIRST-GENERATION NICOTINE VACCINES

Animal data supporting nicotine vaccine efficacy are robust. A variety of nicotine vaccines have been shown to reduce the distribution to the brain of single, clinically relevant nicotine doses by up to 90% (Cerny et al., 2002; Maurer et al., 2005; Pravetoni et al., 2011; Satoskar et al., 2003). With repeated nicotine dosing simulating 1–2 packs of cigarettes per day, nicotine distribution to the brain is reduced to a lesser extent but each nicotine dose reaches the brain more slowly and is presumably less reinforcing (Hieda, Keyler, Ennifar, Fattom, & Pentel, 2000; Pentel, Dufek, Roiko, Lesage, & Keyler, 2006). Nicotine vaccines readily block or attenuate many nicotine addiction-related behaviors including the acquisition, maintenance, and reinstatement of nicotine self-administration (LeSage, Keyler, Hieda, et al., 2006; Lindblom et al., 2002). These general results have been reproduced in many laboratories with different vaccines, adding confidence to the findings.

Clinical trial results of nicotine vaccines, although some are available only as press releases, have not mirrored the strong preclinical findings (Hartmann-Boyce, Cahill, Hatsukami, & Cornuz, 2012). Except for one phase II clinical trial of 3′-AmNic-rEPA (NicVAX) (Hatsukami et al., 2011), overall efficacy for smoking cessation has not been greater than with placebo vaccine (Fahim, Kessler, & Kalnik, 2013). The follow-up phase III trials of NicVAX failed to confirm the earlier finding of the overall efficacy. However, the phase II trials of both NicQb and NicVAX had a similar efficacy signal in subgroup analyses; one-third of subjects with the highest serum antibody concentrations or titers showed an approximately doubled smoking cessation rate compared to controls (Cornuz et al., 2008; Hatsukami et al., 2011). A phase II trial of another conjugate vaccine, Niccine, reported no such efficacy signal but antibody levels were uniformly low and efficacy would not be expected (Tonstad et al., 2013). These data suggest that improved vaccines that consistently generate higher antibody levels could be effective therapies.

3. LIMITATIONS OF FIRST-GENERATION NICOTINE VACCINES

3.1. Importance of achieving high antibody levels

Vaccines generate antibodies that bind nicotine and alter its access to the brain. Vaccine effects on nicotine pharmacokinetics correlate closely with the amount of antibody generated, as estimated by the serum nicotine-specific antibody concentration or the antibody titer (a functional measure that is sensitive to both antibody concentration and antibody affinity for nicotine) (Keyler et al., 2005; Maurer et al., 2005; Pravetoni et al., 2011). Because the amount of nicotine consumed by smokers can approach or exceed the binding capacity of the available antibody produced by vaccination, it is critical to generate antibody levels that are as high as possible. In rats or mice, serum IgG antibody concentrations of >100 μg/ml are associated with significant effects on nicotine distribution and attenuation of its behavioral effects, and antibody levels of 100–500 μg/ml can be achieved (Keyler, Roiko, Earley, Murtaugh, & Pentel, 2008; Maurer et al., 2005). High antibody levels are more readily achieved in rodents than in humans because it is possible to use strong or experimental adjuvants that are not suitable for clinical use. It is also possible to use much higher mg/kg immunogen doses in rodents (typical 50–100 μg/kg) than in humans (typical 1–5 μg/kg) because larger ml/kg vaccine volumes are acceptable for use in animals. Acute nicotine exposure in rats does not interfere with nicotine vaccine immunogenicity (Hieda et al., 2000), but smokers have reduced antibody responses to some infectious disease vaccines (Crothers et al., 2011; Finklea et al., 1971; Roseman, Truedsson, & Kapetanovic, 2012; Winter, Follett, McIntyre, Stewart, & Symington, 1994). Therefore, difficulty inducing sufficient antibody levels in humans could be anticipated, and this has proven to be the principal challenge presented by the use of nicotine vaccines for smoking cessation.

Because of limited clinical experience with addiction vaccines, it is difficult to predict the nicotine-specific antibody serum concentration required for clinical efficacy, but initial studies provide an estimate. In phase II clinical trials of the 3′-AmNic-rEPA vaccine, a peak geometric mean serum IgG concentration of 45 μg/ml was associated with higher smoking cessation rates (Hatsukami et al., 2011). In a clinical laboratory study of the same vaccine, subjects with serum antibody levels of 40–160 μg/ml had a significant but minimal (mean of 12%) reduction in occupancy of brain nicotinic cholinergic receptors (nAChRs) compared to controls after receiving a single i.v. dose of nicotine (Esterlis et al., 2013). These data suggest that serum nicotine-specific antibody levels of greater than 50–100 μg/ml provide an approximate minimum target concentration. This estimate is consistent with rat and mouse data showing that mean serum antibody levels of 50–100 μg/ml produce a significant but small reduction in the distribution of clinically relevant nicotine doses to the brain and that effects increase at higher serum antibody levels (Keyler et al., 2008; Maurer et al., 2005). As in animals, higher serum antibody concentrations in the 3′-AmNic-rEPA phase II study appeared to be more effective for smoking cessation (Hatsukami et al., 2011).

To put this estimate in perspective, the whole-body content of nicotine-specific IgG after vaccination, and of nicotine after smoking, can be estimated. Using a volume of distribution for IgG of 70 ml/kg, which indicates that about 2/3 of IgG exists outside of serum, a serum antibody concentration of 100 μg/ml would provide about 6 μmole of binding sites for nicotine (two binding sites per IgG) (Migone et al., 2009). Smoking one cigarette provides an absorbed nicotine dose of about 1–1.5 mg or 5–7 μmol (Gelal et al., 2005). Therefore, the proposed minimum effective serum nicotine-specific antibody concentration of 50–100 μg/ml would provide the binding capacity for at most one cigarette. By this measure, it is not surprising that the 50–100 μg/ml level would allow only minimal efficacy and that higher concentrations might be required for optimal results.

3.2. Variability in vaccine immunogenicity

An additional limitation of first-generation nicotine vaccines, in both animals and humans, is large individual variability in the immune response. Serum nicotine-specific antibody titer or concentration ranges of 30-fold or greater have been reported and appear to be the rule rather than the exception with the nicotine vaccines studied to date (Cornuz et al., 2008; Hatsukami et al., 2011; Tonstad et al., 2013). This wide range reflects in part the underlying variability of immune responses in a population and is also found with cocaine or opioid vaccines and many infectious disease vaccines (Kosten et al., 2002). Large variability results in a substantial number of nonresponders with very low antibody levels that are unlikely to be effective. The goal of next-generation vaccine design must be both to enhance the mean antibody response and to reduce the number of nonresponders by either reducing variability or enhancing mean efficacy enough to raise the lowest responders into an acceptable range.

While most studies have focused on serum antibody concentrations or titers as a surrogate for concentration, antibody affinity for nicotine also influences efficacy in rats (Keyler et al., 2005). Antibody affinity is measured as the dissociation rate constant K_d, with lower values indicating greater affinity for nicotine. The K_d value corresponds with the nicotine concentration at which antibody binding sites are half saturated with nicotine. When the serum nicotine concentration is above the K_d, the antibody is highly saturated and most of its binding capacity is utilized. When the serum nicotine concentration is below the K_d, saturation is low and less of the binding capacity is being utilized. Venous serum nicotine concentrations in smokers are generally around 5–40 ng/ml (30–240 nM), so that antibodies with a K_d near or below the lower end of this range should be most effective. This estimate corresponds well with vaccine or passive immunization experience in rats or mice, where effective antibodies have had K_d's in the range of 10–100 nM (as measured by equilibrium dialysis or soluble radioimmunoassay), and this range provides a target for vaccine or immunotherapy development (Maurer et al., 2005; Moreno et al., 2010; Pentel et al., 2000). The mean affinity of antibodies generated in a phase I study of NicQb was 33 nM, also within the proposed target range (Maurer et al., 2005). The extent of individual variability in antibody affinity was not reported, but we have found a 10-fold range in affinity for nicotine in rats vaccinated with 3'-AmNic-rEPA (unpublished data). Measuring this parameter in clinical trials might add insight into the causes of variability in vaccine efficacy (Orson et al., 2007).

4. LIMITATIONS OF VACCINATION AS A GENERAL STRATEGY FOR TREATING NICOTINE ADDICTION

It is likely that sufficiently immunogenic nicotine vaccines will be effective for enhancing smoking cessation rates. Advances in vaccine design, outlined in Section 6, should substantially enhance vaccine efficacy in the next few years and provide tools for testing this hypothesis. A more general question is how effective even the most immunogenic vaccines can be and which aspects of tobacco addiction they can address.

4.1. Nicotine versus other tobacco components

Nicotine is the principal addictive component of tobacco but other chemicals may contribute to tobacco addiction through their effects on nicotine absorption (e.g., alkali) (Anon, 1988), enhancement of nicotine reinforcement (other tobacco alkaloids and acetaldehyde) (Cao et al., 2007; Clemens, Caille, Stinus, & Cador, 2009), or modulation of mood or cognition (monoamine oxidase inhibitors) (George & Weinberger, 2008). Nicotine vaccines can attenuate only the effects of nicotine and perhaps its active but minor metabolite nornicotine. Whether other components of tobacco or tobacco smoke are sufficient to maintain addiction by themselves or in the presence of the lower concentrations of nicotine that persist even after vaccination is not clear. Addressing the effects of these non-nicotine components may prove helpful or necessary for maximizing the impact of nicotine vaccines.

4.2. Immediate versus long-lasting effects of nicotine exposure

The nicotine-specific antibodies generated by vaccination modify nicotine's access to brain nAChRs by altering its distribution to tissues and its elimination. These actions can only occur when nicotine is present. The primary target of vaccination is therefore the immediate effects of nicotine. Longer-lasting effects of nicotine such as withdrawal and craving, which occur when nicotine is no longer present, cannot be directly altered by vaccination. It is possible that a persistent reduction of nicotine's acute effects may indirectly lead to less subsequent withdrawal or craving (Lindblom et al., 2005), but a role for this in humans is speculative. It is more likely that additional measures, such as counseling or other medications, will be needed to complement vaccination in order to achieve optimal efficacy.

4.3. Quantitative limits on antibody effects

Immunotherapies can reduce but not completely prevent nicotine distribution to the brain. Even if there is sufficient antibody on a molar basis to bind all of the nicotine present, binding is reversible and governed by the dissociation rate constant (K_d). For example, viral vector-directed production of extremely high serum antibody concentration in mice (1 mg/ml) reduced the distribution of a single nicotine dose to the brain by only 85% (Hicks et al., 2012). This is important because even low serum concentrations of nicotine may be sufficient to produce addiction-relevant effects. Smoking just one low-nicotine Quest cigarette (5% of the nicotine content of a standard cigarette) produces 26% occupancy of brain nAChRs (Brody et al., 2009). The serum nicotine concentration estimated from these data to produce 50% nAChR occupancy was 0.75 ng/ml, considerably lower than typical serum nicotine concentration in smokers of 10–40 ng/ml.

It is possible that immunotherapy will benefit from other measures or medications to address the residual effects of low levels of nicotine.

These considerations do not minimize the encouraging results found to date with vaccines or argue against the use of vaccines for nicotine addiction. Rather, they point to the need to consider vaccination in the larger context of addiction treatment and to take advantage of complementary approaches, in addition to optimizing vaccine immunogenicity.

5. DESIGN OF NICOTINE VACCINES

5.1. Types of nicotine vaccines

First-generation nicotine vaccines consist of protein conjugate immunogens (nicotine linked, or conjugated, to a carrier protein) mixed with adjuvant. Next-generation vaccines comprise a diverse array of approaches employing improvements in protein conjugate design, use of novel vaccine components, or vaccine component display on synthetic nanoparticles. The rationale for these designs and innovations derives from advances in understanding how vaccines engage an immune response and elicit antibody production.

5.2. Vaccine immunology

Generation of an effective humoral immune response (Fig. 14.1) requires linked recognition of the antigenic epitopes bound by B and T cells and coordinated interactions among B cells, T cells, and other antigen-presenting cells (APCs) (dendritic cells and macrophages) and follicular dendritic cells, neutrophils, and NKT cells (see McHeyzer-Williams & McHeyzer-Williams, 2005, for a more detailed review). The key components of a conjugate nicotine vaccine are the following: (1) a B cell epitope, in this case nicotine, to bind and engage those B cells that have the capacity to mature into nicotine-specific antibody-producing cells; (2) a T cell epitope, provided by the carrier protein of a conjugate vaccine or by smaller peptides, to bind and engage the T helper cells that assist B cell activation and maturation; and (3) an adjuvant, such as alum, that enhances vaccine immunogenicity. Sections 5 and 6 that follow are not intended to provide a comprehensive summary of humoral immunity, but rather to focus on those aspects most pertinent to vaccine design and performance.

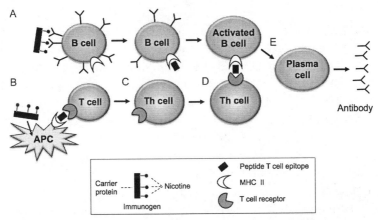

Figure 14.1 Key elements of conjugate vaccine interaction with immune cells that are relevant to nicotine vaccine design. For a more detailed account of humoral immunity, see McHeyzer-Williams and McHeyzer-Williams (2005). Humans have $>10^8$ naive B cells bearing surface antibody (B cell receptor) with different specificities that are capable of binding a wide range of chemical structures, including small molecules such as nicotine. When a nicotine vaccine is administered, (A) the nicotine component (B cell epitope) of the conjugate vaccine binds to those naive B cells that have appropriate surface antibody, and the entire conjugate is internalized. Internalization is enhanced by having multiple nicotine molecules attached to each carrier protein so that many surface antibody interactions take place. The carrier protein is digested within the B cell and peptide fragments (T cell epitopes) are displayed on its surface in association with MHC class II molecules. It is the display of these T cell epitopes that will subsequently allow helper T cells that have encountered the same T cell epitopes to recognize and interact with nicotine-specific B cells. (B) Immunogen is phagocytized by antigen-presenting cells (APCs) such as dendritic cells. This is a nonspecific process (does not involve immunogen receptors) that can be facilitated by the presence of an adjuvant (not shown). Particle uptake is enhanced if it is an appropriate size. APCs digest the carrier protein and display T cell epitope peptides on their surface in association with MHC class II molecules. Only peptides (not nicotine) can serve as T cell epitopes. Some T cells bear surface receptors capable of binding the T cell epitopes presented by APCs. (C) T cell interaction with APCs allows them differentiate into T helper (Th) cells that can provide stimulatory signals to B cells. (D) Those Th cells bearing receptors that are specific for the particular T cell epitope derived from the nicotine immunogen recognize and interact with the correct subset of B cells (those capable of binding nicotine) because those B cells now bear the immunogen's T cell epitope on their surface. It is this specific recognition of T cell epitopes displayed by nicotine-specific B cells that allows Th cells to interact selectively with these B cells. (E) Activated B cells undergo maturation into antibody-secreting cells and memory cells (not shown) that can be activated by subsequent booster doses of vaccine. *Adapted from materials provided by Y. Chang. (For color version of this figure, the reader is referred to the online version of this chapter.)*

5.2.1 B cell epitope

Nicotine serves as the B cell epitope in nicotine vaccines. Nicotine and a source of T cell help (carrier protein or peptide sequences) must be internalized in the same B cell to allow B cell recognition by helper T cells. In protein conjugate vaccines, this is assured by covalently attaching nicotine to a carrier protein through a short linker that allows nicotine to be displayed to the B cell without being buried within the carrier protein surface. To accomplish this, nicotine is modified by adding a chemical "handle" for linker attachment. Linkage of the modified nicotine (hapten) to carrier protein forms the complete immunogen (Fig. 14.2B).

B cells display a transmembrane form of immunoglobulin on their surface (B cell receptor, BCR) and each B cell displays a unique BCR. The naive (nonvaccinated) B cell repertoire for a single individual consists of $>10^8$ B cells, each with its own surface antibody and capacity to recognize and bind certain molecules (Taylor, Jenkins, & Pape, 2012). A small fraction of these naive B cells bear antibodies that can recognize and bind nicotine that is linked to a carrier protein (or nanoparticle), initiating internalization of the immunogen (Pape, Taylor, Maul, Gearhart, & Jenkins, 2011).

Once immunogen is internalized, B cells digest the carrier protein to shorter (12–20 amino acid) peptides, which are then displayed on their surface in association with MHC class II molecules (Fig. 14.1A). Therefore, the role of nicotine on the immunogen is to select and engage just those B cells bearing surface antibody that can bind nicotine, while the carrier protein provides peptide sequences (T cell help) that can subsequently recognize and interact with T cells to obtain the signals needed for maturation into antibody-secreting cells. This interaction takes place primarily in the germinal centers of lymph nodes where B and T cells are abundant and in close proximity to each other.

5.2.2 T cell help peptides

B cells require help from T cells, via direct contact and soluble signals, in order to mature into activated B cells capable of producing high-affinity nicotine-specific antibody. The process of engaging T cell help is initiated when immunogen is taken up nonspecifically, a process not dependent upon the presence of hapten, by APCs consisting primarily of dendritic cells and macrophages (Fig. 14.1B). APCs digest the carrier protein to shorter peptides, which are then displayed on their surface by MHC class II molecules. Some T cells bear surface receptors (structurally similar to antibodies) that can recognize the peptide sequences displayed by APCs. This interaction

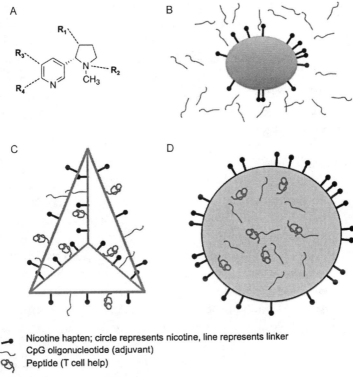

Nicotine hapten; circle represents nicotine, line represents linker
CpG oligonucleotide (adjuvant)
Peptide (T cell help)

Figure 14.2 Immunogen structures, not drawn to scale. (A) Nicotine, with positions commonly used for attachment of linkers indicated as R_{1-4}. (B) Conjugate vaccine. Nicotine is covalently attached to a carrier protein through a short linker that allows the nicotine to be accessible for binding to B cells. Some linkers are illustrated in Fig. 14.3A. A high density of nicotine hapten on the carrier protein facilitates its binding and uptake. Covalently linking nicotine to carrier assures that nicotine hapten and carrier protein will be taken into the same B cell. Conjugate immunogens are generally mixed with adjuvant to enhance antibody generation. (C) Nanoparticle vaccine: Synthetic scaffold (illustration is a DNA tetrahedron) (Liu et al., 2012). Nanoparticle scaffolds allow vaccine components to be covalently linked with readily controlled density and stoichiometry. T cell help can be provided by attachment of either whole protein or shorter peptide sequences. Some molecularly defined adjuvants, such as CpG oligonucleotides, can also be covalently linked to the nanoparticle. (D) Nanoparticle vaccine: Liposome or synthetic vesicle. Vaccine components such as hapten that require interactions with cell surface receptors can be attached to or embedded within the vesicle surface, while components intended for delivery to the cell interior can be encapsulated within. (For color version of this figure, the reader is referred to the online version of this chapter.)

activates those T cells to differentiate into a T helper cell. Because the T helper cell bears surface receptors that recognize peptides derived from the carrier protein, it can now recognize and interact with nicotine-specific B cells displaying this same peptide. This interaction, along with additional surface interactions and release of soluble mediators, activates the nicotine-specific B cell. The B cell then undergoes a complex process of affinity maturation within the germinal center of lymph nodes to select and produce high-affinity nicotine-specific antibodies.

5.2.3 Adjuvant

Adjuvants are a diverse class of distinct chemicals or complex mixtures that can facilitate an immune response (Wilson-Welder et al., 2009). They broadly signal either tissue injury or the presence of something foreign, creating an immune-competent environment at the injection site (Awate, Babiuk, & Mutwiri, 2013). Some adjuvants may also prolong immunogen retention at the injection site or enhance immunogen delivery to regional lymph nodes where the abundance of B and T cells maximizes their opportunity to encounter immunogen and interact. Alum (most often $Al(OH)_3$), the most widely used adjuvant in humans, appears to mimic tissue injury but has other postulated mechanisms of action as well (Spreafico, Ricciardi-Castagnoli, & Mortellaro, 2010). Many newer or experimental adjuvants bind specifically to Toll-like receptors or NOD-like proteins that recognize structural components of bacteria and viruses, for example, CpG oligonucleotides, lipopolysaccharide, and flagellin, or components that are released from injured cells (Klinman, Klaschik, Sato, & Tross, 2009). Some adjuvants have proven more effective than alum for specific immunogens, but it is not clear that any one adjuvant is consistently best. Combining CpG with alum enhances responses to some vaccines, including a nicotine conjugate vaccine (McCluskie et al., 2013), but failed to do so with one other (Bremer & Janda, 2012). Some carrier proteins have intrinsic adjuvant activity but all conjugate addiction vaccines that have advanced to clinical trials to date have used alum as adjuvant.

6. STRATEGIES FOR IMPROVING VACCINE EFFICACY

6.1. Vaccine design: Conjugate immunogens

Many promising improvements in nicotine vaccines have been studied. It is difficult to compare the efficacy of nicotine vaccines to each other from the available literature because (1) the density of hapten on carrier protein, a key determinant of immunogenicity, is often not measured or reported;

(2) immunogenicity is often reported only as antibody titer, a measure that is method-dependent; and (3) many vaccines and adjuvants are proprietary and not available for direct comparison. Nevertheless, some general principles are apparent.

The basic components of nicotine vaccines are summarized in Fig. 14.2. All nicotine vaccines (and cocaine vaccines as well) in clinical trials reported to date have been conjugate vaccines consisting of nicotine linked, or conjugated, to a carrier protein and then mixed with alum adjuvant. Conjugate vaccine development has focused on choosing the most effective (1) site of attachment of linker to nicotine, (2) linker composition and length, (3) number of nicotine molecules linked to each carrier protein (higher ratios are generally more effective), and (4) carrier protein. There are few rules to guide these choices, and design generally proceeds empirically by systematically comparing alternatives.

6.1.1 Nicotine hapten
A variety of positions for linker attachment to nicotine have been used (Fig. 14.2A) and are effective (de Villiers et al., 2010; Isomura, Wirsching, & Janda, 2001; Pravetoni et al., 2012). No one linker position stands out as superior. Linker attachment away from the site of metabolism to its primary metabolite cotinine, keeping this site exposed, should favor production of antibodies with greater specificity for nicotine over cotinine, but many linker positions appear to accomplish this. Because nicotine can rotate about the bond between its pyridine and pyrrolidine rings, a rigid conformationally constrained hapten was studied and found to be more immunogenic than its nonconstrained counterpart (Moreno, Azar, Koob, & Janda, 2012). Whether it is more effective than other nicotine haptens is not clear. Fluorination of drugs, in which a hydrogen is replaced by the sterically similar but more electronegative fluorine, is a common method of enhancing drug–receptor binding and might also affect the binding of haptens to BCRs. Fluorination of a cocaine hapten did not alter the affinity for cocaine of the antibodies produced by vaccination of mice, but modestly increased the mean cocaine-specific serum antibody level (Cai, Tsuchikama, & Janda, 2013). Because ligand fluorination is a general method, it may be useful for other haptens as well.

6.1.2 Linker
The purposes of a linker are to tether nicotine to its carrier or scaffold, provide a geometry that allows binding of nicotine hapten to B cells, and display a high enough density of nicotine haptens to optimize hapten binding to

B cells. The most commonly manipulated variables are linker length and lipophilicity. Published comparisons of linker attributes can be difficult to interpret if the haptenation ratio (number of haptens conjugated to each protein molecule) is not reported. Thus, a linker that forms a conjugate with particularly high immunogenicity might be doing so either because of its ability to effectively present nicotine to B cells or because of the efficiency with which it can be conjugated to protein. Most linkers are 5–15 atoms long and consist of simple unsubstituted chains in order to minimize their own immunogenicity (de Villiers et al., 2010; Pravetoni et al., 2012).

6.1.3 Carrier proteins or peptides

A variety of foreign proteins known to be highly immunogenic have proven useful as carriers for conjugate vaccines. Several proteins, such as keyhole limpet hemocyanin or tetanus toxoid, are generally highly effective and widely used in animal models but it is far from clear that any one protein is best for all haptens or in all species. Carrier proteins used in nicotine conjugate vaccines reaching clinical trials include recombinant *P. aeruginosa* exoprotein A, recombinant cholera toxin B subunit, and tetanus toxoid (Pentel et al., 2000; Tonstad et al., 2013; Anon, 2004). All were immunogenic in rodents but less so in humans. Some viruses are highly immunogenic because they are readily recognized as foreign, and their large size promotes cellular uptake. One vaccine reaching clinical trials, NicQb, consists of a nicotine hapten conjugated to the outer protein capsid of bacteriophage Qb (Maurer et al., 2005). The capsid therefore serves the same function as the protein in a standard conjugate vaccine. This noninfectious construct proved highly immunogenic in animals but, like the conjugate vaccine NicVAX, showed efficacy in clinical trials only in the minority of subjects who achieved the highest antibody levels (Cornuz et al., 2008). Disrupted adenovirus has also proven quite effective as a carrier for nicotine or other haptens in animals but clinical data are not available. Immunogenicity was preserved even in animals with prior exposure to this common virus (De et al., 2013).

Only certain peptide sequences within carrier proteins provide T cell help. Haptens can be linked directly to these peptides rather than to the whole carrier protein, but it is not clear if there is an advantage to this. Peptides may however prove particularly useful in the construction of nanoparticle vaccines (see succeeding text) because they can be more readily and predictably incorporated into these structures. Nicotine haptens have also been linked directly to an agonist of C5a receptors found on APCs, which provides direct adjuvant activity and, presumably, T cell help (Sanderson et al., 2003). This construct is immunogenic, but no more so than standard protein conjugate vaccines.

6.2. Vaccine design: Nanoparticles

Conjugate vaccines are effective but it can be challenging or impossible to reliably achieve the desired hapten density on the protein or to try new designs such as directly attaching other vaccine components (e.g., adjuvant) to the immunogen or to alter the immunogen's size, shape, or chemical composition to enhance cellular uptake or engagement of the initial immune response. Nanoparticle scaffolds have been designed to facilitate these kinds of manipulations and allow a wider range of immunization strategies to be studied (Peek, Middaugh, & Berkland, 2008; Zaman, Good, & Toth, 2013).

One approach under development is the use of liposomes or self-assembling synthetic vesicles constructed from nontoxic biodegradable polymers (Kasturi et al., 2011; Lockner et al., 2013). The outer surface of these particles can be chemically modified with handles for component attachment. Lipophilic components such as monophosphoryl lipid A adjuvant can also be embedded in liposomal membranes, or components can be enclosed within (Matyas et al., 2013; Peek et al., 2008). One such nicotine vaccine consisting of a synthetic vesicle with nicotine haptens linked to its surface, and T cell help peptides and adjuvant packaged within, has proven highly immunogenic in rodents and primates and has advanced to early clinical trials (Kishimoto, Altreuter, Johnston, Keller, & Pittet, 2012). Other scaffolds are in early stages of development for nicotine and other types of vaccines and may provide even greater flexibility and control of composition. DNA scaffolds are of particular interest because they can be fashioned into a wide variety of complex, self-assembling sizes and shapes through DNA origami using base pairing algorithms (Han et al., 2011). Precise control of the number and placement of handles for hapten, T cell peptides, and adjuvant linkage is possible (Liu et al., 2012). This assures control of component density and stoichiometry. Self-assembling peptides are being developed that provide both a scaffold for vaccine components and an intrinsic adjuvant activity (Rudra, Tian, Jung, & Collier, 2010). These and other nanoparticle designs provide a means of more systematically studying novel vaccine components and better defining the qualitative and quantitative determinants of vaccine efficacy.

6.3. Multivalent vaccines (Fig. 14.3A)

It may be possible to enhance nicotine vaccine efficacy by combining two or more effective immunogens. Multivalent vaccines are widely used for the prevention of infectious diseases. Individual immunogens are combined to provide coverage for related pathogens (e.g., a 23-valent pneumococcal vaccine containing capsular polysaccharides from 23 of the most important serotypes of pneumococcus), or unrelated immunogens can be combined as a convenience so that fewer immunization injections are needed (measles, mumps, and rubella vaccine). This is possible because the immune system has the capacity to respond to multiple simultaneous immune challenges. This capacity can be exploited for nicotine vaccines by immunizing animals with two or three structurally distinct nicotine immunogens, containing haptens with linkers at different positions. If these haptens are sufficiently distinct, they can elicit independent immunologic responses by activating different populations of B cells (Keyler et al., 2008; Pravetoni et al., 2012). Each of the immunogens elicits antibodies against nicotine, but the responses involve different populations of B cells and so are independent and additive. The resulting antibody levels are higher than for the same dose of a monovalent vaccine (Fig. 14.3A). The effects of bi- or trivalent nicotine vaccines on nicotine distribution in rats mirror the titers and are also additive (de Villiers, Cornish, Troska, Pravetoni, Pentel, 2013). An additional benefit seen in this study is that some animals with a low response to one immunogen had a high response to another, reducing the number of low or nonresponders. The concept of multivalent vaccines is quite general and not limited to the specific immunogens studied. As newer and more effective immunogens are developed, it may be possible to combine the best of these to further enhance their efficacy. Experience with this approach is limited and it has not entered clinical trials.

6.4. Combining vaccines with medications (Fig. 14.3B)

Because the mechanism of action of nicotine vaccines is unique among tobacco addiction treatments, it should be possible to combine vaccines with other types of smoking cessation medications. This is of interest because both vaccines alone and existing medications alone are only partially effective, combining them might enhance the efficacy of both (Bevins et al., 2008; Orson et al., 2007; Raupach et al., 2012). Vaccines cannot directly block withdrawal or craving, which occur when nicotine is no longer present. However, bupropion and varenicline have activities for

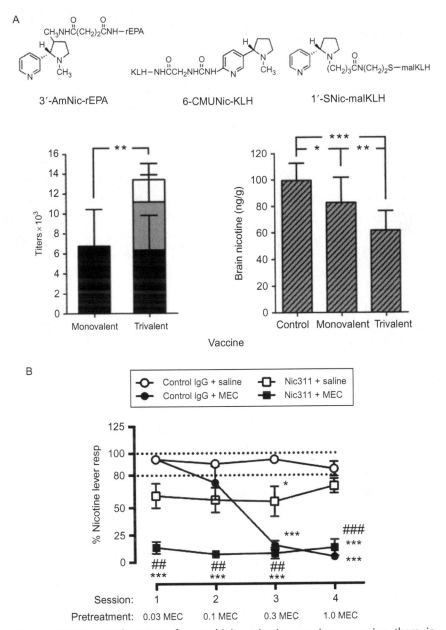

Figure 14.3 Potential options for combining nicotine vaccines or using them in combination with medications. (A) Trivalent nicotine vaccine (de Villiers et al., 2013). Rats were vaccinated with three structurally distinct nicotine immunogens (linkers attached at different positions, carrier proteins; rEPA, recombinant exoprotein A; KLH, keyhole

(Continued)

reducing craving and withdrawal. There are limited clinical data addressing this hypothesis. Two clinical trials of nicotine vaccines plus varenicline failed to find enhanced efficacy but each had limitations. A NicVAX + varenicline trial used a vaccine that is at best minimally effective and provided only a limited period of overlap between varenicline and peak antibody levels (Hoogsteder et al., 2012). It was therefore more of a study of sequential varenicline followed by vaccine than their combined use. A second clinical trial used Niccine vaccine plus varenicline but achieved only very low antibody levels that would not have been expected to show efficacy (Tonstad et al., 2013).

One combination study in rats showed a strong synergistic effect of the nicotine-specific mAb Nic311 in combination with the nicotinic receptor antagonist mecamylamine for reducing nicotine discrimination (LeSage, Shelley, Pravetoni, & Pentel, 2012) (Fig. 14.3B). The mAb Nic311 was used as a surrogate for vaccination. Mecamylamine was used because its blocking of nicotine effects at nAChRs was expected to augment the reduction in nicotine reaching the receptors produced by Nic311. Mecamylamine alone can provide a high degree of receptor blockade but the high doses required cause side effects. The combination blocked nicotine discrimination at mAb Nic311 and mecamylamine doses that by themselves had a modest or no effect, respectively. Although preliminary, these data encourage further study of mechanistically complementary vaccine and medication combinations. They also suggest a potential broader role for vaccines in medication development as a platform for development of pharmacotherapies for tobacco addiction. Vaccines could enhance the efficacy of other types of

---

Figure 14.3—cont'd limpet hemocyanin; malKLH, maleimide activated KLH) or a dose-matched monovalent immunogen s.c. with alum adjuvant. After the last of three vaccine doses, rats received a single i.v. dose of 0.03 mg/kg nicotine. The trivalent immunogen elicited higher nicotine-specific antibody titers and concentrations than the monovalent vaccine (left) and reduced nicotine distribution to the brain to a greater extent (right). $^*p < 0.05$. (B) Combined use of the nicotine-specific mAb Nic311 and mecamylamine to block the subjective effects of nicotine in rats trained in a two-lever nicotine discrimination assay. Each point is the mean ($\pm$SEM)% responding on the nicotine lever during consecutive daily test sessions with the 0.4 mg/kg nicotine training dose in each treatment group following administration of control antibody (IgG) and saline (open circles), Nic311 alone (open squares), ascending doses of MEC alone (solid circles), or both (solid squares). Dashed horizontal lines indicate criterion levels of performance for discrimination of the 0.4 mg/kg nicotine training dose. Significantly different from control IgG + saline, $^*p < 0.05$, $^{***}p < 0.001$. Significantly different from Nic311 + saline, $^{##}p < 0.01$, $^{###}p < 0.001$ (LeSage et al., 2012).

medications by reducing the brain concentrations of nicotine that compete with a medication for binding to nicotinic receptors or for producing other downstream neural effects. To the extent that this lowers the dose of medication required, vaccines could reduce the side effects of that medication. The excellent safety profile, distinct mechanism of action, and potentially low cost of vaccines make them well suited to serving as a medication development platform.

7. ALTERNATIVES TO VACCINATION

7.1. Passive immunization

The principal limitations of vaccination are the magnitude of the mean antibody response and large individual variability. In addition, vaccines require weeks to months to generate an effective level of antibody, requiring careful planning and timing of smoking cessation attempts. Each of these limitations can be circumvented by passive immunization consisting of the administration of preformed antibodies. Because drug-specific antibodies appear to have no important toxicity, arbitrarily high doses can be used and more uniformly high serum antibody levels achieved. Passive immunization with drug-specific monoclonal antibodies (mAbs) can block the effects of very high doses of phencyclidine (Hardin et al., 2002), methamphetamine (Gentry et al., 2006), nicotine (Carrera et al., 2004; Keyler et al., 2005; LeSage et al., 2012), or cocaine (Fox et al., 1996) in rodents, and a methamphetamine mAb has entered clinical trials (ClinicalTrials.gov, 2013).

The principal drawback of passive immunization is the very high cost of the required doses of mAb. mAbs are widely used to treat cancer or immune disorders, but the doses likely needed to treat tobacco addiction (40–160 mg/kg per dose in rats) are 10–100 times higher (Carrera et al., 2004; Keyler et al., 2005; LeSage et al., 2012). Passively administered antibody also has a somewhat shorter elimination half-life (IgG half-life 3 weeks in humans) (Waldmann & Strober, 1969) than the decline in antibody titer after vaccination (approximate half-life 2 months after nicotine or cocaine vaccines in humans) (Hatsukami et al., 2005), and even fully human antibody can elicit the formation of anti-mAb antibodies that reduce its efficacy or half-life (Presta, 2006). The required dose of drug-specific mAb can perhaps be reduced by combining it with vaccination, administering mAb to only those subjects who have insufficient responses to vaccine alone, but even with this strategy, high mAb doses may still be needed (Cornish et al., 2011; Roiko et al., 2008). Passive immunization is highly effective for blocking nicotine effects in animals but has not been studied in humans.

7.2. Gene transfer

An emerging approach that bypasses the need for either active or passive immunization is the administration of viral vectors containing genes for the expression of drug-specific antibody (Brimijoin, Shen, Orson, & Kosten, 2013; Mingozzi & High, 2011). Adeno-associated virus (AAV) vectors with such sequences can be administered parenterally and become incorporated into the cytoplasm of host cells as plasmids that produce fully formed and functional mAb. Expression of very high levels (up to 1 mg/ml) of nicotine-specific antibody has been demonstrated in mice and nonhuman primates that results in a marked decrease in drug distribution and effects (Hicks et al., 2012). The AAV vectors used are nonreplicating, have low rates of insertion into host DNA, and have shown no important toxicity in initial clinical trials of their use for the transfer of other types of genes (Mingozzi & High, 2011). However, in view of its novelty and the unanticipated toxicities associated with some other types of gene transfer therapies, a high degree of confidence in long-term safety will be needed to allow the use of viral vectors for tobacco addiction treatment. Those addictions that have no other medication therapies available, such as cocaine or methamphetamine, may be more attractive initial candidates (Brimijoin et al., 2013).

8. TRANSLATIONAL CONSIDERATIONS
8.1. Adequacy of animal models

Animal models of nicotine vaccines generally involve the administration of nicotine i.v. or s.c. rather than by inhalation and by itself rather than in combination with the thousands of other chemicals present in tobacco and tobacco smoke. One study showed that a nicotine vaccine was equally effective for blocking nicotine distribution to the brain after a single dose of nicotine administered either i.v. or via inhalation of cigarette smoke (Pravetoni et al., 2011). This validates the pharmacokinetic aspects of the i.v. model but does not address the possible behavioral effects of other compounds in tobacco smoke. As such, it is possible that these animal models overestimate the efficacy of vaccines for smoking cessation.

Cigarette smoking occurs in a complex environment of sensory stimuli from smoke inhalation (taste, smell, and "impact" on the respiratory tract), conditioned cues, social influences, and economic and regulatory factors, all of which are important mediators of smoking behavior. Animal models provide only the most basic aspects of some of these, such as a cue light or tone during self-administration procedures. However, all currently approved medications for smoking cessation show activity in animal models of nicotine addiction (Damaj et al., 2010; Le Foll et al., 2012; LeSage, Keyler, Collins, & Pentel, 2003).

There are few data directly addressing whether one or more species of experimental animal is the best predictor of addiction vaccine immunogenicity in humans. Rats and mice are well studied with regard to vaccine immunogenicity and convenient to use for initial vaccine evaluation. It is unclear if, in general, primates offer additional predictive information. Primates are sometimes preferred for infectious disease vaccine studies because the target infections are better modeled in primates than rodents, but nicotine distribution to the brain can be adequately modeled in rats. However, some adjuvants such as certain CpG oligonucleotides are species-specific, and vaccine formulations containing these adjuvants may require testing in primates to better anticipate their immunogenicity in humans (Klinman et al., 2009).

8.2. Design of clinical trials

Phase I clinical trials of nicotine vaccines have focused on establishing an immunogen dose, number of booster doses, and dosing interval. Until the factors controlling vaccine immunogenicity are more fully understood, phase I clinical trials may benefit from examining additional variables such as choice of adjuvant or route of administration. For example, intradermal vaccination is often more immunogenic than intramuscular (La Montagne & Fauci, 2004), and this has now been shown for one nicotine immunogen administered with CpG adjuvant in mice (Chen, Pravetoni, Bhayana, Pentel, & Wu, 2012). Adaptive designs that allow sequential exploration of several of these parameters may prove helpful for optimizing vaccine formulation. Knowing that next-generation vaccines must produce higher serum antibody concentrations than the first-generation vaccines already tested, it is important to identify early in clinical development those immunogens and vaccine formulations with the greatest likelihood of clinical success.

8.3. Individual variability

Strategies for addressing individual variability in vaccine response are needed. With this information, individuals predicted to have a poor response to a particular vaccine could be directed to a different vaccine or to a non-vaccine therapy. No validated predictive biomarkers of nicotine vaccine response are currently available. Cocaine vaccine studies have identified possible effects of HLA type or the presence of low levels of preexisting spontaneous anticocaine antibodies (Orson et al., 2013) as factors in vaccine response. The ability of naive (prevaccination) B cells to bind an opioid hapten *in vitro* correlates with the magnitude of opioid-specific antibody response to vaccination in mice (M. Pravetoni, personal communication). However, these approaches have not been studied for nicotine vaccines.

8.4. Safety

Nicotine conjugate vaccines have been associated with few serious adverse effects in clinical trials. One subject with a history of penicillin allergy had an anaphylactic reaction after initial vaccination with NicVAX (Hatsukami et al., 2011). Reactogenicity (transient adverse effects associated with vaccine administration) was mild with Niccine (conjugated to tetanus toxoid) or NicVAX (conjugated to recombinant *P. aeruginosa* exoprotein A) but more marked with NicQb (conjugated to a viruslike particle) (Cornuz et al., 2008; Hatsukami et al., 2011, 2005; Maurer et al., 2005; Tonstad et al., 2013). Side effects from each of these vaccines were seen in control groups as well, so they were likely due to carrier protein and/or adjuvant rather than immunogen. Because all vaccine side effects have been transient, the nicotine-specific antibodies generated by vaccination, which persist in the blood for months, appear to have no adverse effects. The substantially higher levels of nicotine-specific antibody generated in animals by vaccination (Keyler et al., 2008), passive immunization (Keyler et al., 2005), or gene transfer (Hicks et al., 2012) are also well tolerated. This supports the critical premise that it will be safe to generate the higher serum antibody levels needed for nicotine vaccine efficacy. All vaccines studied in clinical trials used alum as adjuvant. While these data are reassuring, new vaccine platforms, nanoparticles, novel adjuvants, and gene transfer strategies will need to be carefully evaluated to establish their safety.

Vaccination does not precipitate nicotine withdrawal. In rats, neither vaccination (Lindblom et al., 2005) nor a very high bolus dose of nicotine-specific mAb (Roiko, Harris, LeSage, Keyler, & Pentel, 2009) elicited withdrawal signs or elevations in the brain reward threshold. No symptoms of withdrawal have been reported in clinical trials of nicotine vaccines (Hartmann-Boyce et al., 2012).

9. CONCLUSION

Abundant opportunities exist for enhancing nicotine vaccine efficacy through optimization of conjugate vaccine components, the use of nanoparticle scaffolds, combining immunogens in a multivalent vaccine, or combining vaccines with other types of medications. Passive immunization or antibody gene transfer offers potential alternatives to vaccination if concerns about cost and long-term safety can be addressed. It is likely that one or more next-generation vaccines or immunotherapies will reliably provide high enough serum nicotine-specific antibody levels to adequately test their efficacy for smoking cessation.

CONFLICT OF INTEREST

The authors have no conflicts of interest to report.

ACKNOWLEDGMENTS

We thank Yung Chang for helpful discussions of humoral immune response mechanisms. This work is supported by NIDA grants DA10714 and T32-DA07097.

REFERENCES

Anon. (1988). *The health consequences of smoking: Nicotine addiction, a report of the Surgeon General*. Atlanta, GA: U.S. Department of Health and Human Services, Centers for Disease Control and Prevention, Office on Smoking and Health.

Anon. (2004). Trial watch: Xenova's TA-NIC vaccine shows promise. *Expert Review of Vaccines, 3*, 386.

Awate, S., Babiuk, L. A., & Mutwiri, G. (2013). Mechanisms of action of adjuvants. *Frontiers in Immunology, 4*, 114.

Bevins, R. A., Wilkinson, J. L., & Sanderson, S. D. (2008). Vaccines to combat smoking. *Expert Opinion on Biological Therapy, 8*, 379–383.

Bremer, P. T., & Janda, K. D. (2012). Investigating the effects of a hydrolytically stable hapten and a Th1 adjuvant on heroin vaccine performance. *Journal of Medicinal Chemistry, 55*, 10776–10780.

Brimijoin, S., Shen, X., Orson, F., & Kosten, T. (2013). Prospects, promise and problems on the road to effective vaccines and related therapies for substance abuse. *Expert Review of Vaccines, 12*, 323–332.

Brody, A. L., Mandelkern, M. A., Costello, M. R., Abrams, A. L., Scheibal, D., Farahi, J., et al. (2009). Brain nicotinic acetylcholine receptor occupancy: Effect of smoking a denicotinized cigarette. *The International Journal of Neuropsychopharmacology, 12*, 305–316.

Cai, X., Tsuchikama, K., & Janda, K. D. (2013). Modulating cocaine vaccine potency through hapten fluorination. *Journal of the American Chemical Society, 135*, 2971–2974.

Cao, J., Belluzzi, J. D., Loughlin, S. E., Keyler, D. E., Pentel, P. R., & Leslie, F. M. (2007). Acetaldehyde, a major constituent of tobacco smoke, enhances behavioral, endocrine, and neuronal responses to nicotine in adolescent and adult rats. *Neuropsychopharmacology, 32*, 2025–2035.

Carrera, M. R., Ashley, J. A., Hoffman, T. Z., Isomura, S., Wirsching, P., Koob, G. F., et al. (2004). Investigations using immunization to attenuate the psychoactive effects of nicotine. *Bioorganic and Medicinal Chemistry, 12*, 563–570.

Cerny, E. H., Levy, R., Mauel, J., Mpandi, M., Mutter, M., Henzelin-Nkubana, C., et al. (2002). Preclinical development of a vaccine 'against smoking'. *Onkologie, 25*, 406–411.

Chen, X., Pravetoni, M., Bhayana, B., Pentel, P. R., & Wu, M. X. (2012). High immunogenicity of nicotine vaccines obtained by intradermal delivery with safe adjuvants. *Vaccine, 31*, 159–164.

Clemens, K. J., Caille, S., Stinus, L., & Cador, M. (2009). The addition of five minor tobacco alkaloids increases nicotine-induced hyperactivity, sensitization and intravenous self-administration in rats. *The International Journal of Neuropsychopharmacology, 12*, 1355–1366.

ClinicalTrials.gov, (2013). *Safety study of Ch-mAb7F9 for methamphetamine abuse. http:// clinicaltrialsgov/ct2/show/NCT01603147?term=methamphetamine+antibody&rank=4*.

Cornish, K. E., Harris, A. C., LeSage, M. G., Keyler, D. E., Burroughs, D., Earley, C., et al. (2011). Combined active and passive immunization against nicotine: Minimizing monoclonal antibody requirements using a target antibody concentration strategy. *International Immunopharmacology, 11*, 1809–1815.

Cornuz, J., Zwahlen, S., Jungi, W. F., Osterwalder, J., Klingler, K., van Melle, G., et al. (2008). A vaccine against nicotine for smoking cessation: A randomized controlled trial. *PLoS One, 3*, e2547.

Crothers, K., Daly, K. R., Rimland, D., Goetz, M. B., Gibert, C. L., Butt, A. A., et al. (2011). Decreased serum antibody responses to recombinant pneumocystis antigens in HIV-infected and uninfected current smokers. *Clinical and Vaccine Immunology, 18*, 380–386.

Damaj, M. I., Grabus, S. D., Navarro, H. A., Vann, R. E., Warner, J. A., King, L. S., et al. (2010). Effects of hydroxymetabolites of bupropion on nicotine dependence behavior in mice. *Journal of Pharmacology and Experimental Therapeutics, 334*, 1087–1095.

De, B. P., Pagovich, O. E., Hicks, M. J., Rosenberg, J. B., Moreno, A. Y., Janda, K. D., et al. (2013). Disrupted adenovirus-based vaccines against small addictive molecules circumvent anti-adenovirus immunity. *Human Gene Therapy, 24*, 58–66.

de Villiers, S. H., Cornish, K. E., Troska, A. J., Pravetoni, M., & Pentel, P. R. (2013). Increased efficacy of a trivalent nicotine vaccine compared to a dose-matched monovalent vaccine when formulated with alum. *Vaccine, 31*, 6185–6193.

de Villiers, S. H., Lindblom, N., Kalayanov, G., Gordon, S., Baraznenok, I., Malmerfelt, A., et al. (2010). Nicotine hapten structure, antibody selectivity and effect relationships: Results from a nicotine vaccine screening procedure. *Vaccine, 28*, 2161–2168.

Esterlis, I., Hannestad, J. O., Perkins, E., Bois, F., D'Souza, D. C., Tyndale, R. F., et al. (2013). Effect of a nicotine vaccine on nicotine binding to beta2*-nicotinic acetylcholine receptors in vivo in human tobacco smokers. *The American Journal of Psychiatry, 170*, 399–407.

Fahim, R. E., Kessler, P. D., & Kalnik, M. W. (2013). Therapeutic vaccines against tobacco addiction. *Expert Review of Vaccines, 12*, 333–342.

Finklea, J. F., Hasselblad, V., Riggan, W. B., Nelson, W. C., Hammer, D. I., & Newill, V. A. (1971). Cigarette smoking and hemagglutination inhibition response to influenza after natural disease and immunization. *American Review of Respiratory Disease, 104*, 368–376.

Fox, B. S., Kantak, K. M., Edwards, M. A., Black, K. M., Bollinger, B. K., Botka, A. J., et al. (1996). Efficacy of a therapeutic cocaine vaccine in rodent models. *Nature Medicine, 2*, 1129–1132.

Gelal, A., Balkan, D., Ozzeybek, D., Kaplan, Y. C., Gurler, S., Guven, H., et al. (2005). Effect of menthol on the pharmacokinetics and pharmacodynamics of felodipine in healthy subjects. *European Journal of Clinical Pharmacology*, *60*, 785–790.

Gentry, W. B., Laurenzana, E. M., Williams, D. K., West, J. R., Berg, R. J., Terlea, T., et al. (2006). Safety and efficiency of an anti-(+)-methamphetamine monoclonal antibody in the protection against cardiovascular and central nervous system effects of (+)-methamphetamine in rats. *International Immunopharmacology*, *6*, 968–977.

George, T. P., & Weinberger, A. H. (2008). Monoamine oxidase inhibition for tobacco pharmacotherapy. *Clinical Pharmacology and Therapeutics*, *83*, 619–621.

Han, D., Pal, S., Nangreave, J., Deng, Z., Liu, Y., & Yan, H. (2011). DNA origami with complex curvatures in three-dimensional space. *Science*, *332*, 342–346.

Hardin, J. S., Wessinger, W. D., Wenger, G. R., Proksch, J. W., Laurenzana, E. M., & Owens, S. M. (2002). A single dose of monoclonal anti-phencyclidine IgG offers long-term reductions in phencyclidine behavioral effects in rats. *Journal of Pharmacology and Experimental Therapeutics*, *302*, 119–126.

Hartmann-Boyce, J., Cahill, K., Hatsukami, D., & Cornuz, J. (2012). Nicotine vaccines for smoking cessation. *Cochrane Database of Systematic Reviews*, *8*, CD007072.

Hatsukami, D. K., Jorenby, D. E., Gonzales, D., Rigotti, N. A., Glover, E. D., Oncken, C. A., et al. (2011). Immunogenicity and smoking-cessation outcomes for a novel nicotine immunotherapeutic. *Clinical Pharmacology and Therapeutics*, *89*, 392–399.

Hatsukami, D. K., Rennard, S., Jorenby, D., Fiore, M., Koopmeiners, J., de Vos, A., et al. (2005). Safety and immunogenicity of a nicotine conjugate vaccine in current smokers. *Clinical Pharmacology and Therapeutics*, *78*, 456–467.

Hicks, M. J., Rosenberg, J. B., De, B. P., Pagovich, O. E., Young, C. N., Qiu, J. P., et al. (2012). AAV-directed persistent expression of a gene encoding anti-nicotine antibody for smoking cessation. *Science Translational Medicine*, *4*, 140ra87.

Hieda, Y., Keyler, D. E., Ennifar, S., Fattom, A., & Pentel, P. R. (2000). Vaccination against nicotine during continued nicotine administration in rats: Immunogenicity of the vaccine and effects on nicotine distribution to brain. *International Journal of Immunopharmacology*, *22*, 809–819.

Hoogsteder, P. H., Kotz, D., van Spiegel, P. I., Viechtbauer, W., Brauer, R., Kessler, P. D., et al. (2012). The efficacy and safety of a nicotine conjugate vaccine (NicVAX(R)) or placebo co-administered with varenicline (Champix(R)) for smoking cessation: Study protocol of a phase IIb, double blind, randomized, placebo controlled trial. *BMC Public Health*, *12*, 1052.

Isomura, S., Wirsching, P., & Janda, K. D. (2001). An immunotherapeutic program for the treatment of nicotine addiction: Hapten design and synthesis. *Journal of Organic Chemistry*, *66*, 4115–4121.

Kasturi, S. P., Skountzou, I., Albrecht, R. A., Koutsonanos, D., Hua, T., Nakaya, H. I., et al. (2011). Programming the magnitude and persistence of antibody responses with innate immunity. *Nature*, *470*, 543–547.

Keyler, D. E., Roiko, S. A., Benlhabib, E., LeSage, M. G., St Peter, J. V., Stewart, S., et al. (2005). Monoclonal nicotine-specific antibodies reduce nicotine distribution to brain in rats: Dose- and affinity-response relationships. *Drug Metabolism and Disposition*, *33*, 1056–1061.

Keyler, D. E., Roiko, S. A., Earley, C. A., Murtaugh, M. P., & Pentel, P. R. (2008). Enhanced immunogenicity of a bivalent nicotine vaccine. *International Immunopharmacology*, *8*, 1589–1594.

Kishimoto, K., Altreuter, D., Johnston, L., Keller, P., & Pittet, L. (2012). SEL-068 A fully synthetic nanoparticle vaccine for smoking cessation and relapse prevention. In *SRNT 2012 Annual Meeting, Houston*.

Klinman, D. M., Klaschik, S., Sato, T., & Tross, D. (2009). CpG oligonucleotides as adjuvants for vaccines targeting infectious diseases. *Advanced Drug Delivery Reviews*, *61*, 248–255.

Kosten, T. R., Gonsai, K., St Clair Roberts, J., Jack, L., Bond, J., Mitchell, E., et al. (2002). Phase II human study of cocaine vaccine TA-CD. In *CPDD Annual Meeting, Quebec City*.

La Montagne, J. R., & Fauci, A. S. (2004). Intradermal influenza vaccination—Can less be more? *New England Journal of Medicine*, *351*, 2330–2332.

Le Foll, B., Chakraborty-Chatterjee, M., Lev-Ran, S., Barnes, C., Pushparaj, A., Gamaleddin, I., et al. (2012). Varenicline decreases nicotine self-administration and cue-induced reinstatement of nicotine-seeking behaviour in rats when a long pretreatment time is used. *The International Journal of Neuropsychopharmacology*, *15*, 1265–1274.

LeSage, M. G., Keyler, D. E., Collins, G., & Pentel, P. R. (2003). Effects of continuous nicotine infusion on nicotine self-administration in rats: Relationship between continuously infused and self-administered nicotine doses and serum concentrations. *Psychopharmacology*, *170*, 278–286.

LeSage, M. G., Keyler, D. E., Hieda, Y., Collins, G., Burroughs, D., Le, C., et al. (2006). Effects of a nicotine conjugate vaccine on the acquisition and maintenance of nicotine self-administration in rats. *Psychopharmacology*, *184*, 409–416.

LeSage, M. G., Keyler, D. E., & Pentel, P. R. (2006). Current status of immunologic approaches to treating tobacco dependence: Vaccines and nicotine-specific antibodies. *The AAPS Journal*, *8*, E65–E75.

LeSage, M. G., Shelley, D., Pravetoni, M., & Pentel, P. R. (2012). Enhanced attenuation of nicotine discrimination in rats by combining nicotine-specific antibodies with a nicotinic receptor antagonist. *Pharmacology, Biochemistry, and Behavior*, *102*, 157–162.

Lindblom, N., de Villiers, S. H., Kalayanov, G., Gordon, S., Johansson, A. M., & Svensson, T. H. (2002). Active immunization against nicotine prevents reinstatement of nicotine-seeking behavior in rats. *Respiration; International Review of Thoracic Diseases*, *69*, 254–260.

Lindblom, N., de Villiers, S. H., Semenova, S., Kalayanov, G., Gordon, S., Schilstrom, B., et al. (2005). Active immunisation against nicotine blocks the reward facilitating effects of nicotine and partially prevents nicotine withdrawal in the rat as measured by dopamine output in the nucleus accumbens, brain reward thresholds and somatic signs. *Archives of Pharmacology*, *372*, 182–194.

Liu, X., Xu, Y., Yu, T., Clifford, C., Liu, Y., Yan, H., et al. (2012). A DNA nanostructure platform for directed assembly of synthetic vaccines. *Nano Letters*, *12*, 4254–4259.

Lockner, J. W., Ho, S. O., McCague, K. C., Chiang, S. M., Do, T. Q., Fujii, G., et al. (2013). Enhancing nicotine vaccine immunogenicity with liposomes. *Bioorganic & Medicinal Chemistry Letters*, *23*, 975–978.

Matyas, G. R., Mayorov, A. V., Rice, K. C., Jacobson, A. E., Cheng, K., Iyer, M. R., et al. (2013). Liposomes containing monophosphoryl lipid A: A potent adjuvant system for inducing antibodies to heroin hapten analogs. *Vaccine*, *31*, 2804–2810.

Maurer, P., Jennings, G. T., Willers, J., Rohner, F., Lindman, Y., Roubicek, K., et al. (2005). A therapeutic vaccine for nicotine dependence: Preclinical efficacy, and Phase I safety and immunogenicity. *European Journal of Immunology*, *35*, 2031–2040.

McCluskie, M. J., Pryde, D. C., Gervais, D. P., Stead, D. R., Zhang, N., Benoit, M., et al. (2013). Enhancing immunogenicity of a 3′aminomethylnicotine-DT-conjugate antinicotine vaccine with CpG adjuvant in mice and non-human primates. *International Immunopharmacology*, *16*, 50–56.

McHeyzer-Williams, L. J., & McHeyzer-Williams, M. G. (2005). Antigen-specific memory B cell development. *Annual Review of Immunology*, *23*, 487–513.

Migone, T. S., Subramanian, G. M., Zhong, J., Healey, L. M., Corey, A., Devalaraja, M., et al. (2009). Raxibacumab for the treatment of inhalational anthrax. *The New England Journal of Medicine, 361*, 135–144.

Mingozzi, F., & High, K. A. (2011). Therapeutic in vivo gene transfer for genetic disease using AAV: Progress and challenges. *Nature Reviews Genetics, 12*, 341–355.

Moreno, A. Y., Azar, M. R., Koob, G. F., & Janda, K. D. (2012). Probing the protective effects of a conformationally constrained nicotine vaccine. *Vaccine, 30*, 6665–6670.

Moreno, A. Y., Azar, M. R., Warren, N. A., Dickerson, T. J., Koob, G. F., & Janda, K. D. (2010). A critical evaluation of a nicotine vaccine within a self-administration behavioral model. *Molecular Pharmaceutics, 7*, 431–441.

Orson, F. M., Kinsey, B. M., Singh, R. A., Wu, Y., Gardner, T., & Kosten, T. R. (2007). The future of vaccines in the management of addictive disorders. *Current Psychiatry Reports, 9*, 381–387.

Orson, F. M., Rossen, R. D., Shen, X., Lopez, A. Y., Wu, Y., & Kosten, T. R. (2013). Spontaneous development of IgM anti-cocaine antibodies in habitual cocaine users: Effect on IgG antibody responses to a cocaine cholera toxin B conjugate vaccine. *The American Journal on Addictions, 22*, 169–174.

Pape, K. A., Taylor, J. J., Maul, R. W., Gearhart, P. J., & Jenkins, M. K. (2011). Different B cell populations mediate early and late memory during an endogenous immune response. *Science, 331*, 1203–1207.

Peek, L. J., Middaugh, C. R., & Berkland, C. (2008). Nanotechnology in vaccine delivery. *Advanced Drug Delivery Reviews, 60*, 915–928.

Pentel, P. R., Dufek, M. B., Roiko, S. A., Lesage, M. G., & Keyler, D. E. (2006). Differential effects of passive immunization with nicotine-specific antibodies on the acute and chronic distribution of nicotine to brain in rats. *The Journal of Pharmacology and Experimental Therapeutics, 317*, 660–666.

Pentel, P. R., Malin, D. H., Ennifar, S., Hieda, Y., Keyler, D. E., Lake, J. R., et al. (2000). A nicotine conjugate vaccine reduces nicotine distribution to brain and attenuates its behavioral and cardiovascular effects in rats. *Pharmacology, Biochemistry, and Behavior, 65*, 191–198.

Pravetoni, M., Keyler, D. E., Pidaparthi, R. R., Carroll, F. I., Runyon, S. P., Murtaugh, M. P., et al. (2012). Structurally distinct nicotine immunogens elicit antibodies with non-overlapping specificities. *Biochemical Pharmacology, 83*, 543–550.

Pravetoni, M., Keyler, D. E., Raleigh, M. D., Harris, A. C., Lesage, M. G., Mattson, C. K., et al. (2011). Vaccination against nicotine alters the distribution of nicotine delivered via cigarette smoke inhalation to rats. *Biochemical Pharmacology, 81*, 1164–1170.

Presta, L. G. (2006). Engineering of therapeutic antibodies to minimize immunogenicity and optimize function. *Advanced Drug Delivery Reviews, 58*, 640–656.

Raupach, T., Hoogsteder, P. H., & Onno van Schayck, C. P. (2012). Nicotine vaccines to assist with smoking cessation: Current status of research. *Drugs, 72*, e1–e16.

Roiko, S. A., Harris, A. C., Keyler, D. E., Lesage, M. G., Zhang, Y., & Pentel, P. R. (2008). Combined active and passive immunization enhances the efficacy of immunotherapy against nicotine in rats. *Journal of Pharmacology and Experimental Therapeutics, 325*, 985–993.

Roiko, S. A., Harris, A. C., LeSage, M. G., Keyler, D. E., & Pentel, P. R. (2009). Passive immunization with a nicotine-specific monoclonal antibody decreases brain nicotine levels but does not precipitate withdrawal in nicotine-dependent rats. *Pharmacology, Biochemistry, and Behavior, 93*, 105–111.

Roseman, C., Truedsson, L., & Kapetanovic, M. C. (2012). The effect of smoking and alcohol consumption on markers of systemic inflammation, immunoglobulin levels and immune response following pneumococcal vaccination in patients with arthritis. *Arthritis Research and Therapy*, *14*, R170.

Rudra, J. S., Tian, Y. F., Jung, J. P., & Collier, J. H. (2010). A self-assembling peptide acting as an immune adjuvant. *Proceedings of the National Academy of Sciences of the United States of America*, *107*, 622–627.

Sanderson, S. D., Cheruku, S. R., Padmanilayam, M. P., Vennerstrom, J. L., Thiele, G. M., Palmatier, M. I., et al. (2003). Immunization to nicotine with a peptide-based vaccine composed of a conformationally biased agonist of C5a as a molecular adjuvant. *International Immunopharmacology*, *3*, 137–146.

Satoskar, S. D., Keyler, D. E., LeSage, M. G., Raphael, D. E., Ross, C. A., & Pentel, P. R. (2003). Tissue-dependent effects of immunization with a nicotine conjugate vaccine on the distribution of nicotine in rats. *International Immunopharmacology*, *3*, 957–970.

Shen, X. Y., Orson, F. M., & Kosten, T. R. (2012). Vaccines against drug abuse. *Clinical Pharmacology and Therapeutics*, *91*, 60–70.

Spreafico, R., Ricciardi-Castagnoli, P., & Mortellaro, A. (2010). The controversial relationship between NLRP3, alum, danger signals and the next-generation adjuvants. *European Journal of Immunology*, *40*, 638–642.

Taylor, J. J., Jenkins, M. K., & Pape, K. A. (2012). Heterogeneity in the differentiation and function of memory B cells. *Trends in Immunology*, *33*, 590–597.

Tonstad, S., Heggen, E., Giljam, H., Lagerback, P. A., Tonnesen, P., Wikingsson, L. D., et al. (2013). Niccine(R), a nicotine vaccine, for relapse prevention: A Phase II, randomized, placebo-controlled, multicenter clinical trial. *Nicotine & Tobacco Research*, *15*(9), 1492–1501.

Waldmann, T. A., & Strober, W. (1969). Metabolism of immunoglobulins. *Progress in Allergy*, *13*, 1–110.

Wilson-Welder, J. H., Torres, M. P., Kipper, M. J., Mallapragada, S. K., Wannemuehler, M. J., & Narasimhan, B. (2009). Vaccine adjuvants: Current challenges and future approaches. *Journal of Pharmaceutical Sciences*, *98*, 1278–1316.

Winter, A. P., Follett, E. A., McIntyre, J., Stewart, J., & Symington, I. S. (1994). Influence of smoking on immunological responses to hepatitis B vaccine. *Vaccine*, *12*, 771–772.

Zaman, M., Good, M. F., & Toth, I. (2013). Nanovaccines and their mode of action. *Methods*, *60*, 226–231.

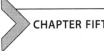

CHAPTER FIFTEEN

Bath Salts, Mephedrone, and Methylenedioxypyrovalerone as Emerging Illicit Drugs That Will Need Targeted Therapeutic Intervention

Richard A. Glennon[1]
Department of Medicinal Chemistry, School of Pharmacy, Virginia Commonwealth University, Richmond, Virginia, USA
[1]Corresponding author: e-mail address: glennon@vcu.edu

Contents

Advances in Pharmacology, Volume 69
ISSN 1054-3589
http://dx.doi.org/10.1016/B978-0-12-420118-7.00015-9

Abstract

The term "synthetic cathinones" is fairly new, but, although the abuse of synthetic cathinones is a recent problem, research on cathinone analogs dates back >100 years. One structural element cathinone analogs have in common is an α-aminophenone moiety. Introduction of amine and/or aryl substituents affords a large number of agents. Today, >40 synthetic cathinones have been identified on the clandestine market and many have multiple "street names." Many cathinone analogs, although not referred to as such until the late 1970s, were initially prepared as intermediates in the synthesis of ephedrine analogs. *The cathinones do not represent a pharmacologically or mechanistically homogeneous class of agents.* Currently abused synthetic cathinones are derived from earlier agents and seem to produce their actions primarily via the dopamine, norepinephrine, and/or serotonin transporter; that is, they either release and/or inhibit the reuptake of one or more of these neurotransmitters. The actions of these agents can resemble those of central stimulants such as methamphetamine, cocaine, and/or empathogens such as 1-(3,4-methylenedioxyphenyl)-2-aminopropane (Ecstasy) and/or produce other effects. Side effects are primarily of a neurological and/or cardiovascular nature. The use of the "and/or" term is emphasized because synthetic cathinones represent a broad class of agents that produce a variety of actions; the agents cannot be viewed as being pharmacologically equivalent. Until valid structure–activity relationships are formulated for each behavioral/mechanistic action, individual synthetic cathinones remain to be evaluated on a case-by-case basis. Treatment of synthetic cathinone intoxication requires more "basic science" research. At this time, treatment is mostly palliative.

ABBREVIATIONS

2-FMC 2-fluoromethcathinone
3-BMC 3-bromomethcathinone
3-FMC 3-fluoromethcathinone
4-BMC 4-bromomethcathinone
4-FMC 4-fluoromethcathinone
4-MEC 4-methylethcathinone
AMPH amphetamine
DA dopamine
DAT dopamine transporter
DiMe AMPH N,N-dimethylamphetamine
DMCN N,N-dimethylcathinone
DOM 1-(2,5-dimethoxy-4-methylphenyl)-2-aminopropane
MAPB buphedrone
MCAT methcathinone

MDA 1-(3,4-methylenedioxyphenyl)-2-aminopropane
MDMA *N*-methyl-1-(3,4-methylenedioxyphenyl)-2-aminopropame
MDMC methylone
MDPBP 3,4-methylenedioxy-α-PBP
MDPV methylenedioxypyrovalerone
METH methamphetamine
MMA 3-methoxyamphetamine
MOPPP 4-methoxy-α-PPP
MPEP 1-phenyl-2-pyrrolidin-1-yl propane
*m*TAP *meta*-tolylaminopropane
NET norepinephrine transporter
NPS new psychoactive substance
OMA 2-methoxyamphetamine
*o*TAP *ortho*-tolylaminopropane
PCA 4-chloroamphetamine
PIA(s) phenylisopropylamine(s)
PMA 4-methoxyamphetamine
PMEA 4-methoxy-*N*-ethylamphetamine
PMMA 4-methoxymethamphetamine
*p*TAP *para*-tolylaminopropane
SAR structure–activity relationships
SERT serotonin transporter
UNODC United Nations Office on Drugs and Crime
VMAT vesicular monoamine transporter
α-PBP α-pyrrolidinobutyrophenone
α-PPP α-(pyrrolidin-1-yl)propiophenone
α-PVP α-(pyrrolidin-1-yl)valerophenone

1. INTRODUCTION

"Synthetic cathinones" represent an emerging drug-abuse problem. Relatively little seems to be known about these "mysterious" new agents and their pharmacology. But, more might be known than (or might be inferred from) what is commonly recognized or acknowledged. What are synthetic cathinones? Where did they come from? Do they really represent something new? Synthetic cathinones constitute a broad category of agents whose individual members produce similar, somewhat similar, dissimilar, and, occasionally, unique effects; hence, their mechanisms of action cannot be identical. What should emerge from this review are the following: (i) synthetic cathinones are structurally (i.e., chemically and stereo-chemically) derived from amphetamine (i.e., *phenylisopropylamine*) analogs, (ii) the actions and mechanisms of action of synthetic cathinones are no

more homogeneous than those of other "amphetamine-related" phenylisopropylamines (PIAs), and (iii) an understanding of amphetamine-
related PIAs and their structure–activity relationships (SARs) will provide
a sound backdrop for understanding the synthetic cathinones.

Synthetic cathinones should not be viewed as an entirely novel class of
drugs of abuse for which no previous literature or prior understanding is
available. Actually, synthetic cathinones are derivatives of an agent (i.e.,
cathinone) that is the active stimulant component of a natural product
(i.e., the khat plant). The use/abuse of khat is many centuries old; however,
cathinone was not specifically identified as its active stimulant constituent
until 1975 (UN Document, 1975). Much can be learned from an examination of earlier literature. In fact, many synthetic cathinones, although it
should be recognized that they were not termed as such at the time of their
initial discovery, have been around for decades; some have been known for
100 years. Unfortunately, complex and inconsistent chemical nomenclature
has often obscured, or at least complicated, a proper understanding or appreciation of these agents.

Prior to just a few years ago, the scientific literature on cathinone, and
cathinone-related analogs (α-aminopropiophenones and chain-extended
derivatives thereof, now termed "synthetic cathinones"), was relatively
meager, quite manageable, and presented an interesting (if somewhat
incomplete) story. In the past, except for a brief period in the early
1980s—coincident with the identification of cathinone as a natural plant-
derived product with abuse potential—there was relatively little scientific
interest in cathinone or cathinone analogs. There was a second wave of
interest in the early 1990s when *methcathinone* (N-methylcathinone or
MCAT) was identified as a potential drug-abuse problem and scheduled
by the US government as a schedule I substance. Since then, the field has
burgeoned tremendously. "Synthetic cathinones" and new "synthetic cannabinoids" are two of the latest global drug-abuse problems, and both seem
to have had a nearly exponential growth rate. The two "problems" are *not*
related from a structural or mechanistic perspective. Only the former will be
discussed here.

Synthetic cathinones, synthetic cannabinoids, and other novel agents—
including some recently introduced LSD-like (i.e., lysergic acid
diethylamide-like) hallucinogenic agents—have been termed "new psychoactive substances" or "NPSs" (UNODC, 2013). This is a "bucket" appel-
lation that is appropriate and well suited for legal purposes (perhaps the goal
for which it was intended) and is a term suitable for the lay press, but it lends

no understanding of the actions and mechanisms of action of the individual agents (or classes of agents) involved. Indeed, several NPSs already have been investigated and they are structurally diverse, produce different effects, and act by different mechanisms. Structurally, synthetic cathinones might be described as "nuevo amphetamines" or, better yet, as "nuevo phenylisopropylamine analogs" because their actions and, particularly, mechanisms of action, are not necessarily identical to that of amphetamine itself.

The roots of the "cathinone story" are >1000 years old, but the bulk of what has been published on synthetic cathinones has occurred only in the past few years. By means of analogy, some parallels can be drawn from the current cocaine-abuse problem. Coca leaf (primarily *Erythroxylum coca*) was (and continues to be) chewed in certain parts of South America as an antifatigue agent. It was not until cocaine was identified as the major active stimulant constituent of coca leaf, and made widely available in pure form (i.e., in the form of cocaine and "crack"), that it became a major, worldwide drug-abuse problem. The same might be said about the khat plant—with cathinone now being considered its most potent central stimulant constituent—but with a twist. Cocaine analogs never became widely available. Why? Difficulty of synthesis of cocaine analogs? Indeed, there are some complex synthetic and stereochemistry problems here. The ready availability of cocaine? In contrast, many novel synthetic cathinone analogs are now flooding clandestine markets. The khat plant is not readily available outside its indigenous area, and it is the *fresh* plant that is desired (i.e., cathinone degrades as the harvested khat plant ages). Pure cathinone, unlike cocaine, has never been heavily trafficked. However, cathinone analogs are relatively easier to synthesize than cocaine analogs, they are generally more stable than cathinone (particularly in solution), and their synthetic precursors are readily available. Some synthetic cathinones are more potent than cathinone itself, can produce a different effect than cathinone, and possess different mechanisms of action (see the succeeding text). Hence, they are fairly simple to synthesize, and a wide variety of analogs is possible. This might explain the rapid shift in market-available synthetic cathinone products, as time goes on, to circumvent legal restrictions.

Structurally, synthetic cathinones are, simply put, β-keto analogs of amphetamine-related structures. Cathinone, for example, is the β-keto analog of amphetamine (AMPH). In theory, each "AMPH analog" can have a synthetic cathinone counterpart. However, some synthetic cathinones represent novel entities whose parent AMPH has never been extensively (or at all) investigated (at least not in a systematic, scientific manner or in human subjects). So, it is not surprising that little is known about many of the new synthetic cathinones. It might appear that the synthetic cathinones are wholly novel and unexpected drug-abuse entities, but a retrospective analysis suggests that there is/was some forethought behind the market introduction of the abused agents we now term synthetic cathinones.

Synthetic cathinones can be viewed from several perspectives. As mentioned earlier, they are β-keto analogs of AMPH (i.e., they are *PIA* analogs). They can also be viewed as oxidation products of *phenylpropanolamines* (i.e., β-hydroxyphenylisopropylamines) such as ephedrine and norephedrine. Cathinone is the oxidized version of norephedrine where the β-hydroxyl group of norephedrine has been oxidized to a carbonyl group.

PIAs *do not* represent a pharmacologically or mechanistically homogeneous class of agents (Glennon & Young, 2011). Hence, there is no reason to assume that synthetic cathinones (or *phenylpropanonamines*) will be any more pharmacologically or mechanistically homogeneous than their PIA parents. These agents need to be investigated on a case-by-case basis (Dal Cason, Young, & Glennon, 1997) until some general SARs can be identified. The pharmacology, SARs, and mechanism(s) of action of PIAs and/or phenylpropanolamines have been the subject of scientific investigation for >100 years now. The alarming increase in the number of new phenylpropanonamines (i.e., synthetic cathinones) appearing on the clandestine market in the past few years will require a considerable catch-up effort by scientists, the medical community, and drug enforcement agencies so that intelligent treatment and legal decisions can be made.

2. PIA ANALOGS: NOMENCLATURE AND PHARMACOLOGICAL ASSAYS

2.1. General nomenclature

Synthetic cathinones are best described as α-aminophenones (i.e., Ar–CO–CH(R_3)–(NR_1R_2) where "Ar" is typically a phenyl or substituted phenyl ring; NR_1R_2 represents a primary, secondary, or tertiary amine; and R_3 is a carbon chain of 0 to several carbon atoms in length).

Amphetamine (1-phenyl-2-aminopropane or 1-phenyl-2-propanamine or AMPH) not only is the structural parent of a large class of agents referred to as PIAs but also is known as phenylisopropylamine itself (i.e., from whence the class derives its name) (Fig. 15.1). That is, the term PIA not only refers to a specific agent (i.e., AMPH) but also refers to a class of agents (i.e., *the* PIAs)—all of which possess a similar structural skeleton. *Substituted phenylisopropylamines* are often referred to as *substituted amphetamines*. The latter (inaccurate) terminology should be resisted because it conjures up "AMPH-like" pharmacology. For example, the PIA DOM (i.e., 1-(2,5-dimethoxy-4-methylphenyl)-2-aminopropane; see later text) is frequently referred to as 2,5-dimethoxy-4-methylamphetamine. The latter name suggests that, pharmacologically, DOM might be an "AMPH-like" agent. This is not the case. DOM is a potent *classical hallucinogen* that lacks central stimulant character and acts via a mechanism that is entirely different from that of AMPH (Glennon & Young, 2011). Many other examples exist. Yet, both AMPH and DOM possess the same PIA backbone. Thus, the actions (and mechanisms of action) of substituted PIAs are not homogeneous; action depends upon pendant substituents. In what follows, the term *AMPH* will be used to refer to amphetamine, *phenylisopropylamines* (or *PIAs*) to refer to the class as a whole, and *AMPH-like action* to represent a pharmacology consistent with that observed following administration of AMPH.

Related PIAs with central stimulant character include β-hydroxyphenylisopropylamines and β-ketophenylisopropylamines. PIA nomenclature is generic; that is, all three types of agents can be considered as being PIAs. All three possess the same structural skeleton. To distinguish among the three structural categories, a more specific nomenclature is employed here. That is, β-hydroxyphenylisopropylamines are more specifically synonymous with *phenylpropanolamines*, and β-ketophenylisopropylamines are more synonymous with *phenylpropanonamines* (or, now, more commonly

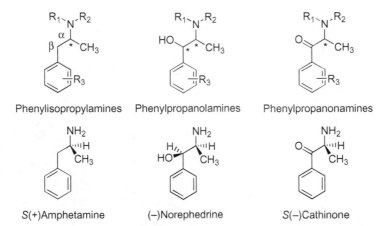

Phenylisopropylamines   Phenylpropanolamines   Phenylpropanonamines

S(+)Amphetamine   (−)Norephedrine   *S*(−)Cathinone

Figure 15.1 General chemical structures of phenylisopropylamines, phenylpropanolamines, and phenylpropanonamines (top row; asterisks indicate chiral centers), and representative examples of such, respectively (bottom row).

referred to as β-ketoamphetamines, bk-amphetamines, bk-AMPHs, β-keto PIAs, bk-PIAs or, simply, "synthetic cathinones"). See Fig. 15.1 for structural detail.

2.2. Stereochemistry

When PIAs possess a chiral center at the α-carbon atom (see Fig. 15.1), two optical isomers are possible: (+) and (−). Their *absolute configuration*, or their three-dimensional structural arrangement, can be designated as R or S. For example, AMPH exists as S(+)AMPH and R(−)AMPH. An equal mixture of two optical isomers (the most frequently encountered form for many agents) is designated a racemate or the (±) form; if no stereochemical descriptor is provided, it must be assumed that the racemate is being referred to. Hence, (±)AMPH and AMPH (unless the term is being used in the most generic sense, such as in "AMPH-like agents" or "AMPH-like action") refer, by definition, to racemic AMPH. When making stereochemical comparisons, it is the absolute configuration (i.e., R or S) that is to be compared; optical rotation (i.e., + and −) does not allow accurate structural comparisons to be made between agents. For greater detail, see Glennon and Young (2011).

Certain PIAs, specifically the phenylpropanolamines, can, depending upon their specific substituents, possess two chiral centers; hence, four optical isomers might be possible. For example, the simplest phenylpropanolamines are norephedrine and pseudonorephedrine (aka Ψ-norephedrine); each has two possible isomers (Fig. 15.2) (Glennon, 2008). Oxidation of the benzylic (or β-) alcohol of the phenylpropanolamines to a β-keto (i.e., carbonyl) group eliminates stereochemical considerations at this position and the resultant phenylpropanonamines exist only as a pair of (+) and

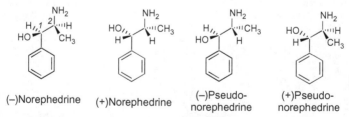

(−)Norephedrine   (+)Norephedrine   (−)Pseudo-norephedrine   (+)Pseudo-norephedrine

Figure 15.2 Structures of the four simplest phenylpropanolamines: (1R,2S)(−) norephedrine, (1S,2R)(+)norephedrine, (1R,2R)(−)pseudonorephedrine, and (1S,2S)(+) pseudonorephedrine or cathine. Introduction of an N-methyl group would afford the corresponding four optical isomers of ephedrine.

(−) isomers. For example, the structure of $S(−)$cathinone, the oxidation product of both (−)norephedrine and (+)pseudonorephedrine, is shown in Fig. 15.1.

2.3. Pharmacological assays

A variety of animal assays have been employed to examine AMPH-like agents (and PIAs in general). The most common among them are (i) drug discrimination, (ii) self-administration, (iii) locomotor activity, and (iv) stereotypy. These assays are so widely used that they deserve a brief description here because they are quite pertinent to what follows. In *drug discrimination* studies, animals (typically rodents, but sometimes pigeons, monkeys, or humans) are trained to respond (e.g., in a two-lever operant chamber—for rodents) to a given dose of a specific (i.e., training) agent; in subsequent tests of "stimulus generalization," the subjects are administered doses of a novel agent. Stimulus generalization implies that the novel agent produces stimulus effects common to the training agent—though not necessarily via an identical mechanism of action (Glennon & Young, 2011). Stimulus generalization provides evidence for commonality (*not* identity) of effect. *Self-administration* is another type of operant behavior where the novel agent is the "reward"; a high frequency of self-administration suggests that a drug might be rewarding (i.e., possess abuse potential) (Negus & Banks, 2011). It is well known that AMPH-related stimulants produce *hyperlocomotion* (i.e., an increase in locomotor action) in rodents, and this is thought to be related to increased dopamine neurotransmission in the nucleus accumbens (Ljungberg & Ungerstedt, 1985). AMPH-like stimulants can also produce *stereotypy* in rodents; that is, AMPH-like agents produce an increase in rodent locomotor action but, at some higher dose(s), cause the animals to make certain repetitive behaviors (i.e., "stereotypy") that result in decreased locomotor action. Certainly, other assays have been employed (and a few will be mentioned).

3. CATHINONE ANALOGS: HISTORICAL PERSPECTIVES

3.1. Ephedra and khat

Where did the synthetic cathinones come from? What follows is neither a comprehensive nor exhaustive treatment of the subject. Rather, it is meant to describe some early studies and put the subject in proper historical perspective; citations to some additional review articles are provided for those with greater interest.

Although the term "cathinone" is only about 40 years old, its lineage can be traced to two distinct shrubby parents: ephedra and khat. The ephedra plant (primarily *Ephedra sinica*, ma huang) has been used by the Chinese for thousands of years for its cardiovascular, bronchodilator, mild stimulant, and other effects (Lee, 2011). The major stimulant component of ephedra is (−)ephedrine. Ephedra was a "wonder drug" of the late 1800s and early 1900s and, during this time, its chemistry and pharmacology were being investigated in many laboratories. There were synthetic and stereochemistry problems (ephedrine and norephedrine have two chiral centers and four isomeric phenylpropanolamines exist for each; see Fig. 15.2). An apparent ephedra shortage in the 1920s spurred the chemical synthesis of ephedrine and novel ephedrine analogs; laboratories rose to the challenge and numerous patent applications were submitted. One such patent emanating from these studies was that for amphetamine. At the time, Chen and Kao (1926) wrote that "the success in the synthesis of ephedrine and pseudoephedrine marks one of the triumphs in the field of synthetic organic chemistry."

According to Alles, Fairchild, and Jensen (1961), the first written record concerning khat was in the 1300s, although khat use most certainly predates that time. The fresh leaves of the shrub *Catha edulis* are chewed in the Arabian Peninsula and in certain regions of Eastern Africa for their central stimulant effects. Occasionally, they are brewed as a tea. The leaves and preparations are known by nearly 100 different names—perhaps an indication of their popularity—including khat, k'at, kat, kath, gat, miraa, qat, tschat, Abyssinian tea, Arabian tea, and Somali tea (UN Document, 1979). The League of Nations considered the khat problem in 1935, and the United Nations (UN)/World Health Organization (WHO) considered it again in the 1960s and, later, in the 1970s (UN Document, 1979). Khat is still used on a regular basis, and the concept of *"cultural drug dependence"* has been introduced to explain its popularity and frequent use in certain geographic regions (Kennedy, Teague, & Fairbanks, 1980). The khat literature has been reviewed (e.g., Al-Hebshi & Skaug, 2002; Anderson & Carrier, 2011; Fitzgerald, 2009; Halbach, 1972; Kalix & Braeden, 1985; Kennedy et al., 1980).

3.2. Cathine and cathinone

What is the active central stimulant component of khat? The norephedrine isomer (+)pseudonorephedrine (aka "cathine") was first isolated from the khat plant in 1930 (Wolfes, 1930) and later by Alles et al. (1961) and Ristic and Thomas (1962). Alles et al. (1961) found cathine to possess central stimulant character. Given the popular interest in psychoactive substances at that time, khat and cathine were the subject of a major New York Times article (Fellows, 1967). But, soon after cathine was reported to be a central stimulant, it was found to be less potent than fresh khat extract (Friebel & Brilla, 1963). This led to speculation that khat might contain other stimulant components. In a series of studies culminating in the eventual identification of "more than forty alkaloid [khat leaf] components" (UN Document, 1979), a UN working group isolated $(-)\alpha$-aminopropiophenone from fresh khat leaves in 1975 and termed the substance "cathinone" (UN Document, 1975). $(-)$Cathinone (Schorno & Steinegger, 1978) and racemic or $(\pm)$ cathinone and its optical antipode were synthesized (UN Document, 1978), and the UN made samples available to various investigators.

$(-)$Cathinone was found to be a more potent AMPH-like locomotor stimulant in rodents than $(\pm)$cathinone, $(+)$cathinone, and/or cathine (Glennon & Showalter, 1981; Kalix, 1980a; Knoll, 1979; Rosecrans, Campbell, Dewey, & Harris, 1979; Yanagita, 1979) and produced AMPH-like stereotypic behavior in rats at high doses (Berardelli et al., 1980). Interestingly, van der Schoot, Ariens, van Rossum, and Hurkmans (1962)) had found nearly 20 years earlier (i.e., prior to cathinone being identified as a constituent of khat or before the term "cathinone" was introduced) in a random screen of a large number of PIA analogs that this aminopropiophenone produced locomotor stimulation in mice. As with its structural cousin AMPH, $(-)$cathinone also produced hyperthermia in rabbits that could be blocked by the dopamine antagonist haloperidol (Kalix, 1980b). Other studies (reviewed by Kalix & Braeden, 1985) also confirmed that cathinone is a potent AMPH-like substance; indeed, Kalix was probably the first to refer to $(-)$cathinone as "natural amphetamine" (Kalix, 1992). Furthermore, $(-)$cathinone was found, as was previously reported for $(+)$AMPH, to act as a dopamine (DA)-releasing agent (e.g., Kalix, 1981; Kalix & Glennon, 1986).

In drug discrimination studies employing rats trained to discriminate $(+)$ AMPH from vehicle, both isomers of cathinone substituted for training drug, with relative potencies of $S(-)$cathinone $\geq S(+)$AMPH $> (\pm)$ cathinone $> R(+)$cathinone (Glennon, Young, Hauck, & McKenney, 1984), and stimulus generalization could be blocked by the dopamine receptor antagonist haloperidol (Glennon, 1986). Cathinone, itself, has been used as a training drug in drug discrimination studies with rats (Glennon,

Schechter, & Rosecrans, 1984; Schechter & Glennon, 1985). In these, and other, investigations $S(-)$cathinone was consistently found to be more potent than $R(+)$cathinone just as $S(+)$AMPH is more potent than $R(-)$ AMPH (Glennon, Young, Martin, & Dal Cason, 1995).

3.3. Methcathinone

In a structure–activity investigation, several analogs of cathinone were prepared and examined. One of these was N-monomethyl cathinone (termed "methcathinone" by analogy to the N-monomethyl analog of AMPH, METH) (Glennon, Yousif, Naiman, & Kalix, 1987). Methcathinone (MCAT) might be considered the first synthetic cathinone. MCAT was found to be at least as potent as METH as a locomotor stimulant, as a DA-releasing agent, and in tests of stimulus generalization using rats trained to discriminate either $(+)$AMPH or cocaine from vehicle (Glennon et al., 1995; Young & Glennon, 1993). As expected, $S(-)$MCAT was found to be more potent than its $R(+)$enantiomer. Rats were subsequently trained to discriminate $S(-)$MCAT from vehicle and the stimulus was potently blocked by haloperidol (Young & Glennon, 1998). The S-isomer of MCAT was also more potent than its R-enantiomer as a locomotor stimulant in mice (Glennon et al., 1995). All evidence suggested that $S(-)$MCAT was a potent AMPH-like central stimulant. Methcathinone has now been found on the clandestine markets of various countries and is referred to as CAT, MCAT, and M-CAT.

As an aside, several phenylpropanonamines, including the substance now termed MCAT (and what is now known as cathinone), were initially synthesized by Eberhard in 1915 and again in 1920 (Eberhard, 1915, 1920) and by Fourneau and Kanao (1924) as synthetic intermediates in the preparation of ephedrine and norephedrine. Several other investigators repeated these syntheses (with slight modifications—and these synthetic routes are still employed today for the synthesis of synthetic cathinones), but the most commonly acknowledged synthesis is that by Roger Adams and his students in 1928 (Hyde, Browning, & Adams, 1928), which is a replicate of the Eberhard (1920) synthesis. MCAT, using today's terminology, has been around for 100 years, but it was prepared as a precursor for ephedrine synthesis and as a potential cardiovascular agent—that is, its central stimulant properties were not evaluated at the time. This same substance, and both of its optical isomers, was also patented in Germany in 1936 as synthetic precursors for the preparation of ephedrine analogs (Bockmuhl & Gorr, 1936).

"N-Methyl-β-ketoamphetamine" (now termed MCAT) was later patented by Parke-Davis as an analeptic agent (L'Italien, Park, & Rebstock, 1957). It was also shown, serendipitously, to be one of a number of several dozen PIA-related agents that act as locomotor stimulants in mice (van der Schoot et al., 1962). These studies never seemed to go any farther than to become historical footnotes.

In 1992, it was learned that what we had termed methcathinone was a very widely abused substance (under the name of *ephedrone*) in the former Soviet Union (*personal written communication* from Dr. I. Philippov, Lensoviet Technological Institute to R. A. Glennon dated August 18, 1992). A USSR Interior Ministry document released in 1989 (Savenko, Semkin, Sorokin, & Kazankov, 1989) reported that "In our country, the most widely used amphetamine derivatives obtained from ephedrine are ephedron and pervitin [i.e., pervitin = methamphetamine]." "The first pervitin synthesis for illegal distribution in the U.S.S.R. was in 1979 in Moscow and later in Leningrad." It might be noted that the chemical reduction (i.e., hydrogenolysis) of ephedrine results in METH, whereas the oxidation of ephedrine results in MCAT. Ephedrone (now recognized as being synonymous with MCAT) "surfaced in Leningrad for the first time in 1982" and was being prepared by the oxidation of ephedrine (Savenko et al., 1989). However, this report was not available until years later. The first mention of ephedrone in the Western literature was as a technical note in a forensic science journal (Zhingel, Dovensky, Crossman, & Allen, 1991) and the agent was probably not immediately recognized by most, at the time, as being synonymous with methcathinone.

3.4. Methylone

Another early synthetic cathinone was methylenedioxymethcathinone (MDMC or methylone). The agent was independently prepared by two groups of investigators in the mid-1990s (Dal Cason et al., 1997; Jacob & Shulgin, 1996). Methylone is the β-keto analog of N-methyl-1-(3,4-methylenedioxyphenyl)-2-aminopropane (MDMA).

3.5. Newer synthetic cathinones and "bath salts"

Although investigations with cathinone-related analogs occasionally appeared in the scientific literature, there was relatively little scientific interest in synthetic cathinones until Iversen (2010) prepared a report for the UK Home Office entitled *Consideration of the Cathinones*. About two dozen synthetic cathinones were identified as becoming an abuse problem in the European community. One preparation receiving particular attention at the time was *bath salts*, which, presumably, included mephedrone, methylenedioxypyrovalerone (MDPV), and/or methylone (MDMC).[1]

Mephedrone is the *para*-methyl analog of MCAT or the beta-keto analog of *p*TAP (*para*-tolylaminopropane) (see later text); methylone was described earlier. MDPV was, seemingly, something novel. The first report on the possible abuse of MDPV appeared in 2007 (Fuwa et al., 2007). Today, dozens of synthetic cathinones are available; they are sold under the general names of, for example, bath salts, plant food, stain removers, insect repellants, glass cleaners, and room deodorizers and are usually labeled "not for human consumption" (e.g., Kelly, 2011; UNODC, 2013).

4. AMPHETAMINE (I.E., PHENYLISOPROPYLAMINE) ANALOGS

Because synthetic cathinones or β-ketoamphetamines are structurally related to AMPH-like structures, a very brief overview on some simple phenylisopropylamines, or AMPH analogs, will provide a backdrop on what is to come in the subsequent section. Furthermore, it might be noted that certain AMPH analogs (sometimes, even long-known AMPH analogs) are now appearing on the clandestine market as "new" designer drugs. Indeed, although AMPH analogs and synthetic cathinones do not necessarily produce identical effects, they are inextricably linked. An appreciation of AMPH analogs will assist the understanding of the synthetic cathinones and will also provide some understanding of their structural evolution.

4.1. Structural modifications

AMPH and its *N*-monomethyl analog, METH, are well-established central stimulants with an extensive history. But, what happens when minor structural alterations are made to these structures? The simplest structural

---

[1] There is anecdotal information that "bath salts" initially contained one, two, or more of these agents (perhaps in combination with other agents). Three synthetic cathinones were scheduled (US schedule I) in 2011 with the statement that "Mephedrone, methylone, and MDPV are falsely marketed as . . . 'bath salts'" (Federal Register, 2011); the exact composition of "bath salts" was not specified. Spiller, Ryan, Weston, and Jansen (2011) have used the term collectively to refer to individual synthetic cathinones and to combinations of these agents. Indeed, the term "bath salts" has morphed into a generic term that now encompasses nearly any synthetic cathinone, alone, or in combination with other agents. The term "bath salts" does not refer to a specific agent or an unvarying combination of agents.

modification of AMPH analogs involves introduction of a single new substituent. For example, *N,N*-dimethylamphetamine (DiMe AMPH; Fig. 15.3), the *N*-methyl analog of METH, has been found on the clandestine market since the early 1990s, but its abuse has never been particularly widespread. At one time, it was thought that DiMe AMPH was merely an impurity in the clandestine synthesis of METH. DiMe AMPH has been examined in drug discrimination studies and in self-administration studies employing monkeys. In general, DiMe AMPH seems to be an AMPH-like agent but is at least 10-fold less potent than AMPH or METH (Dal Cason et al., 1997; Katz, Ricaurte, & Witkin, 1992; Young & Glennon, 1986), and *S*(+)DiMe AMPH is the more potent of the two isomers.

S(+)DiMe AMPH preferentially undergoes demethylation to *S*(+) METH (Lee, Yoo, In, Jin, & Kim, 2013); hence, some of the actions of DiMe AMPH might be attributed to the formation of this metabolite. Where investigated, this seems to be a common theme; that is, *N,N*-dimethyl PIAs generally undergo demethylation to their *N*-monomethyl products and/or their primary amines (though other routes of metabolism are also possible). In fact, for a series of *N*-substituted and *N,N*-disubstituted AMPH derivatives, it was found that, given the same lipophilicity, (i) tertiary amines are excreted faster than secondary amines, which are, in turn, excreted faster than primary amines, and (ii) the rate of N–dealkylation

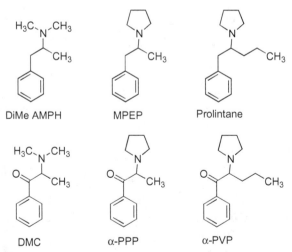

Figure 15.3 The structures of several basic (i.e., AMPH-like) phenylisopropylamines (top row) and their respective β-ketophenylisopropylamine (i.e., synthetic cathinone) counterparts (bottom row) demonstrating their structural similarity.

increases with the lipophilicity of the agent but decreases with increasing bulk of the leaving N-substituent (Testa & Salvesen, 1980). In other words, tertiary amine analogs of AMPH can be converted to their secondary amine counterparts, and this is most true when the N,N-dialkyl AMPH analog possesses small, sterically unhindered alkyl groups (such as a methyl or ethyl group). The metabolism of PIAs has been extensively investigated (reviewed by Kraemer & Maurer, 2002). Typical pathways involve N-demethylation or N-dealkylation of N-substituted AMPHs (at least of N-methyl and N-ethyl AMPHs) and O-demethylation of methoxy- or methylenedioxy-substituted AMPHs. Depending upon structure, the O-demethylated AMPHs can undergo further O-methylation by catecholamine O-methyltransferase. Some of these metabolites retain psychoactive character (see specific cases) (Kraemer & Maurer, 2002).

Other N,N-disubstituted AMPH analogs are known, but are uncommon. It is recognized that homologation (i.e., extension) of the N-methyl group of METH to an ethyl, n-propyl, or n-butyl group results in a progressive decrease in potency/action as determined in self-administration studies with rhesus monkeys (Woolverton, Shybut, & Johanson, 1980). Given that conversion of METH to its tertiary amine DiMe AMPH counterpart results in at least a 10-fold potency decrease in AMPH-like action, it is perhaps not surprising that there is relatively little literature on N,N-diethyl AMPH or its higher N,N-disubstituted homologs or agents with very bulky terminal amine substituents.

Conjoining the termini of the two ethyl groups of N,N-diethyl AMPH by a carbon–carbon single bond results in the pyrrolidine derivative MPEP (compare the structure of N,N-diethyl AMPH in Fig. 15.4 with the structure of MPEP in Fig. 15.3). MPEP possesses central stimulant action. Aminoketones, including what is now termed α-pyrrolidinopropiophenone (α-PPP) (Fig. 15.3—discussed later), were prepared as intermediates or synthetic precursors *en route* to the preparation of their corresponding phenylpropanolamine analogs that were being explored at the time as ephedrine-like (i.e., as sympathomimetic) agents. Reduction of the phenylpropanonamines provided the desired phenylpropanolamines. Overreduction (i.e., hydrogenolysis of the resulting phenylpropanolamines— not a particularly desired consequence of these studies) resulted in PIAs (including, e.g., MPEP) (Heinzelman & Aspergren, 1953). Shortly thereafter, several of these PIA analogs (including MPEP) were patented for their central stimulant actions (Thomae, 1959).

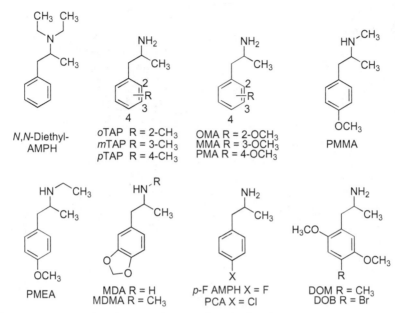

Figure 15.4 Some phenylisopropylamines described in this section.

Extension of the α-methyl group of MPEP to an *n*-propyl group results in prolintane (Fig. 15.3). The agent, patented in 1959 (Thomae, 1959), has seen clinical application as a stimulant (although not in the United States) for the treatment of, for example, fatigue. Several studies have demonstrated the AMPH-like central stimulant character of prolintane (Hollister & Gillespie, 1970; Kuitunen, Kärkkäinen, & Ylitalo, 1984; Nicholson, Stone, & Jones, 1980). Now, there are recent reports of prolintane abuse (Gaulier, Canal, Pradeille, Marquet, & Lachâtre, 2002; Kyle & Daley, 2007; Payá, Guisado, Vaz, & Crespo-Facorro, 2002).

Up to this point, discussion has been focused on the terminal amine and the α-alkyl group of the PIAs. Certainly, other amine substituents can be introduced, and the length and nature of the α-alkyl chain can be varied (i.e., shortened, lengthened, and branched). Indeed, a wide variety of such analogs was patented more than 50 years ago (e.g., Thomae, 1959).

AMPH-like agents can also possess substituents on the aromatic ring. For example, there are three monomethyl analogs of AMPH, known as *ortho*-tolylaminopropane (*o*TAP), *meta*-tolylaminopropane (*m*TAP), and *p*TAP (Fig. 15.4). In drug discrimination studies, only *o*TAP fully substituted in

(+)AMPH-trained rats and was about 10-fold less potent than (+)AMPH itself (Higgs & Glennon, 1990); mTAP and pTAP disrupted the animals' behavior (i.e., no conclusions could be drawn). However, both mTAP and pTAP (oTAP was not examined) were self-administered by rhesus monkeys (Wee et al., 2005), indicating at least some potential for abuse liability. There are three monomethoxy analogs of AMPH: the ortho-methoxy analog OMA (2-methoxyamphetamine), the meta-methoxy analog MMA, and the para-methoxy analog PMA (4-methoxyamphetamine) (Fig. 15.4); all three substituted in rats trained to discriminate (+)AMPH from vehicle in tests of stimulus generalization (Glennon, Young, & Hauck, 1985). That is, these agents were able to produce AMPH-like stimulus effects in animals. Dimethoxy and trimethoxy analogs failed to substitute. PMA and its N-monomethyl analog, para-methoxymethamphetamine (PMMA) (Fig. 15.4), have been abused and are responsible for a number of deaths over the years (see Zaitsu et al., 2008), and now, a homolog of PMMA, 4-methoxy-N-ethylamphetamine (PMEA) (Fig. 15.4), has appeared as a new designer drug (Zaitsu et al., 2008). Methylenedioxy analogs of AMPH have been known for some time. A rather interesting PIA is 1-(3,4-methylenedioxyphenyl)-2-aminopropane or MDA (Fig. 15.4). Its $S(+)$-isomer behaves as a central stimulant, whereas its $R(-)$-isomer acts more like a classical hallucinogen (Young & Glennon, 1996). Its N-monomethyl homolog is the well-known empathogen MDMA (Fig. 15.4).

A variety of halogenated AMPH analogs have been studied. For example, the meta-fluoro and para-fluoro (i.e., p-F AMPH; Fig. 15.4) analogs of AMPH were self-administered in rhesus monkeys (Wee et al., 2005) and both compounds, including the para-fluoro analog (and the para-fluoro analogs of METH, N-ethylamphetamine and α-ethylamphetamine), have been encountered on the clandestine market (Rösner, Quednow, Girreser, & Junge, 2005). The para-chloro analog of AMPH (i.e., PCA; Fig. 15.4) has also appeared on the illicit market (Lin, Lin, & Lua, 2011) as has the 5-fluoro analog of OMA and the 3-fluoro analog of PMA (Rösner et al., 2005). Numerous combinations and permutations of aryl-substituted, N-substituted phenylisopropylamines are possible. Many have been examined (e.g., Shulgin & Shulgin, 1991), quite a few have been encountered on the clandestine market, and, undoubtedly, more are likely to appear.

The number of potential psychoactive PIAs, or chain-extended PIAs, is staggering. Certainly, many PIA analogs lack AMPH-like stimulant properties. This does not necessarily mean they are inactive. For example, depending on the number and type of substituents, certain PIAs are *classical hallucinogens* (Glennon, 1996); these types of agents, typified by DOM and DOB (Fig. 15.4), will not be described here. The discussion earlier was simply meant to be a sampling of the types of PIAs that have been investigated, and nearly all have been found on the clandestine market. This discussion serves as an introduction to the synthetic cathinones; recall that introduction of a β-keto group to a PIA converts it to a phenylpropanonamine. In the section that follows, many of the same substitution patterns described earlier will be reencountered.

5. SYNTHETIC CATHINONES: SPECIFIC AGENTS

5.1. Simple structural modifications

The simplest modified cathinone or MCAT analog is dimethylcathinone (DMCN or N,N-dimethylcathinone), or the β-keto analog of DiMe AMPH. The agent, synthesized in 1954 (Iwao, Kowaki, & Rakemi, 1954) and later patented as an anorectic agent together with diethylpropion and several related structures in 1961 (Schütte, 1961), is known by a number of names including dimethylpropion, dimepropion, and metamfepramone. There are some anecdotal reports of its abuse. It has also been identified by the United Nations Office on Drugs and Crime (UNODC, 2013). Dimethylcathinone is metabolized to MCAT and methylpseudoephedrine (Markantonis, Kyroudis, & Beckett, 1989). This has led to recent efforts to differentiate among the three substances using instrumental methods (Thevis et al., 2009). (It might be noted that most of the terminology and acronyms used herein are those used by the UNODC (2013); for the most part, these were not those originally used to describe the agents when they were first reported in the scientific or patent literature.)

Another simple structural modification of MCAT is homologation of the *N*-methyl substituent to an *N*-ethyl group (i.e., ethcathinone; Fig. 15.5). Aromatic substituents, similar to those described earlier for the AMPH analogs, have been incorporated into cathinone and MCAT. For example, the 4-methyl analog of MCAT is known as mephedrone (4-methylmethcathinone or 4-MMC), whereas its corresponding 4-methoxy analog is termed methedrone (4-methoxymethcathinone or PMMC, by analogy to *para*-methoxymethamphetamine or PMMA). Mephedrone is the most widely seized synthetic cathinone by European law enforcement officials

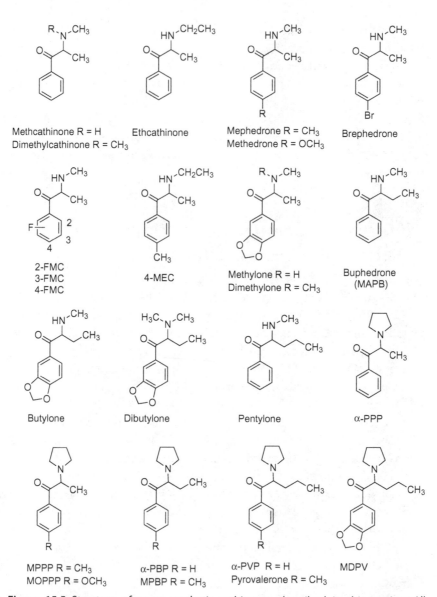

Figure 15.5 Structure of some synthetic cathinones described in this section. All (including about two dozen others) have been reported by the United Nations Office on Drugs and Crime (UNODC, 2013).

(UNODC, 2013). Other aryl-substituted cathinone analogs include 4-bromomethcathinone (brephedrone or 4-BMC), all three positional isomers of fluoromethcathinone (2-FMC, 3-FMC, and 4-FMC), and the 3,4-methylenedioxy analog of MCAT (methylone or MDMC) (Fig. 15.5).

5.2. Complex structural modifications

Terminal amine and aryl modifications can appear in the same agent. For example, the 4-methyl counterpart of ethcathinone is 4-methylethcathinone or 4-MEC, whereas the 3,4-methylenedioxy counterpart of dimethylcathinone is dimethylone. The latter agent (Iwao et al., 1954) and 3,4-dimethoxy- and 4-methoxydimethylcathinone were first investigated in the 1950s as sympathomimetic agents, but their central stimulant properties were not examined (Shapiro, 1950).

A common molecular modification among the synthetic cathinones is homologation of the α-methyl group. Perhaps the first "extended" cathinone analog is what is now termed buphedrone (MAPB) (Hyde et al., 1928). Buphedrone-related agents include butylone and dibutylone. Further extension of the chain results in pentylone (Hyde et al., 1928) (Fig. 15.5). Here, too, their stimulant character was not a subject of investigation at the time.

Constraint of the ethyl substituents of N,N-diethyl AMPH (Fig. 15.4) by conversion to a pyrrolidine ring afforded MPEP (Fig. 15.3). A similar strategy in the cathinone series results in α-PPP. α-PPP and its 4-methoxy analog (now known as MOPPP) (Fig. 15.5) were first prepared by Heinzelman and Aspergren (1953) as precursors for the synthesis of sympathomimetic amines. Replacement of the pyrrolidine ring of α-PPP with a piperidine ring affords its piperidinyl counterpart (Iwao et al., 1954). Several years later, α-PPP was one of a number of agents (including 1-piperidynyl, morpholinyl, and N-methylpiperazinyl derivatives) patented as anorectic agents (Schütte, 1961). Extension of the α-PPP side chain to an ethyl group results in α-pyrrolidinobutyrophenone (α-PBP), and further extension to an *n*-propyl group results in α-pyrrolidinovalerophenone (α-PVP) (Fig. 15.5); both agents (including 4-methyl, 4-methoxy, and 4-chloro α-PVP) were patented in 1964 as central stimulants (Seeger, 1964). The 4-methyl analog of α-PVP, pyrovalerone, and a number of related analogs have been recently prepared (Meltzer, Butler, Deschamps, & Madras, 2006). α-PVP and its 4-methyl, 4-methoxy, and 4-chloro derivatives were patented earlier as central stimulants (Wander, 1963), but no pharmacological data were provided. Methylenedioxypyrovalerone (MDPV), an occasional component of "bath salts," was patented as a central stimulant in 1969 (Boehringer Ingelheim, 1969; Köppe, Ludwig, & Zeile, 1969).

5.3. Metabolism

It is rather remarkable that many agents now termed synthetic cathinones were initially examined as anorectic agents or central stimulants (patented, primarily, by the pharmaceutical industry) in the 1960s or earlier. It might also be noted that novel synthetic cathinones (and phenylpropanolamines) can result from the metabolism of known synthetic cathinones and become a potential source of new drugs of abuse. For example, one of the metabolites of MCAT is cathinone (Beyer, Peters, Kraemer, & Maurer, 2007; Paul & Cole, 2001), and cathinone is pharmacologically active as a central stimulant. In addition, cathinone can be further metabolized to norephedrine or cathine, depending upon the cathinone isomer ingested, and cathine, too, is a known (although weak) central stimulant. The pharmacology (and toxicology) of most synthetic cathinone metabolites has yet to be studied.

Typically, cathinones undergo N-dealkylation (as mentioned earlier for AMPH-related agents) and reduction of the carbonyl group to an alcohol (i.e., a phenylpropanolamine). When a 3,4-methylenedioxy group is present, it undergoes ring opening to afford a dihydroxy intermediate that is eventually converted to its corresponding 3-hydroxy-4-methoxy and/or 4-hydroxy-3-methoxy counterparts; with pyrrolidine-containing compounds, the pyrrolidine ring can either be oxidized to a lactam (that, in some cases, undergoes ring opening) or is converted to an iminium salt that is subsequently hydrolyzed to the corresponding ketone. The metabolism of many of the synthetic cathinones shown in Fig. 15.5 has been examined, including cathinone (Beyer et al., 2007; Brenneisen, Geisshüsler, & Schorno, 1986), MCAT (Beyer et al., 2007; Paul & Cole, 2001), methylone (Kamata et al., 2006), 3-FMC (Pawlik, Plässer, Mahler, & Daldrup, 2012), butylone (Zaitsu et al., 2009), α-PPP (Meyer, Du, Schuster, & Maurer, 2010; Springer, Fritschi, & Maurer, 2003b) and its 3,4-methylenedioxy counterpart (Springer, Fritschi, & Maurer, 2003a), MPPP (Springer, Fritschi, & Maurer, 2003b; Springer, Paul, Staack, Kraemer, & Maurer, 2003; Springer, Peters, Fritschi, & Maurer, 2002), MOPPP (Springer, Staack, Paul, Kraemer, & Maurer, 2003), MPBP (Westphal et al., 2007), α-PVP (Springer, Staack, Paul, Kraemer, & Maurer, 2003), and MDPV (Meyer et al., 2010; Strano-Rossi, Cadwallader, de la Torre, & Botrè, 2010). Ammanna, McLaren, Gerostamoulos, and Beyer (2012) had also examined 25 synthetic cathinone analogs in an attempt to develop instrumental assays that can differentiate among them. More such studies are required to separate and/or identify newer cathinones and cathinone metabolites.

6. SYNTHETIC CATHINONES: MECHANISMS OF ACTION AND BEHAVIORAL STUDIES

Many of the "new" synthetic cathinones have not been extensively investigated and only very recently has attention been focused on these agents. Hence, potency comparisons are elusive (and, for reasons to be discussed later, are often difficult to make). Mechanistic data are scant. That is, although there is some new information on what a few specific synthetic cathinone analogs might "do" (transporter-wise, receptor-wise, and behaviorally), for the most part, their behavioral actions (in the few cases where such data are available) have not been specifically related to specific mechanisms of action.

6.1. Transporter studies

Cathinone and MCAT were shown quite some time ago to cause release of DA (Glennon et al., 1987). Subsequently, $S(-)$MCAT was found to act at NET, DAT, and SERT (serotonin transporter) and displayed potencies similar to $S(+)$METH (i.e., NET≈DAT>SERT) (Rothman et al., 2003). Notable is that reduction of the keto group of $S(-)$MCAT, to afford $(-)$ ephedrine and $(+)$pseudoephedrine, resulted in decreased potency at NET and DAT and loss of activity at SERT. Others have since found that MCAT is nearly equipotent as a DA-releasing agent and reuptake inhibitor, whereas cathinone was severalfold more potent as a releasing agent (Simmler et al., 2012). Both agents were more potent at releasing NE than DA, and neither agent had a significant effect at SERT. MCAT and methylone were substantially less potent as inhibitors of the vesicular monoamine transporter (bovine VMAT2) than at inhibiting transmembrane reuptake by serotonin (human platelets), DAT, and NET (expressed in human glial cells) (Cozzi, Sievert, Shulgin, Jacob, & Ruoho, 1999).

Among the newer synthetic cathinones, two of the first to be examined were mephedrone and MDPV. Using a frog oocyte preparation transfected with hDAT, mephedrone produced DA-like depolarization, whereas MDPV produced cocaine-like hyperpolarization (Cameron, Kolanos, Solis, Glennon, & De Felice, 2013; Cameron, Kolanos, Vekariya, De Felice, & Glennon, 2013; Kolanos, Cameron, Vekariya, De Felice, & Glennon, 2011). These are signatures of a releasing agent and a reuptake inhibitor, respectively. Simmler et al. (2012) found mephedrone to be nearly equipotent as an inhibitor and releaser of DA and 5-HT; it was substantially more potent as an inhibitor of NET. In contrast, MDPV was a potent inhibitor of DAT and NET, a very weak inhibitor of SERT, but neither released DA or 5-HT (Simmler et al., 2012). Others (Eshleman et al., 2013) reported comparable results. A study of butylone, methylone, ethylone, flephedrone pyrovalerone, MDPV, and several other agents concluded that all of the cathinone analogs were inhibitors of the three monoamine transporters but with varying selectivities; most of the compounds (with the exception of methylone, pyrovalerone, and MDPV) were substrate releasers (Simmler et al., 2012). These same agents displayed low affinity for 5-HT_{1A}, 5-HT_{2A}, 5-HT_{2C}, D_1, D_2, D_3, and H_1 histamine receptors and $\alpha 1A$- and $\alpha 2A$-adrenoceptors (Simmler et al., 2012). Pyrovalerone and several related agents had been found earlier to act as DAT/NET inhibitors, to have little effect at SERT, and to lack affinity for 5-HT_{1A}, 5-HT_{1B}, 5-HT_{2C}, D_1, D_2, or D_3 receptors (Meltzer et al., 2006). Mephedrone displayed low micromolar affinity for 5-HT_2 receptors and even lower affinity for DA receptors (Martínez-Clemente, Escubedo, Pubill, & Camarasa, 2012). An examination of a series of cathinone analogs revealed that 4-FMC, mephedrone, and methylone, but not butylone or MDPV, generally induced release of neurotransmitter from DAT, NET, and SERT; these agents were also shown bind with low (i.e., μM) affinity at 5-HT_{1A}, 5-HT_{2A}, and 5-HT_{2C} receptors, with little to no affinity for DA receptors (Eshleman et al., 2013). Iversen et al. (2013) examined the binding of several synthetic cathinones (including mephedrone, 4-MEC, and four others not discussed here) at 49 receptors and transporters. Except for the transporters, and a modest affinity ($pK_i = 6.1$) for mephedrone at 5-HT_{2B} receptors, the agents typically displayed, at best, micromolar affinity. Synthetic cathinones currently being abused seem to produce their actions primarily at the DA, norepinephrine (NE), and/or serotonin (5-HT) transporter; that is, they either release and/or block the reuptake of one or more of these neurotransmitters. Simmler et al. (2012) suggested a classification of various cathinone analogs, based on their transporter profiles, as (i) cocaine–MDMA mixed cathinones, (ii) methamphetamine-like cathinones, and (iii) pyrovalerone cathinones. Additional agents will need to be examined, and careful SAR studies need to be performed, but transporter profiles will certainly be a key to unraveling the behavioral (and other) actions of these agents. In a recent study, for example, it was demonstrated that both the extended chain and the pyrrolidine moiety of pyrovalerone- or MDPV-type agents need not be present for the agents to function as hyperpolarizing agents at DAT expressed in frog oocytes; for example, dimethylone, 3,4-methylenedioxy-α-PPP, and N-methyl-3,4-methylenedioxypentylone all produced MDPV-like hyperpolarization (i.e., cocaine-like DAT inhibition) (Kolanos, Solis, Sakloth, De Felice, & Glennon, 2013).

6.2. Locomotor studies

Like AMPH, METH, and cathinone (*vide supra*), some synthetic cathinones can increase rodent locomotor activity. Racemic MCAT produced locomotor stimulation in mice similar to that produced by cathinone itself (Glennon et al., 1987; van der Schoot et al., 1962); the rank order of potency of its optical isomers was $S(-)MCAT > S(+)AMPH \geq R(+)MCAT$ (Glennon et al., 1995). Likewise, mephedrone and methylone produced hyperlocomotion in rats (Baumann et al., 2012; Kehr et al., 2011; Marusich, Grant, Blough, & Wiley, 2012; Motbey, Hunt, Bowen, Artiss, & McGregor, 2011) and mephedrone produced a similar effect in mice (Angoa-Perez et al., 2012). Mephedrone, methylone, and butylone produced hyperlocomotion in mice (potency: METH > butylone > methylone ≥ mephedrone) (López-Arnau, Martinez-Clemente, Pubill, Escubedo, & Camarasa, 2012), and mephedrone increased wheel-running activity in rats (Huang et al., 2012). Mephedrone and MDMA induced the release both of DA and 5-HT in rat nucleus accumbens that was accompanied by increased locomotor activity (Kehr et al., 2011).

MDPV was reported to "exhibit extraordinarily powerful central nervous system stimulating activities in warm-blooded animals" (Köppe et al., 1969), but no data were provided, and oral administration of a single dose of MDPV increased mouse locomotor activity (Fuwa et al., 2007). Huang et al. (2012) found that MDPV behaved in a manner similar to that of (+)METH in a wheel-turning locomotor assay but differently than that of mephedrone, suggesting that different mechanisms of action might be involved. Others have found that MDPV is a locomotor stimulant in mice and that its effects are potentiated by warm ambient temperatures (Fantegrossi, Gannon, Zimmerman, & Rice, 2013).

Marusich et al. (2012) compared the hyperlocomotor actions of six synthetic cathinones (including mephedrone, methylone, methedrone, MDPV, 3-FMC, and 4-FMC) in rats; all were locomotor stimulants with MDPV being among the most potent and methedrone being the least potent. MDPV was found to be comparable in potency to (+)METH as a locomotor stimulant (Aarde, Huang, Creehan, Dickerson, & Taffe, 2013). Another mouse locomotor study examined six synthetic cathinones and resulted in the following order of potency: $S(+)$METH > MDPV ≅ mephedrone > methylone > flephedrone > butylone > cocaine > naphylone; the stimulant actions of MDPV were long-lasting (i.e., 250–300 min depending upon dose) (Gatch, Taylor, & Forster, 2013).

AMPH-related stimulants produce hyperlocomotion in rodents that is related to increased DA transmission (Ljungberg & Ungerstedt, 1985). Although weaker than AMPH, PMA, the *para*-methoxy analog of AMPH, is a locomotor stimulant; its actions seem to be mediated through a serotonergic rather than dopaminergic mechanism (Loh & Tseng, 1978). N-Monomethylation of PMA to PMMA results in a loss in locomotor stimulant action (Glennon, Ismaiel, Martin, Poff, & Sutton, 1988). However, introduction of a β-keto group, converting PMMA to methedrone, reintroduces hyperlocomotor character. It has been reported that 5-HT (i.e., 5-HT_{2A}) receptors play a role in DA release and locomotor responses to AMPH (Auclair, Drouin, Cotecchia, Glowinski, & Tassin, 2004). Indeed, pretreatment of mice with the 5-HT_2 antagonist ketanserin or the DA antagonist haloperidol blocked the hyperlocomotor actions of methylone and butylone and partially inhibited the actions of mephedrone; pretreatment with a 5-HT_{1B} antagonist reduced the actions of butylone but failed to inhibit the locomotor actions of methylone or butylone (López-Arnau et al., 2012).

Bupropion, the N-*tert*-butyl analog of 3-chlorocathinone, is a clinically employed antidepressant. In a comparison of rat locomotor action, several cathinone analogs produced hyperlocomotor effects with relative potencies of MCAT > 3-bromomethcathinone (3-BMC) > bupropion (Foley & Cozzi, 2003). The 4-bromo positional isomer of 3-BMC, 4-BMC, was inactive at the highest dose evaluated, but the deschloro analog of bupropion produced an effect comparable to that of a similar dose of bupropion (Foley & Cozzi, 2003). 4-(Trifluoromethyl)methcathinone failed to increase rat horizontal motor action (Cozzi et al., 2013). Compared to methcathinone, all three possible trifluoromethyl analogs were less potent at releasing or blocking the reuptake of DA, NE, and 5-HT, but introduction of a ring substituent at the 3- or 4-positions increased their potency at SERT and decreased potency at DAT and NET, resulting in agents with enhanced SERT selectivity (Cozzi et al., 2013). In another recent study, the hyperlocomotor potencies of six cathinone analogs were found to correlate with their binding at VMAT2 and inhibition of NE uptake by VMAT2 (Gatch et al., 2013).

6.3. Drug discrimination studies

Few cathinone analogs have been examined in drug discrimination studies, and even fewer have been used as training drugs. In (+)AMPH-trained rats, cathinone and its individual optical isomers substituted (S-cathinone was more potent than R-cathinone), but α-desmethylcathinone failed to generalize (Glennon, Schechter, et al., 1984; Glennon, Young, et al., 1984; Kalix & Glennon, 1986). Lacking an α-methyl group, α-desmethylcathinone might not readily penetrate the blood–brain barrier. S(−)Cathinone (the R-isomer was not examined) also substituted in cocaine-trained rats (Woolverton, 1991). Racemic MCAT and both of its optical isomers substituted for (+)AMPH (Glennon et al., 1995, 1987) and for cocaine (Young & Glennon, 1993). α-Desmethylcathinone and β-aminopropiophenone failed to substitute (Kalix & Glennon, 1986). S(−)Dimethylcathinone, (±)dimethylcathinone, ethcathinone, N-n-propylcathinone, and methylone (listed in decreasing order of potency) substituted in (+)AMPH-trained rats, but 3,4-methylenedioxycathinone (i.e., the N-desmethyl counterpart of methylone) did not (Dal Cason et al., 1997). S(−)Methcathinone, but not S(+)METH, substituted in (−) ephedrine-trained rats (Bondareva, Young, & Glennon, 2002). With racemic cathinone as the training drug, stimulus generalization occurred to both cathinone optical isomers (S > R), cathine, (+)AMPH, METH, and cocaine, but not to α-desmethylcathinone, 4-hydroxycathinone, 4-methoxycathinone, or 4-chlorocathinone (Glennon, Schechter, et al., 1984; Glennon, Young, et al., 1984; Schechter & Glennon, 1985), nor 4-fluorocathinone (unpublished data). Likewise, (+)AMPH, cocaine, cathine, but not α-desmethylcathinone, substituted in cathinone-trained rats (Goudie, Atkinson, & West, 1986). S(−)MCAT-trained rats recognized (±)MCAT, S(+)METH, cathinone, R(−)MCAT, cocaine, and several other central stimulants (Young & Glennon, 1998). Clearly, cathinone and MCAT produce stimulus effects similar to those of other central stimulants, and alteration of structure influences their potency and actions. Furthermore, the S(−)MCAT stimulus was potently antagonized by the DA antagonist haloperidol (Young & Glennon, 1998). However, MDMA substituted in rats trained to discriminate mephedrone, but full substitution failed to occur with METH or cocaine; furthermore, the mephedrone stimulus could not be antagonized by pretreatment of the animals with haloperidol (Varner et al., 2012). It was recently demonstrated, using mice trained to discriminate MDPV from saline, that substitution occurred following administration of (±)METH and (±)MDMA (Fantegrossi et al., 2013), suggesting similarities among the stimulus actions of the three agents. In rats trained to discriminate S(+)METH from vehicle, each of the following agents was found to substitute, with relative potencies of S(+)-METH > MDPV > mephedrone > butylone ≅ methylone ≅ flephedrone ≅ naphylone, whereas in cocaine-trained rats, their relative potencies were MDPV > mephedrone ≅ methylone > naphylone ≅ cocaine ≅ flephedrone > butylone (Gatch et al., 2013). Clearly, additional studies are required to better understand the complex stimulus properties of the synthetic cathinones. Nevertheless, it would appear that these agents do not represent a behaviorally homogeneous class.

6.4. Other studies

MDPV, but not mephedrone, produced stereotypic behavior in rats (Aarde et al., 2013; Huang et al., 2012), and MDPV produced stereotypy in mice (Fantegrossi et al., 2013). Mephedrone was self-administered and increased core body temperature (rats) (Hadlock et al., 2011). MDPV had only a negligible effect on body temperature (Aarde et al., 2013). In mice, hyperthermia following MDPV administration was observed only at warm ambient temperatures (Fantegrossi et al., 2013). MDPV was also self-administered by rats (Aarde et al., 2013; Watterson et al., 2013) and was more potent and efficacious than S(+)METH. MCAT, methylone, mephedrone, and MDPV facilitated intracranial self-stimulation (ICSS) in rats; MCAT displayed the highest efficacy and mephedrone the lowest (Bonano, Glennon, De Felice, Banks, and Negus (2013). Several studies have examined the "binge-like" actions of methedrone by administration of multiple doses (Angoa-Perez et al., 2012; Hadlock et al., 2011). In one such study, it was shown that mephedrone enhanced the hyperthymic action of (+) METH and enhanced the neurotoxic actions of (+)AMPH and MDMA on DA nerve endings (Angoa-Perez et al., 2012).

7. SYNTHETIC CATHINONES: HUMAN STUDIES

The desired effects of synthetic cathinones apparently include euphoria, mental alertness, talkativeness, sexual arousal, a focused mind, and overall positive feelings; the effects generally occur within 30–45 min following administration and last from 1 to 3 h (Marinetti & Antonides, 2013). The undesirable effects, primarily neurological and cardiovascular, can last for hours to days (Marinetti & Antonides, 2013). This is probably a fairly accurate, if not somewhat generalized, statement. No controlled clinical studies have been performed with synthetic cathinones. What makes descriptions of the human pharmacology of specific synthetic cathinones particularly difficult is that (i) the various preparations are known by dozens of names, (ii) some preparations contain multiple constituents—up to as many as 10 (Gil, Adamowicz, Skulska, Tokarczyk, & Stanaszek, 2013), (iii) the constituents are constantly changing (even if a "brand name" does not), and (iv) individuals presenting at emergency departments typically are unaware of specifically what they have taken. Another confounding factor is the route of administration. For example, synthetic cathinone preparations can be administered orally, rectally, intramuscularly, intravenously, or by inhalation (Prosser & Nelson, 2012); route of administration will likely influence potency, rate of onset, duration of action, and metabolism. Self-reported doses range from a few milligrams to >1 g (and, of course, certain synthetic cathinones are more potent than others given a common route of administration). Because users cannot be certain of the contents or purity of the drug, self-reporting results can be highly variable (Prosser & Nelson, 2012).

To illustrate the complexity of the problem, a few examples are provided. Samples of 24 products sold as *Energy* (e.g., NRG-1, NRG-2) in the United Kingdom were analyzed and 70% contained mixtures of cathinones including mephedrone, butylone, flephedrone, and MDPV (Brandt, Sumnall, Measham, & Cole, 2010). A follow-up study additionally identified pentylone, MPPP, and MDPBP (i.e., the 3,4-methylenedioxy analog of α-PBP) (Brandt, Freeman, Sumnall, Measham, & Cole, 2011). A similar study conducted in the United States on 15 "brand-name" products identified single-component preparations (e.g., mephedrone, MDPV, and methylone) and mixtures of synthetic cathinones (e.g., mephedrone + MDPV + methylone and MDPV + methylone); in two instances, products occurring with the same "brand name" and packaging consisted of different synthetic cathinones (Spiller et al., 2011).

A retrospective analysis of 236 poison center records for "bath salts" exposure revealed 39 separate "brand names" from patient histories; of these, the two most frequently cited were *Cloud 9* and *White Lightening* (Spiller et al., 2011). The most common symptoms included agitation, violent behavior, tachycardia, hallucinations, and paranoia. Perhaps the first study to report analytically confirmed mephedrone intoxication was that by Wood et al. (2010), who found that the clinical features were consistent with an acute sympathomimetic toxidrome (e.g., hypertension, tachycardia, and agitation). An analysis of 32 cases of presumed synthetic cathinone use in Ohio, including 23 postmortem studies, quantitatively identified MDPV, methylone, pentylone, pyrovalerone, α-PVP, and methedrone (Marinetti & Antonides, 2013).

In a case series, it was suggested that a consumed "bath salt" product consisted of mephedrone (Kasick, McKnight, & Kilsovic, 2012); in another study, it was argued that because MDPV, but not mephedrone, can produce a false-positive for phencyclidine (a finding common to both studies), the substance consumed in the first study might have been MDPV (Penders, Gestring, & Vilensky, 2012). Both studies found that the agents produced an extreme degree of psychomotor agitation and violent behavior (referred to as *excited delirium syndrome* or ExDS). In another case study describing similar symptoms, both MDPV and flephedrone were identified in blood and urine, and an analysis of the actual powdered material showed a nearly equal mixture of the two agents (Thornton, Gerona, & Tomaszewski, 2012). A clearer case study described a patient exhibiting unusual behavior, severe agitation, altered mental status, tachycardia, hypertension, and ultimately multiorgan failure, who tested positive for MDPV and negative for about three dozen other drugs of abuse including mephedrone (Borek & Holstege, 2012).

A case series identified 4-MEC in powdered form, and in two of the three cases, the subjects' blood and/or urine 4-MEC levels were measured; in two cases, subjects had a high blood-alcohol level, whereas in the third case, resulting in death, AMPH, PMA, and PMMA were also identified (Gil et al., 2013).

Some studies on the acute clinical/subjective effects (with route of administration and duration of action) of mephedrone, methylone, MDPV, methedrone, and butylone have been reviewed (Karila & Reynaud, 2010; Kelly, 2011; Prosser & Nelson, 2012).

Treatment for patients with exposure to synthetic cathinones is primarily supportive and consists of benzodiazepines to control agitation and seizures (e.g., Borek & Holstege, 2012; Prosser & Nelson, 2012). Haloperidol (Kasick et al., 2012) and droperidol (Thornton et al., 2012) also have been used. The health risks of mephedrone (Dybdal, Holder, Ottoson, Sweeney, & Williams, 2013) and MDPV (Coppola & Mondola, 2012) have been reviewed. Specific treatments have also been recently reviewed (Zawilska & Wojcieszak, 2013).

A problem, likely restricted to MCAT abuse alone, due to a method of preparation—oxidation of ephedrine with potassium permanganate—is manganism caused by manganese in impure samples. The Parkinsonian-like extrapyramidal syndrome of manganism is irreversible and unresponsive to treatment with levodopa (e.g., Sikk et al., 2013).

8. CONCLUSION

Synthetic cathinones are either β-keto analogs of known PIAs or chain-extended derivatives thereof. Many so-called synthetic cathinones have been known for quite some time in the scientific or patent literature (although they were never termed such), and some are simply derived from the application of AMPH-like or PIA-like SAR to cathinone or MCAT. PIAs do not represent a functional or mechanistically homogeneous class of agents! Thus, there is no reason to suspect that phenylpropanonamines (i.e., synthetic cathinones) will be any more homogeneous in their actions or mechanisms of action. We indicated, more than 15 years ago, that cathinone analogs will need to be examined on a case-by-case basis (Dal Cason et al., 1997). The results presented above now echo this sentiment. Much can be learned about synthetic cathinones by examining their corresponding AMPH-like counterparts. But, the addition of a β-keto group can influence function in unexpected ways. Some synthetic cathinones (e.g., MCAT) function as might be expected—that is, the resulting agent is simply a more selective and potent stimulant (and DA-releasing agent) than its corresponding AMPH counterpart—METH. Other synthetic cathinones, due to minor tweaks in their ability to release or block the reuptake of 5-HT, DA, and/or NE, possess different qualities. Some inroads have been made, but much more needs to be done to understand this large, and growing, class of agents. For the most part, these agents either block or release the reuptake of DA, 5-HT, and/or NE. Selectivity profiles remain to be fully investigated. And such studies are ongoing. None of the agents, thus far, show any significant affinity for the various neurotransmitter receptors at which they have been examined (at least, no trend has yet been identified), except for their affinity at the various transporters.

To conclude, synthetic cathinones represent a heterogeneous class of psychoactive agents that likely act, primarily, at one or more of three major neurotransmitter transporters, by release, reuptake inhibition, or both, and require much more investigation on a case-by-case basis.

CONFLICT OF INTEREST

The author has no conflicts of interest to declare.

ACKNOWLEDGMENTS

Work from our laboratories described earlier was supported by DA01642 and DA033930.

REFERENCES

Aarde, S. M., Huang, P. K., Creehan, K. M., Dickerson, T. J., & Taffe, M. A. (2013). The novel recreational drug 3,4-methylenedioxypyrovalerone (MDPV) is a potent psychomotor stimulant: Self-administration and locomotor activity in rats. *Neuropharmacology*, 71, 130–140.

Al-Hebshi, N. N., & Skaug, N. (2002). Khat (*Catha edulis*)—An updated review. *Addiction Biology*, 10, 299–307.

Alles, G. A., Fairchild, M. D., & Jensen, M. (1961). Chemical pharmacology of *Catha edulis*. *Journal of Medicinal and Pharmaceutical Chemistry*, 3, 323–352.

Ammanna, D., McLaren, J. M., Gerostamoulos, D., & Beyer, J. (2012). Detection and quantification of new designer drugs in human blood: Part 2—Designer cathinones. *Journal of Analytical Toxicology*, 36, 381–389.

Anderson, D. M., & Carrier, N. C. M. (2011). Khat: Social harms and legislation. A literature review. U. K. Home Office Report. ISBN: 978-1-84987-494-6.

Angoa-Perez, M., Kane, M. J., Fracescutti, D. M., Sykes, K. E., Shah, M. M., Mohammed, A. M., et al. (2012). Mephedrone, and abused psychoactive component of "bath salts" and methamphetamine congener, does not cause neurotoxicity to dopamine nerve endings of the striatum. *Journal of Neurochemistry*, 120, 1097–1107.

Auclair, A., Drouin, C., Cotecchia, S., Glowinski, J., & Tassin, J. P. (2004). 5-HT$_{2A}$ and α1B adrenergic receptors entirely mediate dopamine release, locomotor response and behavioural sensitization to opiates and psychostimulants. *European Journal of Neuroscience*, 20, 3073–3084.

Baumann, M. H., Ayestas, M. A., Jr., Partilla, J. S., Sink, J. R., Shulgin, A. T., Daley, P. F., et al. (2012). The designer methcathinone analogs, mephedrone and methylone, are substrates for monoamine transporters in brain tissue. *Journal of Neuropsychopharmacology*, 37, 1192–1203.

Berardelli, A., Capocaccia, L., Pacitti, C., Tancredi, V., Quinteri, F., & Elmi, A. (1980). Behavioural and EEG effects induced by an amphetamine-like substance (cathinone) in rats. *Pharmacological Research Communications*, 12, 959–964.

Beyer, J., Peters, F. T., Kraemer, T., & Maurer, H. H. (2007). Detection and validated quantification of nine herbal phenalkylamines and methcathinone in human blood plasma by LC-MS/MS with electrospray ionization. *Journal of Mass Spectrometry*, 42, 150–160.

Bockmuhl, M., & Gorr, G. (1936). Verfahren zur Darstellung von optisch active 1-aryl-2-amino-1-propanolen. German patent 639,126. November 28, 1936.

Boehringer Ingelheim. (1969). α-Substituted-ketones and processes for their preparation. British patent 1,149,366. April 23, 1969.

Bonano, J., Glennon, R. A., De Felice, L. J., Banks, M., & Negus, S. S. (2013). Abuse-related and abuse-limiting effects of methcathinone, and the synthetic "bath salts" cathinone analogs methylenedioxypyrovalerone (MDPV), methylone and mephedrone on intracranial self-stimulation in rats. *Psychopharmacology*, in press.

Bondareva, T. S., Young, R., & Glennon, R. A. (2002). Central stimulants as discriminative stimuli: Asymmetric generalization between (-)ephedrine and (S+)methamphetamine. *Pharmacology, Biochemistry, and Behavior*, 74, 157–162.

Borek, H. A., & Holstege, C. P. (2012). Hyperthermia and multiorgan failure after abuse of "bath salts" containing 3,4-methylenedioxypyrovalerone. *Annals of Emergency Medicine*, *60*, 103–105.

Brandt, S. D., Freeman, S., Sumnall, H. R., Measham, F., & Cole, J. (2011). Analysis of NRG 'legal highs' in the UK: Identification and formation of novel cathinones. *Drug Testing and Analysis*, *3*, 569–575.

Brandt, S. D., Sumnall, H. R., Measham, F., & Cole, J. (2010). Analyses of second-generation 'legal highs' in the UK: Initial findings. *Drug Testing and Analysis*, *2*, 377–382.

Brenneisen, R., Geisshüsler, S., & Schorno, X. (1986). Metabolism of cathinone to (-)-norephedrine and (-)-norpseudoephedrine. *Journal of Pharmacy Pharmacology*, *38*, 298–300.

Cameron, K. N., Kolanos, R., Solis, E., Glennon, R. A., & De Felice, L. J. (2013). Bath salts components mephedrone and methylenedioxypyrovalerone (MDPV) act synergistically at the human dopamine transporter. *British Journal of Pharmacology*, *68*, 1750–1757.

Cameron, K., Kolanos, R., Vekariya, R., De Felice, L., & Glennon, R. A. (2013). Mephedrone and methylenedioxypyrovalerone (MDPV), major constituents of "bath salts", produce opposite effects at the human dopamine transporter. *Psychopharmacology*, *227*, 493–499.

Chen, K. K., & Kao, C. H. (1926). Ephedrine and pseudoephedrine, their isolation, constitution, isomerism, properties, derivatives, and synthesis. *Journal of the American Pharmaceutical Association*, *15*, 625–639.

Coppola, M., & Mondola, R. (2012). 3.4-Methylenedioxypyrovalerone (MDPV): Chemistry, pharmacology and toxicology of a new designer drug of abuse marketed online. *Toxicology Letters*, *208*, 12–15.

Cozzi, N. V., Brandt, S. D., Daley, P. F., Partilla, J. S., Rothman, R. B., Tulzer, A., et al. (2013). Pharmacological examination of trifluoromethyl ring-substituted methcathinone analogs. *European Journal of Pharmacology*, *699*, 180–187.

Cozzi, N. V., Sievert, M. K., Shulgin, A. T., Jacob, P., III, & Ruoho, A. E. (1999). Inhibition of plasma membrane monoamine transporters by β-ketoamphetamines. *European Journal of Pharmacology*, *381*, 63–69.

Dal Cason, T. A., Young, R., & Glennon, R. A. (1997). Cathinone: An investigation of several *N*-alkyl and methylenedioxy analogs. *Pharmacology, Biochemistry, and Behavior*, *58*, 1109–1116.

Dybdal, N. F., Holder, N. D., Ottoson, P. E., Sweeney, M. D., & Williams, T. (2013). Mephedrone: Public health risk, mechanisms of action, and behavioral effects. *European Journal of Pharmacology*, *714*, 32–40.

Eberhard, A. (1915). Ueber das Ephedrine und verwante Verbindugen. *Archivs die Pharmazie*, *253*, 62–91.

Eberhard, A. (1920). Ueber die Synthese des inaktiven Ephedrine bez. Pseudoephedrins. *Archivs die Pharmazie*, *258*, 97–129.

Eshleman, A. J., Wofrum, K. M., Hatfield, M. G., Johnson, R. A., Murphy, K. V., & Janowsky, A. (2013). Substituted methcathinones differ in transporter and receptor interactions. *Biochemical Pharmacology*, *85*, 1803–1815.

Fantegrossi, W. E., Gannon, B. M., Zimmerman, S. M., & Rice, K. C. (2013). In vivo effects of abused 'bath salt' constituent 3,4-methylenedioxypyrovalerone (MDPV) in mice: Drug discrimination, thermoregulation, and locomotor activity. *Neuropsychopharmacology*, *38*, 563–573.

Federal Register, (2011). Schedules of controlled substances: Temporary placement of three synthetic cathinones into Schedule I. *Federal Register*, *76*, 65371–65375.

Fellows, L. (1967). East Africa turns on with khat. *New York Times, July 9*, 1967.

Fitzgerald, J. (2009). Khat: A literature review. http://www.ceh.org.au/downloads/khat_report_final.pdf.

Foley, K. F., & Cozzi, N. V. (2003). Novel aminopropiophenones as potential antidepressants. *Drug Development Research, 60,* 252–260.

Fourneau, E., & Kanao, S. (1924). Sur la synthese l'ephedrine. *Bulletin de la Sociétée chimique de France, 35,* 614–625.

Friebel, H., & Brilla, R. (1963). Über den zentralerregenden Wirkstoff der frischen Blätter und Zweigspitzen von *Catha edulis* Forskal. *Naturwissenschaften, 50,* 354–355.

Fuwa, T., Fukumori, N., Tanaka, T., Kubo, Y., Ogata, A., Uehara, S., et al. (2007). Microdialysis study of drug effects on central nervous system: Changes of dopamine levels in mice striatum after oral administration of methylenedioxypyrovalerone. *Annual Report Tokyo Metropolitan Institute of Public Health, 58,* 287–292.

Gatch, M. B., Taylor, C. M., & Forster, M. J. (2013). Locomotor stimulant and discriminative stimulus effects of "bath salt" cathinones. *Behavioral Pharmacology, 24,* 437–447.

Gaulier, J. M., Canal, M., Pradeille, J. L., Marquet, P., & Lachâtre, G. (2002). New drugs at "rave parties": Ketamine and prolintane. *Acta Clinica Belgica. Supplementum,* 41–46.

Gil, D., Adamowicz, P., Skulska, A., Tokarczyk, B., & Stanaszek, R. (2013). Analysis of 4-MEC in biological and non-biological material-three case reports. *Forensic Science International, 228,* e11–e15.

Glennon, R. A. (1986). Discriminative stimulus properties of phenylisopropylamine derivatives. *Drug and Alcohol Dependence, 17,* 119–134.

Glennon, R. A. (1996). Classical hallucinogens. In C. R. Schuster & M. J. Kuhar (Eds.), *Handbook of experimental pharmacology: Pharmacological aspects of drug dependence* (pp. 343–371). Basel, Switzerland: Springer Verlag.

Glennon, R. A. (2008). Hallucinogens, stimulants, and related drugs of abuse. In D. A. Williams, T. L. Lempke, V. F. Roche, & S. W. Zito (Eds.), *Foye's principles of medicinal chemistry* (pp. 631–651) (5th ed.) Baltimore, MD: Lippincott, Williams & Wilkins.

Glennon, R. A., Ismaiel, A. M., Martin, B., Poff, D., & Sutton, M. (1988). A preliminary behavioral investigation of PMMA, the 4-methoxy analog of methamphetamine. *Pharmacology, Biochemistry, and Behavior, 31,* 9–13.

Glennon, R. A., Schechter, M. D., & Rosecrans, J. A. (1984). Discriminative stimulus properties of *S*(-)- and *R*(+)-cathinone, (+)-cathine and several structural modifications. *Pharmacology, Biochemistry, and Behavior, 21,* 1–3.

Glennon, R. A., & Showalter, D. (1981). The effect of cathinone and several related derivatives on locomotor activity. *Research Communications on Substance Abuse, 2,* 186–192.

Glennon, R. A., & Young, R. (2011). *Drug discrimination: Applications to medicinal chemistry and drug studies.* Hoboken: John Wiley and Sons, Inc.

Glennon, R. A., Young, R., & Hauck, A. E. (1985). Structure-activity studies on methoxy-substituted phenylisopropylamines using drug discrimination methodology. *Pharmacology, Biochemistry, and Behavior, 22,* 723–729.

Glennon, R. A., Young, R., Hauck, A. E., & McKenney, J. D. (1984). Structure-activity studies of amphetamine analogs using drug discrimination methodology. *Pharmacology, Biochemistry, and Behavior, 21,* 895–901.

Glennon, R. A., Young, R., Martin, B. R., & Dal Cason, T. A. (1995). Methcathinone ("Cat"): An enantiomeric potency comparison. *Pharmacology, Biochemistry, and Behavior, 50,* 601–606.

Glennon, R. A., Yousif, M., Naiman, N. A., & Kalix, P. (1987). Methcathinone: A new and potent amphetamine-like agent. *Pharmacology, Biochemistry, and Behavior, 26,* 547–551.

Goudie, A. J., Atkinson, J., & West, C. R. (1986). Discriminative properties of the psychostimulant dl-cathinone in a two lever operant task. Lack of evidence for dopaminergic mediation. *Neuropharmacology, 25,* 85–94.

Hadlock, G. C., Webb, K. M., McFadden, L. M., Chu, P. W., Ellis, J. D., Allen, S. C., et al. (2011). 4-Methylmethcathinone (mephedrone): Neuropharmacological effects of a designer stimulant of abuse. *The Journal of Pharmacology and Experimental Therapeutics*, *339*, 530–536.

Halbach, H. (1972). Medical aspects of the chewing of khat leaves. *Bulletin of the World Health Organization*, *47*, 21–29.

Heinzelman, R. V., & Aspergren, D. B. (1953). Compounds containing the pyrrolidine ring: Analogs of sympathomimetic amines. *Journal of the American Chemical Society*, *75*, 3409–3413.

Higgs, R. A., & Glennon, R. A. (1990). Stimulus properties of ring-methyl amphetamine analogs. *Pharmacology, Biochemistry, and Behavior*, *37*, 835–837.

Hollister, L. E., & Gillespie, H. K. (1970). A new stimulant, prolintane hydrochloride, compared with dextroamphetamine in fatigued volunteers. *The Journal of Clinical Pharmacology*, *10*, 103–109.

Huang, P. K., Aarde, S. M., Angrish, D., Houseknecht, K. L., Dickerson, T. J., & Taffe, M. A. (2012). Contrasting effects of d-methamphetamine, 3,4-methylenedioxymethamphetamine, 3,4-methylenedioxypyrovalerone, and 4-methylmethcathinone on wheel activity in rats. *Drug and Alcohol Dependence*, *126*, 168–175.

Hyde, J. F., Browning, E., & Adams, R. (1928). Synthetic homologs of d,l-ephedrine. *Journal of the American Chemical Society*, *50*, 2287–2292.

Iversen, L. E. (2010). Consideration of the cathinones. Advisory Council on the Misuse of Drugs. A report submitted to the Home Secretary of the UK (March 31, 2010).

Iversen, L., Gibbons, S., Treble, R., Setola, V., Huang, X. P., & Roth, B. L. (2013). Neurochemical profiles of some novel psychoactive substances. *European Journal of Pharmacology*, *700*, 147–151.

Iwao, J., Kowaki, C., & Rakemi, H. (1954). Studies on alkanolamines. II. Synthesis of N-methylephedrone and its derivatives. Application of the Viogt reaction. *Yakugaku Zasshi*, *74*, 551–553.

Jacob, P., & Shulgin, A. T. (1996). Novel N-substituted 2-amino-3',4'-methylenedioxypropiophenones. WO patent 9639133. December 12, 1996.

Kalix, P. (1980a). Hypermotility of the amphetamine type induced by a constituent of khat leaves. *British Journal of Pharmacology*, *68*, 11–13.

Kalix, P. (1980b). Hyperthermic response to (-)cathinone, an alkaloid of *Catha edulis* (khat). *Journal of Pharmacy and Pharmacology*, *32*, 662–663.

Kalix, P. (1981). Cathinone, an alkaloid from khat leaves with an amphetamine-like releasing effect. *Psychopharmacology*, *74*, 269–270.

Kalix, P. (1992). Cathinone, a natural amphetamine. *Pharmacology and Toxicology*, *70*, 77–86.

Kalix, P., & Braeden, O. (1985). Pharmacological aspects of the chewing of khat leaves. *Pharmacological Reviews*, *37*, 149–164.

Kalix, P., & Glennon, R. A. (1986). Further evidence for an amphetamine-like mechanism of action of the alkaloid cathinone. *Biochemical Pharmacology*, *35*, 3015–3019.

Kamata, H. T., Shima, N., Zaitsu, K., Kamata, T., Miki, A., Nishikawa, M., et al. (2006). Metabolism of the recently encountered designer drug, methylone, in humans and rats. *Xenobiotica*, *36*, 709–723.

Karila, L., & Reynaud, M. (2010). GHB and synthetic cathinones: Clinical effects and potential consequences. *Drug Testing and Analysis*, *3*, 552–559.

Kasick, D. P., McKnight, C. A., & Kilsovic, E. (2012). "Bath salt" ingestion leading to severe intoxication delirium: Two cases and a brief review of the emergence of mephedrone use. *Clinical Toxicology*, *38*, 176–180.

Katz, J. L., Ricaurte, G. A., & Witkin, J. M. (1992). Reinforcing effects of enantiomers of N,N-dimethylamphetamine in squirrel monkeys. *Psychopharmacology*, *107*, 315–318.

Kehr, J., Ichinose, F., Yoshitake, S., Goiny, M., Sievertsson, T., Nyberg, F., et al. (2011). Mephedrone, compared with MDMA (ecstasy) and amphetamine, rapidly increases both dopamine and 5-HT levels in nucleus accumbens of awake rats. *British Journal of Pharmacology, 164,* 1949–1958.

Kelly, J. P. (2011). Cathinone derivatives: A review of their chemistry, pharmacology and toxicology. *Drug Testing and Analysis, 3,* 439–453.

Kennedy, J. G., Teague, J., & Fairbanks, L. (1980). Qat use in North Yemen and the problem of addiction: A study in medical anthropology. *Culture, Medicine and Psychiatry, 4,* 311–344.

Knoll, J. (1979). Studies on the central effects of (-)cathinone. *NIDA Research Monograph, 27,* 322–323.

Kolanos, R., Cameron, K. N., Vekariya, R. H., De Felice, L. J., & Glennon, R. A. (2011). "Bath salts": An imitation of methamphetamine plus cocaine? In *Southeast Regional Meeting of American Chemical Society (SERMACS), Richmond VA, October 26–29.*

Kolanos, R., Solis, E., Sakloth, F., De Felice, L. J., & Glennon, R. A. (2013). 'Deconstruction' of the abused synthetic cathinone methylenedioxypyrovalerone (MDPV) and an examination of effects at the human dopamine transporter. *ACS Chemical Neuroscience,* in press. Unpublished data, manuscript submitted for publication.

Köppe, H., Ludwig, G., & Zeile, K. (1969). 1-(3′4′-Methylenedioxy-phenyl)-2-pyrrolidino-alkanones-(1). U.S. Patent 3,478,050, November 11, 1969.

Kraemer, T., & Maurer, H. H. (2002). Toxicokinetics of amphetamines: Metabolism and toxicokinetic data of designer drugs, amphetamine, methamphetamine, and their N-alkyl derivatives. *Therapeutic Drug Monitoring, 24,* 277–289.

Kuitunen, T., Kärkkäinen, S., & Ylitalo, P. (1984). Comparison of the acute physical and mental effects of ephedrine, fenfluramine, phentermine and prolintane. *Methods and Findings in Experimental and Clinical Pharmacology, 6,* 265–270.

Kyle, P. B., & Daley, W. P. (2007). Domestic abuse of the European rave drug prolintane. *Journal of Analytical Toxicology, 31,* 415–418.

Lee, M. R. (2011). The history of ephedra (ma-huang). *The Journal of the Royal College of Physicians of Edinburg, 41,* 78–84.

Lee, S., Yoo, H. H., In, M. K., Jin, C., & Kim, D. H. (2013). Stereoselectivity in the cytochrome P450-dependent N-demethylation and flavin monooxygenase-dependent N-oxidation of N,N-dimethylamphetamine. *Archives of Pharmacal Research, 36,* 1385–1391.

Lin, T. C., Lin, D. L., & Lua, A. C. (2011). Detection of p-chloroamphetamine in urine samples with mass spectrometry. *Journal of Analytical Toxicology, 35,* 205–210.

L'Italien, Y. J., Park, H., & Rebstock, L. C. (1957). Methylaminopropiophenone compounds and methods for producing the same. US patent 2,802,865, August 13, 1957.

Ljungberg, T., & Ungerstedt, U. (1985). A rapid and simple behavioural screening method for simultaneous assessment of limbic and striatal blocking effects of neuroleptic drugs. *Pharmacology, Biochemistry, and Behavior, 23,* 479–485.

Loh, H. H., & Tseng, L.-F. (1978). Role of biogenic amines in the actions of methoxyamphetamines. In R. C. Stillman & R. E. Willette (Eds.), *The psychopharmacology of hallucinogens* (pp. 13–22). New York: Pergamon Press.

López-Arnau, R., Martinez-Clemente, J., Pubill, D., Escubedo, E., & Camarasa, J. (2012). Comparative neuropharmacology of three psychostimulant cathinone derivatives: Butylone, mephedrone and methylone. *British Journal of Pharmacology, 167,* 407–420.

Marinetti, L. J., & Antonides, H. M. (2013). Analysis of synthetic cathinones commonly found in bath salts in human performance and postmortem toxicology: Method development, drug distribution and interpretation of results. *Journal of Analytical Toxicology, 37,* 135–146.

Markantonis, S. L., Kyroudis, A., & Beckett, A. H. (1989). The in vitro reduction of dimethylpropion. *Biochemical Medicine and Metabolic Biology, 42,* 1–8.

Martínez-Clemente, J., Escubedo, E., Pubill, D., & Camarasa, J. (2012). Interaction of mephedrone with dopamine and serotonin targets in rats. *European Neuropsychopharmacology*, 22, 231–236.

Marusich, J. A., Grant, K. R., Blough, B. E., & Wiley, J. L. (2012). Effects of synthetic cathinones contained in "bath salts" on motor behavior and a functional observational battery in mice. *NeuroToxicology*, 33, 1305–1313.

Meltzer, P. C., Butler, D., Deschamps, J. R., & Madras, B. K. (2006). 1-(4-Methylphenyl)-2-pyrrolidin-1-yl-pentan-1-one (pyrovalerone) analogs. A promising class of monoamine uptake inhibitors. *Journal of Medicinal Chemistry*, 49, 1420–1432.

Meyer, M. R., Du, P., Schuster, F., & Maurer, H. H. (2010). Studies on the metabolism of the α-pyrrolidinophenone designer drug methylenedioxy-pyrovalerone (MDPV) in rat and human urine and human liver microsomes using GC-MS and LC-high-resolution MS and its detectability in urine by GC-MS. *Journal of Mass Spectrometry*, 45, 1426–1442.

Motbey, C. P., Hunt, G. E., Bowen, M. T., Artiss, S., & McGregor, I. S. (2011). Mephedrone (4-methylmethcathinone, 'meow'): Acute behavioural effects and distribution of Fos expression in adolescent rats. *Addiction Biology*, 17, 409–422.

Negus, S. S., & Banks, M. L. (2011). Making the right choice: Lessons from drug discrimination, for research on drug reinforcement and drug self-administration. In R. A. Glennon & R. Young (Eds.), *Drug discrimination: Applications to medicinal chemistry and drug studies* (pp. 361–388). Hoboken: John Wiley and Sons, Inc.

Nicholson, A. N., Stone, B. M., & Jones, M. M. (1980). Wakefulness and reduced rapid eye movement sleep: Studies with prolintane and pemoline. *British Journal of Clinical Pharmacology*, 10, 465–472.

Paul, B. D., & Cole, K. A. (2001). Cathinone (Khat) and methcathinone (CAT) in urine specimens: A gas chromatographic-mass spectrometric detection procedure. *Journal of Analytical Toxicology*, 25, 525–530.

Pawlik, E., Plässer, G., Mahler, H., & Daldrup, T. (2012). Studies on the phase I metabolism of the new designer drug 3-fluoromethcathinone using rabbit liver slices. *International Journal of Legal Medicine*, 126, 231–240.

Payá, B., Guisado, J. A., Vaz, F. J., & Crespo-Facorro, B. (2002). Visual hallucinations induced by the combination of prolintane and diphenhydramine. *Pharmacopsychiatry*, 35, 24–25.

Penders, T. M., Gestring, R. E., & Vilensky, D. A. (2012). Intoxication delirium following use of synthetic cathinone derivatives. *Clinical Toxicology*, 38, 616–617.

Prosser, J. M., & Nelson, L. S. (2012). The toxicology of bath salts: A review of synthetic cathinones. *Journal of Medical Toxicology*, 8, 33–42.

Ristic, S., & Thomas, A. (1962). On the constituents of Catha edulis. *Archives die Pharmazie*, 295, 524–525.

Rosecrans, J. A., Campbell, O. L., Dewey, W. L., & Harris, L. S. (1979). Discriminative stimulus and neurochemical mechanism of cathinone: A preliminary study. *NIDA Research Monograph*, 27, 328–329.

Rösner, P., Quednow, B., Girreser, U., & Junge, T. (2005). Isomeric fluoro-methoxy-phenylalkylamines: A new series of controlled-substance analogues (designer drugs). *Forensic Science International*, 148, 143–156.

Rothman, R. B., Vu, N., Partilla, J. S., Roth, B. L., Hufeisen, S. J., Compton-Toth, B. A., et al. (2003). In vitro characterization of ephedrine-related stereoisomers at biogenic amine transporters and the receptorome reveals selective actions as norepinephrine transporter substrates. *The Journal of Pharmacology and Experimental Therapeutics*, 307, 138–145.

Savenko, V. G., Semkin, E. P., Sorokin, V. I., & Kazankov, S. P. (1989). Expert examination of narcotic substances obtained from ephedrine. Ministry of the Interior, All-Union Scientific Research Institute Report, pp. 1–22.

Schechter, M. D., & Glennon, R. A. (1985). Cathinone, cocaine and methamphetamine: Similarity of behavioral effects. *Pharmacology, Biochemistry, and Behavior, 22*, 913–916.

Schorno, X., & Steinegger, E. (1978). The phenylalkylamines of *Catha edulis* Forsk. The absolute configuration of cathinone. United Nations Laboratory document MNAR/7/1978, GE. 78-3956.

Schütte, J. (1961). Anorexigenic propiophenones. U. S. patent 3,001,910. September 26, 1961.

Seeger, E. (1964). Verfahren zur Herstellung von α-Pyrrolidinoketonen und deren Salzen. German patent 1,161,274. January 16, 1964.

Shapiro, D. (1950). Benzoisoquinoline studies. Part I. Open-ring models of 4-benzylisoquinolines. *Journal of Organic Chemistry, 15*, 1027–1036.

Shulgin, A., & Shulgin, A. (1991). *Pihkal*. Berkeley, CA: Transform Press.

Sikk, K., Haldre, S., Aquilonius, S. M., Asser, A., Paris, M., Roose, A., et al. (2013). Manganese-induced parkinsonism in methcathinone abusers: Bio-markers of exposure and follow-up. *European Journal of Neurology, 20*, 915–920.

Simmler, L. D., Buser, T. A., Donzelli, M., Schramm, Y., Dieu, L.-H., Huwyler, J., et al. (2012). Pharmacological characterization of designer cathinones in vitro. *British Journal of Pharmacology, 168*, 458–470.

Spiller, H. A., Ryan, M. L., Weston, R. G., & Jansen, J. (2011). Clinical experience with and analytical confirmation of "bath salts" and "legal highs" (synthetic cathinones) in the United States. *Clinical Toxicology, 49*, 499–505.

Springer, D., Fritschi, G., & Maurer, H. H. (2003a). Metabolism and toxicological detection of the new designer drug 3,4-methylenedioxy-α-pyrrolidinopropiophenone studied in urine using gas chromatography-mass spectrometry. *Journal of Chromatography B, 793*, 377–388.

Springer, D., Fritschi, G., & Maurer, H. H. (2003b). Metabolism of the new designer drug alpha-pyrrolidinopropiophenone (PPP) and the toxicological detection of PPP and 4-methyl-alpha-pyrrolidinopropiophenone (MPPP) studied in rat urine using gas chromatography-mass spectrometry. *Journal of Chromatography B, Analytical Technologies in the Biomedical and Life Sciences, 796*, 253–266.

Springer, D., Paul, L. D., Staack, R. F., Kraemer, T., & Maurer, H. H. (2003). Identification of cytochrome P450 enzymes involved in the metabolism of 4-methyl-α-pyrrolidinopropiophenone, a novel scheduled designer drug, in human liver microsomes. *The American Society for Pharmacology and Experimental Therapeutics, 31*, 979–982.

Springer, D., Peters, F. T., Fritschi, G., & Maurer, H. H. (2002). Studies on the metabolism and toxicological detection of the new designer drug 4-methyl-α-pyrrolidinopropiophenone in urine using gas chromatography-mass spectrometry. *Journal of Chromatography B, 773*, 25–33.

Springer, D., Staack, R. F., Paul, L. D., Kraemer, T., & Maurer, H. H. (2003). Identification of cytochrome P450 enzymes involved in the metabolism of 4′-methoxy-α-pyrrolidinopropiophenone (MOPPP), a designer drug, in human liver microsomes. *Xenobiotica, 33*, 989–998.

Strano-Rossi, S., Cadwallader, A. B., de la Torre, X., & Botrè, F. (2010). Toxicological determination and *in vitro* metabolism of the designer drug methylenedioxypyrovalerone (MPDV) by gas chromatography/mass spectrometry and liquid chromatography/ quadrupole time-of-flight mass spectrometry. *Rapid Communications in Mass Spectrometry, 24*, 2706–2714.

Testa, B., & Salvesen, B. (1980). Quantitative structure-activity relationships in drug metabolism and disposition: Pharmacokinetics of N-substituted amphetamines in humans. *Journal of Pharmaceutical Sciences, 69*, 497–501.

Thevis, M., Sigmund, G., Thomas, A., Gougoulidis, V., Rodchenkov, G., & Schanzer, W. (2009). Doping control analysis of metamfepramone and two major metabolites using liquid chromatography-tandem mass spectrometry. *European Journal of Mass Spectrometry*, *15*, 507–515.

Thomae, K. (1959). Improvements in or relating to tertiary amines and their salts and the production thereof. UK patent GB814153. May 27, 1959.

Thornton, S. L., Gerona, R. R., & Tomaszewski, C. A. (2012). Psychosis from a bath salt product containing flephedrone and MDPV with serum, urine, and product quantification. *Journal of Medical Toxicology*, *8*, 310–313.

UN Document. (1975). Studies on the chemical composition of khat. III. Investigations on the phenylalkylamine fraction. United Nations Laboratory document MNAR/11/75, GE. 75-1264.

UN Document. (1978). Note on the synthesis of cathinone and its "dimer" (3,6-dimethyl-2,5-diphenylpyrazine). United Nations Laboratory document MNAR/3/1978, GE. 78-1836.

UN Document. (1979). The botany and chemistry of khat. United Nations Laboratory document MNAR/3/1979, GE. 79-10365.

UNODC. (2013). The challenge of new psychoactive substances. A report from the United Nations Office on Drugs and Crime. Vienna, Austria, pp 1–56.

van der Schoot, J. B., Ariens, E. J., van Rossum, J. M., & Hurkmans, J. A. T. M. (1962). Phenylisopropylamine derivatives, structure and action. *Arznemittel-Forschung*, *12*, 902–907.

Varner, K. J., Daigle, K., Weed, P. F., Lewis, P. B., Mahne, S. E., Sankaranarayanan, A., et al. (2012). Comparison of the behavioral and cardiovascular effects of mephedrone with other drugs of abuse in rats. *Psychopharmacology (Berlin)*, *225*, 675–685.

Wander, A. (1963). α-Pyrrolidino-valerophenones. British patent 927,475. May 29, 1963.

Watterson, L. R., Kufahl, P. R., Nemirovsky, N. E., Sewalia, K., Grabenauer, M., Thomas, B. F., et al. (2013). Potent rewarding and reinforcing effects of the synthetic cathinone 3,4-methylenedioxypyrovalerone (MDPV). *Addiction Biology*, http://dx.doi.org/10.1111/j.1369-1600.2012.00474.x.

Wee, S., Anderson, K. G., Baumann, M. H., Rothman, R. B., Blough, B. E., & Woolverton, W. L. (2005). Relationship between the serotonergic activity and reinforcing effects of a series of amphetamine analogs. *The Journal of Pharmacology and Experimental Therapeutics*, *313*, 848–854.

Westphal, F., Junge, T., Rösner, P., Fritschi, G., Klein, B., & Girreser, U. (2007). Mass spectral and NMR spectral data of two new designer drugs with an α-aminophenone structure: 4'-Methyl-α-pyrrolidinohexanophenone and 4'-methyl-α-pyrrolidinobutyrophenone. *Forensic Science International*, *169*, 32–42.

Wolfes, O. (1930). Über das Vorkommen von *d*-nor-iso-Ephedrin in Catha edulis. *Archives die Pharmazie*, *268*, 81–83.

Wood, D. M., Davies, S., Greene, S. L., Button, J., Holt, D. W., Ramsey, J., et al. (2010). Case series of individuals with analytically confirmed acute mephedrone toxicity. *Clinical Toxicology*, *48*, 924–927.

Woolverton, W. L. (1991). Discriminative stimulus effects of cocaine. In R. A. Glennon, T. U. C. Jarbe, & J. Frankenheim (Eds.), *Drug discrimination: Applications to drug abuse research* (pp. 61–74). Rockville, MD: National Institute on Drug Abuse.

Woolverton, W. L., Shybut, G., & Johanson, C. E. (1980). Structure-activity relationships among some d-N-alkylated amphetamines. *Pharmacology, Biochemistry, and Behavior*, *13*, 869–876.

Yanagita, T. (1979). Studies on cathinones: Cardiovascular and behavioral effects in rats and self-administration experiment in Rhesus monkeys. *NIDA Research Monograph*, *27*, 326–327.

Young, R., & Glennon, R. A. (1986). Discriminative stimulus properties of amphetamine and structurally related phenalkylamines. *Medicinal Research Reviews*, *6*, 99–130.

Young, R., & Glennon, R. A. (1993). Cocaine-stimulus generalization to two new designer drugs: Methcathinone and 4-methylaminorex. *Pharmacology, Biochemistry, and Behavior, 45,* 229–231.

Young, R., & Glennon, R. A. (1996). A three-lever operant procedure differentiates the stimulus effects of R(-)-MDA from S(+)-MDA. *Journal of Pharmacology and Experimental Therapeutics, 276,* 594–601.

Young, R., & Glennon, R. A. (1998). Discriminative stimulus effects of S(-)-methcathinone (CAT): A potent stimulant drug of abuse. *Psychopharmacology, 140,* 250–256.

Zaitsu, K., Katagi, M., Kamata, H. T., Kamata, T., Shima, N., Miki, A., et al. (2009). Determination of the metabolites of the new designer drugs bk-MBDB and bk-MDEA in human urine. *Forensic Science International, 188,* 131–139.

Zaitsu, K., Katagi, M., Kamata, T., Kamata, H., Shima, N., Tsuchihashi, H., et al. (2008). Determination of a newly encountered designer drug "p-methoxyethylamphetamine" and its metabolites in human urine and blood. *Forensic Science International, 177,* 77–84.

Zawilska, J. B., & Wojcieszak, J. (2013). Designer cathinones—An emerging class of novel recreational drugs. *Forensic Science International, 231,* 42–53.

Zhingel, K. Y., Dovensky, W., Crossman, A., & Allen, A. (1991). Ephedrone: 2-Methylamino-1-phenylpropan-1-one. *Journal of Forensic Sciences, 36,* 915–920.

INDEX

Note: Page numbers followed by "*f*" indicate figures and "*t*" indicate tables.